Surgical Oncology: Fluorescence-Guided Surgery

Surgical Oncology: Fluorescence-Guided Surgery

Editor: Jaime Allison

AMERICAN
MEDICAL PUBLISHERS
www.americanmedicalpublishers.com

AMERICAN
MEDICAL PUBLISHERS
www.americanmedicalpublishers.com

Cataloging-in-Publication Data

Surgical oncology : fluorescence-guided surgery / edited by Jaime Allison.
p. cm.
Includes bibliographical references and index.
ISBN 979-8-88740-480-6
1. Cancer--Surgery. 2. Cancer--Laser surgery. 3. Tumors--Surgery. 4. Lasers in surgery.
5. Oncology. I. Allison, Jaime.
RD651 .S87 2023
616.994 059--dc23

American Medical Publishers,
41 Flatbush Avenue,
1st Floor, New York,
NY 11217, USA

ISBN 979-8-88740-480-6 (Hardback)

Contents

Preface

This book was inspired by the evolution of our times; to answer the curiosity of inquisitive minds. Many developments have occurred across the globe in the recent past which has transformed the progress in the field.

Fluorescence-guided surgery (FGS) is a type of surgery that is performed with the guidance of fluorescence imaging. It has emerged as a new approach to detect the primary tumor, tumor margins, and metastatic lymph nodes. A major cause of tumor recurrence is the presence of residual tumor cells after surgery. Therefore, it is necessary to have a negative tumor margin to ensure a successful cancer resection. Despite widespread use of preoperative imaging techniques such as computed tomography (CT) scan, magnetic resonance imaging (MRI) scan, and positron emission tomography (PET) scan, the surgical margin positive rate failed to reflect remarkable improvement. The plausible reason for this failure is the reliance of surgeons on the visual inspection and intraoperative histopathological analysis of the frozen tissue specimen. FGS is now emerging as an effective tool to guide the surgical oncologists by generating real time fluorescence images of the surgical region. It reduces the possibility of recurrence of cancer. This book strives to provide a fair idea about the fluorescence-guided surgery and to help develop a better understanding of the latest advances related to this medical procedure. It is a vital tool for all researching and studying fluorescence-guided surgery as it gives incredible insights into the emerging trends and concepts.

This book was developed from a mere concept to drafts to chapters and finally compiled together as a complete text to benefit the readers across all nations. To ensure the quality of the content we instilled two significant steps in our procedure. The first was to appoint an editorial team that would verify the data and statistics provided in the book and also select the most appropriate and valuable contributions from the plentiful contributions we received from authors worldwide. The next step was to appoint an expert of the topic as the Editor-in-Chief, who would head the project and finally make the necessary amendments and modifications to make the text reader-friendly. I was then commissioned to examine all the material to present the topics in the most comprehensible and productive format.

I would like to take this opportunity to thank all the contributing authors who were supportive enough to contribute their time and knowledge to this project. I also wish to convey my regards to my family who have been extremely supportive during the entire project.

Editor

1

Optical Molecular Imaging of Inflammatory Cells in Interventional Medicine

Gavin P. Birch[1,2*], *Thane Campbell*[2*], *Mark Bradley*[1] *and Kevin Dhaliwal*[2]

[1] *EaStChem School of Chemistry, University of Edinburgh, Edinburgh, United Kingdom,* [2] *Centre for Inflammation Research, University of Edinburgh, Edinburgh, United Kingdom*

***Correspondence:**
Gavin P. Birch
gavin.birch@ed.ac.uk
Thane Campbell
s1003032@sms.ed.ac.uk

The optical molecular imaging of inflammation is an emerging strategy for interventional medicine and diagnostics. The host's inflammatory response and adaptation to acute and chronic diseases provides unique signatures that have the potential to guide interventions. Thus, there are emerging a suite of molecular imaging and sensing approaches for a variety of targets in this area. This review will focus on two key cellular orchestrators that dominate this area, neutrophils and macrophages, with recent developments in molecular probes and approaches discussed.

Keywords: molecular imaging, inflammation, interventional medicine, optical imaging, macrophage, neutrophil

INTRODUCTION

Recent developments in optical molecular imaging are enabling the identification and evaluation of inflammatory cells such as macrophages and neutrophils in a variety of imaging scenarios. This is important as these leukocytes are an important part of host defense and immune homeostasis. Their pivotal roles as professional phagocytes in acute and chronic inflammatory disease may allow their use as versatile interventional biomarkers and as such fluorescent imaging of these cells has the potential to advance disease treatment and management, by producing sub-cellular information in real-time.

Intrinsic tissue autofluorescence adds further value when the structures of extracellular matrix or metabolic activities are of interest. The predominant modality of fluorescence intensity measurements, coupled with recent technological developments such as label-free non-linear optical images and Raman analyses (1, 2), have opened up the possibility of giving the surgeon functional images of the surgical site in real time. Furthermore, exciting developments are resulting from the integration of cell classification and machine learning techniques, allowing deeper analysis of the richness of imaging datasets.

Macroscopic widefield open fluorescence systems and high-resolution endomicroscopy are the predominant systems that have been used clinically to detect optical molecular tracers. The recent advances in imaging technology mean that fluorescence guided surgery is becoming a reality for cancer resection (3). Complete tumor removal is crucial for patient outcomes, but difficult to ensure by conventional microscopy as visual characteristics and palpitation are inadequate to determine tumor-free margin. With fluorescence systems, surgeons have the future ability to assess the extent of tumor excision and local metastases in real-time using a fluorescent label that "lights-up" the tumor and hence delineates its margins. Optical endomicroscopy (OEM) enables optical imaging at high resolution typically via a bundle of optical fibers (although rapidly being replaced by chip-on-tip technologies) to enable imaging with microscopic resolution, with the added ability to explore within a variety of cavities. Recently fiber-bundle endomicroscopy has been used in the lung to assess alveolar structure in emphysema, neoplastic changes in epithelial cells and real-time *in vivo* detection of bacteria (4–6). As well as in the GI tract, where it has been used to detect changes associated with squamous cell carcinoma and colorectal polyps (7). There are a range of OEM platforms, spanning clinical use and developmental systems (6, 8), although standardization is necessary to generate meaningful diagnostic data (9).

Alongside the devices that enable real-time fluorescence imaging capability, optical molecular probes are required that provide contrast and are suitable for use *in vivo*. Although extensive libraries of optical agents for many targets have been developed (10, 11), none have been licensed for routine clinical use. This review will focus on fluorescent molecular probes for inflammatory cells, in particular neutrophils and macrophages. Recent agents allow the identification of these cells, as well as providing information on dynamic cellular processes such as enzymatic activity, redox processes, and phagocytic ability; processes that impact pathophysiology. Overall, inflammatory cell imaging creates an ideal paradigm for patient-specific disease monitoring and intervention (**Table 1**). Recent advances in the fluorescent and Raman imaging are enabling macrophage and neutrophil burden and activity to be described non-invasively and dynamically with tissue-level resolution.

TABLE 1 | Evidence for the role of neutrophils and macrophages as biomarkers in various diseases.

Cell	Information	Disease	References
Neutrophil	Disease stage	Gastrointestinal tumors	(12)
		Solid tumors	(13)
		Inflammatory bowel disease	(14)
	Disease onset	Bacteremia	(15)
		Sepsis-induced acute kidney injury	(16)
	Critical event	Cardiovascular	(17)
		Diabetic neuropathy	(18)
		Chronic obstructive pulmonary disease	(19)
		Pesticide poisoning	(20)
Macrophage	Disease stage	Solid tumors	(21)
		Sentinel lymph node metastasis (breast cancer)	(22)
		Rheumatoid arthritis	(23)
		Liver fibrosis	(24)

Data referenced to meta-analyses or patient studies in the literature.

NEUTROPHILS AS BIOMARKERS

As cells that migrate to diseased tissues and accumulate, both over the course of a disease and due to chemotactic stimuli, neutrophils can provide meaningful prognostic data just by their enumeration. Neutrophil counts have long been used to stratify patients by scoring disease, for example in ulcerative colitis (25). Several large patient studies and systematic reviews show the neutrophil to lymphocyte ratio is useful in staging inflammatory bowel disease (IBD) and numerous solid tumors (13, 14), as well as predicting cardiovascular disease, diabetic neuropathy, sepsis-induced acute kidney injury, glaucoma and bacteremia (15–19, 26). Simple neutrophil enumeration may even resolve the controversial question of when to intervene in carotid artery disease (27). Using explanted human tissues Ionita et al. evidenced correlations between neutrophil count and several critical factors in atherosclerotic plaque stability (28).

Of course, more sophisticated insights can be drawn from considering the viability status of neutrophils and quantifying neutrophil extracellular traps (NETs) independently of neutrophils in altered activation states. The accumulation of neutrophils on the ocular surface in dry-eye disease (DED) is thought to result in pathological NET formation (29). With the recent success of a phase I/II study evaluating DNase treatment for DED, NET burden is becoming an important clinical parameter in this disease (30). Also, neutrophil nuclei undergo morphological changes in DED that can assist the detection of DED-related hyperosmolarity (31). Due to the abundance of human neutrophil elastase (HNE) in NETs (32) and this enzyme's stimulatory role in mucin production (33), HNE may allow diagnostic disease monitoring in DED. Beyond the conjunctiva, neutrophil infiltration is inversely correlated with neuroprotection D1 and their pro-inflammatory activity has clear implications in retinal vascular and neural degeneration (34). Tumor associated neutrophils (TANs) play a wide array of roles and their investigation can reveal where they act in opposition. For example, in early stage lung cancer TANs were shown to help limit disease progression however animal models have elucidated several pro-tumoral mechanisms (35, 36). Some of the heterogeneity measured may come from relying on the expression of TAN markers which can vary in different tumor microenvironments and no suitable marker exists for distinguishing between the N1 and N2 phenotypes (37).

Another layer of insight may be accessible via measurement of neutrophil activity, as studies of patients with inflammatory bowel disease have demonstrated. Patient studies found changes in fecal lactoferrin, calprotectin and the protease HNE were significantly correlated with endoscopy and could be used to distinguish between mild disease, mucosal healing and clinical remission, and even predict flare onset (38). HNE is further implicated in IBD treatment by cleaving therapeutic monoclonal antibodies Infliximab, Adalumimab, Vedolizumab (39). The varied and clear benefits of such simple and direct analyses highlight the precision of the inflammatory response and the diagnostic potential of optical probes for neutrophil imaging.

NEUTROPHIL IMAGING PROBES

Neutrophils are the first leukocytes to be recruited to an inflammatory site. Their capacities to respond en masse and

Abbreviations: DiD, A lipophilic carbocyanine dye; FAM, Carboxyfluorescein; FITC, Fluorescein isothiocyanate; FLIM, Fluorescence lifetime imaging microscopy; FRET, Förster resonant energy transfer; FR, Folate receptor; HNE/NE, (Human) neutrophil elastase; IBD, Inflammatory bowel disease; MMP, Matrix metalloproteinase; MMR, Macrophage mannose receptor; NIR, Near infrared; OEM, Optical endomicroscopy; PET, Positron emission tomography; TPEM, Two-photon endomicroscopy; UC, Ulcerative colitis.

TABLE 2 | Overview of optical probes for imaging neutrophils.

Target	Molecule class	Optical modality	Models	References
Serprocidins	Quenched dendrimeric probe	Fluorescence	Human cells *ex vivo*	(40)
HNE	Quenched probe	Fluorescence	Mouse	(41)
	Quenched dendrimeric probe	Fluorescence	Sheep, human	(42)
FPR1	Peptide	Fluorescence	Human	(43)
	Radioactive nanoparticle	Dual PET/MRI	Mouse	(44)
Nucleus	Label-free	Raman	Human cells *ex vivo*	(45)
	Label-free	2-photon FLIM	Human	(46)

rapidly underscore their potential as biomarkers capable of producing large readouts in short time-frames—properties that are particularly desirable for surgical guidance. The relatively short neutrophil half-life acts to limit any off-target consequences of labeling to days or hours, whilst the persistence of the neutrophilic influx in inflamed tissues makes neutrophil readouts useful over the entire disease monitoring period, irrespective of its duration. Overall, neutrophil imaging creates an ideal paradigm for patient-specific disease monitoring and intervention. Recent advances in the fluorescent and Raman spectroscopic modes of optical imaging are, for the first time, enabling neutrophil burden and activity to be described non-invasively and dynamically with tissue-level resolution (**Table 2**).

Proteases

Human neutrophil elastase (HNE) is a serprocidin stored at millimolar concentrations in the azurophil granules of neutrophils (47). Although HNE is chiefly a microbicidal protease, its broad substrate specificity allows neutrophils to use it intracellularly, extracellularly and in membrane-bound form for a variety of purposes. Phagocytosis, extravasation (48), extracellular matrix remodeling (49–51), cell-signaling (52), mucus production (53), mucociliary function, (54), and NETosis (55) all have roles for HNE and a host of further interactions give the enzyme utility for other cell-types including monocytes, endothelial, and adenocarcinoma cells. When released by activated neutrophils HNE can be used to destroy pathogens and promote neovascularization as part of tissue repair, however sustained HNE release contributes to the pathophysiological sequalae of acute respiratory distress syndrome, lung adenocarcinoma, atherosclerosis and other chronic inflammatory diseases.

Craven et al. recently reported a probe that revealed neutrophil activation. This was designed to detect the serine proteases (serprocidins) using a pan-serprocidin substrate. A tribranched probe was developed which maintains an optically super-silent ground state with a methyl red and fluorescein FRET pair on each of its three branches (**Figure 1A**) (40). The structure facilitates internalization by activated neutrophils and once in the phagolysosome, active serprocidins cleave the peptide sequences to remove the methyl red quenchers and generate a large fold increase in fluorescence (**Figure 1B**). The probe generates bright intracellular puncta, in human neutrophils, within seconds of activation with pharmacological stimulus or bacterial co-incubation. By adding the probe to whole blood in a simple, no-wash, no-lyse, flow cytometric assay, activated neutrophils could be profiled (**Figure 1C**). Combining rapid signal generation and detailed cell-type specific analysis situates this pan-serprocidin probe as a promising patient-stratification biomarker for several chronic inflammatory diseases.

The neutrophil elastase probe NE680 is a near-infrared multi-branched probe which is sensitive to cleavage by murine NE and HNE, amongst others (**Figure 2**) (41). It consists of a peptide sequence (PMAVVQSVP) flanked by NIR fluorophores and conjugated to a polylysine dendrimer, which lengthens its plasma and tissue half-lives and results in internal quenching. Upon cleavage by proteases, NIR fluorescence emission is generated. NE680's quantification of NE activity was demonstrated by incubating lung sections, from LPS/fMLF challenged mice, in increasing doses of the NE-specific inhibitor, sivelestat (**Figures 2C,D**). Non-invasive, quantitative NE imaging was demonstrated using fluorescence molecular tomography (41). Wang et al. demonstrated a similar dose dependent reduction in NIR fluorescence of NE680 could be achieved under more physiologically relevant conditions, using recombinant alpha 1-antiproteinase (a1PI) instead of sivelestat (56). Further studies using NE680 have revealed roles for NE in promoting neutrophil accumulation in atherosclerotic plaques, insulin resistance and arthritic pain, in murine models (57–59). Although NE680 cleavage by HNE has been demonstrated *in vitro*, structural differences between the murine and human NE active sites and functional differences between murine and human neutrophils mean the clinical utility of NE680 has yet to be demonstrated.

Although a wealth of neutrophil probes have not reached *in vivo* studies, exciting developments in optical probe design provide discriminatory power between related proteases. Despite their concomitant release from degranulating neutrophils, the various serprocidins perform distinct molecular functions (60). Screening combinations of natural and unnatural amino acids by their kinetic affinity and rate constants, Kasperkiewicz et al. designed a HNE probe with a 100-fold sensitivity over the previous champion substrate designed by Korkmaz et al. (61). The group's combinatorial substrate library technique generated substrate-based activatable probes and inhibitory, targeted probes and their approach included counter selection which biases against the interference of substrate cleavage from

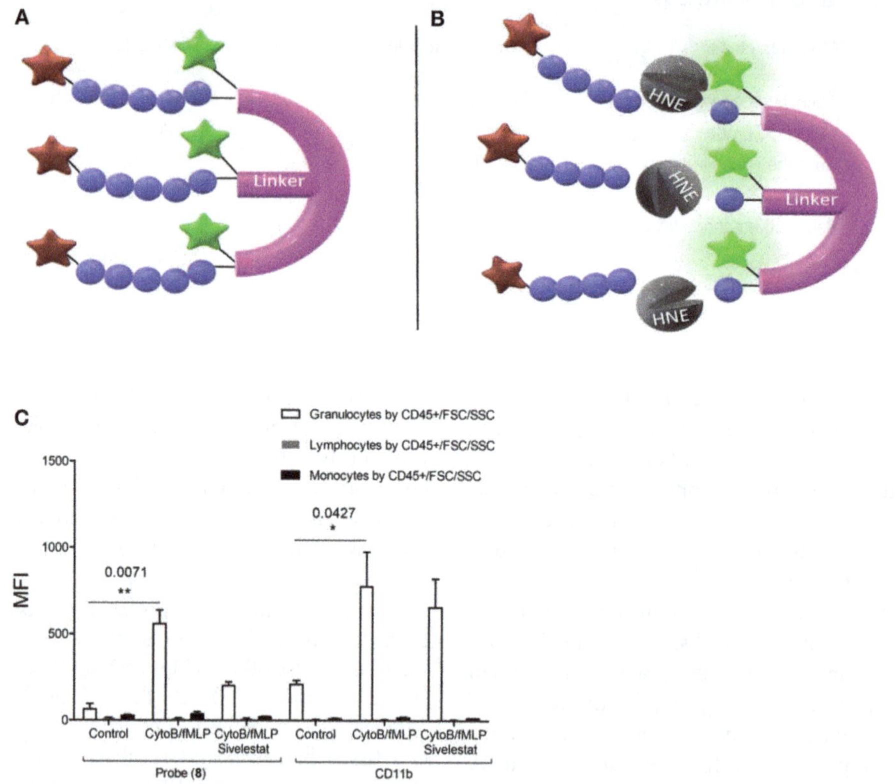

FIGURE 1 | Structure of Craven's neutrophil probe **(A)** before and **(B)** after cleavage by active HNE and indicating the resulting FAM fluorescence. **(C)** In a no-wash, no-lyse whole blood flow cytometric assay, neutrophils activated with bacterial products take up Probe (8) and upregulate CD11b. Fluorescent signal is blocked in activated neutrophils with 100 μM sivelestat co-incubation. MFI = Geometric mean fluorescent index. $^{*}P < 0.05$, $^{**}P < 0.01$, exact multiplicity adjusted *p* values are shown with the figure. **(C)** Reproduced under the CC BY 4.0 license (40).

similar protease families (62, 63). Finally, the recently synthesized fluorogenic toolbox contained unique substrate-fluorophore combinations for each of the four neutrophil serine proteases (HNE, proteinase 3, cathepsin G and neutrophil serine protease 4) and revealed for the first time their uneven distributions in azurophil granules (64).

To enable clinical, functional neutrophil imaging via HNE activity at inflammatory sites a Neutrophil Activation Probe (NAP) was developed (42). Using static quenching NAP's tribranched structure holds fluorescein moieties in close proximity limiting fluorescence. Each of these SmartProbe's three branches contain an HNE substrate sequence cleaved by the active enzyme to generate large fold increases in fluorescent intensity. Encouraging results with NAP came from synthesizing the SmartProbe to GMP standards and endomicroscopically imaging neutrophil activation in ventilated and perfused *ex vivo* human lungs (37). Craven et al. found NAP to be dequenched within the phagolysosome specifically in response to NE and this lead to a successful phase 1 clinical study (NCT01532024) (42). The ability of NAP to inform clinical decision making is currently being investigated in the phase 2 clinical study, SNAP-IT (number: NCT02804854). SNAP-IT will evaluate the utility of imaging NAP-illumined neutrophils, endomicroscopically, in intensive care unit patients.

Formyl Peptide Receptor 1

NIR imaging is often superior to other wavelengths as tissue autofluorescence is lowest in this region of the visible spectrum. Zhou et al. synthesized a NIR fMLF receptor 1 targeting nanoprobe for imaging inflammation (**Figure 3**) (43). The issue of inflammatory site access was solved by building the labeling (cFLFLF) and fluorophore (Oyster-800) components onto a hydrophilic 8-arm PEG scaffold. There are many benefits to using the cFLFLF ligand: its high affinity FPR1 binding (K_d = 2 nM) generates a sensitive readout of leukocyte distribution (65). The ability of cFLFLF probes to access inflammatory sites with either PET (^{64}Cu, ^{99m}Tc) or NIR (Cy5, Cy7) labels has also been demonstrated. However FPR1 is not cell-type specific and these probes bound macrophages (66) and neutrophils (67, 68). cFLFLF probes may generate a useful readout when information on inflammatory cell accumulation is sought in broad terms but may fail to clarify whether clinical intervention should focus on altering neutrophil or macrophage activity.

Pellico et al. created neutrophil-specific radiotracers with dual PET and MRI signals by coating gallium-doped nanoparticles with cFLFLF for FPR1 labeling (44). Coating with peptide can produce significant probe hydrophobicity which has prevented other radiotracers from reaching the inflammatory site. By citrate-coating nanoparticles, the relatively large nanoparticle

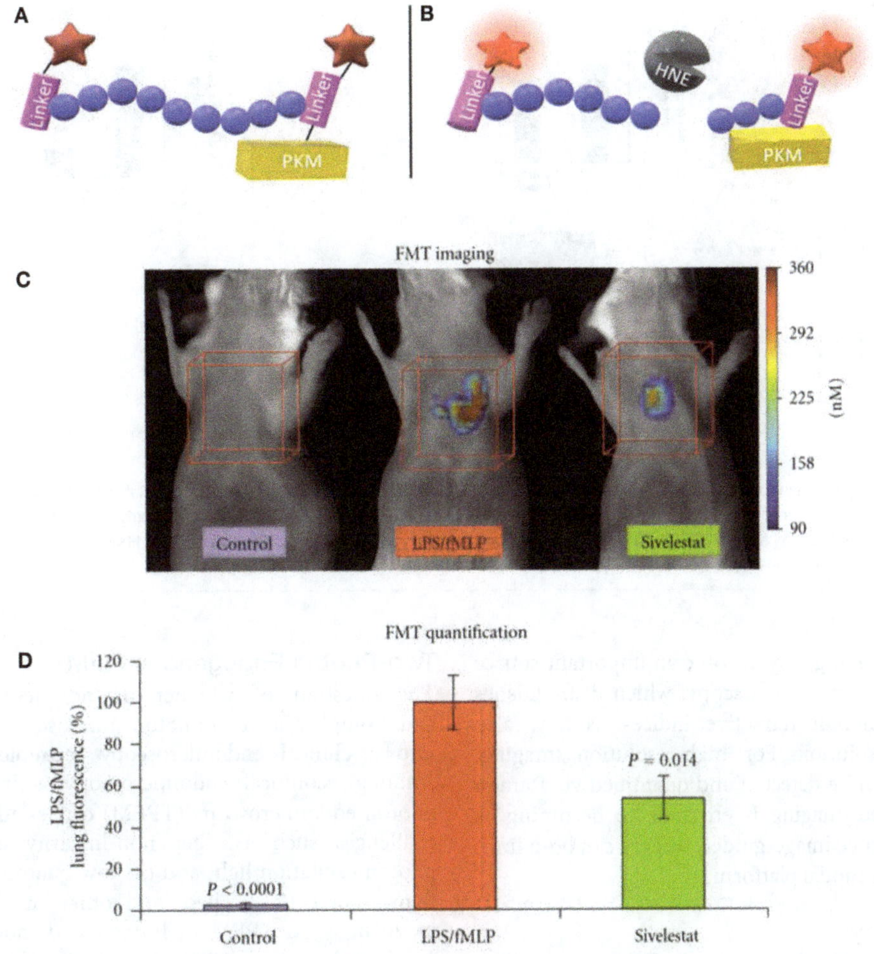

FIGURE 2 | Schematic representation of NE680 FAST before **(A)** and after **(B)** cleavage by active NE which alleviates fluorescence quenching. **(C)** Fluorescence molecular tomography of NE680 FAST (4 nM intranasal) instilled into control, LPS/fMLP and LPS/fMLP mice treated with inhibitor. NIR signal is absent in untreated controls and reduced in sivelestat (5 mg/kg intranasal) treated controls **(D)** and mean concentration of fluorescence (in nM) was quantified in the lung area ROIs (orange cubes) for control ($N = 12$), LPS/fMLP ($N = 16$), and sivelestat ($N = 12$) groups. **(C,D)**

surface confers the necessary solubility for targeting neutrophils *in vivo*. Although neutrophil depletion was capable of removing signal, it also removes important cross-talk from the LPS inflammatory response.

A truly neutrophil specific target has proved elusive. Instead neutrophil specificity has arisen from combinatorial strategies exploiting the unique confirmations of certain targets within neutrophils. For example, HNE reaches such high concentrations in neutrophils that most systems will fail to detect the minority of HNE positive monocytes which bares far lower quantities of the enzyme. Neutrophil specific functions can also be exploited by careful probe design. Phagolysosome alkalinisation does not occur in monocytes and enhance the fluorescence signal of some fluorophores. The super-silent FRET probe combines these structural and functional cellular characteristics to achieve neutrophil specificity. Label-free methods of cell identification have also sought neutrophils using targets found in other cell types but uniquely arranged in neutrophils.

Label Free Neutrophil Imaging

Neutrophil imaging in the context of inflammatory research has aimed at understanding the relevance of cellular components to cell function. Questions of molecular colocalization and characterization are well-served by fluorescent labels for elucidating the spatiotemporal relationships of cells and subcellular structures without altering the processes for investigation. As translational research influences surgical guidance questions of long-term cytotoxicity and ease-of-adoption are more important. Label free imaging, which may seem imprecise for research purposes, is often cheaper, safer and does not require the considerable translation effort of alternative techniques. Molecules such as NADH, elastin, and hemoglobin have been claimed to provide intracellular and extracellular autofluorescence, but signals from cells will always be an amalgamation of signatures of multiple and complex analytes. There is still much characterization to generate clinically meaningful autofluorescence imaging and techniques such as

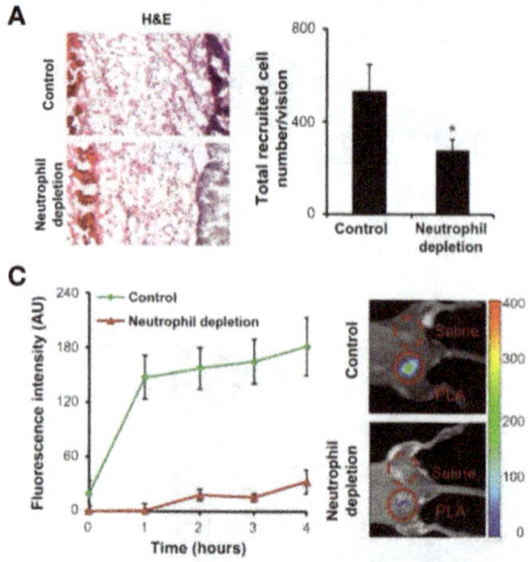

FIGURE 3 | fMLF receptor targeting nanoprobes were implanted in control and neutrophil depleted mice, neutrophils were labeled and quantified. **(A)** Image of hematoxylin and eosin staining and quantification of inflammatory cells. **(B)** Immunohistochemistry and quantification of neutrophils. **(C)** Fluorescence intensities over 4 h post-injection showing the diminished accumulation of the nanoprobe in neutrophil depleted mice compared to control. H&E, hematoxylin and eosin; IHC, immunohistochemistry; PLA, poly(lactic acid); $^{*}P < 0.05$, $^{**}P < 0.01$.

fluorescence lifetime imaging may become an important source of differentiation. Reflectance microscopy, which distinguishes between matter of different refractive indices, is now also capable of cellular resolution. For high-resolution imaging, individual molecules can be detected and quantified via Raman spectroscopy. Label free imaging is en route to becoming as informative as fluorescence image-guided surgery can be, a limit it may exceed in a multi-modal platform.

Raman Spectroscopy

By measuring the minute proportion of photons which interact with molecules inelastically, Raman spectroscopy can, non-destructively, describe the chemical composition of unlabeled matter. The first look at a leukocyte using Raman spectroscopy was when Puppels et al. compared eosinophils and Chinese hamster lung cells (69). The group found nuclei spectroscopically distinct from cytoplasm and that distinctions between granulocytes may be made on the basis of their cytoplasmic contents (70). In 1998, Otto et al. collected the first Raman spectrum of activated neutrophils (71). More recently, Ramoji et al. demonstrated the ability to discern between lymphocytes and neutrophils with concomitant Raman mapping of nuclear morphology (45). Using principal components analysis, cells could be classified with 94% accuracy in the validation dataset and predicted with 81% accuracy in a new dataset from a completely different donor. As Raman spectroscopy can describe intracellular contents it may be better suited to quantifying cell function. Instead of identifying cells, Harz et al. used spectrally distinct Raman and fluorescence excitation wavelengths to successfully multiplex these spectroscopic and microscopic techniques (2). Particularly in such a multiplexed system, intracellular localization and oxidation states of functionally significant molecules may be revealed through Raman mapping to imitate whether or not neutrophils are effecting processes such phagocytosis and to what extent (72).

Two-Photon Endogenous FLIM

The question of whether or not technology as nascent and complex as two-photon microscopy can be translated into a clinical endomicroscopy technology is unanswered. Although confocal endomicroscopy is in clinical use, two-photon endomicroscopy (TPEM) carries additional fiber optics challenges such as fiber non-linearity distorting the two-photon excitation light and the low quantum yields of intrinsic fluorophores (73). These and other hurdles were overcome in 2008, when TPEM of human and mouse sarcomeres was conducted using a GRIN lens (74). The technique involved a minimally-invasive needle clad fiber capable of imaging directly beneath the skin. *In vivo* TPEM was performed laparoscopically with a "stick" lens which avoids GRIN lens associated spherical aberrations revealing ovarian cancer through a laparoscopic procedure, centimeters into the body (75). However murine tissues were investigated *in vivo* with a flexible FLIM endomicroscope, of working distance 135 µm in 2011, and the field continues to rapidly improve this label-free technology (76).

Using two-photon excited fluorescence (TPEF), Zeng et al. characterized blood cells by their endogenous fluorescence lifetime signals (**Figure 4**). TPEF fluorescence lifetime imaging can detect differences in bound and unbound NADH such erythrocytes, agranulocytes and granulocytes are distinguishable (46). As proportions of bound and free NADH vary by the dominant metabolic pathway employed by the cell—TPEF FLIM is functional imaging. Metabolic functional imaging may be able to identify granulocytes undergoing phagocytosis but whether or not phagocytosis and other factors affecting the NAD/NADH ratio, such as oxygen availability, can be disentangled remains unclear. By visualizing cytoplasmic protein, TPEF FLIM can identify the size and shape of cells and, by exclusion, their nuclei—detailing the characteristic lobular structure of granulocyte nuclei. With neutrophils comprising 95% of the granulocytes population, these morphological distinctions give TPEF FLIM neutrophil-specificity to rival the

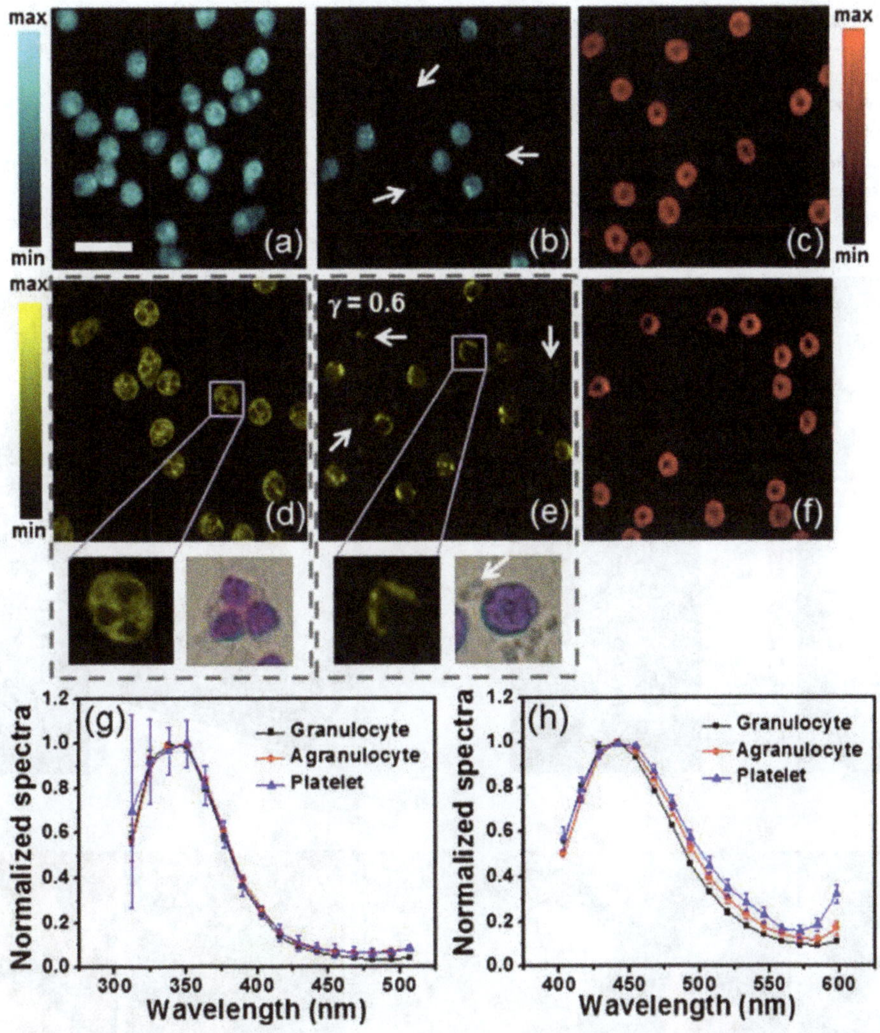

FIGURE 4 | TPEF showing granulocytes, agranulocytes with platelets (white arrows) and erythrocytes **(a–c)** under 600 nM excitation and **(d–f)** under 700 nM excitation, with bright field images in **(d)** and **(e)** showing blood smears granulocytes and agranulocytes with platelets. Normalized spectra of blood cell autofluorescence under 600 nm (5 mW) and 720 nm (10 mW) excitation, are seen in **(g)** and **(h)**, respectively. The acquisition time for each TPEF image: 32 s; resolution: 128 × 128 pixels; scale bar: 20 μm; γ is the gamma value in the gamma correction of **(e)**.

best ligand-based, fluorescent probes. Although the distinction between phagocytic and untreated neutrophils is subtle, this technique can separate untreated from activated neutrophils on morphological grounds. Quiescent neutrophils have a rounded morphology but membrane ruffling characteristic of neutrophil activation was visualized when neutrophils phagocytosed *E. coli* (46).

MACROPHAGES AS BIOMARKERS

Macrophages are readily found at the site of inflammation or infection, forming the first defense against pathogens. Although they play a key role in the initiation of defensive inflammation, recent literature suggests they are also responsible for the resolution of inflammation and repair processes (77). Several large studies show the role of macrophages in solid tumors, sentinel lymph node metastasis, rheumatoid arthritis and liver fibrosis (21–24). In ophthalmology, macrophages have been shown to play a role in preventing ocular infection (78) and contribute to corneal wound healing (79) and biomarkers of macrophage activity have been linked to primary open angle glaucoma and dry eye disease (80, 81).

Macrophages have been broadly classified into two different phenotypes—M1 and M2, with further subsets M2a, M2b, M2c identified, and they display plasticity by moving between these phenotypes (82). Generally, the M1 "classically activated" macrophages are seen as pro-inflammatory and exhibit killing mechanisms against microorganisms, while M2 "alternatively activated" macrophages are anti-inflammatory and exhibit wound healing functions. Further evidence shows that they

TABLE 3 | Overview of optical probes for imaging macrophages.

Target	Molecule class	Optical modality	Models	References
FR-β	Small molecule	SPECT/CT, *in vivo* imaging	Mice/Human (RA)	(85, 86)
CD206	Nanobody (sdAb)	PET	Mice	(87)
	Peptide	Fluorescence	Mice	(88)
MMP-12	Peptidomimetic	Fluorescence	Mice	(89)
Cathepsins	Quenched polymer probe	Fluorescence	Rat	(90)
	Peptide—activity probe	PET/CT and Fluorescence	Mice, Human (PET in IPF patients)	(91)

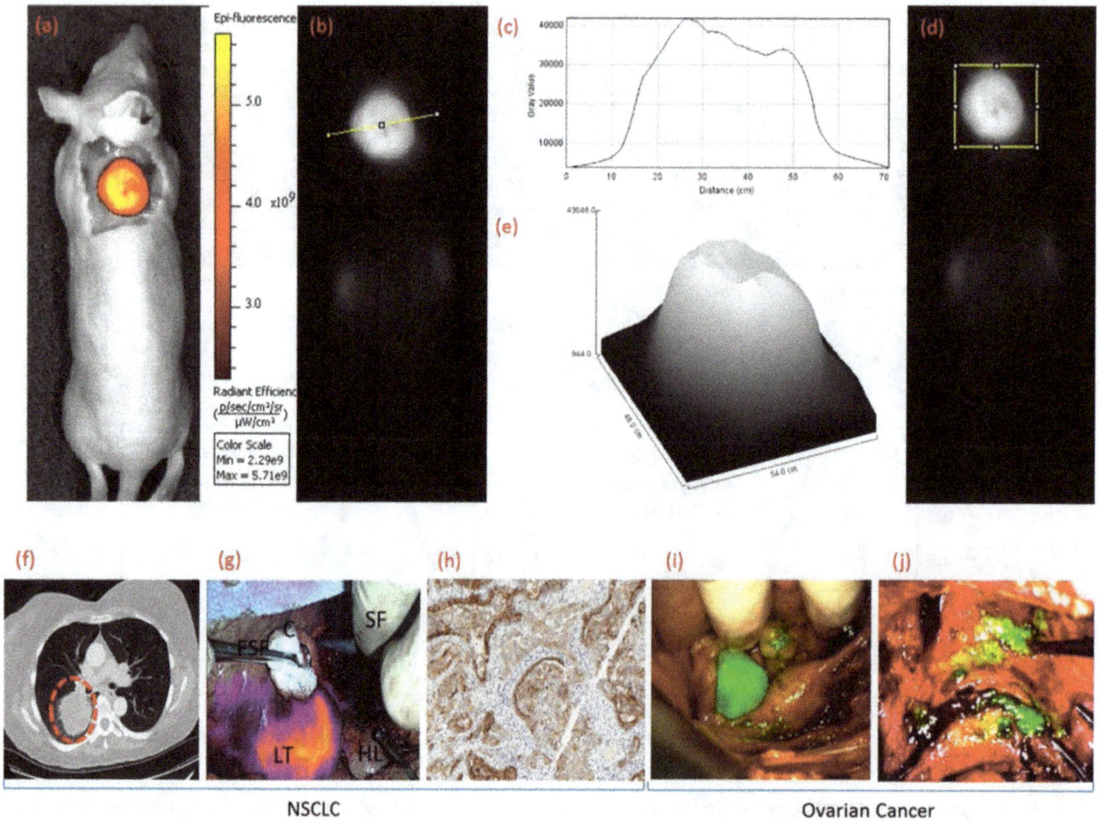

FIGURE 5 | Clinical uses of OTL38 showing whole body fluorescence imaging of a mouse bearing a FRα$^+$ KB tumor in color **(a)** and grayscale **(b,d)** 2 h after administering OTL38. Analysis of gray value vs. distance **(c,e)** [across the line from **(b)** or within the box from **(d)**]. Representative fluorescence images NSCLC and ovarian cancer during image-guided surgery 2 h after administering OTL38. **(f)** Preoperative CT image of pulmonary tumor nodal, **(g)** overlay of fluorescence image over white light image of pulmonary tumor nodal, and **(h)** immunohistochemical (IHC) staining of resected pulmonary tumor nodal indicating tumor is FRα+. Representative fluorescence images over white light images of primary and metastatic ovarian tumors in **(i)** uterine adnexa and **(j)** uterus and bladder peritoneum. LT, lung tumor; HL, healthy lung; FSF, Foerster sponge forceps; SF, surgeons fingers; C, cotton.

do not rest in one polarization state, instead they may be reactivated into a different state. The ability to understand the crosstalk between macrophage activation signals and how this alters their phenotypes would be valuable in characterizing disease phenotypes. In oncology, tumor associated macrophages (TAMs) represent a significant imaging target due to their recruitment in the microenvironment of a tumor (83). Their presence contributes to the invasiveness of tumors as they have been linked to angiogenesis, cell proliferation, invasion and immune suppression (84). Targets to visualize macrophages include MMP-12, cathepsin S, the macrophage mannose receptor (CD206), and folate receptor beta (FR-β) (**Table 3**).

Folate Receptor Beta

Folate receptor (FR) targeting is a promising method for visualization of cells that overexpress the folate receptor. Recently, a demonstration of the capabilities of folate targeting during fluorescence guided surgery of cancer was described by Mahalingam (92). OTL-38 is an NIR labeled folate that accumulates in cancer tissue, has a high target affinity and enables the visualization of cancer tissue using image-guided surgery (**Figure 5**). This agent has completed Phase I and II trials for ovarian and lung cancers, and is now in Phase III clinical trials for the detection of FR$^+$ ovarian cancer (NCT03180307). For inflammatory cells, the β isoform (FR-β) is expressed on

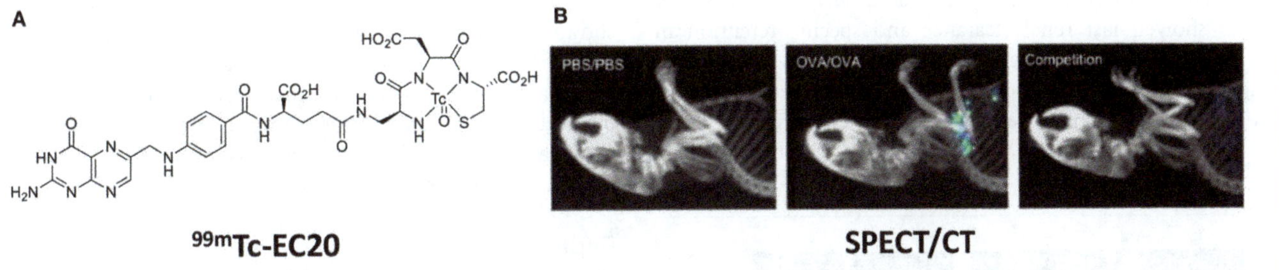

FIGURE 6 | (A) Chemical structure of EC20—a folate radiolabel. **(B)** SPECT/CT images ^{99m}Tc-EC20 uptake in the lung of OVA-induced asthmatic mice, competition experiment with ^{99m}Tc-EC20 plus 100-fold excess folate-glucosamine.

activated macrophages and has a high affinity for its ligand folic acid ($K_d = 10^{-10}$ M) (93). Its identification on synovial macrophages in patients with rheumatoid arthritis was first described by Nakashima-Matsushita et al. (94). Studies on both rheumatoid and osteoarthritis in dogs, horses, rats, mice, and humans have demonstrated that essentially all joints experiencing active inflammation uptake folate conjugates (93). A number of studies have reported on the cellular uptake of FR targeted molecules by activated monocytes (95) and macrophages in a number of different diseases (85, 86, 96).

Xia et al. investigated the presence of the folate receptor on activated macrophages from arthritic patients (85). Fluorescence imaging was used to show that the folate receptor was a valid marker for activated macrophages, while non-activated macrophages did not express the folate receptor. After characterizing that bacteria-recruited murine macrophages expressed FR and that these were activated (upregulation of Ly-6C/G, CD80, and CD86), folate-FITC was incubated with the synovial fluid of patients with diagnosed rheumatoid arthritis. A subset of the CD11b$^+$ macrophages was found to uptake folate-FITC, and competition experiments showed that this uptake could be inhibited with the non-conjugated folic acid—showing FR specificity. Finally, a technetium-radiolabelled folate (FolateScan: EC20) was utilized to perform SPECT imaging of human inflamed joints in a Phase II trial (NCT00588393).

In murine models of asthma, Shen et al. showed that *ex vivo* lung macrophages with an M2 phenotype (arginase$^+$, CD206$^+$) bound the green fluorescent probe, folate-Oregon Green. Further, SPECT/CT imaging of ^{99m}Tc-EC20 showed uptake in ovalbumin induced asthmatic lungs, while there was no uptake in the lungs of healthy mice (**Figure 6**) (86).

Recent work by Poh et al. showed that a folate liposome could act as a specific method of targeting FR$^+$ immune cells, specifically in mouse models of colitis and atherosclerosis (97). This study used fluorescent DiD liposomes, labeled with folate, as a demonstration of the ability to deliver payloads via the folate receptor which can accumulate in inflamed tissues. Atherosclerotic mice (ApoE$^{-/-}$ mice fed a high fat diet) were injected via the tail vein with 2 mg/kg of NT-liposome-DiD or Fol-liposome-DiD, respectively. Fluorescence imaging showed selective uptake of Fol-liposomes in the atherosclerotic mice.

To further our understanding of the clinical applicability of folate targeted imaging agents, the field should aim to evaluate their performance in human inflammatory models. It is however also worth mentioning an observation from this field; the use of folate depleted media is necessary for any folate targeting cell studies due to high levels of folic acid in routine media formulations.

CD206

CD206, also known as the macrophage mannose receptor (MMR), is a well-reported marker of M2 differentiated macrophages (82). Its functional role is to recognize mannose lectins found on pathogens. A number of different approaches to probe design have been taken against CD206$^+$ macrophages, from antibodies to a more recent report of a target-binding peptide. The Manocept concept of nanomolecule imaging agents targeting the lectin domain of CD206 has resulted in the FDA approval of γ-Tilmanocept, a ^{99m}Tc-labeled radiolabelled tracer for the imaging of sentinel lymph nodes (98). A similar strategy was applied by Kim et al. who developed a near-infrared MMR targeting polymer and utilized using OCT-NIRF imaging to visualize carotid atheroma plaques (99). However, mannose derivatives are not specific to CD206 and can be recognized by other mannose receptors (100). Therefore, there is a need to develop ligands that are more specific for CD206 which are more suitable for use in the clinic.

Targeted Nanobodies

The most advanced agents for CD206 targeting are labeled nanobodies, which have shown promise as molecular imaging agents (101). Nanobodies (Nb) have been developed as imaging tracers against a number of targets in oncology and inflammation due to their high affinities and small size compared to antibodies (102). Movahedi et al. produced a ^{99m}Tc-labeled nanobody against MMR with an affinity of 2 nM determined by SPR and validated its use for SPECT/micro-CT imaging of tumor-associated macrophages in preclinical models (103). SPECT/CT imaging in tumor-bearing mice showed uptake of the Nb which was significantly higher than uptake of the control Nb with analysis of the dissected tissue confirming these findings.

This nanobody was further developed by Blykers et al. as an ^{18}F-PET tracer for the detection of macrophages in tumor stroma (87). Tumor associated macrophages (TAMs) with upregulated CD206 were found to be tumor promoting. *In vitro* studies with the ^{18}F-fluorobenzoic acid (FB) labeled nanobody (anti-MMR 3.49) showed that it had a high affinity for human MMR (K_D = 1.8 nM), while *in vivo* biodistribution studies showed fast renal clearance and specific retention in the tumor and MMR-expressing tissue. In a small animal PET imaging study, the nanobody was specifically recognized by MMR in 3LL-R tumor bearing mice, when compared with the uptake in MMR-deficient mice (**Figure 7**). This ligand shows promise as a radiopharmaceutical, while in future it could be developed as an optical probe for highlighting M2 macrophages by fluorescence guided surgery. As noted by Debie et al., the fluorophore chosen and method of conjugation should be carefully considered when developing labeled nanobodies (104).

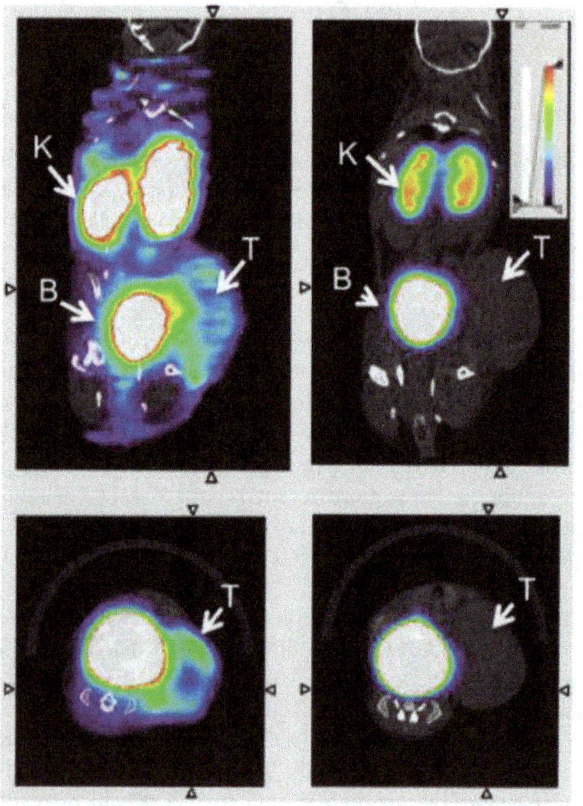

FIGURE 7 | Transverse and coronal PET/CT images of WT (left) vs. MMR-deficient (right) 3LL-R tumor–bearing mice scanned 3 h after injection of ^{18}F-FB-anti MMR 3.49. Arrows point to tumor (T), kidney (K), and bladder (B).

Peptides

Fluorescent peptides are a widely utilized method for labeling receptors and a number of peptidic agents are under clinical investigation for cancer and bacterial infection imaging (10). Recently, Scodeller et al. showed that M2-like TAMs could be targeted by a "FAM-UNO" fluorescent peptide [sequence: 5(6)-FAM-Ahx-CSPGAKVRC] (88). The peptide sequence was identified by *in vivo* phage display of peptides that bound peritoneal macrophages in 4T1 tumor-bearing mice. FAM-UNO was found to target M2-like TAMs via the CD206 receptor (**Figure 8**) and this binding was confirmed by fluorescence anisotropy. Cargos were delivered to TAMs by coating polymer vesicles with the FAM-UNO peptide and these could be used as a contrast agent for sentinel lymph node imaging. Although this agent is yet to be translated to humans, it could be an attractive method for imaging TAMs. However, green autofluorescence of human tissues means alternative fluorophores may need to be considered to make a case for future clinical applications.

MMP-12

The matrix metalloproteinases (MMPs) are a family of proteases that play a key role in ECM structure, function and remodeling. In the tumor microenvironment macrophages have been found to be potent producers of MMP 2 and 9 (105). It is important to note the pioneering work of the Tsien lab and Avelas Biosciences in advancing activatable cell penetrating peptides (ACPPs) for imaging protease activity. In 2004, the lab demonstrated that an MMP-2 cleavable ACPP could detect tumor cells in resected tissue (106). More recently, Miampamba et al. developed AVB-620, a ratiometric ACPP

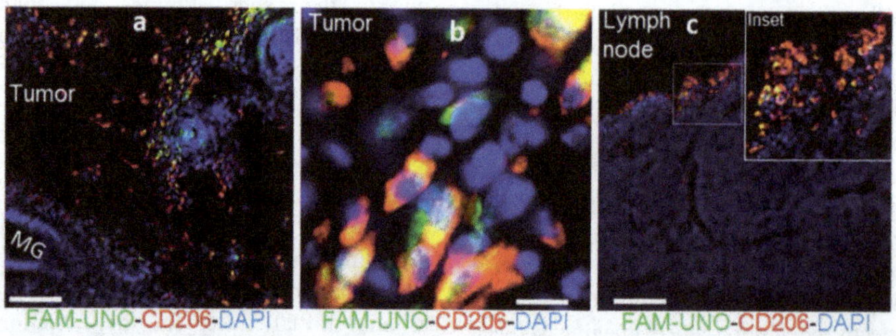

FIGURE 8 | FAM-UNO accumulates in CD206$^+$, TIE2$^+$ macrophages in breast tumors **(a,b)** and lymph nodes **(c)**. 4T1 tumor bearing mice were injected i.v. with FAM-UNO (30 nmol), mice were sacrificed after 2 h and tumor tissues were analyzed by immunofluorescence: rabbit anti-FAM (green), rat anti-CD206 (red) antibodies and counterstained with DAPI. Scale: 100 μm.

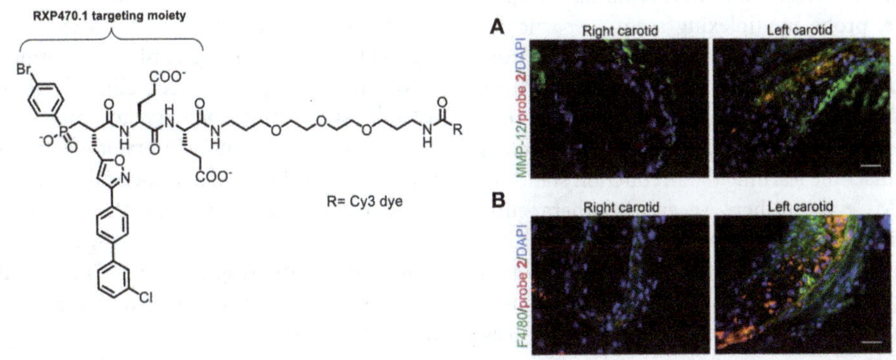

FIGURE 9 | Left: Structure of the Cy3-labeled MMP-12 probe 2. Right: Immunostaining demonstrating that the Cy3-labeled probe 2 (red) binds to carotid arteries and co-localizes with an MMP-12 antibody (**A**, green) and F4/80 positive cells (**B**, green). Nuclei are stained with DAPI (blue). Scale: 50 μm. Reproduced under the CC BY 4.0 license (89).

with Cy5 and Cy7 fluorophores that is a substrate for MMP-2 and -9 (107). This agent has completed Phase I clinical trials for imaging breast cancer tumors in patients undergoing surgery (NCT02391194).

While there are many non-selective imaging agents for MMPs, there is a lack of selective MMP tracers and this may hamper the understanding of the role of a specific MMP in disease. For example MMP-12, macrophage elastase, is responsible for the breakdown of elastin and it is associated with a number of inflammatory pathologies such as aortic aneurysm, emphysema, and rheumatoid arthritis (108). It has been characterized as having a protective role during wound healing in injury models (109).

Bordenave et al. reported the synthesis and evaluation of a Cy5 MMP-12 probe based on a pseudopeptide (RXP470.1) which had previously been shown to inhibit atherosclerotic plaque growth *in vivo* (110). This study noted that the fluorophore used was important to the blood clearance rate and biodistribution of this probe, a factor that has been highlighted by other groups working on the development of fluorescent probes. Further optimization lead to a zwitterionic labeled probe which had good affinity to MMP-12 and fast blood clearance (89). The selectivity of this MMP inhibitor should give advantages over other pan-MMP probes in showing the specific MMP implicated in a disease. Immunostaining showed an analog (probe 2) bound to MMP-12$^+$ and F4/80 macrophages (**Figure 9**). The probe was used for imaging active forms of MMP-12 in murine models. Using a sponge implantation model of sterile inflammation, increased cell infiltration was seen which correlated with mannose receptor positive macrophages. The study was also interested in the role that MMP-12 plays in aneurysm. In a model of carotid aneurysm, significant upregulation of MMP-12 was seen, along with significantly higher signal for the probe, compared to the control (**Figure 9**). Although this was only demonstrated in a mouse model, because of this probe's high selectivity and the clinical relevance of the experimental setup could allow this probe to be used in an intraoperative setting.

Cathepsins

TAMs remodel the extracellular matrix (ECM) through MMPs and cathepsins, specifically during tumor invasion (111). Onda et al. used a commercial NIR fluorescent protease-activatable probe (ProSense), in which they demonstrated imaging of cathepsin activity and confirmed its localization to macrophages. Using *in vivo* and *ex vivo* models of colon cancer they showed that infiltrating TAMs initiate tissue remodeling at the tumor margins by secreting cathepsins. ProSense signal at the tumor margin was shown to be due to cathepsin B$^+$ macrophage infiltration in a rat colon model (90). However, large probes such as ProSense suffer from slow tumor uptake leading to slow rates of activation, as well as demonstrating off-target activation by other proteases which limits their applicability as a fluorescence diagnostic tool.

A number of alternative cathepsin activatable probes are under development (112, 113). Withana et al. investigated the role that macrophages play in idiopathic pulmonary fibrosis (IPF) by staining human biopsy tissue from IPF patients. The optical probe BMV109 is broadly activated by cathepsins B, S, L, and X, was used to validate pan-cathepsin labeling of sectioned frozen tissue. This showed that macrophages expressing active cathepsins were at fibrotic sites in comparison to healthy tissue which showed no cathepsin activity (91). To date, this probe has only been demonstrated in the topical labeling of IPF tissue, further investigation would be necessary to show its utility in fluorescence based diagnostics in the clinic.

CONCLUSION

The nascent field of optical molecular imaging of inflammatory cells appears to be a vibrantly innovative arena full of early-stage biomarkers that offer promise of patient benefits. Targeting neutrophils and macrophages may deliver previously inaccessible measures of disease activity across common and life-threatening diseases. Whilst, in this review, the current stage of neutrophil and macrophage imaging has been discussed, clearly other inflammatory cells such as T cells play major role in interventional medicine. With many non-redundant targets and readouts available, probe multiplexing seems a particular advantage of this field with the potential to matching monitoring and treatment with immunological precision. As well as being informative in its own right, parallel label-free imaging may become a rapid means of interpreting labeled techniques across multiple contexts and machine learning data-reduction stands to push the power of OMI even further. An exciting therapeutic potential lies in the how imaging agents can impact the drug discovery process—with immune cells. These new technologies stand to enrich assay outputs, accelerate drug development decisions and clinical outputs, and enable better direct drug response metrics in trials.

Future studies will demonstrate the translatability of imaging agents into clinically useful optical probes. Despite the plethora of novel reagents advancing with *in vitro* investigations very few have begun the translational journey. This inertia is perhaps not surprising as the technical demands of translating novel imaging methods can become overwhelming, especially within an academic environment. Probes must be innovative enough to meet clinical needs, yet synthetically feasible and complementary to imaging systems. This is a fiercely interdisciplinary pursuit from start to finish and nearly impossible without optical imaging device standards, as all technologies must meet safety and efficacy standards. Without standardization, investigators risk underestimating translation-ready reagents with "sub-standard" apparatus, or unnecessarily pursue doomed reagents with poor selectivity and specificity (114).

AUTHOR CONTRIBUTIONS

GB and TC wrote the manuscript. KD and MB assisted with proofreading and preparation for publication.

REFERENCES

1. Sun Y, You S, Tu H, Spillman DR, Chaney EJ, Marjanovic M, et al. Intraoperative visualization of the tumor microenvironment and quantification of extracellular vesicles by label-free nonlinear imaging. *Sci Adv.* (2018) 4:eaau5603. doi: 10.1126/sciadv.aau5603
2. Harz M, Kiehntopf M, Stckel S, Rsch P, Deufel T, Popp J. Analysis of single blood cells for CSF diagnostics via a combination of fluorescence staining and micro-Raman spectroscopy. *Analyst.* (2008) 133:1416–23. doi: 10.1039/b716132h
3. Zhang RR, Schroeder AB, Grudzinski JJ, Rosenthal EL, Warram JM, Pinchuk AN, et al. Beyond the margins: real-time detection of cancer using targeted fluorophores. *Nat Rev Clin Oncol.* (2017) 14:347–64. doi: 10.1038/nrclinonc.2016.212
4. Yserbyt J, Dooms C, Janssens W, Verleden GM. Endoscopic advanced imaging of the respiratory tract: exploring probe-based confocal laser endomicroscopy in emphysema. *Thorax.* (2018) 73:188–90. doi: 10.1136/thoraxjnl-2016-209746
5. Fuchs FS, Zirlik S, Hildner K, Schubert J, Vieth M, Neurath MF. Confocal laser endomicroscopy for diagnosing lung cancer *in vivo*. *Eur Respir J.* (2013) 41:1401–8. doi: 10.1183/09031936.00062512
6. Krstajić N, Akram AR, Choudhary TR, McDonald N, Tanner MG, Pedretti E, et al. Two-color widefield fluorescence microendoscopy enables multiplexed molecular imaging in the alveolar space of human lung tissue. *J Biomed Opt.* (2016) 21:046009. doi: 10.1117/1.JBO.21.4.046009
7. East JE, Vleugels JL, Roelandt P, Bhandari P, Bisschops R, Dekker E, et al. Advanced endoscopic imaging: European Society of Gastrointestinal Endoscopy (ESGE) Technology Review. *Endoscopy.* (2016) 48:1029–45. doi: 10.1055/s-0042-118087
8. Thiberville L, Moreno-Swirc S, Vercauteren T, Peltier E, Cavé C, Bourg Heckly G. *In vivo* imaging of the bronchial wall microstructure using fibered confocal fluorescence microscopy. *Am J Respir Crit Care Med.* (2007) 175:22–31. doi: 10.1164/rccm.200605-684OC
9. Koch M, Symvoulidis P, Ntziachristos V. Tackling standardization in fluorescence molecular imaging. *Nat Photonics.* (2018) 12:505–15. doi: 10.1038/s41566-018-0221-5
10. Staderini M, Megia-Fernandez A, Dhaliwal K, Bradley M. Peptides for optical medical imaging and steps towards therapy. *Biorg Med Chem.* (2018) 26:2816–26. doi: 10.1016/j.bmc.2017.09.039
11. Garland M, Yim JJ, Bogyo M. A bright future for precision medicine: advances in fluorescent chemical probe design and their clinical application. *Cell Chem Biol.* (2016) 23:122–36. doi: 10.1016/j.chembiol.2015.12.003
12. Bowen RC, Ann N, Little B, Harmer JR, Ma J, Mirabelli LG, et al. Neutrophil-to-lymphocyte ratio as prognostic indicator in gastrointestinal cancers: a systematic review and meta-analysis. *Oncotarget.* (2017) 8:32171–89. doi: 10.18632/oncotarget.16291
13. Templeton AJ, McNamara MG, eruga B, Vera-Badillo FE, Aneja P, Ocaa A, et al. Prognostic role of neutrophil-to-lymphocyte ratio in solid tumors: a systematic review and meta-analysis. *J Natl Cancer Inst.* (2014) 106:dju124. doi: 10.1093/jnci/dju124
14. Zhao C, Ding C, Xie T, Zhang T, Dai X, Wei Y, et al. Validation and optimization of the Systemic Inflammation-Based modified Glasgow Prognostic Score in predicting postoperative outcome of inflammatory bowel disease: preliminary data. *Sci Rep.* (2018) 8:747. doi: 10.1038/s41598-017-18771-3
15. de Jager CPC, van Wijk PTL, Mathoera RB, de Jongh-Leuvenink J, van der Poll T, Wever PC. Lymphocytopenia and neutrophil-lymphocyte count ratio predict bacteremia better than conventional infection markers in an emergency care unit. *Crit Care.* (2010) 14:R192. doi: 10.1186/cc9309
16. Yilmaz H, Cakmak M, Inan O, Darcin T, Akcay A. Can neutrophil-lymphocyte ratio be independent risk factor for predicting acute kidney injury in patients with severe sepsis? *Renal Fail.* (2015) 37:225–9. doi: 10.3109/0886022X.2014.982477
17. Angkananard T, Anothaisintawee T, Thakkinstian A. Neutrophil lymphocyte ratio and risks of cardiovascular diseases: a systematic review and meta-analysis. *Atherosclerosis.* (2017) 263:e159–60. doi: 10.1016/j.atherosclerosis.2017.06.507
18. Xu T, Weng Z, Pei C, Yu S, Chen Y, Guo W, et al. The relationship between neutrophil-to-lymphocyte ratio and diabetic peripheral neuropathy in Type 2 diabetes mellitus. *Medicine.* (2017) 96:e8289. doi: 10.1097/MD.0000000000008289
19. Teng F, Ye H, Xue T. Predictive value of neutrophil to lymphocyte ratio in patients with acute exacerbation of chronic obstructive pulmonary disease. *PLoS ONE.* (2018) 13:e0204377. doi: 10.1371/journal.pone.0204377
20. Dundar ZD, Ergin M, Koylu R, Ozer R, Cander B, Gunaydin YK. Neutrophil-lymphocyte ratio in patients with pesticide poisoning. *J Emerg Med.* (2014) 47:286–93. doi: 10.1016/j.jemermed.2014.01.034
21. Zhang QW, Liu L, Gong CY, Shi HS, Zeng YH, Wang XZ, et al. Prognostic significance of tumor-associated macrophages in solid tumor: a meta-analysis of the literature. *PLoS ONE.* (2012) 7:e50946. doi: 10.1371/journal.pone.0050946
22. Sondak VK, King DW, Zager JS, Schneebaum S, Kim J, Leong SPL, et al. Combined analysis of phase III trials evaluating [^{99}mTc]tilmanocept and vital blue dye for identification of sentinel lymph nodes in clinically node-negative cutaneous melanoma. *Ann Surg Oncol.* (2013) 20:680–8. doi: 10.1245/s10434-012-2612-z
23. Cook AD, Hamilton JA. Investigational therapies targeting the granulocyte macrophage colony-stimulating factor receptor-α in rheumatoid arthritis: focus on mavrilimumab. *Ther Adv Musculoskeletal Dis.* (2018) 10:29–38. doi: 10.1177/1759720X17752036

24. Friedman SL, Ratziu V, Harrison SA, Abdelmalek MF, Aithal GP, Caballeria J, et al. A randomized, placebo-controlled trial of cenicriviroc for treatment of nonalcoholic steatohepatitis with fibrosis. *Hepatology.* (2018) 67:1754–67. doi: 10.1002/hep.29477
25. Bressenot A, Salleron J, Bastien C, Danese S, Boulagnon-Rombi C, Peyrin-Biroulet L. Comparing histological activity indexes in UC. *Gut.* (2015) 64:1412–8. doi: 10.1136/gutjnl-2014-307477
26. Li S, Cao W, Han J, Tang B, Sun X. The diagnostic value of white blood cell, neutrophil, neutrophil-to-lymphocyte ratio, and lymphocyte-to-monocyte ratio in patients with primary angle closure glaucoma. *Oncotarget.* (2017) 8:68984–95. doi: 10.18632/oncotarget.16571
27. Biller J, Thies WH. When to operate in carotid artery disease. *Am Fam Physician.* (2000) 61:400–6. Available online at: https://www.aafp.org/afp/2000/0115/p400.html
28. Ionita MG, van den Borne P, Catanzariti LM, Moll FL, de Vries JP, Pasterkamp G, et al. High neutrophil numbers in human carotid atherosclerotic plaques are associated with characteristics of rupture-prone lesions. *Atertio Thromb Vasc Biol.* (2010) 30:1842–8. doi: 10.1161/ATVBAHA.110.209296
29. Sonawane S, Khanolkar V, Namavari A, Chaudhary S, Gandhi S, Tibrewal S, et al. Ocular surface extracellular DNA and nuclease activity imbalance: a new paradigm for inflammation in dry eye disease. *Invest Ophthalmol Vis Sci.* (2012) 53:8253–63. doi: 10.1167/iovs.12-10430
30. Mun C, Gulati S, Tibrewal S, Chen Y-F, An S, Surenkhuu B, et al. A Phase I/II placebo-controlled randomized pilot clinical trial of recombinant deoxyribonuclease (DNase) eye drops use in patients with dry eye disease. *Transl Vis Sci Technol.* (2019) 8:10. doi: 10.1167/tvst.8.3.10
31. Tibrewal S, Ivanir Y, Sarkar J, Nayeb-Hashemi N, Bouchard CS, Kim E, et al. Hyperosmolar stress induces neutrophil extracellular trap formation: implications for dry eye disease. *Invest Ophthalmol Vis Sci.* (2014) 55:7961–9. doi: 10.1167/iovs.14-15332
32. Yoo D-g, Winn M, Pang L, Moskowitz SM, Malech HL, Leto TL, et al. Release of cystic fibrosis airway inflammatory markers from Pseudomonas aeruginosa-stimulated human neutrophils involves NADPH oxidase-dependent extracellular DNA trap formation. *J Immunol.* (2014) 192:4728–38. doi: 10.4049/jimmunol.1301589
33. Kohri K, Ueki IF, Nadel JA. Neutrophil elastase induces mucin production by ligand-dependent epidermal growth factor receptor activation. *Am J Physiol Lung Cell Mol Physiol.* (2002) 283:L531–40. doi: 10.1152/ajplung.00455.2001
34. Bazan NG. Neuroprotectin D1-mediated anti-inflammatory and survival signaling in stroke, retinal degenerations, and Alzheimer's disease. *J Lipid Res.* (2009) 50(Suppl.):S400–5. doi: 10.1194/jlr.R800068-JLR200
35. Gregory AD, McGarry Houghton A. Tumor-associated neutrophils: new targets for cancer therapy. *Cancer Res.* (2011) 71:2411–6. doi: 10.1158/0008-5472.CAN-10-2583
36. Gong L, Cumpian AM, Caetano MS, Ochoa CE, De la Garza MM, Lapid DJ, et al. Promoting effect of neutrophils on lung tumorigenesis is mediated by CXCR2 and neutrophil elastase. *Mol Cancer.* (2013) 12:154. doi: 10.1186/1476-4598-12-154
37. Wu L, Saxena S, Awaji M, Singh KR. Tumor-associated neutrophils in cancer: going pro. *Cancers.* (2019) 11:E564. doi: 10.3390/cancers11040564
38. Langhorst J, Boone J, Lauche R, Rueffer A, Dobos G. Faecal lactoferrin, calprotectin, PMN-elastase, CRP, and white blood cell count as indicators for mucosal healing and clinical course of disease in patients with mild to moderate ulcerative colitis: *post-hoc* analysis of a prospective clinical trial. *J Crohns Colitis.* (2016) 10:786–94. doi: 10.1093/ecco-jcc/jjw044
39. Kok K, Curciarello R, Soband T, Jones S, Docena G, MacDonald T. Human neutrophil elastase degrades the therapeutic monoclonal antibodies effective in IBD. *J Crohns Colitis.* (2018) 12(Suppl. 1):S146. doi: 10.1093/ecco-jcc/jjx180.232
40. Craven TH, Avlonitis N, McDonald N, Walton T, Scholefield E, Akram AR, et al. Super-silent FRET sensor enables live cell imaging and flow cytometric stratification of intracellular serine protease activity in neutrophils. *Sci Rep.* (2018) 8:1–10. doi: 10.1038/s41598-018-31391-9
41. Kossodo S, Zhang J, Groves K, Cuneo GJ, Handy E, Morin J, et al. Noninvasive *in vivo* quantification of neutrophil elastase activity in acute experimental mouse lung injury. *Int J Mol Imaging.* (2011) 2011:1–11. doi: 10.1155/2011/581406
42. Craven T, Walton T, Akram A, McDonald N, Scholefield E, Walsh T, et al. *In-situ* imaging of neutrophil activation in the human alveolar space with neutrophil activation probe and pulmonary optical endomicroscopy. *Lancet.* (2016) 387:S31. doi: 10.1016/S0140-6736(16)00418-9
43. Zhou J, Tsai YT, Weng H, Tang EN, Nair A, Dav. Real-time detection of implant-associated neutrophil responses using a formyl peptide receptor-targeting NIR nanoprobe. *Int J Nanomed.* (2012) 7:2057–68. doi: 10.2147/IJN.S29961
44. Pellico J, Lechuga-Vieco AV, Almarza E, Hidalgo A, Mesa-Nuez C, Fernndez-Barahona I, et al. *In vivo* imaging of lung inflammation with neutrophil-specific 68Ga nano-radiotracer. *Sci Rep.* (2017) 7:1–10. doi: 10.1038/s41598-017-12829-y
45. Ramoji A, Neugebauer U, Bocklitz T, Foerster M, Kiehntopf M, Bauer M, et al. Toward a spectroscopic hemogram: Raman spectroscopic differentiation of the two most abundant leukocytes from peripheral blood. *Anal Chem.* (2012) 84:5335–42. doi: 10.1021/ac3007363
46. Zeng Y, Yan B, Sun QQ, Teh SK, Zhang W, Wen ZL, et al. Label-free *in vivo* imaging of human leukocytes using two-photon excited endogenous fluorescence. *J Biomed Opt.* (2013) 18:040504. doi: 10.1117/1.JBO.18.4.040504
47. Hirche TO, Benabid R, Deslee G, Gangloff S, Achilefu S, Guenounou M, et al. Neutrophil elastase mediates innate host protection against Pseudomonas aeruginosa. *J Immunol.* (2008) 181:4945. doi: 10.4049/jimmunol.181.7.4945
48. Young RE, Thompson RD, Larbi KY, La M, Roberts CE, Shapiro SD, et al. Neutrophil elastase (NE)-deficient mice demonstrate a nonredundant role for NE in neutrophil migration, generation of proinflammatory mediators, and phagocytosis in response to zymosan particles *in vivo*. *J Immunol.* (2004) 172:4493–502. doi: 10.4049/jimmunol.172.7.4493
49. Ferry G, Lonchampt M, Pennel La. Activation of MMP-9 by neutrophil elastase in an *in vivo* model of acute lung injury. *FEBS Lett.* (1997) 402:111–5. doi: 10.1016/S0014-5793(96)01508-6
50. Jackson PL, Xu X, Wilson L, Weathington NM, Clancy JP, Blalock JE, et al. Human neutrophil elastase-mediated cleavage sites of MMP-9 and TIMP-1: implications to cystic fibrosis proteolytic dysfunction. *Mol Med.* (2010) 16:159–66. doi: 10.2119/molmed.2009.00109
51. Oltmanns U, Sukkar MB, Xie S, John M, Chung KF. Induction of human airway smooth muscle apoptosis by neutrophils and neutrophil elastase. *Am J Respir Cell Mol Biol.* (2005) 32:334–41. doi: 10.1165/rcmb.2004-0321OC
52. Benabid R, Wartelle J, Malleret L, Guyot N, Gangloff S, Lebargy F, et al. Neutrophil elastase modulates cytokine expression: contribution to host defense against pseudomonas aeruginosa-induced pneumonia. *J Biol Chem.* (2012) 287:34883–94. doi: 10.1074/jbc.M112.361352
53. Shao MXG, Nadel JA. Neutrophil Elastase Induces MUC5AC mucin production in human airway epithelial cells via a cascade involving protein kinase C, reactive oxygen species, and TNF- -converting enzyme. *J Immunol.* (2005) 175:4009–16. doi: 10.4049/jimmunol.175.6.4009
54. Smallman LA, Hill SL, Stockley RA. Reduction of ciliary beat frequency *in vitro* by sputum from patients with bronchiectasis: a serine proteinase effect. *Thorax.* (1984) 39:663–7. doi: 10.1136/thx.39.9.663
55. Papayannopoulos V, Metzler KD, Hakkim A, Zychlinsky A. Neutrophil elastase and myeloperoxidase regulate the formation of neutrophil extracellular traps. *J Cell Biol.* (2010) 191:677–91. doi: 10.1083/jcb.201006052
56. Wang M, Zhan Y, Chen J, Rong H, O'Neil SP, Ghosh B, et al. Understanding lung deposition of alpha-1 antitrypsin in acute experimental mouse lung injury model using fluorescence microscopy. *Int J Mol Imaging.* (2016) 2016:1–11. doi: 10.1155/2016/5768312
57. Glinzer A, Ma X, Prakash J, Kimm MA, Lohfer F, Kosanke K, et al. Targeting elastase for molecular imaging of early atherosclerotic lesions. *Atertio Thromb Vasc Biol.* (2017) 37:525–33. doi: 10.1161/ATVBAHA.116.308726
58. Talukdar S, Oh DY, Bandyopadhyay G, Li D, Xu J, McNelis J, et al. Neutrophils mediate insulin resistance in mice fed a high-fat diet through secreted elastase. *Nat Med.* (2012) 18:1407–12. doi: 10.1038/nm.2885
59. Muley MM, Reid AR, Botz B, Blcskei K, Helyes Z, McDougall JJ. Neutrophil elastase induces inflammation and pain in mouse knee joints via activation of proteinase-activated receptor-2. *Br J Pharmacol.* (2016) 173:766–77. doi: 10.1111/bph.13237
60. Wiedow O, Meyer-Hoffert U. Neutrophil serine proteases: potential key regulators of cell signalling during inflammation. *J Intern Med.* (2005)

257:319–28. doi: 10.1111/j.1365-2796.2005.01476.x
61. Kasperkiewicz P, Poreba M, Snipas SJ, Parker H, Winterbourn CC, Salvesen GS, et al. Design of ultrasensitive probes for human neutrophil elastase through hybrid combinatorial substrate library profiling. *Proc Natl Acad Sci USA.* (2014) 111:2518–23. doi: 10.1073/pnas.1318548111
62. Kasperkiewicz P, Kot S, Janiszewski T, Groborz K, Porba M, Snipas SJ, et al. Determination of extended substrate specificity of the MALT1 as a strategy for the design of potent substrates and activity-based probes. *Sci Rep.* (2018) 8:1–10. doi: 10.1038/s41598-018-34476-7
63. Poreba M, Solberg R, Rut W, Lunde Ngoc N, Kasperkiewicz P, Snipas Scott J, et al. Counter selection substrate library strategy for developing specific protease substrates and probes. *Cell Chem Biol.* (2016) 23:1023–35. doi: 10.1016/j.chembiol.2016.05.020
64. Kasperkiewicz P, Altman Y, D'Angelo M, Salvesen GS, Drag M. Toolbox of fluorescent probes for parallel imaging reveals uneven location of serine proteases in neutrophils. *J Am Chem Soc.* (2017) 139:10115–25. doi: 10.1021/jacs.7b04394
65. Locke LW, Chordia MD, Zhang Y, Kundu B, Kennedy D, Landseadel J, et al. A novel neutrophil-specific PET imaging agent: cFLFLFK-PEG-64Cu. *J Nucl Med.* (2009) 50:790–7. doi: 10.2967/jnumed.108.056127
66. Yang X, Chordia MD, Du X, Graves JL, Zhang Y, Park YS, et al. Targeting formyl peptide receptor 1 of activated macrophages to monitor inflammation of experimental osteoarthritis in rat. *J Orth Res.* (2016) 34:1529–38. doi: 10.1002/jor.23148
67. Xiao L, Zhang Y, Berr SS, Chordia MD, Pramoonjago P, Pu L, et al. A novel near-infrared fluorescence imaging probe for *in vivo* neutrophil tracking. *Mol Imaging.* (2012) 11:372–82. doi: 10.2310/7290.2011.00054
68. Xiao L, Zhang Y, Liu Z, Yang M, Pu L, Pan D. Synthesis of the Cyanine 7 labeled neutrophil-specific agents for noninvasive near infrared fluorescence imaging. *Bioorg Med Chem Lett.* (2010) 20:3515–7. doi: 10.1016/j.bmcl.2010.04.136
69. Puppels GJ, de Mul FF, Otto C, Greve J, Robert-Nicoud M, Arndt-Jovin DJ, et al. Studying single living cells and chromosomes by confocal Raman microspectroscopy. *Nature.* (1990) 347:301–3. doi: 10.1038/347301a0
70. Puppels GJ, Garritsen HS, Segers-Nolten GM, de Mul FF, Greve J. Raman microspectroscopic approach to the study of human granulocytes. *Biophys J.* (1991) 60:1046–56. doi: 10.1016/S0006-3495(91)82142-7
71. Otto C, Sijtsema NM, Greve J. Confocal Raman microspectroscopy of the activation of single neutrophilic granulocytes. *Eur Biophys J.* (1998) 27:582–9. doi: 10.1007/s002490050169
72. van Manen HJ, van Bruggen R, Roos D, Otto C. Single-cell optical imaging of the phagocyte NADPH oxidase. *Antioxidants Redox Signall.* (2006) 8:1509–22. doi: 10.1089/ars.2006.8.1509
73. Ducourthial G, Leclerc P, Mansuryan T, Fabert M, Brevier J, Habert R, et al. Development of a real-time flexible multiphoton microendoscope for label-free imaging in a live animal. *Sci Rep.* (2015) 5:1–9. doi: 10.1038/srep 18303
74. Llewellyn ME, Barretto RPJ, Delp SL, Schnitzer MJ. Minimally invasive high-speed imaging of sarcomere contractile dynamics in mice and humans. *Nature.* (2008) 454:784–8. doi: 10.1038/nature07104
75. Williams RM, Flesken-Nikitin A, Ellenson LH, Connolly DC, Hamilton TC, Nikitin AY, et al. Strategies for high resolution imaging of epithelial ovarian cancer by laparoscopic nonlinear microscopy. *Transl Oncol.* (2010) 3:181–94. doi: 10.1593/tlo.09310
76. Brown CM, Rivera DR, Pavlova I, Ouzounov DG, Williams WO, Mohanan S, et al. *In vivo* imaging of unstained tissues using a compact and flexible multiphoton microendoscope. *J Biomed Opt.* (2012) 17:040505. doi: 10.1117/1.JBO.17.4.040505
77. Pollard JW. Trophic macrophages in development and disease. *Nat Rev Immunol.* (2009) 9:259–70. doi: 10.1038/nri2528
78. Liyanage SE, Gardner PJ, Ribeiro J, Cristante E, Sampson RD, Luhmann UFO, et al. Flow cytometric analysis of inflammatory and resident myeloid populations in mouse ocular inflammatory models. *Exp Eye Res.* (2016) 151:160–70. doi: 10.1016/j.exer.2016.08.007
79. Liu J, Xue Y, Dong D, Xiao C, Lin C, Wang H, et al. CCR2- and CCR2+ corneal macrophages exhibit distinct characteristics and balance inflammatory responses after epithelial abrasion. *Mucosal Immunol.* (2017) 10:1145–59. doi: 10.1038/mi.2016.139
80. Boehm N, Riechardt AI, Wiegand M, Pfeiffer N, Grus FH. Proinflammatory cytokine profiling of tears from dry eye patients by means of antibody microarrays. *Invest Ophthalmol Vis Sci.* (2011) 52:7725–30. doi: 10.1167/iovs.11-7266
81. Sawada H, Fukuchi T, Tanaka T, Abe H. Tumor necrosis factor-α concentrations in the aqueous humor of patients with glaucoma. *Invest Ophthalmol Vis Sci.* (2010) 51:903–6. doi: 10.1167/iovs.09-4247
82. Hussell T, Bell TJ. Alveolar macrophages: plasticity in a tissue-specific context. *Nat Rev Immunol.* (2014) 14:81–93. doi: 10.1038/nri3600
83. Conway EM, Pikor LA, Kung SHY, Hamilton MJ, Lam S, Lam WL, et al. Macrophages, inflammation, and lung cancer. *Am J Respir Crit Care Med.* (2015) 193:116–30. doi: 10.1164/rccm.201508-1545CI
84. Lewis CE, Pollard JW. Distinct role of macrophages in different tumor microenvironments. *Cancer Res.* (2006) 66:605–12. doi: 10.1158/0008-5472.CAN-05-4005
85. Xia W, Hilgenbrink AR, Matteson EL, Lockwood MB, Cheng JX, Low PS. A functional folate receptor is induced during macrophage activation and can be used to target drugs to activated macrophages. *Blood.* (2009) 113:438–46. doi: 10.1182/blood-2008-04-150789
86. Shen J, Chelvam V, Cresswell G, Low PS. Use of folate-conjugated imaging agents to target alternatively activated macrophages in a murine model of asthma. *Mol Pharm.* (2013) 10:1918–27. doi: 10.1021/mp3006962
87. Blykers A, Schoonooghe S, Xavier C, D'Hoe K, Laoui D, D'Huyvetter M, et al. PET imaging of macrophage mannose receptor-expressing macrophages in tumor stroma using 18F-radiolabeled camelid single-domain antibody fragments. *J Nucl Med.* (2015) 56:1265–71. doi: 10.2967/jnumed.115.156828
88. Scodeller P, Simón-Gracia L, Kopanchuk S, Tobi A, Kilk K, Säälik P, et al. Precision targeting of tumor macrophages with a CD206 binding peptide. *Sci Rep.* (2017) 7:14655. doi: 10.1038/s41598-017-14709-x
89. Razavian M, Bordenave T, Georgiadis D, Beau F, Zhang J, Golestani R, et al. Optical imaging of MMP-12 active form in inflammation and aneurysm. *Sci Rep.* (2016) 6:38345. doi: 10.1038/srep38345
90. Onda N, Kemmochi S, Morita R, Ishihara Y, Shibutani M. *In vivo* imaging of tissue-remodeling activity involving infiltration of macrophages by a systemically administered protease-activatable probe in colon cancer tissues. *Transl Oncol.* (2013) 6:628–37. doi: 10.1593/tlo.13430
91. Withana NP, Ma X, McGuire HM, Verdoes M, van der Linden WA, Ofori LO, et al. Non-invasive imaging of idiopathic pulmonary fibrosis using cathepsin protease probes. *Sci Rep.* (2016) 6:19755. doi: 10.1038/srep19755
92. Mahalingam SM, Kularatne SA, Myers CH, Gagare P, Norshi M, Liu X, et al. Evaluation of novel tumor-targeted near-infrared probe for fluorescence-guided surgery of cancer. *J Med Chem.* (2018) 61:9637–46. doi: 10.1021/acs.jmedchem.8b01115
93. Low PS, Henne WA, Doorneweerd DD. Discovery and development of folic-acid-based receptor targeting for imaging and therapy of cancer and inflammatory diseases. *Acc Chem Res.* (2008) 41:120–9. doi: 10.1021/ar7000815
94. Nakashima-Matsushita N, Homma T, Yu S, Matsuda T, Sunahara N, Nakamura T, et al. Selective expression of folate receptor β and its possible role in methotrexate transport in synovial macrophages from patients with rheumatoid arthritis. *Arthritis Rheum.* (2001) 42:1609–16. doi: 10.1002/1529-0131(199908)42:8<1609::AID-ANR7>3.0.CO;2-L
95. Shen J, Hilgenbrink AR, Xia W, Feng Y, Dimitrov DS, Lockwood MB, et al. Folate receptor-beta constitutes a marker for human proinflammatory monocytes. *J Leukoc Biol.* (2014) 96:563–70. doi: 10.1189/jlb.2AB07 13-372R
96. Han W, Zaynagetdinov R, Yull FE, Polosukhin VV, Gleaves LA, Tanjore H, et al. Molecular imaging of folate receptor β-positive macrophages during acute lung inflammation. *Am J Respir Cell Mol Biol.* (2015) 53:50–9. doi: 10.1165/rcmb.2014-0289OC
97. Poh S, Chelvam V, Ayala-López W, Putt KS, Low PS. Selective liposome targeting of folate receptor positive immune cells in inflammatory diseases. *Nanomedicine.* (2018) 14:1033–43. doi: 10.1016/j.nano.2018.01.009
98. Azad AK, Rajaram MVS, Metz WL, Cope FO, Blue MS, Vera DR, et al. γ-tilmanocept, a new radiopharmaceutical tracer for cancer sentinel lymph nodes, binds to the mannose receptor (CD206). *J Immunol.* (2015) 195:2019–29. doi: 10.4049/jimmunol.1402005

99. Kim JB, Park K, Ryu J, Lee JJ, Lee MW, Cho HS, et al. Intravascular optical imaging of high-risk plaques *in vivo* by targeting macrophage mannose receptors. *Sci Rep.* (2016) 6:22608. doi: 10.1038/srep22608
100. Geijtenbeek TBH, Torensma R, van Vliet SJ, van Duijnhoven GCF, Adema GJ, van Kooyk Y, et al. Identification of DC-SIGN, a novel dendritic cell-specific ICAM-3 receptor that supports primary immune responses. *Cell.* (2000) 100:575–85. doi: 10.1016/S0092-8674(00)80693-5
101. Chakravarty R, Goel S, Cai W. Nanobody: the "magic bullet" for molecular imaging? *Theranostics.* (2014) 4:386–98. doi: 10.7150/thno.8006
102. Devoogdt N, Xavier C, Hernot S, Vaneycken I, D'Huyvetter M, De Vos J, et al. Molecular imaging using nanobodies: a case study. In: Saerens D, Muyldermans S, editors. *Single Domain Antibodies. 911. Methods in Molecular Biology.* Totowa, NJ: Humana Press (2012). p. 559–67. doi: 10.1007/978-1-61779-968-6_35
103. Movahedi K, Schoonooghe S, Laoui D, Houbracken I, Waelput W, Breckpot K, et al. Nanobody-based targeting of the macrophage mannose receptor for effective *in vivo* imaging of tumor-associated macrophages. *Cancer Res.* (2012) 72:4165–77. doi: 10.1158/0008-5472.CAN-11-2994
104. Debie P, Van Quathem J, Hansen I, Bala G, Massa S, Devoogdt N, et al. Effect of dye and conjugation chemistry on the biodistribution profile of near-infrared-labeled nanobodies as tracers for image-guided surgery. *Mol Pharm.* (2017) 14:1145–53. doi: 10.1021/acs.molpharmaceut.6b01053
105. Kessenbrock K, Plaks V, Werb Z. Matrix metalloproteinases: regulators of the tumor microenvironment. *Cell.* (2010) 141:52–67. doi: 10.1016/j.cell.2010.03.015
106. Jiang T, Olson ES, Nguyen QT, Roy M, Jennings PA, Tsien RY. Tumor imaging by means of proteolytic activation of cell-penetrating peptides. *Proc Natl Acad Sci USA.* (2004) 101:17867–72. doi: 10.1073/pnas.0408191101
107. Miampamba M, Liu J, Harootunian A, Gale AJ, Baird S, Chen SL, et al. Sensitive *in vivo* visualization of breast cancer using ratiometric protease-activatable fluorescent imaging agent, AVB-620. *Theranostics.* (2017) 7:3369–86. doi: 10.7150/thno.20678
108. Parks WC, Shapiro SD. Matrix metalloproteinases in lung biology. *Respir Res.* (2000) 2:3. doi: 10.1186/rr33
109. Dean RA, Cox JH, Bellac CL, Doucet A, Starr AE, Overall CM. Macrophage-specific metalloelastase (MMP-12) truncates and inactivates ELR+ CXC chemokines and generates CCL2, −7, −8, and−13 antagonists: potential role of the macrophage in terminating polymorphonuclear leukocyte influx. *Blood.* (2008) 112:3455–64. doi: 10.1182/blood-2007-12-129080
110. Bordenave T, Helle M, Beau F, Georgiadis D, Tepshi L, Bernes M, et al. Synthesis and *in vitro* and *in vivo* evaluation of MMP-12 selective optical probes. *Bioconj Chem.* (2016) 27:2407–17. doi: 10.1021/acs.bioconjchem.6b00377
111. Afik R, Zigmond E, Vugman M, Klepfish M, Shimshoni E, Pasmanik-Chor M, et al. Tumor macrophages are pivotal constructors of tumor collagenous matrix. *J Exp Med.* (2016) 213:2315–31. doi: 10.1084/jem.20151193
112. Ofori LO, Withana NP, Prestwood TR, Verdoes M, Brady JJ, Winslow MM, et al. Design of protease activated optical contrast agents that exploit a latent lysosomotropic effect for use in fluorescence-guided surgery. *ACS Chem Biol.* (2015) 10:1977–88. doi: 10.1021/acschembio.5b00205
113. Verdoes M, Edgington LE, Scheeren FA, Leyva M, Blum G, Weiskopf K, et al. A nonpeptidic cathepsin S activity-based probe for noninvasive optical imaging of tumor-associated macrophages. *Chem Biol.* (2012) 19:619–28. doi: 10.1016/j.chembiol.2012.03.012
114. Sevick-Muraca EM, Zhu B. The need for performance standards in clinical translation and adoption of fluorescence molecular imaging. *Med Phys.* (2013) 40:040402. doi: 10.1118/1.4789499

2

The Role of 5-ALA in Low-Grade Gliomas and the Influence of Antiepileptic Drugs on Intraoperative Fluorescence

Sergey A. Goryaynov[1], Georg Widhalm[2], Maria F. Goldberg[3], Danil Chelushkin[1], Aldo Spallone[4,5], Kosta A. Chernyshov[3], Marina Ryzhova[1], Galina Pavlova[6], Alexander Revischin[6], Ludmila Shishkina[1], Vadim Jukov[1], Tatyana Savelieva[7,8], Loschenov Victor[7] and Alexander Potapov[7]*

[1] N. N. Burdenko Scientific Research Neurosurgery Institute, Moscow, Russia, [2] Department of Neurosurgery, Medical University of Vienna, Vienna, Austria, [3] I.M. Sechenov First Moscow State Medical University, Moscow, Russia, [4] NCL-Institute of Neurological Sciences, Rome, Italy, [5] Department of Biomedicine, University of Rome Tor Vergata, Rome, Italy, [6] Institute of Gene Biology, Russian Academy of Science, Moscow, Russia, [7] Prokhorov General Physics Institute, Russian Academy of Sciences, Moscow, Russia, [8] National Research Nuclear University, Moscow Engineering Physics Institute, Moscow, Russia

***Correspondence:**
Sergey A. Goryaynov
sgoraynov@nsi.ru

Objectives: Intraoperative tumor visualization with 5-aminolevulinic acid (5-ALA) induced protoporphyrin IX (PpIX) fluorescence is widely applied for improved resection of high-grade gliomas. However, visible fluorescence is present only in a minority of low-grade gliomas (LGGs) according to current literature. Nowadays, antiepileptic drugs (AEDs) are frequently administered to LGG patients prior to surgery. A recent *in-vitro* study demonstrated that AEDs result in significant reduction of PpIX synthesis in glioma cells. The aim of this study was thus to investigate the role of 5-ALA fluorescence in LGG surgery and the influence of AEDs on visible fluorescence.

Patients and Methods: Patients with resection of a newly diagnosed suspected LGG after 5-ALA (25 mg/kg) administration were initially included. During surgery, the presence of visible fluorescence (none, mild, moderate, or bright) within the tumor and intratumoral fluorescence homogeneity (diffuse or focal) were analyzed. Tissue samples from fluorescing and/or non-fluorescing areas within the tumor and/or the assumed tumor border were collected for histopathological analysis (WHO tumor diagnosis, cell density, and proliferation rate). Only patients with diagnosis of LGG after surgery remained in the final study cohort. In each patient, the potential preoperative intake of AEDs was investigated.

Results: Altogether, 27 patients with a histopathologically confirmed LGG (14 diffuse astrocytomas, 6 oligodendrogliomas, 4 pilocytic astrocytomas, 2 gemistocytic astrocytomas, and one desmoplastic infantile ganglioglioma) were finally included. Visible fluorescence was detected in 14 (52%) of 27. In terms of fluorescence homogeneity ($n = 14$), 7 tumors showed diffuse fluorescence, while in 7 gliomas focal fluorescence was noted. Cell density ($p = 0.03$) and proliferation rate ($p = 0.04$) was significantly higher in fluorescence-positive than in fluorescence-negative samples. Furthermore, 15 (56%)

of 27 patients were taking AEDs before surgery. Of these, 11 patients (73%) showed no visible fluorescence. In contrast, 10 (83%) of 12 patients without prior AEDs intake showed visible fluorescence. Thus, visible fluorescence was significantly more common in patients without AEDs compared to patients with preoperative AED intake (OR = 0,15 (CI 95% 0.012–1.07), $p = 0.046$).

Conclusions: Our study shows a markedly higher rate of visible fluorescence in a series of LGGs compared to current literature. According to our preliminary data, preoperative intake of AEDs seems to reduce the presence of visible fluorescence in such tumors and should thus be taken into account in the clinical setting.

Keywords: low-grade glioma, 5-aminolevulinic acid, protoporphyrin IX, fluorescence, antiepileptic drugs

INTRODUCTION

Gliomas are the most common intracranial tumors representing approximately 70% of all primary brain tumors (1, 2). It is well-known that gross-total resection correlates with improved progression-free and overall survival in patients with low-grade gliomas (LGGs) (3–6). Thus, maximum safe resection of LGGs is regarded nowadays as the recommended primary treatment to delay potential malignant transformation (7, 8). However, such maximum safe resection is only achieved in the minority of LGGs due to their infiltrative growth and undefined borders (9).

Surgery using 5-aminolevulinic acid (ALA) induced protoporphyrin IX (PpIX) fluorescence has been introduced to the neurosurgical field for improved intraoperative tumor visualization (10). In the last two decades, such fluorescence-guided resections were especially applied to optimize surgery of high-grade gliomas (HGGs) (11). In this sense, 5-ALA fluorescence-guided surgery results in a significantly higher frequency of complete resections and a prolonged progression-free survival in HGGs (12–17). In the last years, 5-ALA was also increasingly investigated during surgery of radiologically suspected LGGs (3, 7, 11, 13, 18–21). According to the data of these first clinical studies, 5-ALA induced fluorescence is a powerful marker to identify potential regions of malignant transformation (anaplastic foci) during surgery of suspected LGG and thus to avoid histopathological undegrading. However, the majority of pure LGGs cannot be visualized by visible fluorescence according to the current literature (3, 7, 11, 13, 18, 19, 21, 22).

The exact mechanisms of PpIX accumulation and thus the presence or absence of visible 5-ALA induced fluorescence in gliomas are still unclear. A large variety of factors were suspected to influence visible 5-ALA fluorescence such as increased metabolism and up-regulation of porphyrin-producing enzymes (23), reduced iron metabolism within neoplastic cells (24), and reduction of activity of the ferrochelatase enzyme that converts fluorescing PpIX into heme (25). Recently, an *in-vitro* study reported that antiepileptic drugs (AEDs) result in an injury of the mitochondrial membrane and thus lead to inhibition of PpIX synthesis in glioma cells (26). Nowadays, AEDs are frequently administered to patients suffering from LGG prior to surgery. We hypothesize that administration of AEDs might influence the presence of visible fluorescence in LGGs during surgical resection.

The aim of the present study was thus to investigate the role of 5-ALA induced fluorescence in LGG surgery and analyze the influence of AEDs on the presence of visible fluorescence.

MATERIALS AND METHODS

Patient Population

Patients that underwent resection of a newly diagnosed suspected LGG at the Burdenko Neurosurgical Institute after 5-ALA administration between March 2014 and March 2016 were recruited. In our study, altogether 27 patients with a histopathologically confirmed LGG were finally included. Our study cohort included 19 men and eight women with a median age of 33 years (range: 18–66 year). According to our histopathological analysis, 14 diffuse astrocytomas, 6 oligodendrogliomas, 4 pilocytic astrocytomas, 2 gemistocytic astrocytomas, and one desmoplastic infantile ganglioglioma were diagnosed. The application of 5-ALA during surgery was feasible in all 27 patients. In none of our patients, any significant 5-ALA related side effects occurred in our study. Informed consent for the surgical procedure and administration of 5-ALA was obtained from all patients. The study was approved by the local ethics committee of the N. N. Burdenko National Medical Research Center of Neurosurgery (Moscow, Russia).

Inclusion and Exclusion Criteria

Inclusion criteria for enrolment into this study were age ≥18 years, MRI-suspected LGG, possible gross total resection (GTR) (i.e., >90%) as judged by preoperative surgical estimation, absence of any known history of liver disease or signs of significant hepatic dysfunction and Karnofsky scale ≥70. Exclusion criteria for the administration of 5-ALA were history of photosensitivity, patient, or family history of porphyria, pregnancy, and breast-feeding. Only patients with diagnosis of LGG after surgery remained in the final study cohort.

Surgical Procedure

Patients were administered orally 25 mg/kg bodyweight 5-ALA ("Alasence" NIOPIK, Moscow, Russia) dissolved in 100 ml of water ~3 h before surgery. Depending on the tumor localization, intraoperative neuromonitoring with sensory/motor evoked potentials, and/or direct stimulation (Viking Select, Nicolet; $n = 21$ patients) as well as awake surgery ($n = 2$ patients) was performed. A modified neurosurgical microscope (Carl Zeiss OPMI Pentero, Germany) equipped with a fluorescent 400 nm UV light module and specific filters were used. Microsurgical tumor removal was performed using primarily standard white light microscopy with assistance of neuronavigation in most cases ($n = 20$ patients). During surgery, the microscope was switched to violet-blue excitation light repeatedly to visualize potential fluorescence.

Fluorescence intensity was visually assessed by a surgeon and determined as "weak" with only a small tumor part showing pink fluorescence with its bulk not fluorescing at all, "moderate" with more than half of the tumor revealing pink fluorescence, and "bright" with the major part of the tumor looking bright red. Spectroscopy-assisted Fluorescence was quantitatively assessed in 12 patients. The level of fluorescence varied from 0 values up to 15 arbitrary units (after data normalization) regarding the intact brain. We specially did not highlight the role of spectroscopy, as it was performed only in some of our patients. Furthermore, also the intratumoral fluorescence homogeneity of each tumor was determined. In this sense, diffuse fluorescence was defined as homogeneous glowing of the whole tumor. In contrast, focal fluorescence was defined as a circumscribed area of fluorescence within an otherwise non-fluorescing tumor. In the course of surgery, tissue samples from fluorescing and/or non-fluorescing areas within the tumor and/or the assumed tumor border were subsequently collected for histopathological analysis. To avoid potential phototoxicity related to 5-ALA, all patients were protected from strong light sources for at least 24 h after drug administration.

Histopathology

All formalin-fixed, paraffin-embedded tissue samples were processed for hematoxylin and eosin (H & E) staining. Tumor diagnosis was established by an experienced neuropathologist according to the current World Health Organization (WHO) histopathological criteria (27). In our study, cell density and proliferation rate (Ki-67 labeling index) was investigated in each of the collected tissue samples.

Preoperative Intake of AEDs

Since the main focus of our study was to investigate the potential influence of AEDs on 5-ALA induced fluorescence, we documented in each patient if AEDs were administered prior to surgery (yes or no). Patients were ingested average AED dosages: valproic acid (up to 1.5 mg per day), levetiracetam (800 mg per day). We did not study each drug separately, as the general series was not large.

Postoperative Course

The neurological status of each patient was investigated before and after surgery to detect potential postoperative deterioration of neurological symptoms. Additionally, the extent of resection was judged according to the results of an early (up-to 72 h post-surgery) post-operative MRI: (1) GTR was present if at least 90% of the tumor mass was removed, (2) subtotal resection if more than 50% of the tumor mass was resected, and (3) partial resection if <50% of the tumor was removed.

Statistical Analysis

Data processing was performed using R software for statistical computing (version 3.4.4). The continuous variables were compared in groups using Mann–Whitney U-test. To analyze the relationship between the categorical variables, a Fisher exact test was applied. A logistic regression analysis was performed to adjust for confounders when testing the effect of AED on fluorescence. The results were considered statistically significant for $p < 0.05$.

RESULTS

5-ALA Induced Fluorescence and Histopathological Diagnosis

We observed visible fluorescence during surgery in 14 (52%) of 27 cases, whereas no fluorescence was detected in the remaining 13 cases (48%).

According to the histopathological tumor diagnosis, all 4 pilocytic astrocytomas, all 2 gemistocytic astrocytomas, and the only desmoplastic infantile ganglioglioma showed visible fluorescence. Furthermore, visible fluorescence was found in 4 (29%) of 14 diffuse astrocytomas, and 3 (50%) of 6 oligodendrogliomas. According to the intratumoral fluorescence homogeneity ($n = 14$ cases), 7 tumors had "diffuse" visible fluorescence, while the other 7 gliomas had "focal" sites of visible fluorescence. Details on the fluorescence data of our cohort are provided in **Table 1** and illustrative cases in **Figure 1**.

5-ALA Induced Fluorescence and Histological Parameters

Altogether, 80 tissue samples were collected during surgery from the 27 patients (median: 3 samples; range 1–12 specimens per patient). Of these, visible fluorescence was found in 21 samples (26%), whereas 59 samples (74%) showed no visible fluorescence. Cell density was significantly higher in fluorescence-positive samples (2,180 mm^2) than in fluorescence-negative samples (1,510 mm^2; $p = 0.03$). Additionally, the proliferation rate assessed by Ki-67 labeling index was also significantly higher in fluorescence-positive samples (2.52%) than in fluorescence-negative samples (0.41%; $p = 0.04$).

5-ALA Induced Fluorescence and AEDs

Due to a prior history of preoperative seizures, 15 patients (56%) of our study cohort were taking AEDs before surgery (finlepsin, levetiracetam, trileptal, and/or valproid acid). Of the 15 patients with preoperative AED intake, 11 patients (73%) showed no visible fluorescence during the resection. In contrast, 10 (83%) of the remaining 12 patients without prior AEDs intake showed visible fluorescence. Thus, visible fluorescence was significantly more common in patients without AEDs intake as compared to patients with preoperative AED intake [OR = 0.15 (CI 95% 0.012–1.07), $p = 0.046$]. The AED showed to be a significant factor ($p =$ 0,048) influencing the probability of

TABLE 1 | Intraoperative fluorescence characteristics.

Histopathology	Fluorescence					
	Visible fluorescence					Absence of fluorescene
	Fluorescence grade			Fluorescence homogeneity		
	1-Mild	2-Moderate	3-Bright	Diffuse	Focal	
Diffuse astrocytoma	1 (3.7%)	2 (7.4%)	1 (3.7%)	2 (7.4%)	2 (7.4%)	10 (37%)
Oligodendroglioma	1 (3.7%)	1 (3.7%)	1 (3.7%)	1 (3.7%)	2 (7.4%)	3 (11.1%)
Gemistocytic atrocytoma	–	–	2 (7.4%)	2 (7.4%)	0	0
Pilocytic astrocytoma	2 (7.4%)	1 (3.7%)	1 (3.7%)	1 (3.7%)	3 (11.1%)	0
Desmoplastic infantile ganglioglioma	–	1 (3.7%)	–	1 (3.7%)	0	0
In total:	4 (14.8%)	5 (18.5%)	5 (18.5%)	7 (25.9%)	7 (25.9%)	13 (48.1%)
In total:		14 (52%)			14 (51.8%)	13 (48%)
In total:				27 (100%)		

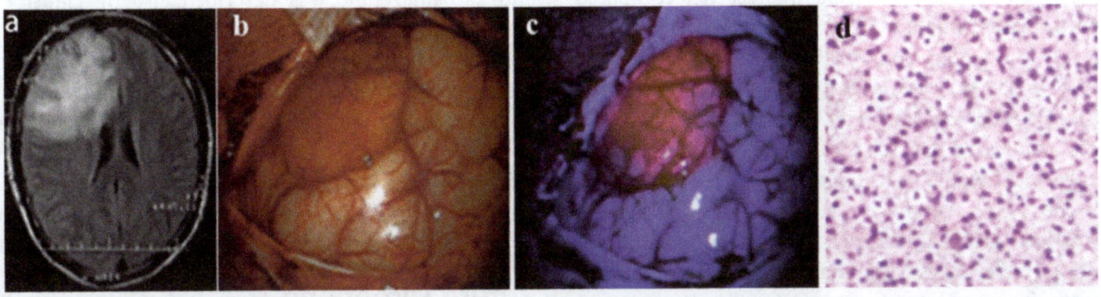

FIGURE 1 | Illustrative case No. 16 (Diffuse fluorescence type). Oligodendroglioma WHO Grade II of the right frontal lobe. **(A)**–Preoperative FLAIR images show a large hyperintense lesion, **(B)**–White light microscopy shows distint cortical abnormalities; **(C)**–The tumor reveals moderate fluorescence with violet-blue excitation light; **(D)**–Histology reveals tumor tissue of a oligodenroglioma WHO grade II. Informed consent has been obtained from the patient for the publication of data, including images.

intraoperative fluorescence when adjusted for other potential confounders (astrocytoma/non-astrocytoma, frontal localization, dexamethasone dose) in a logistic regression model. The other factors included in the model did not show a significant relationship with the fluorescence ($p > 0.05$).

Postoperative Course

After surgery, 21 patients showed stable and four patients improved neurological symptoms. In contrast, deterioration of neurological symptoms was found in the remaining two patients. According to early postoperative MRI, gross total resection was achieved in 16 patients (59%), subtotal resection in 8 patients (30%), and partial resection in three patients (11%). Fluorescence did not correlate with extent of resection.

DISCUSSION

The use 5-ALA induced fluorescence is becoming increasingly popular with the aim of maximizing the extent of resection especially in HGGs and thus improving postoperative patient prognosis. In this sense, fluorescence-guided surgery demonstrated to significantly improve the rate of complete resections in HGGs as compared to microsurgery alone, and this innovative technique also almost doubled the 6-months progression free-survival (16). Recently, visible PpIX fluorescence was found also in other brain lesions such as meningiomas (19), and metastatic tumors (18, 28).

Current Literature: 5-ALA Fluorescence in LGG

So far, the value of 5-ALA induced fluorescence in LGG was only investigated in few studies. In this sense, Ishihara et al. first described in 2007 the application of 5-ALA in two LGG and did not find any visible fluorescence in the multiple collected tissue samples (29). Additionally, Ruge et al. published in 2009 a case report of a 9-year-old girl who underwent fluorescence-guided resection of a pleomorphic xanthoastrocytoma of the right temporal lobe and detected visible fluorescence of the tumor (20). Moreover, Stockhammer et al. published in 2009 a case report of a diffuse astrocytoma WHO grade II with moderate cellular density, higher microvascular density, and visible fluorescence (30). Cases of fluorescence of pilomyxoid astrocytoma and pilocytic astrocytoma were published by Bernal Garcia et al. (31) and Choo et al. (32), respectively. The first series of patients with LGG and 5-ALA was published by Widhalm et al. (33). In this study, all eight diffusely infiltrating WHO grade II gliomas did not show any visible 5-ALA induced fluorescence during surgery. In a further study, Ewelt et al. reported in 2011 visible fluorescence in only one (8%) of 13 LGGs during surgery (7). Three years after the first patient series, Widhalm et al. published a larger series in 2013 and found visible fluorescence in 4 (9%) of 33 LGGs (34). In another study by Marbacher et al., 8 (40%) of 20 LGGs showed visible fluorescence (18). In 2015, Valdes founded visible fluorescence in 4 (33%) of 12 analyzed LGGs (35). Finally, Jaber et al. found in 2016 in the largest series to date visible fluorescence in 13 (16%) of 82 LGGs (36). Thus, according to the current literature visible fluorescence is observed only in a minority of patients with LGGs.

Current Study: 5-ALA Fluorescence in LGG

Despite of these other studies available in the current literature, our data showed the presence of visible fluorescence in more than half of our cases during surgery. One possible explanation for the higher rate of LGGs with visible fluorescence compared to the current literature might be that we used a slightly higher dose of 5-ALA (25 mg/kg bodyweight) as compared to the other studies (18, 33, 34). However, Stummer et al. compared different doses of 5-ALA in malignant glioma surgery (0.2, 2, 20 mg/kg) and concluded that usage of 5-ALA doses more than 20 mg/kg bodyweight would probably not result in an improved fluorescence effect (37). Another explanation might be that we included also other tumor entities apart from diffusely infiltrating gliomas such as pilocytic astrocytomas or one ganglioglioma. Our promising findings have to be confirmed, however, in independent multicenter studies including a larger cohort of patients suffering from LGG.

Interestingly, we did observe visible fluorescence not only in focal intratumoral areas as previously described (33, 34), but also diffuse fluorescence with homogeneous glowing of the whole tumor. We assume that presence of focal visible fluorescence in LGG might represent areas of potential future malignant transformation. Furthermore, future studies should clarify if the extent of resection could be optimized especially in LGGs with a diffuse fluorescence pattern.

5-ALA Fluorescence and Histopathology

In our study, we observed significantly higher levels of cell density and proliferation in samples with visible fluorescence as compared to no fluorescence. This is in line with the two previous studies by Widhalm et al (33, 34). Similarly, Widhalm et al found a significantly higher mitotic rate, cell density, and nuclear pleomorphism in fluorescing samples as compared to non-fluorescing specimens. Furthermore, the proliferation index assessed by MIB-1 LI was significantly higher in samples with visible fluorescence as compared to non-fluorescing specimens. In this sense, these previous data indicate that visible fluorescence is capable to identify anaplastic foci according to the WHO histopathological criteria (33, 34). Since we also found a significantly higher cell density and proliferation rate in areas of visible fluorescence in a series of LGG, we believe that 5-ALA might serve as an early marker of ongoing malignant transformation of an initial LGG. Future studies with sufficient data on follow-up are needed to clarify this important issue.

5-ALA Fluorescence and AEDs

Nowadays, it is common practice for patients with LGG to have medical treatment of epileptic seizures (38–40). Hefti et al. demonstrated in an *in-vitro* study that the PpIX synthesis was reduced by up to 45% in glioma cells under the effect of phenytoin, but not levetiracetam (26). In our study, we found that visible fluorescence was significantly more common in patients without AEDs intake as compared to patients with preoperative AED intake ($r = 0.56$; $p = 0.045$). Of the 15 patients with preoperative AED intake, 11 patients (73%) showed no visible fluorescence during the resection. In contrast, 10 (83%) of the remaining 12 patients without prior AEDs intake showed visible fluorescence. The underlying mechanisms for the observed influence of AEDs on visible fluorescence is unclear so far. The influence of AEDs on activities of 5-aminolevulinic acid dehydrase and uroporphyrinogen I synthetase in erythrocytes of a Vitamin B6-deficient epileptic boy given valproic acid and carbamazepine was described also by Haust et al. from University of Western Ontario, Canada in 1989 (41). One possible hypothesis might be that AEDs have an influence on the enzyms of the PpIX synthesis in the mitochondria of glioma cells and thus result in presence or absence of fluorescence in LGG. A further study on glioblastoma cell lines found that AEDs (phenytoin/valproates) and dexamethasone may inhibit PpIX synthesis (10). The exact mechanisms for the influence of AEDs on visible fluorescence have to be clarified in future studies.

Future Directions

In future, our first observations should be confirmed in further independent studies with a large cohort of patients. Such larger studies allow also the possibility to analyze the influence of different types of AED separately. Furthermore, the influence of AEDs should also be investigated in HGGs. In cases with lack of visual fluorescence, quantitative detection methods might be useful for improved visualization of LGG tissue. In this sense, confocal microscopy is also a powerful tool to visualize cellular 5-ALA-induced tumor fluorescence within LGGs and at the brain-tumor interface (21). However, convincing data of confocal microscopy in a large cohort of patients with LGG are still missing so far. Another method represents the spectroscopic analysis of PpIX accumulation with specific probes. By this approach, Valdes et al. found that accumulation of PpIX can be detected quantitatively despite the poor diagnostic accuracy of visual fluorescence in LGGs (35, 42). Consequently, this promising approach warrants further investigation in future studies.

CONCLUSIONS

In the present study, we investigated the role of 5-ALA in LGGs and the influence of antiepileptic drugs on intraoperative fluorescence. According to our data, we observed a markedly higher rate of visible fluorescence in our series of LGGs (52%) compared to current literature. Furthermore, increased cell density and proliferation was noted in areas of visible fluorescence. Thus, 5-ALA induced fluorescence might also improve intraoperative visualization of a subgroup of LGGs and might be also a useful marker for optimized detection of histopathological heterogeneity during surgery of LGGs. Furthermore, preoperative intake of AEDs seems to reduce the presence of visible fluorescence in such tumors according to our preliminary data and thus this issue should be taken into account in the clinical setting. Further, independent multicenter studies including a larger cohort of LGG patients are required to confirm the promising data of this present study.

LIMITATIONS

We understand that the analysis of factors influencing Fluorescence should be multifold. To reach that, we used the model of logistic regression. AED proved to be a significant factor influencing the probability of intraoperative fluorescence, when adjusted for other potential confounders (astrocytoma/non-astrocytoma, frontal localization, dexamethasone dose, IDH1-mutation) in a logistic regression model. The cell density and Ki67 index were revealed only in patients with multiple biopsies (10 patients). It was concluded, that cell density, and Ki67 index were higher for the biopsy samples taken from the fluorescing zone compared to the non-fluorescing one. We've got little evidence on cell density for the rest 17 patients, with their Ki67 index making up mainly 4–5%. As this is a retrospective analysis enrolling 27 patients, we did not plan to study cell density and Ki67 index. Unfortunately, we've got no complete dataset for Ki67 and cell density to include into a logistic regression model.

ETHICS STATEMENT

This study was carried out local committee of the N. N. Burdenko National Medical Research Center of Neurosurgery (Moscow, Russia) with written informed consent from all subjects. All subjects gave written informed consent in accordance with the Declaration of Helsinki. The protocol was approved by the local committee of the N. N. Burdenko National Medical Research Center of Neurosurgery (Moscow, Russia).

AUTHOR CONTRIBUTIONS

SG, GW, and AP designed the study. LS, VJ, and MR collected the date. TS, VL, GP, and AR worked out the technical details. MG and DC analyzed the data and wrote the paper with input from all authors. AS and AP edited the text. KC analyzed the data and wrote the paper with input from all authors.

ACKNOWLEDGMENTS

We wish to acknowledge the help provided by our colleagues: Danilov G. V., MD, Ph.D., N. N. Burdenko Scientific Research Neurosurgery Institute, Moscow, Russia for statistic support.

REFERENCES

1. DeAngelis LM. Brain tumors. *N Engl J Med.* (2001) 344:114–23. doi: 10.1056/NEJM200101113440207
2. Ostrom QT, Bauchet L, Davis FG, Deltour I, Fisher JL, Langer CE, et al. The epidemiology of glioma in adults: a "state of the science" review. *Neuro Oncol.* (2014) 16:896–913.doi: 10.1093/neuonc/nou087
3. McGirt MJ, Chaichana KL, Attenello FJ, Weingart JD, Than K, Burger PC, et al. Extend of surgical resection is independently associated with survival in patients with hemispheric infiltraiting low-grade gliomas. *Neurosurgery.* (2008) 63:700–8. doi: 10.1227/01.NEU.0000325729.41085.73
4. Sanai N, Berger MS. Glioma extent of resection and its impact on patient outcome. *Neurosurgery.* (2008) 62:753–66. doi: 10.1227/01.neu.0000318159.21731.cf
5. Schomas DA, Laack NNI, Rao RD, Meyer FB, Shaw EG, O'Neill BP, et al. Intracranial low-grade gliomas in adults: 30-year experience with long-term follow-up at Mayo clinic. *Neuro Oncol.* (2009) 11:437–45. doi: 10.1215/15228517-2008-102
6. Smith JS, Chang EF, Lamborn KR, Chang SM, Prados MD, Cha S, et al. Role of extent of resection in the long-term outcome of low-grade hemispheric gliomas. *J Clin Oncol.* (2008) 26:1338–45. doi: 10.1200/JCO.2007.13.9337
7. Ewelt C, Floeth FW, Felsberg J, Steiger HJ, Sabel M, Langen K-J, et al. Finding the anaplastic focus in diffuse gliomas: the value of Gd-DTPA enhanced MRI, FET-PET, and intraoperative, ALA-derived tissue fluorescence. *Clin Neurol Neurosurg.* (2011) 113:541–7. doi: 10.1016/j.clineuro.2011.03.008
8. Soffietti R, Baumert BG, Bello L, Von Deimling A, Duffau H, Frénay M, et al. Guidelines on management of low-grade gliomas: report of an EFNS-EANO* task force. *Eur J Neurol.* (2010) 17:1124–33. doi: 10.1111/j.1468-1331.2010.03151.x
9. Opoku-Darko M, Lang ST, Artindale J, Cairncross JG, Sevick RJ, Kelly JJP. Surgical management of incidentally discovered diffusely infiltrating low-grade glioma. *J Neurosurg.* (2018) 129:19–26. doi: 10.3171/2017.3.JNS17159
10. Lawrence JE, Steele CJ, Rovin RA, Belton RJ, Winn RJ. Dexamethasone alone and in combination with desipramine, phenytoin, valproic acid or levetiracetam interferes with 5-ALA-mediated PpIX production and cellular retention in glioblastoma cells. *J Neurooncol.* (2016) 127:15–21. doi: 10.1007/s11060-015-2012-x
11. Stummer W, Molina ES. Fluorescence imaging/agents in tumor resection. *Neurosurg Clin.* (2017) 28:569–83. doi: 10.1016/j.nec.2017.05.009
12. Nabavi A, Thurm H, Zountsas B, Pietsch T, Lanfermann H, Pichlmeier U, et al. Five-aminolevulenic acid for fluorescence-guided resection of recurrent malignant gliomas. *Neurosurgery.* (2009) 65:1070–7. doi: 10.1227/01.NEU.0000360128.03597.C7
13. Pichlmeier U, Bink A, Schackert G, Stummer W. Resection and survival in glioblastoma multiforme: an RTOG recursive partitioning analysis of ALA study patients. *Neuro Oncol.* (2008) 10:1025–34. doi: 10.1215/15228517-2008-052
14. Roberts DW, Valdés PA, Harris BT, Hartov A, Fan X, Ji S, et al. Glioblastoma multiforme treatment with clinical trials for surgical resection (aminolevulinic acid). *Neurosurg Clin.* (2012) 23:371–7. doi: 10.1016/j.nec.2012.04.001
15. Roberts DW, Valdés PA, Harris BT, Fontaine KM, Hartov A, Fan X, et al. Coregistered fluorescence-enhanced tumor resection of malignant glioma: relationships between δ-aminolevulinic acid–induced protoporphyrin IX fluorescence, magnetic resonance imaging enhancement, and neuropathological parameters. *J Neurosurg.* (2011) 114:595–603. doi: 10.3171/2010.2.JNS091322
16. Stummer W, Pichlmeier U, Meinel T, Wiestler OD, Zanella F, Reulen H-J. Fluorescence-guided surgery with 5-aminolevulinic acid for resection of malignant glioma: a randomised controlled multicentre phase III trial. *Lancet Oncol.* (2006) 7:392–401. doi: 10.1016/S1470-2045(06)70665-9
17. Stummer W, Reulen H-J, Meinel T, Pichlmeier U, Schumacher W, Tonn J-C, et al. Extend of resection and survival in glioblastoma multiforme. *Neurosurgery.* (2008) 62:564–76. doi: 10.1227/01.neu.0000317304.31579.17
18. Marbacher S, Klinger E, Schwyzer L, Fischer I, Nevzati E, Diepers M, et al. Use of fluorescence to guide resection or biopsy of primary brain tumors and brain metastases. *Neurosurg Focus.* (2014) 36:E10. doi: 10.3171/2013.12.FOCUS13464
19. Potapov AA, Goryaynov SA, Okhlopkov VA, Shishkina L V, Loschenov VB, Savelieva TA, et al. Laser biospectroscopy and 5-ALA fluorescence navigation

as a helpful tool in the meningioma resection. *Neurosurg Rev.* (2016) 39:437–47. doi: 10.1007/s10143-015-0697-0
20. Ruge JR, Liu J. Use of 5-aminolevulinic acid for visualization and resection of a benign pediatric brain tumor: case report. *J Neurosurg Pediatr.* (2009) 4:484–6. doi: 10.3171/2009.6.PEDS08428
21. Sanai N, Snyder LA, Honea NJ, Coons SW, Eschbacher JM, Smith KA, et al. Intraoperative confocal microscopy in the visualization of 5-aminolevulinic acid fluorescence in low-grade gliomas. *J Neurosurg.* (2011) 115:740–8. doi: 10.3171/2011.6.JNS11252
22. Zhang C, Boop FA, Ruge J. The use of 5-aminolevulinic acid in resection of pediatric brain tumors: a critical review. *J Neurooncol.* (2018) 141: 567–73. doi: 10.1007/s11060-018-03004-y
23. Peng Q, Warloe T, Berg K, Moan J, Kongshaug M, Giercksky K-E, et al. 5-Aminolevulinic acid-based photodynamic therapy. *Cancer.* (1997) 79:2282–308.
24. Qian ZM, Chang YZ, Leung G, Du JR, Zhu L, Wang Q, et al. Expression of ferroportin1, hephaestin and ceruloplasmin in rat heart. *Biochim Biophys Acta.* (2007) 1772:527–32. doi: 10.1016/j.bbadis.2007.02.006
25. Kondo M, Hirota N, Takaoka T, Kajiwara M. Heme-biosynthetic enzyme activities and porphyrin accumulation in normal liver and hepatoma cell lines of rat. *Cell Biol Toxicol.* (1993) 9:95–105. doi: 10.1007/BF00755143
26. Hefti M, Albert I, Luginbuehl V. Phenytoin reduces 5-aminolevulinic acid-induced protoporphyrin IX accumulation in malignant glioma cells. *J Neurooncol.* (2012) 108:443–50. doi: 10.1007/s11060-012-0857-9
27. Louis DN, Perry A, Reifenberger G, von Deimling A, Figarella-Branger D, Cavenee WK, et al. The 2016 World Health Organization classification of tumors of the central nervous system: a summary. *Acta Neuropathol.* (2016) 131:803–20. doi: 10.1007/s00401-016-1545-1
28. Kamp MA, Fischer I, Bühner J, Turowski B, Frederick Cornelius J, Steiger H-J, et al. 5-ALA fluorescence of cerebral metastases and its impact for the local-in-brain progression. *Oncotarget.* (2016) 7:66776–89. doi: 10.18632/oncotarget.11488
29. Ishihara R, Katayama Y, Watanabe T, Yoshino A, Fukushima T, Sakatani K. Quantitative spectroscopic analysis of 5-aminolevulinic acid-induced protoporphyrin IX fluorescence intensity in diffusely infiltrating astrocytomas. *Neurol Med Chir.* (2007) 47:53–7. doi: 10.2176/nmc.47.53
30. Stockhammer F, Misch M, Horn P, Koch A, Fonyuy N, Plotkin M. Association of F18-fluoro-ethyl-tyrosin uptake and 5-aminolevulinic acid-induced fluorescence in gliomas. *Acta Neurochir.* (2009) 151:1377. doi: 10.1007/s00701-009-0462-7
31. Bernal García LM, Cabezudo Artero JM, García Moreno R, Marcelo Zamorano MB, Mayoral Guisado C. Fluorescence guided resection with 5-aminolevulinic acid of a pilomyxoid astrocytoma of the third ventricle. *Neurocirugia.* (2017) 28:251–6. doi: 10.1016/j.neucir.2017.03.002
32. Choo J, Takeuchi K, Nagata Y, Ohka F, Kishida Y, Watanabe T, et al. Neuroendoscopic cylinder surgery and 5-aminolevulinic acid photodynamic diagnosis of deep-seated intracranial lesions. *World Neurosurg.* (2018) 116:e35–41. doi: 10.1016/j.wneu.2018.03.112
33. Widhalm G, Wolfsberger S, Minchev G, Woehrer A, Krssak M, Czech T, et al. 5-Aminolevulinic acid is a promising marker for detection of anaplastic foci in diffusely infiltrating gliomas with nonsignificant contrast enhancement. *Cancer Interdiscip Int J Am Cancer Soc.* (2010) 116:1545–52. doi: 10.1002/cncr.24903
34. Widhalm G, Kiesel B, Woehrer A, Traub-Weidinger T, Preusser M, Marosi C, et al. 5-Aminolevulinic acid induced fluorescence is a powerful intraoperative marker for precise histopathological grading of gliomas with non-significant contrast-enhancement. *PLoS ONE.* (2013) 8:e76988. doi: 10.1371/journal.pone.0076988
35. Valdés PA, Jacobs V, Harris BT, Wilson BC, Leblond F, Paulsen KD, et al. Quantitative fluorescence using 5-aminolevulinic acid-induced protoporphyrin IX biomarker as a surgical adjunct in low-grade glioma surgery. *J Neurosurg.* (2015) 123:771–80. doi: 10.3171/2014.12.JNS14391
36. Jaber M, W?lfer J, Ewelt C, Holling M, Hasselblatt M, Niederstadt T, et al. The value of 5-aminolevulinic acid in low-grade gliomas and high-grade gliomas lacking glioblastoma imaging features. *Neurosurgery.* (2016) 78:401–11. doi: 10.1227/NEU.0000000000001020
37. Stummer W, Stepp H, Wiestler OD, Pichlmeier U. Randomized, prospective double-blinded study comparing 3 different doses of 5-aminolevulinic acid for fluorescence-guided resections of malignant gliomas. *Neurosurgery.* (2017) 81:230–9. doi: 10.1093/neuros/nyx074
38. Hirsch LJ. Seizures in patients undergoing resection of low-grade gliomas. *Epilepsy Curr.* (2009) 9:98–100. doi: 10.1111/j.1535-7511.2009.01305.x
39. Kurzwelly D, Herrlinger U, Simon M. Seizures in patients with low-grade gliomas — incidence, pathogenesis, surgical management, and pharmacotherapy. In: Schramm J, editor. *Low-Grade Gliomas. Advances and Technical Standards in Neurosurgery*, vol 35. Vienna: Springer. pp. 81–111. doi: 10.1007/978-3-211-99481-8_4
40. Rudà R, Bello L, Duffau H, Soffietti R. Seizures in low-grade gliomas: natural history, pathogenesis, and outcome after treatments. *Neuro Oncol.* (2012) 14(suppl 4):iv55–64. doi: 10.1093/neuonc/nos199.
41. Haust HL, Poon HC, Carson R, VanDeWetering C, Peter F. Protoporphyrinaemia and decreased activities of 5-aminolevulinic acid dehydrase and uroporphyrinogen I synthetase in erythrocytes of a vitamin B6-deficient epileptic boy given valproic acid and carbamazepine. *Clin Biochem.* (1989) 22:201–11.
42. Valdes PA, Leblond F, Paulsen KD, Kim A, Wilson BC, Conde OM, et al. Combined fluorescence and reflectance spectroscopy for *in vivo* quantification of cancer biomarkers in low-and high-grade glioma surgery. *J Biomed Opt.* (2011) 16:116007. doi: 10.1117/1.3646916

3

Application of Indocyanine Green Videoangiography in Aneurysm Surgery: Evidence, Techniques, Practical Tips

Pedro Norat†*, Sauson Soldozy , Mazin Elsarrag, Jennifer Sokolowski, Kaan Yagmurlu, Min S. Park, Petr Tvrdik and M. Yashar S. Kalani**

Department of Neurological Surgery, University of Virginia Health System, Charlottesville, VA, United States

Correspondence:
M. Yashar S. Kalani
kalani@virginia.edu

†*These authors have contributed equally to this work*

Establishing blood vessel patency in neurovascular surgery is an essential component in treating cerebrovascular disorders. Given the difficulty in confirming complete obliteration of the aneurysm sac, ICG videoangiography has emerged as an intraoperative tool that provides neurosurgeons immediate feedback on the status of vessel flow, allowing for surgical modifications to be made without delay. ICG initially emerged as a tool for assessing hepatic, cardiac, and retinovascular function. It is an inert compound with a high affinity for plasma proteins and fluorescence properties making it the ideal candidate for assessment of vessel patency in neurovascular procedures. Requiring only a bolus peripheral vein injection and integration of a near-infrared imaging device into the surgical microscope, ICG can be visualized without disrupting operating room workflow or the surgical field. Quick response time, high-spatial resolution, and low complication rates are features of ICG videoangiography that prove advantageous when compared to the gold standard intra- and postoperative digital subtraction angiography (DSA). Despite this, ICG is not without limitations, specifically in the setting of atherosclerotic vessels, giant, and complex aneurysms. Additionally, there are instances where DSA may prove superior in detecting vessel stenosis and outflow obstruction, prompting the recommendation of ICG as an adjunct to, rather than complete replacement of DSA. In this article, the authors provide a brief overview of the biochemical properties and historical origins of ICG viedoangiography in addition to discussing its current application in aneurysm surgery.

Keywords: cerebral aneurysm, indocyanin green, digital subtraction angiogram, surgical microscope, near infra-red

INTRODUCTION

Indocyanine green (ICG) is a fluorescent compound that has been utilized for decades in a variety of medical applications. Originally approved by the Food and Drug Administration in 1956, ICG was initially used to evaluate cardiac and hepatic function and later gained extensive use in ophthalmology where it was used to enable angiography (1, 2). More recently, it has been used to enhance tissue visualization in oncology, plastic surgery, neurosurgery, and other fields ( ).

Given that the physical properties of ICG may be utilized to facilitate vascular imaging, the utility of ICG angiography in cerebrovascular surgery has become quite apparent.

The first description of ICG angiography for aneurysm surgery was in 2003, where Raabe et al. assessed the feasibility and quality of ICG videoangiography in assessing patency of arterial and venous vessels and exclusion of aneurysm sacs (4). In their study, the ability to visually inspect vessel patency with intraoperative ICG angiography allowed for real-time surgical changes that significantly altered the surgical course in a number of cases. Given the importance of maintaining tissue perfusion in neurovascular surgery and the difficulty associated with ensuring complete obliteration of an aneurysm, a number of studies have since explored and championed the utility of ICG angiography in aneurysm surgery (2, 5–12) as well as in other neurosurgical settings, such as resection of AVMs and AVFs (13–15), vascular bypass surgery (16), and tumor resection (17). With regards to aneurysm surgery, ICG angiography is often contrasted with other intraoperative monitoring techniques such as digital subtraction angiography (DSA) (5), intraoperative computed tomography (6), and microvascular doppler sonography (7), with these studies concluding that ICG angiography should complement rather than replace these alternative imaging methods. In this review, the authors discuss the biochemical properties of ICG dye, provide a brief history of its use in the medical setting, as well as discuss methodology and current applications in aneurysm surgery while considering both the advantages and limitations of this technique.

BIOCHEMICAL PROFILE AND PROPERTIES

Indocyanine green (**Figure 1**) is a water-soluble, odorless or near odorless tricarbocyanine dye with a strong affinity for plasma proteins (primarily albumin and α- and β-lipoproteins) (1, 19, 20). Once administered, ICG remains 98% bound to plasma proteins; this intravascular sequestration of the dye allows blood vessels to be easily visualized using fluorescence imaging techniques. ICG molecules have a spectral absorption range of 750–800 nm, with a peak emission occurring at approximately 832 nm (1, 3, 21). The range of light wavelengths where biological tissue absorption and scattering are minimum is between 650 and 900 nm, otherwise known as the biological "optical window" (3, 22). As a result, light has maximal tissue penetration at this range of wavelengths. As both the excitation and fluorescence wavelengths of ICG lie within the tissue optical window, the dye may be seen beneath several layers of tissue (3, 21). Furthermore, due to minimal light absorption at this wavelength, tissues have a low degree of near infra-red (NIR) autofluorescence in comparison with ICG, resulting in stark contrast of the dye.

ICG is a relatively safe, nontoxic compound with a lethal dosage (LD_{50}) of 50–80 mg/kg. With a typical ICG angiography dose of 0.2–0.5 mg/kg (21), adverse events are seen in <0.1% of patients (primarily hypotension, tachycardia, and urticarial reactions in iodide allergic patients). The dye is quickly removed from circulation by the liver, mostly clearing within 10–20 min (1, 2). Experiments suggest that ICG is excreted exclusively by the liver into bile with no known metabolites (23).

HISTORICAL CONTEXT

Originally introduced for NIR photography by Kodak research laboratories in 1955, ICG was approved for clinical use by the FDA just a year later in 1956 (23). ICG was initially utilized for quantitative measurements in assessing liver function, in the field of cardiology for determining cardiac output in valvular and septal defects (24), and eventually in the field of ophthalmology beginning in the 1970s (3). The first application of ICG in cerebrovascular angiography was experimentally performed on exposed dog brain, reported by Kogure et al. (25). In this study, a wide parietotemporal craniotomy was performed with ICG dye being injected into the left thyroid artery allowing for gross visualization of the middle cerebral artery (MCA) distribution. The authors heralded the "simplicity of technique and employment of standard equipment" noting "it is entirely feasible that a photographic setup such as described in this article could be easily moved into the neurosurgical operating suite." Their prediction would reign true and was made even more feasible given the technological advancements that occurred in the following decades since their experiment was performed. This includes visualizing ICG fluorescence through a surgical microscope as described by Kuroiwa et al. (26), where they reported clear visualization of human brain surface vessels through the dura mater after intravenous injection of ICG.

The first description of NIR videoangiography using ICG dye for intraoperative visualization in aneurysm surgery was described in 2003. Raabe et al. (4) noted that in three cases, the ICG angiographic findings significantly changed the course of the surgical procedure, thereby suggesting that this technique may be implemented as an adjunct in neurovascular procedures (**Figure 2**). In addition, the ICG angiography results were noted to be comparable to DSA in elucidating patency of all vessel types, including small and perforating arteries (<0.05 mm). The integration of NIR technology into the operating microscope would set the stage for ICG videoangiography in neurovascular surgery in the twenty-first century.

TECHNIQUE

Dosage

The recommended dose of ICG injected peripherally for angiography is between 0.2 and 0.5 mg/kg, not to exceed a maximum dose of 5 mg/kg. The standard dose is injected into a peripheral vein as a bolus of 25 mg dissolved in 5 ml of water (2, 3). Within 1–2 s following injection, the ICG dye binds to plasma proteins and has a plasma half-life of 3–4 min. After 10 min, a repeat dose can be administered or until after the ICG dye clears (2). Caloric restriction has been shown to increase plasma clearance at doses below 0.5 mg/kg (27).

Microscopy

The technical integration of ICG videoangiography into the optical path of the surgical microscope was first described

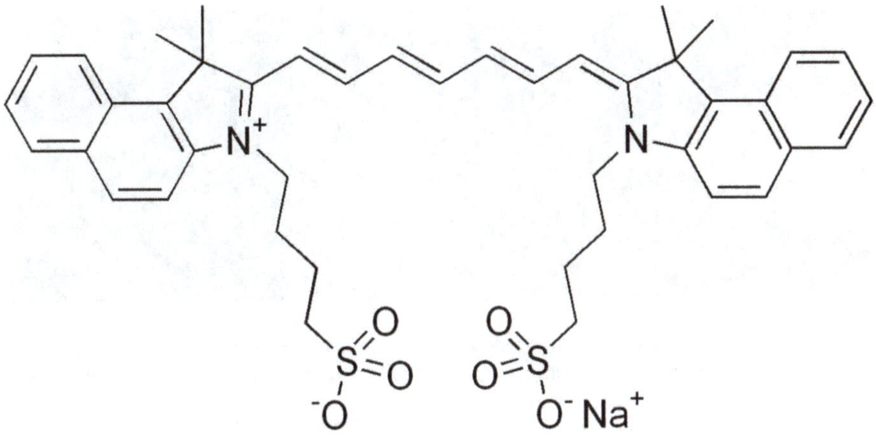

FIGURE 1 | Chemical structure of indocyanine green. Reproduced from File:Indocyanine green.png (18).

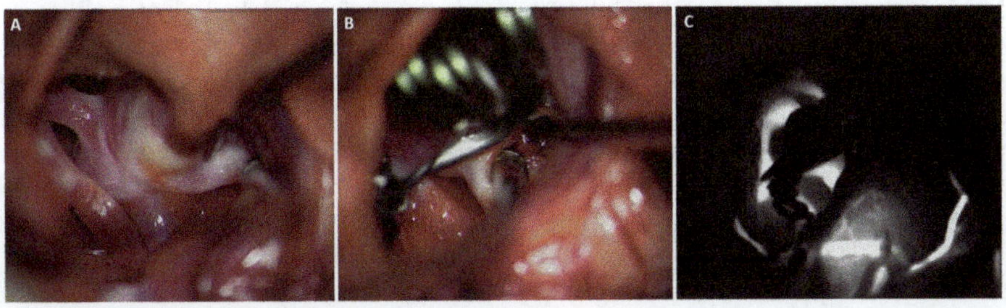

FIGURE 2 | Middle cerebral artery aneurysm with the neck dissected and clear view of the parent vessel, and its two branches **(A)**, after retraction showing the neck of the clipped MCA aneurysm **(B)**, and intraoperative ICG videoangiography showing the patency of the branches of the MCA and complete exclusion of the aneurysm from the circulation **(C)**.

by Raabe et al. (21) and implemented by Carl Zeiss Co. (Oberkochen, Germany). Given that its fluorescent wavelength is in the near-infrared (NIR) spectrum (700–2,500 nm), the dye cannot be seen by the naked eye, and a NIR imaging device must be available to allow vessel visualization. A simple ICG device consists of a NIR light source, an NIR sensitive sensor, and filters used to block light at other wavelengths (3, 21). This allows users to obtain high-resolution NIR images without ambient and excitation light interference. A light source illuminating the operative field has a wavelength comprising the ICG absorption band (range 700–850 nm, peak 805 nm). The setup entails a uniquely designed dielectric filter that allows passage of light in the NIR wavelength that fits the exact absorption band of ICG. An integrated beam splitter in the microscope directs the ICG fluorescence light (range 780–950 nm, peak 835 nm) toward a black-and-white camera, with an observation band-pass filter being used to detect the ICG fluorescence (21).

CURRENT APPLICATIONS

The neurosurgeon's goal for aneurysm surgery is complete exclusion of the aneurysm from the circulation while preserving the parent, perforating, and branching vessels. To achieve this, many intraoperative monitoring techniques, such as microvascular Doppler, monitoring of somatosensory and motor evoked potentials, DSA, and more recently ICG videoangiography, may be utilized. Since the publication of Raabe et al. (4), ICG has been greatly studied and many publications have shown its importance in the microsurgical management of aneurysms; consequently, ICG has become a widely commonplace tool for identification of mis-clipping in aneurysm surgery despite DSA being considered the gold standard technique for intraoperative monitoring in aneurysmal clipping (2, 11, 21, 28, 29). However, intraoperative DSA may be challenging to implement in many centers worldwide due to its requirement of large logistical support, high cost burden, prolonged time frame, and invasive nature. In contrast, ICG is noninvasive with a lower cost burden and quicker image acquisition.

In a prospective two-center trial published in 2005, Raabe et al. (2) directly compared surgical microscope-based ICG videoangiography with intra- or postoperative DSA after aneurysm clipping. The authors described several advantages, including a lower complication rate (0.1% vs. 0.4–2.6%), a faster time frame of 2 min, and higher-spatial resolution that allows for observation of small perforators or cortical arteries of submillimeter diameter that cannot be assessed

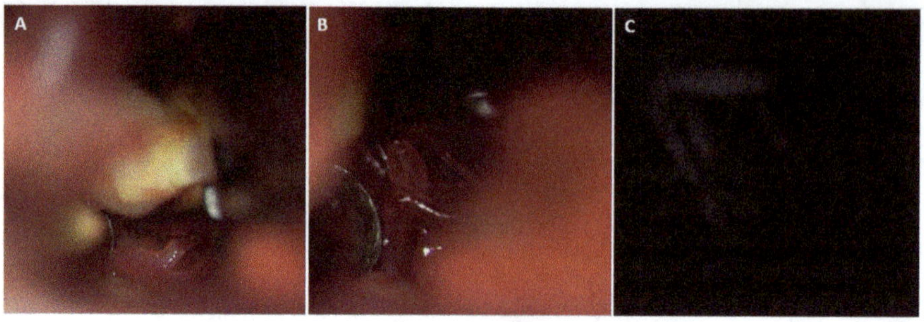

FIGURE 3 | This basilar tip aneurysm was exposed using a modified orbitozygomatic approach. The perforators arising from the posterior aspect of the basilar apex and P1 can be visualized **(A)**. These perforators are dissected from the aneurysm dome and excluded from the clip construct **(B)**. Post clip ICG demonstrates preservation of the perforators **(C)**.

with intraoperative DSA. ICG angiography was reported to be limited in the setting of atherosclerotic or calcified vessels, thrombosed aneurysms, and giant or complex aneurysms; although, ICG disclosed remnant aneurysms mainly in atherosclerotic aneurysms ($p < 0.05$) (30). In cases where ICG angiography missed stenotic vessels, they were found to be likely hemodynamically irrelevant as seen on postoperative DSA. Overall, a correlation of 90% was reported between ICG and DSA, with the authors reporting no cases where inconsistent findings on postoperative DSA lead to reopening and repositioning of the clip (2).

One major utility of ICG is its ability to confirm microsurgical anatomy in a variety of aneurysm cases. de Oliveira et al. (31) have described their experience with 93 ICG videoangiography studies for monitoring the flow in perforating arteries (**Figure 3**) during intracranial aneurysm surgery. They concluded that ICG videoangiography was able to visualize, during the surgical procedure, the small perforating arteries that cannot be detected by intraoperative DSA (31). In addition, Nagai et al. (32) reported a rare case of a ruptured dissecting aneurysm in the A1 segment. Using ICG, the lateral and medial groups of the basal perforating arteries of the anterior communicating artery complex of the ACA were identified prior to clipping, thereby minimizing the risk of complications related to occluding perforator vessels. Other series have been published that further corroborate these findings (8–14, 16, 17, 28, 33–35).

ADVANTAGES AND LIMITATIONS

In concordance with the benefits stated earlier, Sharma et al. (11) demonstrated in 112 patients an 8% clip repositioning rate during surgery after the use of ICG videoangiography, elucidating the clear advantage of having ICG available for use. Despite this, a disagreement between ICG and DSA was observed in 4% of the cases (5 cases—2 patients with anterior communicating aneurysms and ophthalmic ICA aneurysms and 1 middle cerebral artery bifurcation), with discordance being significant higher in ophthalmic ICA when compared with other aneurysm locations ($p = 0.04$; OR = 10.8). Dashti et al. (36) in their series of 239 patients found the rate of unexpected neck residuals to be about 6%; however, neck residuals were significantly more frequent in deep-sited aneurysms (64%). They ultimately concluded that ICG videoangiography is a reliable intraoperative tool for aneurysm surgery, with the exception of giant, complex, and deep-sited aneurysms.

Limitations of ICG videoangiography include trouble visualizing aneurysm residuals after clipping when compared with DSA, inability to visualize areas outside the field of the microscope, and difficulty visualizing of arteries at the depth of the surgical field and residual neck in calcified and thrombosed aneurysms. While Raabe et al. (2) report ICG videoangiography can be used as an independent form of angiography, the majority of other studies recommend this technique as an alternative to or as complementary to intraoperative DSA during aneurysm surgery. In fact, a recent systematic review meta-analysis concluded that ICG videoangiography should serve only a complementary role to DSA rather than fully replace it given a 6.1% rate of mis-clippings not detected by ICG angiography among 1,465 clipped aneurysms as compared to a 4.5% rate of mis-clippings not detected by DSA among 849 clipped aneurysms (5). While not as precise as DSA, the greatest advantage of ICG videoangiography is that it provides real-time information regarding aneurysmal exclusion from the circulation, as well as patency of parent and branch vessels. If necessary, clip repositioning can be performed within minutes given the immediate visual feedback of ICG. Additionally, ICG is susceptible to false negatives further pointing toward its role as an adjunct to DSA (37–39).

FUTURE DIRECTIONS

Given the advantages and ease of use of ICG videoangiography, the dearth of studies examining its utility in other neurovascular procedures suggests that it may be underutilized for these procedures. Examples of these surgeries include ablation of arteriovenous malformations and fistulas along with manipulation and resection of highly vascularized tumors and lesions. The scarcity of data examining ICG videoangiography for these procedures may be a result of their infrequent incidence. Nonetheless, reports on the nuances of employing ICG videoangiography in these procedures may help to further define its specific roles and situational uses. We encourage groups to publish their techniques and experiences with ICG videoangiography in these areas.

One limitation of ICG videaoangiography is its inability to provide information on unexposed vessels. In order to bypass this limitation, several groups have interfaced the indocyanine NIR imaging technology to neuroendoscopes (8, 40–43). The ICG videoangiography-neuroendoscope may extend the benefits of ICG videoangiography to deep seated lesions and other difficult to visualize vessels without expanding the dissection. Cho et al. (41) report higher detection rates of branch orifices and more exact clip position with the ICG videoangiography-neurendoscope compared with commercial microscopic ICG videoangiography. Another mechanism by which the line of sight limitation has been addressed is with integration of ICG angiography and robotic surgery. The union of ICG angiography with robotic surgery has proven to be valuable in other disciplines such as surgical oncology, (44) demonstrating that this technology is feasible.

In addition to extending ICG videoangiography to lesions and vessels not readily exposed, the robotic system has other benefits which could improve aneurysm surgery. The computer of the robotic console allows additional information to be integrated and simultaneously displayed intraoperatively (44), and the increased precision of movements and ability to navigate narrow anatomical cavities may allow access to deep seated lesions while minimizing brain retraction and dissection. Thus, the expansion of robotics into neurosurgery may be a novel method to incorporate NIR imaging technology and use ICG videoangiography to examine vasculature that is not immediately exposed.

A known drawback to ICG videoangiography is its poor ability to visualize thrombosed, calcified, and buried vessels and aneurysms. This may be in part due to the relatively modest tissue penetration by light at these wavelengths in comparison to other wavelengths. Contrast between ICG and surrounding tissue indeed stems from the fluorescent wavelengths of ICG lying within the tissue optical window. However, Smith et al. (45) discuss the existence of a second optical window, with the first window spanning from 650 to 950 nm and the second from 1,000–1,350 nm. They further state that the first window may not be optimal due to tissue autofluorescence producing substantial background noise and the tissue penetration depth being limited to between 1 and 2 cm. Indocyanine green fluorescing in this first window may significantly detract from the visual quality of ICG angiography. Image acuity may therefore be optimized by utilizing compounds that fluoresce in second optical window. Smith et al. (45) cite simulations and modeling studies suggesting that improvement of signal-to-noise ratios by over 100-fold is possible by using quantum dot fluorophores that emit light at 1,320 nm as opposed to 850 nm. However, currently tested compounds that fluoresce at this range are limited due to safety and toxicity as well as technical challenges associated with imaging technology. Nonetheless, the development of both effective and biologically compatible fluorescent substances that operate within the second optical window may have the potential to greatly enhance fluorescent imaging.

Many of the advantages of ICGVA derive from its safety, convenience and cost effectiveness; preservation of these qualities is necessary for a contrast agent to function optimally. Currently, ICG is the only FDA approved near-infrared dye (3, 22). Investigators have explored both structural analogs of indocyanine as well as novel NIR contrast agents (3). Other areas of improvement include enhancements in NIR imaging technology to capture the broad fluorescence peak of ICG while also effectively filtering out background noise. Lastly, technical developments in flow dynamics analysis may improve visualization after multiple indocyanine loads, since rapid ICG reinjections generally suffer from lower contrast due to residual ICG inside the vessels (3). In addition, the versatility of ICG allows it to be paired with multiple intraoperative monitoring techniques such as somatosensory evoked potential (SSEP) and motor evoked potential (MEP) (46). Overall, there is much that remains to be explored in the field of fluorescent angiography and refinements in technology are inevitable.

CONCLUSION

In this article, the authors review the mechanism of action of ICG angiography and examine the evolution of its applications over time, nuances in technique, and clinical implementation. The reviewed data demonstrates that ICG angiography is indeed quite helpful in vascular mapping for cerebral aneurysm surgery and may certainly alter intraoperative decision making. However, its exact role depends on anatomic features of the particular lesion being treated and the technology is ultimately limited by lower accuracy compared to the gold-standard of digital subtraction angiography. Based on these findings, the highest degree of imaging accuracy may be achieved by employing multiple imaging technologies, and we encourage surgeons to use multimodal imaging when possible during aneurysm clipping surgery.

AUTHOR CONTRIBUTIONS

MK, PN, and SS: conception and design. PN, SS, and ME: acquisition of data and drafting the article. All authors critically revising the article. All authors reviewed submitted version of manuscript. MK approved the final version of the manuscript on behalf of all authors.

REFERENCES

1. Reinhart MB, Huntington CR, Blair LJ, Heniford BT, Augenstein VA. Indocyanine green:historical context, current applications, and future considerations. *Surg Innov.* (2016) 23:166–75. doi: 10.1177/1553350615604053
2. Raabe A, Nakaji P, Beck J, Kim LJ, Hsu FPK, Kamerman JD et al. Prospective evaluation of surgical microscope—integrated intraoperative near-infrared

indocyanine green videoangiography during aneurysm surgery. *J Neurosurg.* (2005) 103:982–9. doi: 10.3171/jns.2005.103.6.0982
3. Alander JT, Kaartinen I, Laakso A, Pätilä T, Spillmann T, Tuchin VV, et al. A review of indocyanine green fluorescent imaging in surgery. *Int J Biomed Imaging.* (2012) 2012:940585. doi: 10.1155/2012/940585
4. Raabe A, Beck J, Gerlach R, Zimmermann M, Seifert V. Near-infrared indocyanine green video angiography: a new method for intraoperative assessment of vascular flow. *Neurosurgery.* (2003) 52:132–9. doi: 10.1227/00006123-200301000-00017
5. Riva M, Amin-Hanjani S, Giussani C, De Witte O, Bruneau M. Indocyanine green videoangiography in aneurysm surgery: systematic review and meta-analysis. *Neurosurgery.* (2018) 83:166–180. doi: 10.1093/neuros/nyx387
6. Schnell O, Morhard D, Holtmannspötter M, Reiser M, Tonn JC, Schichor C. Near-infrared indocyanine green videoangiography (ICGVA) and intraoperative computed tomography (iCT): are they complementary or competitive imaging techniques in aneurysm surgery? *Acta Neurochir.* (2012) 154:1861–8. doi: 10.1007/s00701-012-1386-1
7. Fischer G, Stadie A, Oertel JMK. Near-infrared indocyanine green videoangiography versus microvascular Doppler sonography in aneurysm surgery. *Acta Neurochir.* (2010) 152:1519–25. doi: 10.1007/s00701-010-0723-5
8. Nishiyama Y, Kinouchi H, Senbokuya N, Kato T, Kanemaru K, Yoshioka H, et al. Endoscopic indocyanine green video angiography in aneurysm surgery: an innovative method for intraoperative assessment of blood flow in vasculature hidden from microscopic view. *J Neurosurg.* (2012) 117:302–8. doi: 10.3171/2012.5.JNS112300
9. Washington CW, Zipfel GJ, Chicoine MR, Derdeyn CP, Rich KM, Moran CJ, et al. Comparing indocyanine green videoangiography to the gold standard of intraoperative digital subtraction angiography used in aneurysm surgery. *J Neurosurg.* (2013) 118:420–7. doi: 10.3171/2012.10.JNS11818
10. Özgiray E, Aktüre E, Patel N, Baggott C, Bozkurt M, Niemann D, et al. How reliable and accurate is indocyanine green video angiography in the evaluation of aneurysm obliteration? *Clin Neurol Neurosurg.* (2013) 115:870–8. doi: 10.1016/j.clineuro.2012.08.027
11. Sharma M, Ambekar S, Ahmed O, Nixon M, Sharma A, Nanda A, et al. The utility and limitations of intraoperative near-infrared indocyanine green videoangiography in aneurysm surgery. *World Neurosurg.* (2014) 82:e607–13. doi: 10.1016/j.wneu.2014.05.033
12. Roessler K, Krawagna M, Dörfler A, Buchfelder M, Ganslandt O. Essentials in intraoperative indocyanine green videoangiography assessment for intracranial aneurysm surgery: conclusions from 295 consecutively clipped aneurysms and review of the literature. *Neurosurg Focus.* (2014) 36:E7. doi: 10.3171/2013.11.FOCUS13475
13. Schuette AJ, Cawley CM, Barrow DL. Indocyanine green videoangiography in the management of dural arteriovenous fistulae. *Neurosurgery.* (2010) 67:658–62. doi: 10.1227/01.NEU.0000374721.84406.7F
14. Hänggi D, Etminan N, Steiger HJ. The impact of microscope-integrated intraoperative near-infrared indocyanine green videoangiography on surgery of arteriovenous malformations and dural arteriovenous fistulae. *Neurosurgery.* (2010) 67:1094–4. doi: 10.1227/NEU.0b013e3181eb5049
15. Shah KJ, Cohen-Gadol AA. The application of FLOW 800 ICG videoangiography color maps for neurovascular surgery and intraoperative decision making. *World Neurosurg.* (2019) 122:e186–e197. doi: 10.1016/j.wneu.2018.09.195
16. Schuette AJ, Dannenbaum MJ, Cawley CM, Barrow DL. Indocyanine green videoangiography for confirmation of bypass graft patency. *J Korean Neurosurg Soc.* (2011) 50:23–9. doi: 10.3340/jkns.2011.50.1.23
17. Belykh E, Martirosyan NL, Yagmurlu K, Miller EJ, Eschbacher JM, Izadyyazdanabadi M, et al. Intraoperative fluorescence imaging for personalized brain tumor resection: current state and future directions. *Front Surg.* (2016) 3:55. doi: 10.3389/fsurg.2016.00055
18. File:Indocyanine green.png. *Wikimedia Commons, the Free Media Repository.* (2017). Available online at: https://commons.wikimedia.org/w/index.php?title=File:Indocyanine_green.png&oldid=260065692 (retrieved June 11, 2019).
19. Osol A, Hoover JE. Remington's pharmaceutical sciences. *J Pharm Sci.* (1976) 65:933. doi: 10.1002/jps.2600650641
20. Williams M. The merck index: an encyclopedia of chemicals, drugs, and biologicals. *Drug Dev Res.* (2013) 74:339. doi: 10.1002/ddr.21085
21. Raabe A, Beck J, Seifert V. Technique and image quality of intraoperative indocyanine green angiography during aneurysm surgery using surgical microscope integrated near-infrared video technology. *Zentralbl Neurochir.* (2005) 66:1–6. doi: 10.1055/s-2004-836223
22. Mérian J, Gravier J, Navarro F, Texier I. Fluorescent nanoprobes dedicated to *in vivo* imaging: from preclinical validations to clinical translation. *Molecules.* (2012) 17:5564–91. doi: 10.3390/molecules17055564
23. Engel E, Schraml R, Maisch T, Kobuch K, Konig B, Szeimies RM, et al. Light-induced decomposition of indocyanine green. *Investig Opthalmology Vis Sci.* (2008) 49:1777. doi: 10.1167/iovs.07-0911
24. Yannuzzi LA. Indocyanine green angiography: a perspective on use in the clinical setting. *Am J Ophthalmol.* (2011) 151:745–751.e1. doi: 10.1016/j.ajo.2011.01.043
25. Kogure K, Choromokos E. Infrared absorption angiography. *J Appl Physiol.* (1969) 26:154–7. doi: 10.1152/jappl.1969.26.1.154
26. Kuroiwa T, Kajimoto Y, Ohta T. Development and clinical application of near-infrared surgical microscope: preliminary report. *Minim Invasive Neurosurg.* (2001) 44: 240–2. doi: 10.1055/s-2001-19929
27. Ohkubo H, Musha H, Okuda K. Effects of caloric restriction on the kinetics of indocyanine green in patients with liver diseases and in the rat. *Am J Dig Dis.* (1978) 23:1017–24. doi: 10.1007/BF01263102
28. Chiang VL, Gailloud P, Murphy KJ, Rigamonti D, Tamargo RJ. Routine intraoperative angiography during aneurysm surgery. *J Neurosurg.* (2002) 96:988–992. doi: 10.3171/jns.2002.96.6.0988
29. Gruber A, Dorfer C, Standhardt H, Bavinzski G, Knosp E. Prospective comparison of intraoperative vascular monitoring technologies during cerebral aneurysm surgery. *Neurosurgery.* (2011) 68:657–73. doi: 10.1227/NEU.0b013e31820777ee
30. Della Puppa A, Rossetto M, Volpin F, Rustemi O, Grego A, Gerardi A, et al. Microsurgical clipping of intracranial aneurysms assisted by neurophysiological monitoring, microvascular flow probe, and ICG-VA: outcomes and intraoperative data on a multimodal strategy. *World Neurosurg.* (2018) 113:e336–e344. doi: 10.1016/j.wneu.2018.02.029
31. de Oliveira JG, Beck J, Seifert V, Teixeira MJ, Raabe A. Assessment of flow in perforating arteries during intracranial aneurysm surgery using intraoperative near-infrared indocyanine green videoangiography. *Neurosurgery.* (2008) 62:63–73. doi: 10.1227/01.NEU.0000333795.21468.D4
32. Nagai Y, Goto M, Toda H, Nishida N, Yoshimoto N, Iwasaki K. Indocyanine green videoangiography for surgery of a ruptured dissecting aneurysm in the precommunicating anterior cerebral artery: a technical case report. *Oper Neurosurg.* (2017) 13:E14–E18. doi: 10.1093/ons/opx028
33. Jing Z, Ou S, Ban Y, Tong Z, Wang Y. Intraoperative assessment of anterior circulation aneurysms using the indocyanine green video angiography technique. *J Clin Neurosci.* (2010) 17:26–8. doi: 10.1016/j.jocn.2009.03.034
34. He M, You C, Lan Z, Li J. Assessment of microscope-integrated indocyanine green angiography during intracranial aneurysm surgery: a retrospective study of 120 patients. *Neurol India.* (2009) 57:453. doi: 10.4103/0028-3886.55607
35. Xianli L, Zhongxue W, Sun S, Wang Y, Zang P. Indocyanine green videoangiography in clipping of paraclinoid aneurysms. *Turk Neurosurg.* (2012) 24: 319–22. doi: 10.5137/1019-5149.JTN.6284-12.1
36. Dashti R, Laakso A, Niemelä M, Porras M, Hernesniemi J. Microscope-integrated near-infrared indocyanine green videoangiography during surgery of intracranial aneurysms: the Helsinki experience. *Surg Neurol.* (2009) 71:543–50. doi: 10.1016/j.surneu.2009.01.027
37. Caplan JM, Sankey E, Yang W, Radvany MG, Colby GP, Coon AL, et al. Impact of indocyanine green videoangiography on rate of clip adjustments following intraoperative angiography. *Neurosurgery.* (2014) 75:437–44. doi: 10.1227/NEU.0000000000000468
38. Wang S, Liu L, Zhao Y, Zhang D, Yang M, Zhao J. Evaluation of surgical microscope-integrated intraoperative near-infrared indocyanine green videoangiography during aneurysm surgery. *Neurosurg Rev.* (2011) 34:209–15. doi: 10.1007/s10143-010-0305-2
39. Ma C-Y, Shi J-X, Wang H-D, Hang C-H, Cheng H-L, Wu W. Intraoperative indocyanine green angiography in intracranial aneurysm surgery: microsurgical clipping and revascularization. *Clin Neurol Neurosurg.* (2009) 111:840–6. doi: 10.1016/j.clineuro.2009.08.017

40. Cho W-S, Kim JE, Kim SH, Kim HC, Kang U, Lee D-S. Endoscopic fluorescence angiography with indocyanine green: a preclinical study in the swine. *J Kor Neurosurg Soc.* (2015) 58:513. doi: 10.3340/jkns.2015.58.6.513
41. Cho WS, Kim JE, Kang HS, Son YJ, Bang JS, Oh CW. Keyhole Approach and Neuroendoscopy for Cerebral Aneurysms. *J Korean Neurosurg Soc.* (2017) 60:275–81. doi: 10.3340/jkns.2017.0101.002
42. Bruneau M, Appelboom G, Rynkowski M, Cutsem N, Mine B, Witte O. Endoscope-integrated ICG technology: first application during intracranial aneurysm surgery. *Neurosurg Rev.* (2012) 36:77–84. doi: 10.1007/s10143-012-0419-9
43. Mielke D, Malinova V, Rohde V. Comparison of intraoperative microscopic and endoscopic ICG angiography in aneurysm surgery. *Neurosurgery.* (2014) 10:418–25. doi: 10.1227/NEU.0000000000000345
44. Daskalaki D, Aguilera F, Patton K, Giulianotti PC. Fluorescence in robotic surgery. *J Surg Oncol.* (2015) 112:250–6. doi: 10.1002/jso.23910
45. Smith AM, Mancini MC, Nie S. Bioimaging: second window for in vivo imaging. *Nat Nanotechnol.* (2009) 4:710–1. doi: 10.1038/nnano.2009.326
46. Lin J, Zhao J, Zhao Y, Zhang D, Wang R, Qiao H, et al. Multiple Intraoperative monitoring-assisted microneurosurgical treatment for anterior circulation cerebral aneurysm. *J Int Med Res.* (2011) 39:891–903. doi: 10.1177/147323001103900323

4

Robotic-Assisted Sentinel Lymph Node Mapping with Indocyanine Green in Pelvic Malignancies

Yuqing Wu [1,2†], Jibo Jing [1,2†], Jinfeng Wang [3†], Bin Xu [1], Mulong Du [4,5*] and Ming Chen [1*]*

[1] Department of Urology, Affiliated Zhongda Hospital of Southeast University, Nanjing, China, [2] Surgical Research Center, School of Medicine, Institute of Urology, Southeast University, Nanjing, China, [3] Department of Urology, School of Medicine, Affiliated Yancheng Hospital, Southeast University, Yancheng, China, [4] Jiangsu Key Laboratory of Cancer Biomarkers, Department of Environmental Genomics, Prevention and Treatment, Collaborative Innovation Center for Cancer Personalized Medicine, Nanjing Medical University, Nanjing, China, [5] Department of Biostatistics, Center for Global Health, School of Public Health, Nanjing Medical University, Nanjing, China

***Correspondence:**
Bin Xu
njxb1982@126.com
Mulong Du
drdumulong@njmu.edu.cn
Ming Chen
mingchenseu@126.com

† These authors have contributed equally to this work

Objective: Newer technologies such as near-infrared (NIR) imaging of the fluorescent dye indocyanine green (ICG) and daVinci Xi Surgical System have become promising tools for sentinel lymph node (SLN) mapping. This meta-analysis was conducted to comprehensively evaluate the diagnostic value of SLN in assessing lymph nodal metastasis in pelvic malignancies, using ICG with NIR imaging in robotic-assisted surgery.

Materials and Methods: A literature search was conducted using PubMed for studies in English before April 2019. The detection rate, sensitivity of SLN detection of metastatic disease, and factors associated with successful mapping (sample size, study design, mean age, mean body mass index, type of cancer) were synthesized for meta-analysis.

Results: A total of 17 articles including 1,059 patients were finally included. The reported detection rates of SLN ranged from 76 to 100%, with a pooled average rate of 95% (95% CI: 93–97; 17 studies). The sensitivity of SLN detection of metastatic disease ranged from 50 to 100% and the pooled sensitivity was 86% (95% CI: 75–94; 8 studies). There were no complications related to ICG administration reported.

Conclusions: NIR imaging system using ICG in robotic-assisted surgery is a feasible and safe method for SLN mapping. Due to its promising performance, it is considered to be an alternative to a complete pelvic lymph node dissection.

Keywords: indocyanine green, robotic surgery, pelvic, sentinel lymph node, cancer

INTRODUCTION

Pelvic lymphadenectomy (PLND), which remains the most accurate procedure for the detection of lymph node metastasis (LNM) in malignant pelvic tumors, plays an important role in surgical management of endometrial and prostate cancers (1, 2). However, the data from a prospective study suggests that lymphadenectomy is associated with the increasing operative time, blood loss and risk for surgical morbidity (e.g., blood vessel and nerve damage, lymphedema, and lymphocyst formation) (3, 4). Thus, novel nodal assessment techniques should be developed to improve the accuracy of LNM detection with lower surgical morbidity.

The biopsy of SLN which is defined as the first node to receive the drainage from the primary tumor, has been described by Canbanas in 1977 (5). The utility of SLN mapping can avoid the unnecessary LND when the SLN turns out to be negative (6). The different methods used in SLN mapping, such as blue dye, technetium, and ICG with NIR imaging have been investigated, among which ICG has been used clinically for over two decades with an excellent safety profile (7). Also, as one of four fluorochromes approved by US Food and Drug Administration, ICG may be of significant use in pelvic surgery due to its properties (8).

The NIR fluorescence imaging system in daVinci Xi Surgical System (Intuitive Surgical, Sunnyvale, CA, USA) with Firefly technology provides intraoperative ICG near-infrared fluorescence, especially for ICG at low concentrations in lymphatic mapping. While the high concentrations of ICG can be seen directly in green in color on a background of a grayscale image. Moreover, it brings surgeons great convenience to control the scope completely which the infrared and visible light systems are built in.

Nevertheless, although ICG-NIF imaging in SLN detection appears to be superior, there are few studies of meta-analysis on SLN mapping outcomes, and most of them focused on specific one or two types of cancer, especially on endometrial and cervical cancer. Thus, we performed this meta-analysis to evaluate the detection rates and sensitivity of SLN mapping in malignant pelvic tumors, including endometrial, cervical, bladder and prostate cancers.

MATERIALS AND METHODS

Search Strategy

The literature search was conducted on PubMed, only English language studies before April 2019 included. The search terms used are as follow: (robotic OR robot) AND (indocyanine green OR ICG) AND lymph. In addition, the references of included studies were reviewed as supplement.

Inclusion and Exclusion Criteria

Studies were included with the following inclusion criteria: (1) At least 10 patients diagnosed with pelvic malignancies; (2) Robotic-assisted surgery as the surgical approach; (3) Pelvic with or without other lymph node dissection as reference standard; (4) Pathological examination was taken, including hematoxylin-eosin (H&E) staining, immunohistochemistry (IHC) or ultrastaging; (5) ICG was used for SLN mapping; (6) Reported detection rate of SLN. The studies published as reviews and case reports were excluded.

Study Quality Assessment

The quality of enrolled studies was assessed using the QUADAS-2 (Quality Assessment of Diagnostic Accuracy Studies-2) (9) tool by two reviewers independently. The items are shown in the Appendix Table 1 (**Supplementary Material**).

Data Extraction

The following items were collected from each article: (1) authors; (2) year of publication; (3) sample size; (4) study design; (5) type of cancer; (6) injection site; (7) reference standard; (8) pathology assessment; (9) mean patient age and body mass index (BMI); (10) available outcome data.

The overall detection rate was estimated as the proportion of patients with at least 1 SLN identified among all the patients going though PLND. When assessing sensitivity and specificity, the patients who failed in SLN mapping were excluded, and sensitivity is defined as the percentage of patients with positive SLN divided by all patients with positive lymph nodes. The specificity is defined as the percentage of patients with negative SLN divided by all patients with negative lymph nodes. Studies in which the calculation of sensitivity was based on the number of removed node packets but not on the patients were excluded during assessment.

Statistical Analysis

The Stata 15.0 and meta-disc were used to conduct all data analysis. The overall detection rate was calculated using a random-effects model under meta-analysis. The sensitivity of detection rates of SLN was evaluated using summary receiver operating characteristic curve (SROC). The I^2 index was used to detect the heterogeneity among the studies. The Funnel plots, Egger's regression intercepts were used for the evaluation of publication bias. The univariate meta-regression was applied for the association of SLN detection rate and study characteristics, including sample size, study design, mean age, mean BMI, and type of cancer.

RESULTS

Characteristics of Enrolled Studies

Of the 78 abstracts screened, 17 articles including 1,059 patients with pelvic malignancies were eligible for inclusion as demonstrated in **Figure 1**. The sample size of each study ranged from 10 to 197. SNL was evaluated for endometrial cancer in 9 articles, cervical cancer in 1, prostate cancer in 3 and bladder cancer in 1, with the other 3 articles dedicated in both endometrial cancer, and cervical cancer (10–26) (**Table 1**).

An overall mean of 3.5 SLNs was removed per patient (13 studies). All the studies conducted PLND with or without para-aortic LND, and the mean non-SLNs identified per person was 17.9 (5 studies). The mean age of 1,059 patients was 62 years (17

Abbreviations: SLN, sentinel lymph node; ICG, indocyanine green; NIR, near-infrared; LND, lymph node dissection; PLND, pelvic lymphadenectomy; CI, confidence interval.

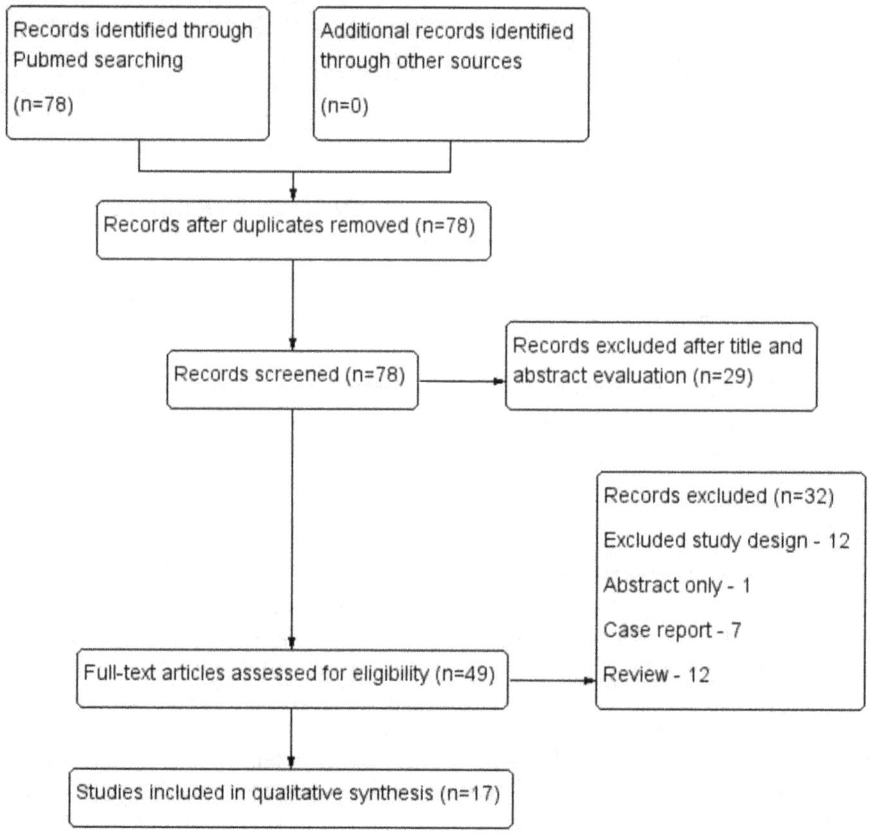

FIGURE 1 | Flow diagram of studies identified, included, and excluded.

studies) and mean BMI was 31.1 kg/m^2 (13 studies) (**Table 1**). No complications, among all 17 articles, were described related to ICG administration.

Data Analysis for the Detection Rate and Diagnostic Accuracy of SLN Mapping

The detection rates of SLN ranged from 76 to 100%, with a pooled average of 95% (95% CI: 93–97; 17 studies) with heterogeneity $I^2 = 56.2\%$ (**Figure 2**). The funnel plot of the pooled overall SLN detection rate is shown in **Figure 3**. The Egger's regression intercept was -4.65 ($p = 0.000$).

Sensitivity of SLN mapping ranged from 50 to 100%. The pooled sensitivity of SLN detection of metastatic disease was 86% (95% CI: 75–94; 8 studies) (**Figure 4**). The funnel plot of the pooled sensitivity is shown in **Figure 3**. The Egger's regression intercept was found out to be -4.85 ($p = 0.003$). The pooled specificity and diagnostic odds ratio were 1.00 (95%Cl: 0.99–1.00) and 381.92 (95%Cl: 111.19–1311.85). The combined positive likelihood ratio and negative likelihood ratio were 67.31 (95% CI: 25.08–180.64) and 0.25 (95% CI: 0.15–0.40), respectively, [Appendix Figure 1 (**Supplementary Material**)]. According to SROC curve, AUC is found to be 0.9971 which is close to 1, showing the high value of ICG in diagnosing lymph node metastasis in pelvic malignancies (**Figure 5**).

Test of Heterogeneity

Due to the heterogeneity I^2 was found to be 56.2% in detection rate a sub-group analysis was conducted to find the reasons for the observed heterogeneity. Univariate meta-regression of SLN detection rate and study characteristics showed that study size, study method, mean patient age, mean patient BMI, and type of cancer were not significantly associated with detection rates (**Table 2**).

DISCUSSION

SLN mapping has been the standard of care for breast cancer and melanoma for a long time (27) and achieved success in many other types of cancer. During the process of assessing the value of SLN mapping, detection rate is taken into consideration in the very first place. Most of meta-analyses on diagnostic efficacy of SLN mapping were focused on uterine cancers, and to our knowledge, this is the first meta-analysis of that in pelvic malignancies.

It should be mentioned that in these previous meta-analyses, studies using both robotic-assisted system and indocyanine green fluorescence tracer in the meantime have not been analyzed statistically before. Compared with prior meta-analyses which studied on tracers including blue dye, ICG and/or 99mTc in

TABLE 1 | Characteristics of included studies.

Author, year	Sample size	Study design	Type of cancer	Injection site	Mean age	Mean BMI (kg/m^2)	Mean number of SLNs detected	Mean number of non-SLNs removed	Reference standard	Pathology assessment	Detection rate	Sensitivity
Rossi et al. (10)	20	Prospective	Endometrium/ cervix	Cervical	61	31	4.5	23.5	Pelvic and para-aortic LND by guidelines	NR	85.0%	50.0%
Holloway et al. (25)	35	Retrospective	Endometrium	Cervical	63	33.1	NR	NR	Complete pelvic and common-iliac LND, aortic LND in high-grade EC	H&E, IHC, ultrastaging	100.0%	90.0%
Manny et al. (11)	50	Prospective	Prostate	Prostate	66	NR	NR	NR	Extended PLND	NR	76.0%	100.0%
Jewell et al. (12)	197	Retrospective	Endometrium/ cervix	Cervical	60	30.2	3	NR	Pelvic and para-aortic LND by guidelines	H&E, ultrastaging	95.0%	NR
Manny et al. (26)	10	Prospective	Bladder	Bladder	71	NR	NR	NR	Complete pelvic and peri-aortic LND	NR	90.0%	100.0%
Sinno et al. (13)	38	Prospective	Endometrium	Cervical	65	31.1	4.8	NR	Complete pelvic and para-aortic LND if preoperative grade 3 endometrioid, serous, clear cell, or carcinosarcoma	H&E, ultrastaging	92.1%	100.0%
Paley et al. (14)	123	Prospective	Endometrium	Cervical	63	32	3	NR	Pelvic and peri-aortic LND if high risk	H&E	96.7%	100.0%
Ehrisman et al. (15)	20	Retrospective	Endometrium	Cervical	67	32.3	2	22	Complete pelvic LND or Memorial Sloan Kettering algorithm	H&E	90.0%	NR
Chennamsetty et al. (16)	20	Prospective	Prostate	Prostate	64	NR	5	NR	Extended PLND	NR	100.0%	NR
Beavis et al. (17)	31	Retrospective	Cervix	Cervical	43	26.5	4	14	Complete pelvic LND, para-aortic LND at surgeon discretion	H&E, IHC, ultrastaging	100.0%	100.0%
Hagen et al. (18)	108	Prospective	Endometrium	Cervical	66	27.5	NR	NR	Surgeon-discretion LND or Memorial Sloan Kettering algorithm	H&E, ultrastaging	96.0%	NR
Erikssion et al. (19)	56	Retrospective	Endometrium/ cervix	Cervical	62	30.6	3	NR	Memorial Sloan Kettering algorithm	H&E, ultrastaging	95.0%	NR
Mendivil et al. (20)	87	Retrospective	Endometrium	Cervical	62	32.9	2	NR	Complete pelvic LND, para-aortic LND if at high risk	H&E	96.5%	NR
Harke et al. (21)	59	Prospective	Prostate	Prostate	64	NR	9	15	Extended PLND	NR	94.9%	78.0%
Rajanbabu and Agarwal (22)	69	Prospective	Endometrium	Cervical	60	27.9	5	NR	Pelvic and para-aortic LND by guidelines	H&E	95.7%	70.0%
Renz et al. (23)	90	Retrospective	Endometrium	Cervical	61	31	2	19	Complete pelvic LND, para-aortic LND by guidelines	H&E	88.0%	83.3%
Rozenholc et al. (24)	46	Prospective	Endometrium	Cervical	64	45	2.4	NR	Pelvic and para-aortic LND by guidelines	H&E, ultrastaging	89.1%	100.0%

NR, not reported; H&E, hematoxylin-eosin; IHC, immunohistochemistry; BMI, body mass index; LND, lymph node dissection; PLND, pelvic lymph node dissection.

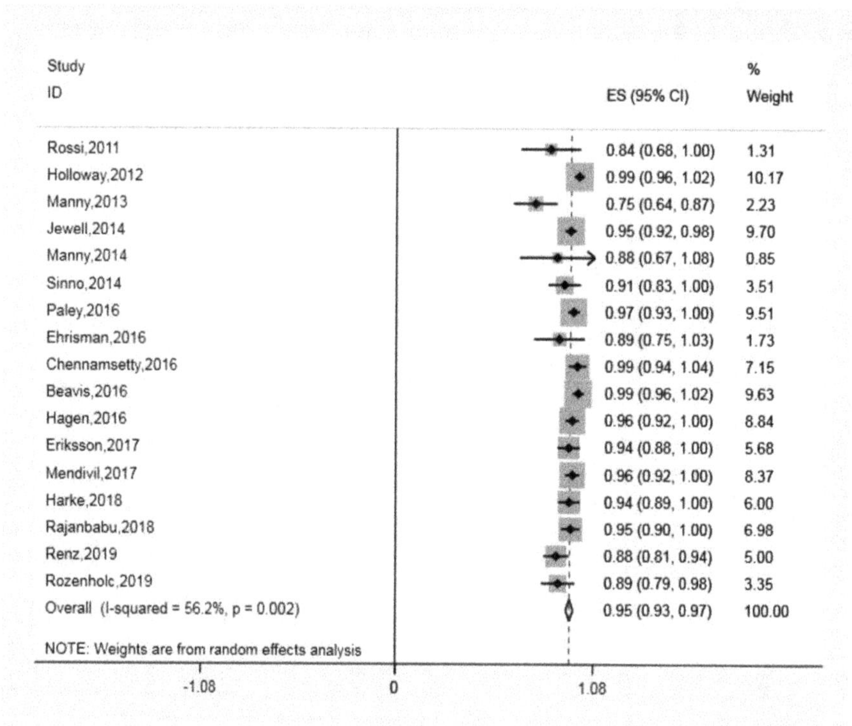

FIGURE 2 | Forest plot of pooled overall detection rate and 95% CI in SLN mapping. CI, confidence interval; SLN, sentinel lymph node.

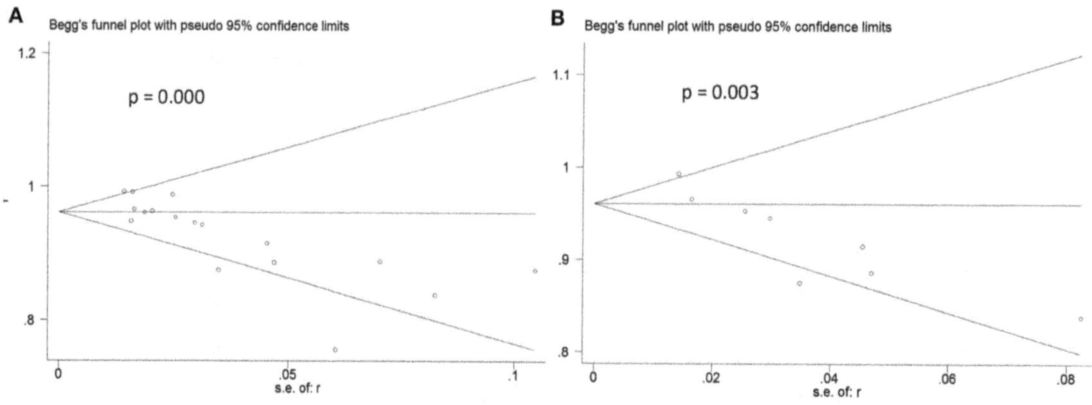

FIGURE 3 | Funnel plot of pooled detection rate and sensitivity. **(A)** Funnel plot of pooled overall detection rate. **(B)** Funnel plot of pooled sensitivity.

endometrial cancer (28–30), this meta-analysis with only ICG used as tracer shows higher detection rate of SLN mapping with detection rate of 95% (95% CI: 93–97), and in study of Lin et al. the detection rate was only 76% (95%: 71–81) with blue dye alone. In their study, detection rates were of 93 and 86% in ICG and 99mTc combined with blue dye, respectively, (28). Moreover, in study of Smith et al. detection rates were found higher of 90.3% in ICG vs. 81% in blue dye (31).

Hybrid image-guided surgery technologies are increasingly gaining interest, such as combined radio- and fluorescence-guidance. In study of KleinJan et al. use of the hybrid tracer ICG-99mTc-nancolloid was evaluated and the detection rate was over 95% (32). Compared with the conventional radioguided SN approach, the additional cost of ICG-99mTc-nancolloid is negligible (33), and use of ICG involves only minor additional costs (34). According to prior studies, the use of ICG also brings several advantages, such as fewer adverse effects, less pain, and quicker transcutaneous real-time visualization (35, 36).

In this meta-analysis, the pooled sensitivity of SLN detection of lymph node metastasis was 86% (95% CI: 75–94). In study of SLN mapping by Rossi et al. there were only two patients with positive lymph nodes in those who had successful mapping

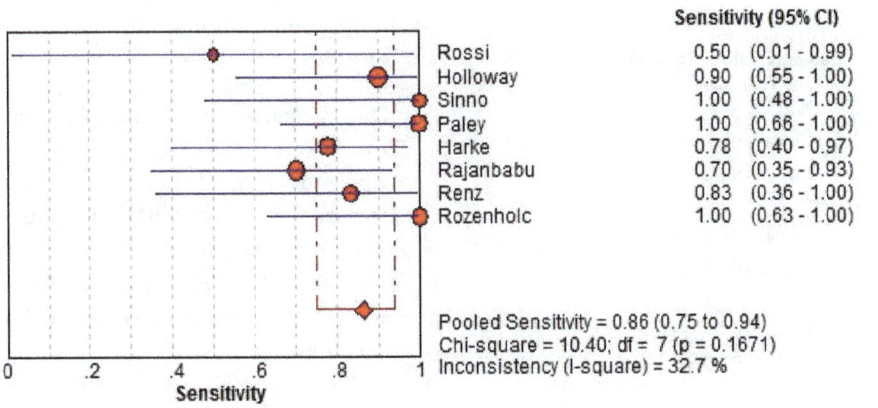

FIGURE 4 | Forest plot of pooled sensitivity of SLN detection and 95% CI in SLN mapping. CI, confidence interval; SLN, sentinel lymph node.

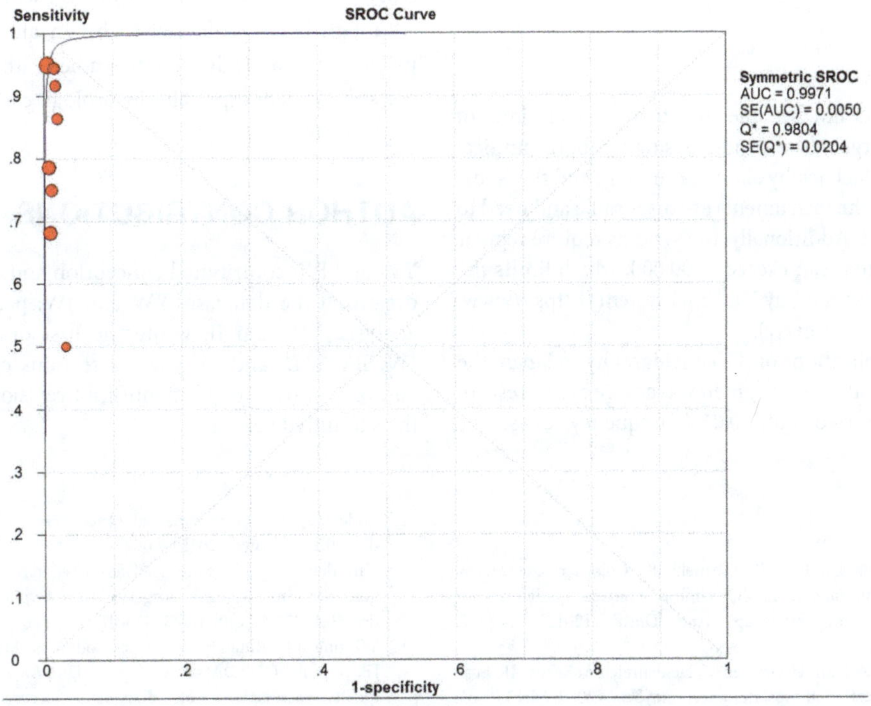

FIGURE 5 | SROC curve. AUC, area under SROC curve; Q* indicates the point at which sensitivity = specificity.

and one of them showed negative SLN, leading to the lowest sensitivity of 50% (10). In other 10 studies with available data, 6 out of them showed the sensitivities of 100% and all of them were over 70% [(11–14, 17, 21–24, 26); **Table 1**]. In previous meta-analyses by Lin et al. and Smith et al. in uterine cancers with several tracers included, sensitivities were found 91% (95% Cl: 87–95) and 96% (95% CI: 93–98), respectively (28, 31).

In pilot meta-analysis, robotic-assisted surgery demonstrated higher detection rates than other modalities. The pilot study conducted by Lin et al. showed that robotic-assisted surgery led to 86% detection rate, when laparoscopy and laparotomy got that of 82 and 77%, respectively, in patients with endometrial cancer (28). In the literature before, a higher BMI is linked to lower detection rate of the SLN (13). However, in the study by Rozenholc et al. there was no difference in the detection rate between surgeries that were robotic (mean BMI 44.6) and laparoscopic (mean BMI 29.4) (24). Moreover, when compared with open surgery, robotic-assisted surgery results in fewer blood transfusions and leads to a slightly shorter hospital stay (37).

However, due to the limitations of robotic-assisted surgery, such as higher costs and the lack of haptic feedback, the current

TABLE 2 | Univariate meta-regression of SLN detection rate and study characteristics.

Characteristics	Detection rate% (95% CI)	*P*-value
Sample size		
<60	0.94 (0.91–0.97)	0.891
≥60	0.95 (0.93–0.97)	
Study design		
Prospective	0.94 (0.91–0.97)	0.456
Retrospective	0.96 (0.93–0.99)	
Mean age		
<63	0.95 (0.92–0.98)	0.985
≥63	0.95 (0.92–0.98)	
Mean BMI		
<32 kg/m^2	0.95 (0.92–0.97)	0.475
≥32 kg/m^2	0.96 (0.94–0.99)	
Type of cancer		
Uterus	0.95 (0.94–0.97)	0.561
Urology	0.91 (0.82–1.00)	

CI, confidence interval; SLN, sentinel lymph node; BMI, body mass index.

robotic technology has not become the standard technique of minimally invasive surgery worldwide. A single robotic surgical system can set a hospital back by about $2 million, and that's just to get started. Some of the instruments are disposable and need to be continually replaced. Additionally, the systems require regular maintenance at rates that can exceed $100,000, which limits the number of hospitals that can buy Da Vinci system (https://www.drugwatch.com/davinci-surgery/).

In a survey of complications of ICG angiography in Japan, the results indicated that indocyanine green was as safe as fluorescein (38), which was reported only 0.05% frequency of severe adverse reactions, such as circulatory shock, bronchospasm, laryngospasm, cardiac arrest, myocardial infarction, and tonic seizure (39).

Our systematic review and meta-analysis has limitations as follow. First, we only included English studies, which may lead to a potential language bias. Second, we didn't have individual patient data, such as age, BMI and so on. The results presented in this study were based on unadjusted estimates. Third, the number of studies included is not sufficient enough so that some subgroup analyses cannot be conducted, and it may contribute to a publication bias.

In conclusion, the NIR imaging system in robotic-assisted surgery with ICG dye is quite easy to master, and the present results confirmed that SLN mapping using ICG alone is a reliable and safe approach that performs well diagnostically when assessing lymph nodal metastasis in pelvic malignancies. Although it is considered to be an alternative to a complete pelvic lymph node dissection, studies with larger patient samples are still needed, especially in urology cancers like prostate and bladder cancer.

AUTHOR CONTRIBUTIONS

YW and BX: contributed conception and design of the study. JJ: organized the database. YW and JW: performed the statistical analysis. YW and JJ: wrote the first draft of the manuscript. JW, BX, MD, and MC: wrote sections of the manuscript. All authors contributed to manuscript revision, read, and approved the submitted version.

REFERENCES

1. Colombo N, Preti E, Landoni F, Carinelli S, Colombo A, Marini C, et al. Endometrial cancer: ESMO clinical practice guidelines for diagnosis, treatment and follow-up. *Ann Oncol.* (2013) 24:33–8. doi: 10.1093/annonc/mdt353
2. Briganti A, Blute ML, Eastham JH, Graefen M, Heidenreich A, Karnes JR, et al. Pelvic lymph node dissection in prostate cancer. *Eur Urol.* (2009) 55:1251–65. doi: 10.1016/j.eururo.2009.03.012
3. Dowdy SC, Borah BJ, Bakkum-Gamez JN, Weaver AL, McGree ME, Haas LR, et al. Prospective assessment of survival, morbidity, and cost associated with lymphadenectomy in low-risk endometrial cancer. *Gynecol Oncol.* (2012) 127:5–10. doi: 10.1016/j.ygyno.2012.06.035
4. Rousseau B, Doucet L, Perrouin Verbe MA, Papin G, Erauso A, Joulin V, et al. Comparison of the morbidity between limited and extended pelvic lymphadenectomy during laparoscopic radical prostatectomy. *Progres En Urologie J.* (2014) 24:114–20. doi: 10.1016/j.purol.2013.07.018
5. Cabanas RM. An approach for the treatment of penile carcinoma. *Cancer.* (1977) 39:456–66. doi: 10.1002/1097-0142(197702)39:2<456::AID-CNCR2820390214>3.0.CO;2-I
6. Wawroschek F, Vogt H, Weckermann D, Harzmann R. The sentinel lymph node concept in prostate cancer-first results of gamma probe-guided sentinel lymph node identifcation. *Eur Urol.* (1999) 36:595–600. doi: 10.1159/000020054
7. How J, Gotlieb WH, Press JZ, Abitbol J, Pelmus M, Ferenczy A, et al. Comparing indocyanine green, technetium, and blue dye for sentinel lymph node mapping in endometrial cancer. *Gynecol Oncol.* (2015) 137:436–42. doi: 10.1016/j.ygyno.2015.04.004
8. Van den Berg NS, van Leeuwen FW, van der Poel HG. Fluorescence guidance in urologic surgery. *Curr Opin Urol.* (2012) 22:109–20. doi: 10.1097/MOU.0b013e3283501869
9. Whiting PF, Rutjes AW, Westwood ME, Mallett S, Deeks JJ, Reitsma JB, et al. QUADAS-2 Group. QUADAS-2: a revised tool for the quality assessment of diagnostic accuracy studies. *Ann Intern Med.* (2011) 155:529–36. doi: 10.7326/0003-4819-155-8-201110180-00009
10. Rossi EC, Ivanova A, Boggess JF. Robotically assisted fluorescence-guided lymph node mapping with ICG for gynecologic malignancies: a feasibility study. *Gynecol Oncol.* (2012) 124:78–82. doi: 10.1016/j.ygyno.2011.09.025
11. Manny TB, Hemal AK. Fluorescence-enhanced robotic radical cystectomy using unconjugated indocyanine green for pelvic lymphangiography, tumor marking, and mesenteric angiography: the initial clinical experience. *Urology.* (2014) 83:824–30. doi: 10.1016/j.urology.2013.11.042
12. Jewell EL, Huang JJ, Abu-Rustum NR, Gardner JR, Brown CL, Sonoda Y, et al. Detection of sentinel lymph nodes in minimally invasive surgery using indocyanine green and near-infrared fluorescence imaging for uterine and cervical malignancies. *Gynecol Oncol.* (2014) 133:274–7. doi: 10.1016/j.ygyno.2014.02.028
13. Sinno AK, Fader AN, Roche KL, Giuntoli RL, Tanner EJ. A comparison of colorimetric versus fluorometric sentinel lymph node mapping during robotic surgery for endometrial cancer. *Gynecol Oncol.* (2014) 134:281–6. doi: 10.1016/j.ygyno.2014.05.022

14. Paley PJ, Veljovich DS, Press JZ, Isacson C, Pizer E, Shah C. A prospective investigation of fluorescence imaging to detect sentinel lymph nodes at robotic-assisted endometrial cancer staging. *Am J Obstet Gynecol.* (2016) 215:117 e1–7. doi: 10.1016/j.ajog.2015.12.046
15. Ehrisman J, Secord AA, Berchuck A, Lee PS, Di Santo N, Lopez-Acevedo M, et al. Performance of sentinel lymph node biopsy in high-risk endometrial cancer. *Gynecol Oncol.* (2016) 17:69–71. doi: 10.1016/j.gore.2016.04.002
16. Chennamsetty A, Zhumkhawala A, Tobis SB, Ruel N, Lau CS, Yamzon J, et al. Lymph node fluorescence during robot-assisted radical prostatectomy with indocyanine green: prospective dosing analysis. *Clin Genitourin Cancer* (2017) 15:e529–34. doi: 10.1016/j.clgc.2016.10.014
17. Beavis AL, Salazar-Marioni S, Sinno AK, Stone RL, Fader AN, Santillan-Gomez A, et al. Sentinel lymph node detection rates using indocyanine green in women with early-stage cervical cancer. *Gynecol Oncol.* (2016) 143:302–6. doi: 10.1016/j.ygyno.2016.08.236
18. Hagen B, Valla M, Aune G, Ravlo M, Abusland AB, Araya E, et al. Indocyanine green fluorescence imaging of lymph nodes during robotic-assisted laparoscopic operation for endometrial cancer. a prospective validation study using a sentinel lymph node surgical algorithm. *Gynecol Oncol.* (2016) 143:479–83. doi: 10.1016/j.ygyno.2016.10.029
19. Eriksson AG, Beavis A, Soslow RA, Zhou Q, Abu-Rustum NR, Gardner GJ, et al. A comparison of the detection of sentinel lymph nodes using indocyanine green and near-infrared fluorescence imaging versus blue dye during robotic surgery in uterine cancer. *Int J Gynecol Cancer.* (2017) 27:743–7. doi: 10.1097/IGC.0000000000000959
20. Mendivil AA, Abaid LN, Brown, JV III, Mori KM, Beck TL, Epstein HD, et al. The safety and feasibility of minimally invasive sentinel lymph node staging using indocyanine green in the management of endometrial cancer. *Eur J Obstet Gynecol Reprod Biol.* (2018) 224:29–32. doi: 10.1016/j.ejogrb.2018.02.027
21. Harke NN, Godes M, Wagner C, Addali M, Fangmeyer B, Urbanova K, et al. Fluorescence-supported lymphography and extended pelvic lymph node dissection in robot-assisted radical prostatectomy: a prospective, randomized trial. *World J Urol.* (2018) 36:1817–23. doi: 10.1007/s00345-018-2330-7
22. Rajanbabu A, Agarwal R. A prospective evaluation of the sentinel node mapping algorithm in endometrial cancer and correlation of its performance against endometrial cancer risk subtypes. *Eur J Obstet Gynecol Reprod Biol.* (2018) 224:77–80. doi: 10.1016/j.ejogrb.2018.03.017
23. Renz M, Marjon N, Devereaux K, Raghavan S, Folkins AK, Karam A. Immediate intraoperative sentinel lymph node analysis by frozen section is predictive of lymph node metastasis in endometrial cancer. *J Robo Surgery.* (2019). doi: 10.1007/s11701-019-00928-z
24. Rozenholc A, Samouelian V, Warkus T, Gauthier P, Provencher D, Sauthier P, et al. Green versus blue: Randomized controlled trial comparing indocyanine green with methylene blue for sentinel lymph node detection in endometrial cancer. *Gynecol Oncol.* (2019) 153:500–4. doi: 10.1016/j.ygyno.2019.03.103
25. Holloway RW, Bravo RA, Rakowski JA, James JA, Jeppson CN, Ingersoll SB, et al. Detection of sentinel lymph nodes in patients with endometrial cancer undergoing robotic-assisted staging: a comparison of colorimetric and fluorescence imaging. *Gynecol Oncol.* (2012) 126:25–9. doi: 10.1016/j.ygyno.2012.04.009
26. Manny TB, Patel M, Hemal AK. Fluorescence-enhanced robotic radical prostatectomy using real-time lymphangiography and tissue marking with percutaneous injection of unconjugated indocyanine green: the initial clinical experience in 50 patients. *Eur Urol.* (2014) 65:1162–8. doi: 10.1016/j.eururo.2013.11.017
27. Mansel RE, Fallowfield L, Kissin M, Goyal A, Newcombe RG, Dixon JM, et al. Randomized multicenter trial of sentinel node biopsy versus standard axillary treatment in operable breast cancer: the ALMANAC Trial. *J Natl Cancer Inst.* (2006) 98:599–609. doi: 10.1093/jnci/djj158
28. Lin H, Ding Z, Kota VG, Zhang X, Zhou J. Sentinel lymph node mapping in endometrial cancer: a systematic review and meta-analysis. *Oncotarget.* (2017) 28:46601–10. doi: 10.18632/oncotarget.16662
29. Kang S, Yoo HJ, Hwang JH, Lim M-C, Seo SS, Park S-Y. Sentinel lymph node biopsy in endometrial cancer: meta-analysis of 26 studies. *Gynecol Oncol.* (2011) 123:522–7. doi: 10.1016/j.ygyno.2011.08.034
30. Ansari M, Rad MAG, Hassanzadeh M, Gholami H, Yousefi Z, Dabbagh VR, et al. Sentinel node biopsy in endometrial cancer: systematic review and meta-analysis of the literature. *Eur J Gynaecol Oncol.* (2013) 34:387–401.
31. Smith BAJ, Fader AN, Tanner EJ. Sentinel lymph node assessment in endometrial cancer: a systematic review and meta-analysis. *Am J Obstet Gynecol.* (2017) 216:459–76. doi: 10.1016/j.ajog.2016.11.1033
32. KleinJan GH, van Werkhoven E, van den Berg NS, Karakullukcu MB, Zijlmans H, van der Hage JA, et al. The best of both worlds: a hybrid approach for optimal pre- and intraoperative identification of sentinel lymph nodes. *Eur J Nucl Med Mol Imaging.* (2018) 45L1915–25. doi: 10.1007/s00259-018-4028-x
33. Lee CM, Park S, Park SH, Jung SW, Choe JW, Sul JY, et al. Sentinel node mapping using a fluorescent dye and visible light during laparoscopic gastrectomy for early gastric cancer: result of a prospective study from a single institute. *Ann Surg.* (2017) 265:766. doi: 10.1097/SLA.0000000000001739
34. Berg NS, Van D, Brouwer OR, Klop WMC, Bari K, Zuur CLI, et al. Concomitant radio- and fluorescence-guided sentinel lymph node biopsy in squamous cell carcinoma of the oral cavity using ICG-(99m)Tc-nanocolloid. *Eur J Nucl Med Mol Imaging.* (2012) 39:1128–36. doi: 10.1007/s00259-012-2129-5
35. Zhang X, Li Y, Zhou Y, Mao F, Lin Y, Guan J, et al. Diagnostic performance of indocyanine green-guided sentinel lymph node biopsy in breast cancer: a meta-analysis. *PLoS ONE.* (2016) 11:e0155597. doi: 10.1371/journal.pone.0155597
36. Ruscito I, Gasparri ML, Braicu EI, Bellati F, Raio L, Sehouli J, et al. Sentinel node mapping in cervical and endometrial cancer: indocyanine green versus other conventional dyes—a meta-analysis. *Ann Surg Oncol.* (2016) 23:3749–56. doi: 10.1245/s10434-016-5236-x
37. Aboumarzouk OM, Bondad J, Ahmed K, Khan MS, Kynaston HG, Dasgupta P, et al. Robotic versus open radical cystectomy for bladder cancer in adults. *Cochrane Database System Rev Ltd.* (2015) 2015: CD011903. doi: 10.1002/14651858.CD011903
38. Obana, A., Miki, T., Hayashi, K., Takeda, M., Kawamura, A., Mutoh, T., et al. Survey of complications of indocyanine green angiography in Japan. *Am J Ophthalmol.* (1994) 118:749–53. doi: 10.1016/S0002-9394(14)72554-1
39. Yannuzzi LA, Rohrer KT, Tindel LJ, Sobel RS, Costanza MA, Shields W, et al. Fluorescein angiography complication survey. *Ophthalmology.* (1986) 93:611–7. doi: 10.1016/S0161-6420(86)33697-2

5

The Utility of Near-Infrared Fluorescence and Indocyanine Green During Robotic Pulmonary Resection

Dana Ferrari-Light[1], *Travis C. Geraci*[1*], *Prabhu Sasankan*[2] *and Robert J. Cerfolio*[1]

[1] *Department of Cardiothoracic Surgery, New York University Langone Health, New York, NY, United States,* [2] *School of Medicine, New York University Langone Health, New York, NY, United States*

Correspondence:
Travis C. Geraci
travis.geraci@nyulangone.org

During minimally invasive pulmonary resection, it is often difficult to localize pulmonary nodules that are small (<2 cm), low-density/subsolid on imaging, or deep to the visceral pleura. The use of near-infrared fluorescence (NIF) imaging for localizing pulmonary nodules using indocyanine green (ICG) contrast is an emerging technology that is increasingly utilized during pulmonary resection. When administered via electromagnetic navigational bronchoscopy (ENB), ICG can accurately localize pulmonary nodules. When injected intravenously (IV), ICG can also help delineate the intersegmental plane. Research is ongoing regarding the utility of ICG for identification of the sentinel lymph node in lung cancer.

Keywords: electromagnetic, fluorescence, localization, navigational bronchoscopy, lung cancer, pulmonary resection, robotic

INTRODUCTION

The use of electromagnetic navigational bronchoscopy (ENB) using near-infrared fluorescence (NIF) with indocyanine green contrast (ICG) has emerged as an accurate and efficient method for localizing pulmonary nodules. Indocyanine green is a fluorophore contrast that illuminates in the near infrared spectrum, has a high signal-to-noise ratio, is inexpensive, and relatively non-toxic (although the potential for patient allergy remains) (1). Indocyanine green is approved by the U.S. Food and Drug Administration as an intravenously (IV) injected drug for angiography studies and sentinel node assessments in various cancers. It is theorized that ICG is retained in malignant tissue by a non-specific inflammatory permeability and retention effect. Importantly, infiltration with ICG will not distort the cellular integrity of tissues and therefore will not interfere with the histopathologic characterization of the target specimen, including tumor margins.

Indocyanine green has been used successfully in many areas of medicine including ophthalmic angiography, cerebral perfusion assessment, and for the identification of sentinel lymph nodes and evaluation of anastomotic perfusion in various oncologic resections. However, its utility in pulmonary resection has only recently been explored.

In this review we discuss the multimodal use of ICG during pulmonary resection—transbronchial injection for localization of the primary tumor, delineation of the intersegmental plane, and identification of regional lymph nodes.

INTRAOPERATIVE LOCALIZATION OF PULMONARY NODULES WITH INDOCYANINE GREEN

The management of pulmonary nodules has evolved in synchrony with technological advancements in chest imaging. The increased precision of modern helical computed tomography

(CT) has led to the detection of small pulmonary lesions, ostensibly creating a window of opportunity for curative surgical resection in patients with early stage lung cancer. In 2011, the National Lung Screening Trial (NLST) reported a 20% relative reduction in mortality from lung cancer in high-risk patients screened with low-dose CT (LDCT) rather than chest radiography (2). Now with an exponentially-increasing rate of patients with screening LDCT scans revealing small, ill-defined pulmonary lesions, they increasingly are referred to thoracic surgeons for management. However, the majority of these indeterminate pulmonary nodules do not represent lung cancer. In the NLST, 96.4% of identified lesions were determined to be false-positive results after three screening rounds (2). These patients are continually followed with serial imaging. A minority of patients with more concerning sequential imaging findings require an invasive biopsy or surgical resection for diagnosis and/or definitive treatment.

The current standard of care for patients with small early-stage non-small cell lung cancer (NSCLC) is pulmonary lobectomy (3). This standard, however, is based on data that is over 20 years old, prior to the routine use of preoperative positron emission tomography scans (PET/CT) and the ascendance of minimally-invasive surgical techniques. Sublobar resection such as anatomic segmentectomy is performed more often in patients with small nodules or reduced cardiopulmonary function. Data regarding the efficacy of lobectomy vs. sublobar resection are mixed. Prospective non-randomized data have shown comparable long-term survival in patients with nodules <2 cm without nodal metastasis (4). Two prospective, randomized clinical trials, the Cancer and Leukemia Group B Trial 140503 and the Japan Clinical Oncology Group 0802/WJOG 4607L and JCOG 1211 Trial, are currently being conducted to help address the oncologic superiority or equality of sublobar resection vs. lobectomy, particularly for patients with small, early-stage lung cancer (5).

During sublobar resection, indeterminate lesions are often difficult to localize, particularly when a minimally invasive approach is performed. Nodule characteristics may also make intraoperative localization more difficult, such as when the lesion is smaller than 2 cm, subsolid and/or of low-density on CT scan, or deep to the visceral pleural surface. If performing a segmental resection, the precise location of the lesion may be difficult to determine on CT imaging alone, particularly if it is located between adjacent segments. Additionally, when performing pulmonary resection with robotic assistance, identifying lesions can be difficult due to the system's lack of haptic feedback and reliance on visual cues. These limitations of surgical technique have prompted the development of intraoperative localization techniques to aid in accurate resection. Additional incisions, conversion to thoracotomy for bimanual palpation, or performing a lobectomy to resect an intraoperative non-identifiable lesion are inefficient and morbid strategies. Intraoperative localization avoids these maneuvers and allows for more precise surgery.

Minimally invasive approaches to pulmonary resection are preferred to reduce perioperative morbidity and length of stay, precluding the standard technique of bimanual palpation. A number of preoperative procedures have been developed to aid localization, including CT-guided placement of metallic wires, coils, or markers (6, 7). While these techniques may be accurate, they require coordination with radiology and/or a hybrid operating room, exposes the patient and staff to radiation, requires a significant amount of time to complete, risk migration of the marker, and may be complicated by parenchymal hematoma or pneumothorax.

In 2001, Sakamoto et al. were the first to describe a method for nodule localization using indigo carmine contrast injected via flexible bronchoscopy near the target lesion (8). This study was followed by a series of studies reporting accurate localization of small pulmonary nodules and regional lymph nodes using electromagnetic navigation bronchoscopy (ENB) with transbronchial injection of blue dyes, most commonly, methylene blue or isosulfan blue (9). While the accuracy of these agents range from 79 to 100%, contrast dyes such as indigo carmine and methylene blue are limited by relatively quick diffusion time thereby limiting precision intraoperative visualization. Additionally, unlike color dyes visualized by white light endoscopy, ICG fluorescence is always detectable regardless of color or texture variation in the pulmonary parenchyma such as regions of anthracotic pigmentation, hematoma, or architectural distortion due to underlying pulmonary disease.

In 2015, Anayama et al. confirmed the feasibility of using NIF for lesion localization via ENB-guided ICG injection in a porcine lung model (10). Both *in vitro* and *ex vivo* studies were performed to assess the tissue penetration and spread of ICG in pulmonary parenchyma and to evaluate intraoperative localization. In the same year, Keating et al. published a case report in a human patient of successful intraoperative localization using NIF imaging with ICG during video-assisted thoracoscopic surgery (VATS) (11). In this study, the patient received an intravenous injection of ICG 24 h prior to surgery. Two lesions were successfully visualized and resected, one of which could not be identified with manual palpation through the thoracoscopic port sites.

A number of groups have since reported institutional studies regarding the accuracy of ENB-guided NIF using ICG for intraoperative localization of pulmonary lesions. In 2015 Okusanya et al. reported localization after administering preoperative intravenous ICG (5 mg/kg) followed by open thoracotomy within 24 h (12). NIF detected 16/18 (88%) nodules compared to manual palpation, which achieved a 100% identification rate. Furthermore, ICG identified five additional malignant subcentimeter nodules not readily apparent on CT imaging, three of which were in different lobes than the primary tumor. The authors found that the sensitivity for detecting nodules with NIF was dependent on tissue depth but independent of nodule size, metabolic activity, histology, or vascularity.

In 2017, Abbas et al. reported their institutional experience with ENB, localizing 54 nodules in 51 patients with a success rate of 98.1% and a false negative rate of 1.9% (13). In the first two patients, methylene blue dye with fiducial markers were used however the markers were found to be of marginal utility and the blue dye diffused quickly, prompting the researchers to switch to an combination of iopamidol (for fluoroscopic identification), methylene blue (for visual identification), and ICG (for fluorescence identification). Two patients required conversion to open thoracotomy for localization and resection due to dense pleural adhesions.

In 2018, Anayama et al. reported a series of 37 patients with nodules <2 cm in size who underwent VATS wedge resection using a mixture of ICG and iopamidol for localization by either CT-guided percutaneous injection or bronchoscopic injection (14). In the CT-guided group, 15/15 (100%) nodules were successfully localized, however a small pneumothorax occurred in three patients (20%) and in one patient this precluded additional marking. In the bronchoscopic group, 20/22 (90.9%) nodules were localized with six patients receiving injections at two anatomic locations. In the two patients unable to be localized, finger palpation was successful after extension of the access port site. The authors concluded that CT-guided localization might not be optimal for patients with multiple nodules, as the risk of pneumothorax may prevent marking of multiple lesions. Additionally, the bronchoscopic method may be preferred for patients with nodules that may be difficult to reach percutaneously, such as lesions adjacent the mediastinum, or posteriorly behind the scapula.

In mid-2019, Chao et al. just recently published their experience with a dual-marker localization technique in a hybrid operating room, using NIF marking with ICG in conjunction with microcoil deployment via CT-guided coaxial needle technique. This dual-marker placement was successful in all 11 patients studied, with a median localization time of 19 min and may be helpful to locate difficult pulmonary nodules (15).

We have recently published our own institutional experience with NIF localization using ICG when administered both via ENB and intravenous injection (16). In our series of patients who underwent planned robotic segmentectomy, 93 were selected for ENB localization with ICG due to small nodule size and/or challenging anatomic location (between segments or deep to the visceral pleural surface). Of the 93 patients undergoing ENB, we successfully identified the pulmonary nodule in 80 patients (86%). We were unable to find a statistically significant variable that would predict success or failure of our method. The most common reasons for localization failure were inaccurate ENB or ICG injection and technical malfunctions of the equipment.

TECHNICAL CONSIDERATIONS FOR ICG LOCALIZATION

At our institution, the decision to use ENB and ICG fluorescence for pulmonary tumor localization is selective. We chose to localize lesions based on size (favored for small lesions <2 cm), lesion morphology (ground-glass opacification), and lesion anatomy (favored in lesions deep to the pleural surface). There is no distance from the pleura that we consider to be an absolute contraindication to lesion localization.

Performing localization starts with a preoperative review of collimated CT scan data using superDimension™ software (Covidien, Minneapolis, MN) to create a virtual bronchoscopic pathway to the target lesion (see **Figure 1**). Identification of the optimal adjacent segmental and/or subsegmental bronchus is important for successful localization. In the operating room, the patient is positioned supine on the operating table and an electromagnetic board is placed beneath. Precordial sensors are attached to the patient which are then registered with the electromagnetic system. The patient is intubated with a single-lumen endotracheal tube. A sensor probe is introduced through the working channel of a flexible bronchoscope and the system is synced with various anatomic coordinates in the proximal and distal airways. Real-time virtual-guided bronchoscopy is then performed to within a goal distance of 1 cm or less to the target lesion (see **Figure 2**). The flexible probe may be extended beyond the end of the bronchoscope, allowing transparenchymal navigation to peripheral lesions and/or those distant from a subsegmental bronchus. In our experience, upper lobe lesions are the most difficult to localize because of the acute bronchoscopic angles required to reach the apical airways. When the lesion is localized, ICG contrast is injected via a bronchoscopic needle. It is prudent to have an assistant hold the bronchoscopic in position during injection to prevent drifting from the target location.

Our method for contrast injection involves an admixture of 10 mL of sterile water in a 25 mg bottled powder of indocyanine green. We inject 0.5 mL of ICG solution followed by a flush of 0.5 mL of sterile water. It is important to use sterile water in the admixture. In our experience, using normal saline will cause the ICG powder to clump and makes it difficult to flush intravenously. The remaining 9.5 mL of ICG solution is given intravenously by the anesthesiologist after control and ligation of the segmental pulmonary artery. During robotic surgery on the Xi version of the da Vinci robotic system, the thoracoscopic camera is equipped with near-infrared technology (Firefly, Intuitive Surgical, Sunnyvale, CA) which illuminates ICG-infiltrated lung parenchyma after peritumoral injection (see **Figure 3**) and ICG-perfused tissue after intravenous administration (see **Figure 4**).

DELINEATION OF THE INTERSEGMENTAL PLANE

During anatomic segmental resection, the corresponding vein, artery, and bronchus are transected and the lung parenchyma is divided with a surgical stapler. During parenchymal division, the surgeon must identify the intersegmental plane while achieving an appropriate tumor margin. Standard techniques for identifying the intersegmental plane such as inflation/deflation of the tissue, are practically cumbersome and may be misleading due to air diffusion through the communicating pores of Kohn. Indocyanine green binds to plasma proteins and when injected intravenously is confined to the vascular compartment. Due to this biochemical property, ICG helps delineate the intersegmental plane after ligation of the segmental artery.

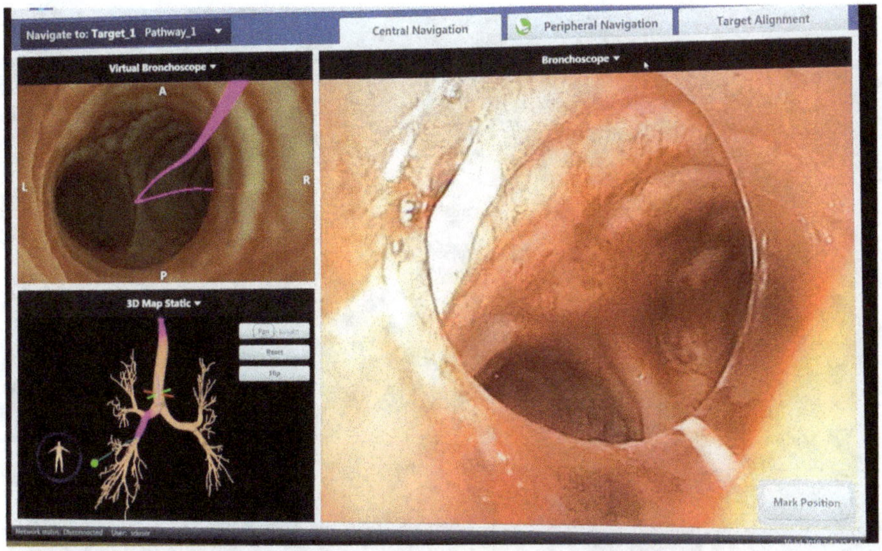

FIGURE 1 | SuperDimension Thoracic Navigation System: electromagnetic bronchoscopic view, showing the pathway to the target nodule in the right lower lobe.

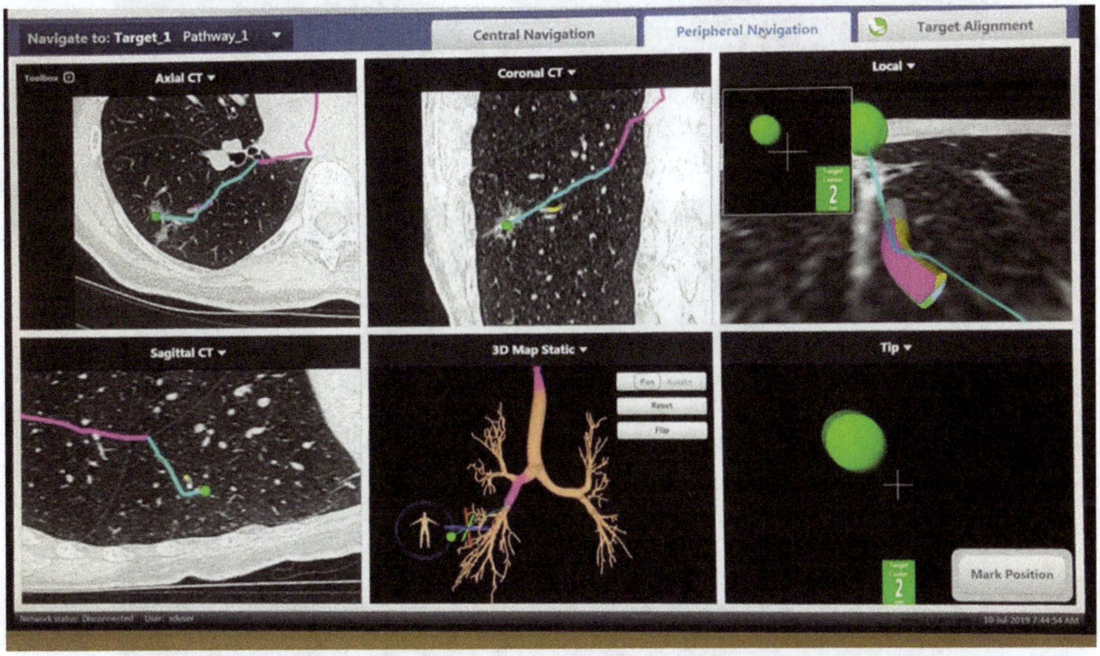

FIGURE 2 | SuperDimension Thoracic Navigation System: image-guided peripheral view, showing electromagnetic probe is 2 cm from the target nodule in the right lower lobe.

Presented in 2017, Mehta et al. conducted a phase II prospective cohort trial evaluating the safety, feasibility, and reproducibility of peripheral venous ICG injection and NIF mapping for delineation of the intersegmental plane during robotic segmental resection (17). Specifically, the researchers assessed whether this technique would increase the oncological margin vs. reliance on visual delineation of the intersegmental plane. In 31 patients who underwent pulmonary resection with ICG injection, 23 (74%) cases resulted in a significant lengthening of the oncologic resection margin. Using a novel 7-point objective rating scale, fluorescent segmental demarcation resulted in an average increase in the oncologic margin of 2.4 cm vs. the predicted plane by a two-surgeon assessment. The long-term significance regarding local control, recurrence, and disease-free survival are unknown, but long-term follow-up is anticipated.

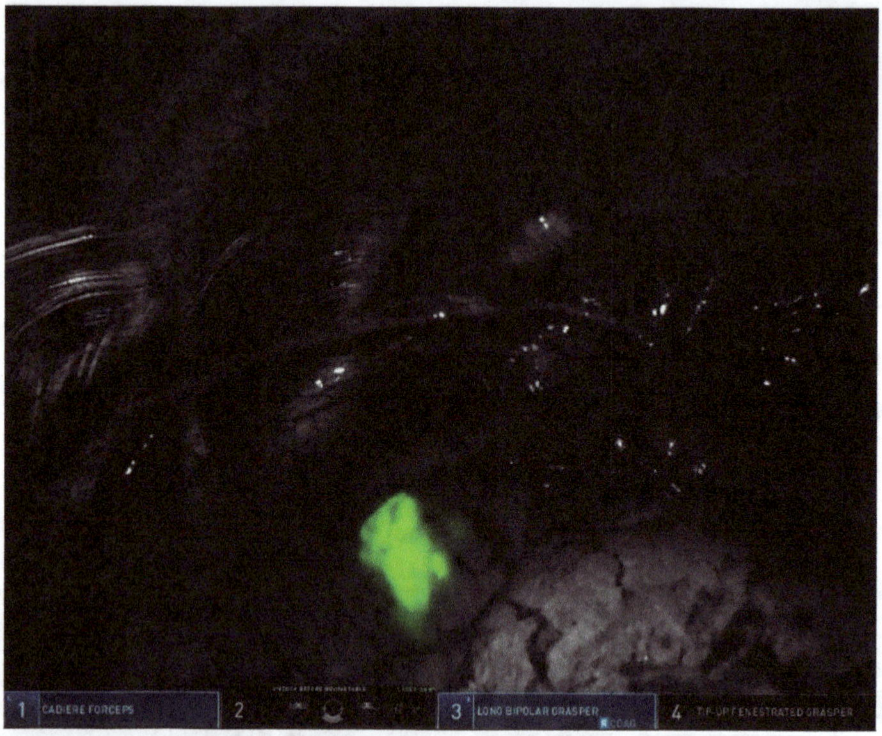

FIGURE 3 | Pulmonary nodule in the left upper lobe, illuminated by ICG fluorescence (firefly mode).

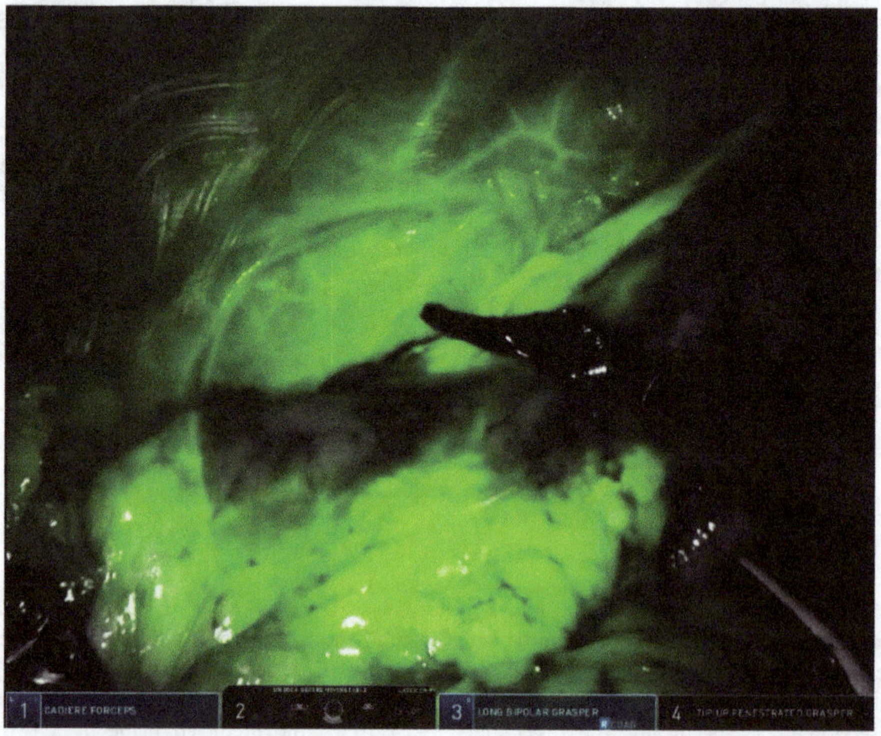

FIGURE 4 | Intravenous ICG delineation of the intersegmental plane between the lingula and the left upper lobe segments during left upper lobe trisegmentectomy. Note the diffusion of ICG contrast around the area of target nodule from **Figure 3**.

In their 2019 report, Sekine et al. report a novel method involving the combined use of 3D image analysis and transbronchial ICG injection to determine surgical margins for pulmonary sublobar resection in patients with early-stage lung cancer. In their method, preoperative 3D image analysis was accomplished using multi-slice enhanced CT imaging to generate pulmonary angiography and virtual bronchoscopy (18). For each case, these virtual models were then used to run several simulations of anatomical sublobar resection in order to determine the appropriate tumor resection margin.

During surgery, transbronchial injection was used to instill ICG into the target segmental bronchus and distribute it throughout the segmental bronchial tree. Following the generation of virtual bronchoscopy from chest CT imaging, sublobar resection simulation was used to identify the segmental area and margins for resection. Intra-operatively, transbronchial ICG injection yielded well-visualized fluorescence and easily definable segmental borders in 55 of 65 cases (84%). A comparison of preoperative simulated resection and postoperative segmental structure found concordance between preoperative virtual segmentectomy and postoperative segmental structures in 54 of the 58 (93.1%) cases. In a propensity-matched comparison of surgical outcomes between patients who underwent fluorescence-guided sublobar resection with patients who underwent traditional VATS segmentectomy, the analysis showed similar operation length, blood loss, length of hospital stay, and postoperative complications.

SENTINEL LYMPH NODE MAPPING

The use of ICG for intraoperative or postoperative identification of the sentinel node is an exciting area of ongoing research, but its role has not been clearly defined in lung cancer. In cancer, the "sentinel node" refers to the lymph node that receives the initial lymphatic flow from a malignant tumor, theoretically representing the first tissue at risk for malignant dissemination of tumor cells. During a resection for certain types of cancer, if a sentinel node is determined to be negative, a less aggressive lymph node dissection is pursued, limiting morbidity. The regional lymph node status is an important prognostic indicator, particularly in lung cancer. Additionally, patients undergoing a lymph node dissection during pulmonary resection may be upstaged based on nodal status and potentially receive adjuvant therapies. However, in the ACOSOG Z4032 multicenter trial of patients undergoing sublobar resection, 35% of patients were found to undergo resection without lymph node assessment (19). With success in identifying the sentinel node in other malignancies using near infrared imaging, there has been progress in the concept of the sentinel lymph node in lung cancer given that ICG often "lights up" an N1 intrasegmental lymph node.

In 2004, Ito et al. utilized sentinel lymph node navigation using ICG in patients with lung cancer, establishing feasibility and safety (20). Presurgical injection of ICG was administered in peritumoral quadrants in 38 patients undergoing pulmonary lobectomy. During lymph node dissection, a sentinel node was identified by visual inspection in 18% of patients. Additionally, sentinel nodes were derived by relative ICG concentration (1.5 × baseline) in 87.5% of patients with a negative predictive rate of 100%. There was a single false-negative result, which the authors posit was due to tumor obstruction of the primary lymphatic flow.

In 2011, Yamashita et al. evaluated the accuracy of ICG to identify the sentinel lymph node in patients with early stage lung cancer undergoing VATS. Peritumoral injection of ICG was performed and a sentinel lymph node was identified with NIF in 25 of 31 patients (80.7%) with a 0% false-negative rate (21). The noted reasons for failure to identify a sentinel lymph node were attributed to intrapleural adhesions or leakage of ICG contrast after injection.

In 2013, Gilmore et al. reported a dose-escalation clinical trial, evaluating the optimal peritumoral injection of ICG to identify sentinel lymph nodes in human patients with lung cancer (22). In 38 patients, the study revealed that sentinel lymph node identification increased with increased dose-response, finding an 89% success rate at a dose of 1,000 μg of ICG. At this dose, 26 sentinel nodes were identified by near infrared imaging in 15 patients, six of which had metastatic disease on histologic analysis. Metastatic nodal disease was not identified in patients with negative sentinel lymph nodes by ICG evaluation.

Recently, Hachey et al. reported a feasibility study using ICG contrast for tumor and sentinel lymph node localization by ENB (23). Performed in 10 patients with early stage NSCLC, the prospective study revealed that ICG accurately and efficiently identifies the target parenchymal lesion by fluorescent flow, with passive drainage to the sentinel lymph node and regional lymph nodes. The technique identified the sentinel node in eight patients (80%) and the sentinel node status was 100% sensitive for overall nodal staging status. Of note, 12.5% of patients were upstaged based on sentinel lymph node mapping.

In a report reviewing the long-term outcomes after NIF-guided sentinel lymph node mapping with peritumoral ICG injection, Digesu et al. compared patients who underwent mediastinal lymph node sampling with or without sentinel lymph node localization (24). Sentinel lymph node mapping was 100% sensitive and specific for local lymph node status; metastatic disease was detected in the sentinel lymph node in all occurrences (7 patients) of positive lymph node disease (pN+) and not detected in the sentinel node in node negative disease. After a median follow-up of nearly 45 months, the study revealed that patients who underwent sentinel node mapping who were found to have pathologic node negative disease (pN0) had an improved estimated overall and disease-free survival than those who were deemed pN0 by lymph node dissection alone (100 vs. 70%, and 100 vs. 66%, respectively). In the non-sentinel lymph node group, 4 of 15 patients (26%) had recurrence of disease despite pN0 status at resection. The authors attribute part of this outcome to improved overall nodal staging with sentinel lymph node mapping, due to the focused histologic analysis of tumor-specific sentinel nodes, thereby shifting patients previously (incorrectly) deemed pN0 to the correct pN+ status.

CONCLUSION

Indocyanine green is emerging as a useful adjunct in the localization of lung nodules and the delineation of the intersegmental plane when given intravenously, via transbronchial injection, or both. There is significant potential for its utility in localizing pulmonary sentinel lymph nodes and its impact on overall and disease-free survival for lung cancer.

AUTHOR CONTRIBUTIONS

DF-L, TG, PS, and RC contributed equally to the formation, writing, and editing of this manuscript.

REFERENCES

1. Alander JT, Kaartinen I, Laakso A, Patila T, Spillmann T, Tuchin VV, et al. A review of indocyanine green fluorescent imaging in surgery. *Int J Biomed Imag.* (2012) 2012:940585. doi: 10.1155/2012/940585
2. Aberle DR, Adams AM, Berg CD, Black WC, Clapp JD, Fagerstrom RM, et al. Reduced lung-cancer mortality with low-dose computed tomographic screening. *N Engl J Med.* (2011) 365:395–409. doi: 10.1056/NEJMoa1102873
3. Ginsberg RJ, Rubinstein LV. Randomized trial of lobectomy versus limited resection for T1 N0 non-small cell lung cancer. Lung Cancer Study Group. *Ann Thorac Surg.* (1995) 60:615–22; discussion: 22–3. doi: 10.1016/0003-4975(95)00537-U
4. Kodama K, Higashiyama M, Okami J, Tokunaga T, Imamura F, Nakayama T, et al. Oncologic outcomes of segmentectomy versus lobectomy for clinical T1a N0 M0 Non-small cell lung cancer. *Ann Thorac Surg.* (2016) 101:504–11. doi: 10.1016/j.athoracsur.2015.08.063
5. Asamura H. Role of limited sublobar resection for early-stage lung cancer: steady progress. *J Clin Oncol.* (2014) 32:2403–4. doi: 10.1200/JCO.2014.56.4203
6. Lin MW, Chen JS. Image-guided techniques for localizing pulmonary nodules in thoracoscopic surgery. *J Thorac Dis.* (2016) 8(Suppl. 9):S749–55. doi: 10.21037/jtd.2016.09.71
7. Zhao ZR, Lau RW, Ng CS. Hybrid theatre and alternative localization techniques in conventional and single-port video-assisted thoracoscopic surgery. *J Thorac Dis.* (2016) 8(Suppl. 3):S319–27. doi: 10.3978/j.issn.2072-1439.2016.02.27
8. Sakamoto T, Takada Y, Endoh M, Matsuoka H, Tsubota N. Bronchoscopic dye injection for localization of small pulmonary nodules in thoracoscopic surgery. *Ann Thorac Surg.* (2001) 72:296–7. doi: 10.1016/S0003-4975(01)02604-2
9. Cuadrado D, Grogan EL. Localization techniques for small lung nodules. *Oper Tech Thoracic Cardiovasc Surg.* (2014) 19:179–98. doi: 10.1053/j.optechstcvs.2014.08.001
10. Anayama T, Qiu J, Chan H, Nakajima T, Weersink R, Daly M, et al. Localization of pulmonary nodules using navigation bronchoscope and a near-infrared fluorescence thoracoscope. *Ann Thorac Surg.* (2015) 99:224–30. doi: 10.1016/j.athoracsur.2014.07.050
11. Keating JJ, Kennedy GT, Singhal S. Identification of a subcentimeter pulmonary adenocarcinoma using intraoperative near-infrared imaging during video-assisted thoracoscopic surgery. *J Thorac Cardiovasc Surg.* (2015) 149:e51–3. doi: 10.1016/j.jtcvs.2014.10.081
12. Okusanya OT, Holt D, Heitjan D, Deshpande C, Venegas O, Jiang J, et al. Intraoperative near-infrared imaging can identify pulmonary nodules. *Ann Thorac Surg.* (2014) 98:1223–30. doi: 10.1016/j.athoracsur.2014.05.026
13. Abbas A, Kadakia S, Ambur V, Muro K, Kaiser L. Intraoperative electromagnetic navigational bronchoscopic localization of small, deep, or subsolid pulmonary nodules. *J Thorac Cardiovasc Surg.* (2017) 153:1581–90. doi: 10.1016/j.jtcvs.2016.12.044
14. Anayama T, Hirohashi K, Miyazaki R, Okada H, Kawamoto N, Yamamoto M, et al. Near-infrared dye marking for thoracoscopic resection of small-sized pulmonary nodules: comparison of percutaneous and bronchoscopic injection techniques. *J Cardiothorac Surg.* (2018) 13:5. doi: 10.1186/s13019-018-0697-6
15. Chao YK, Leow OQY, Wen CT, Fang HY. Image-guided thoracoscopic lung resection using a dual-marker localization technique in a hybrid operating room. *Surg Endosc.* (2019). doi: 10.1007/s00464-019-06883-y. [Epub ahead of print].
16. Geraci TC, Ferrari-Light D, Kent A, Michaud G, Zervos M, Pass H, et al. Technique, outcomes with navigational bronchoscopy using indocyanine green for robotic segmentectomy. *Ann Thorac Surg.* (2019) 108:363–9. doi: 10.1016/j.athoracsur.2019.03.032
17. Mehta M, Patel YS, Yasufuku K, Waddell TK, Shargall Y, Fahim C, et al. Near-infrared mapping with indocyanine green is associated with an increase in oncological margin length in minimally invasive segmentectomy. *J Thorac Cardiovasc Surg.* (2019) 157:2029–35. doi: 10.1016/j.jtcvs.2018.12.099
18. Sekine Y, Itoh T, Toyoda T, Kaiho T, Koh E, Kamata T, et al. Precise anatomical sublobar resection using a 3D medical image analyzer and fluorescence-guided surgery with transbronchial instillation of indocyanine green. *Semin Thorac Cardiovasc Surg.* (2019). doi: 10.1053/j.semtcvs.2019.01.004. [Epub ahead of print].
19. Kent MS, Mandrekar SJ, Landreneau R, Nichols F, Foster NR, DiPetrillo TA, et al. A nomogram to predict recurrence and survival of high-risk patients undergoing sublobar resection for lung cancer: an analysis of a multicenter prospective study (ACOSOG Z4032). *Ann Thorac Surg.* (2016) 102:239–46. doi: 10.1016/j.athoracsur.2016.01.063
20. Ito N, Fukuta M, Tokushima T, Nakai K, Ohgi S. Sentinel node navigation surgery using indocyanine green in patients with lung cancer. *Surg Today.* (2004) 34:581–5. doi: 10.1007/s00595-004-2780-y
21. Yamashita S, Tokuishi K, Anami K, Miyawaki M, Moroga T, Kamei M, et al. Video-assisted thoracoscopic indocyanine green fluorescence imaging system shows sentinel lymph nodes in non-small-cell lung cancer. *J Thorac Cardiovasc Surg.* (2011) 141:141–4. doi: 10.1016/j.jtcvs.2010.01.028
22. Gilmore DM, Khullar OV, Jaklitsch MT, Chirieac LR, Frangioni JV, Colson YL. Identification of metastatic nodal disease in a phase 1 dose-escalation trial of intraoperative sentinel lymph node mapping in non-small cell lung cancer using near-infrared imaging. *J Thorac Cardiovasc Surg.* (2013) 146:562–70; discussion: 9–70. doi: 10.1016/j.jtcvs.2013.04.010
23. Hachey KJ, Digesu CS, Armstrong KW, Gilmore DM, Khullar OV, Whang B, et al. A novel technique for tumor localization and targeted lymphatic mapping in early-stage lung cancer. *J Thorac Cardiovasc Surg.* (2017) 154:1110–8. doi: 10.1016/j.jtcvs.2016.12.058
24. Digesu CS, Hachey KJ, Gilmore DM, Khullar OV, Tsukada H, Whang B, et al. Long-term outcomes after near-infrared sentinel lymph node mapping in non-small cell lung cancer. *J Thorac Cardiovasc Surg.* (2018) 155:1280–91. doi: 10.1016/j.jtcvs.2017.09.150

6

Intraoperative Photodiagnosis for Malignant Glioma Using Photosensitizer Talaporfin Sodium

Jiro Akimoto [1,2*], *Shinjiro Fukami* [1], *Megumi Ichikawa* [1], *Awad Mohamed* [1,3] and *Michihiro Kohno* [1]

[1] *Department of Neurosurgery, Tokyo Medical University, Tokyo, Japan,* [2] *Department of Neurosurgery, Kohsei Chuo General Hospital, Tokyo, Japan,* [3] *Department of Neurosurgery, Sohag University, Sohag, Egypt*

Correspondence:
Jiro Akimoto
jiroaki@gmail.com

Objective: The aim of this study was to demonstrate the clinical feasibility of intraoperative photodiagnosis (PD) of malignant brain tumor using talaporfin sodium (TPS), which is an agent used in photodynamic therapy (PDT) for cancers.

Methods: Forty-seven patients diagnosed with malignant gliomas by preoperative imaging (42 patients with gliomas and 5 patients with other brain tumors) received an intravenous injection of TPS at 40 mg/m^2 24 h before resection. During surgery, these patients were irradiated with diode laser light at 664 nm, and tumor fluorescence was observed. The fluorescence intensity was visually rated on a 3-point rating scale [strong fluorescence, weak fluorescence and no fluorescence]. TPS concentrations in 124 samples from 47 cases were measured by HPLC (High performance liquid chromatography).

Results: The fluorescence intensity was confirmed to be weak in all patients with Grade II gliomas and strong in almost all patients with Grade III or IV gliomas, reflecting the histological grade of malignancy. In patients with non-glioma brain tumors except for 1 patient with a metastatic brain tumor, the fluorescence intensity was strong. The mean TPS concentration in tissues was 1.62 μg/g for strong fluorescence areas, 0.67 μg/g for weak fluorescence areas and 0.19 μg/g for no fluorescence areas.

Conclusions: Establishment of an appropriate fluorescence observation system enabled fluorescence-guided resection of malignant brain tumors using TPS, and the fluorescence intensity of tumors correlated with the TPS concentrations in tissues. These results suggest that TPS is a useful photosensitizer for both intraoperative fluorescence diagnosis and photodynamic therapy.

Keywords: malignant glioma, photodiagnosis, talaporfin sodium, fluorescence guided resection, tissue concentration

INTRODUCTION

The use of photosensitizers (PSs) for malignant gliomas has been aimed mainly at tumor control by photodynamic therapy (PDT). In 1980, a clinical report related to PDT, in which patients with gliomas underwent helium-neon laser irradiation after the administration of Photofrin II, was submitted by Perria et al. (1) Since this report, clinical studies of PDT with dye laser irradiation mainly using hematoporphyrin derivatives (HpDs) have been reported (2–5). The main mechanism of PDT is based on the generation of cytotoxic singlet oxygen in tissues under aerobic conditions, as a result of a photochemical reaction induced by the administration of a non-toxic PS in combination with the irradiation of an excitation laser specific to the PS. The cytotoxic effects of this singlet oxygen cause damage to tumor cells and newly formed blood vessels (6, 7).

After administered to a patient, PS is transformed from the ground state to the excited state by laser irradiation, and immediately returns to the ground state with emitting fluorescence. In 2000, Stummer et al. established a methodology called fluorescence-guided resection (FGR) where tumors are resected using an intraoperative photodiagnosis (PD) of malignant gliomas with the fluorescence as a guide (8, 9). The FGR was acclaimed as a breakthrough methodology where PS is used for purposes other than the original intended use in PDT. A phase III study conducted thereafter proved that the improved extent of resection achieved by FGR would prolong progression free survival (PFS), and FGR has gained recognition as a methodology with a high level of evidence (10–12). The PS they used was 5-aminolevulinic acid (5-ALA), which was thereafter approved as an agent for intraoperative localization of malignant gliomas by the European Medicines Agency in 2007, in Korea in 2011 and also in Japan in 2013. Theoretically, 5-ALA can also be applied to PDT, and basic research and clinical research of PDT using 5-ALA in malignant gliomas have been reported. To date, however, no evidence for the usefulness of 5-ALA in PDT comparable to that in PD has been reported (13, 14).

The authors reported the safety and efficacy of PDT using an HpD, talaporfin sodium (TPS), which is a second-generation photosensitizer, by conducting an *in vitro* study in human glioma cells (15), an *in vivo* study in an experimental model of transplanted C6 glioblastoma in rats (16, 17), and furthermore clinical research including investigator-initiated studies in patients with malignant gliomas (18, 19). Partially because TPS had already been approved as an agent for PDT in patients with early stage lung cancer (20), TPS and an excitation diode laser device specific to TPS were approved for health insurance reimbursement in Japan in 2013 as an agent for PDT in patients with primary malignant brain tumors.

In our previous clinical research on PDT, all patients preoperatively predicted to have malignant gliomas received TPS and underwent FGR (18). Then, PDT was performed only for patients suggested to have residual tumor based on PD. In other words, we found TPS to be useful for both PD and PDT and consider TPS an ideal PS to date in the treatment of malignant brain tumors. In this article, we report the usefulness of PD in the treatment of primary malignant brain tumors with TPS administration and excitation laser irradiation, by presenting actual cases. We also report the correlation between PD, which involves gross assessment, and actual TPS concentrations in brain tumor tissues.

MATERIALS AND METHODS

Talaporfin Sodium and Diode Laser

Talaporfin sodium (TPS: Laserphyrin®, Meiji Seika Pharma Co., Ltd., Tokyo, Japan) is a photosensitizer, a hydrophilic compound manufactured by coupling aspartic acid and chlorine, utilized in PDT, which was approved for use in Japan in 2003 as treatment for early-stage lung cancer, in combination with a diode laser (PD Laser®, Panasonic HealthCare Co., Ltd., Ehime, Japan) at a wavelength of 664 nm (**Figures 1A,B**). TPS is a second-generation photosensitizer that is more quickly excreted from the body than the first-generation porfimer sodium (Photofrin®, Pfizer Japan Inc., Tokyo, Japan). It is characterized by rapid resolution of a skin photosensitivity reaction, which is important with the use of photosensitizers. This has enabled the period of necessary light shielding in a room with measurement of $\leqq$ 500 lux to be reduced to 2 weeks for TPS, whereas porfimer sodium requires patients to stay in a semi-dark ($\leqq$ 300 lux) room for 1 month after administration. A diode laser instrument, a compact system weighing 14 kg, has low power consumption, and can easily be maintained without the need for dye exchange.

Operating Microscope Equipped With Diode Laser (Figure 1)

The PD Laser®(Panasonic HealthCare Co., Ltd.), installed in the MM30 microscope (Mitaka Kohki Co., Ltd., Tokyo, Japan), is combined into a system that provides laser irradiation (664 nm) from the operating microscope from a plane nearly coaxial to the surgical view. The laser light is introduced into the microscope by a quartz fiber, and provides a laser transmission path close to an observation light path using a conventional halogen light. This allows surgeons to accurately identify an irradiation target area during surgery. The wavelength of fluorescence from tumor tissues is 672 nm. To detect this fluorescence, a system was established using a very narrow notch filter (Nitto Optical Co., Ltd., Tokyo, Japan) that can capture an 8-nm difference. The system gathers emitted fluorescence through a cooled charge-coupled device (CCD) and visualizes images on the monitor. The system is designed for enhancing the contrast between the brain surface and the tumor, by mounting 6 white light-emitting diodes (LEDs) as light sources (NSPW500BS and NSPW510BS, Nichia Corporation, Tokushima, Japan) around the objective lens to achieve a clear fluorescence observation by brain surface illumination with LEDs allowing 6-level light intensity control (**Figures 1C–F**).

Phantom Experiment

We conducted an experiment to examine whether this microscopic system allows appropriate intraoperative fluorescence observation during brain tumor surgery. TPS at 3 concentrations of 1, 10, and 100 μg/mL each was mixed with 10% bovine serum albumin (BSA; Wako Pure Chemical Industries Ltd., Osaka, Japan). Then, a cotton ball was moistened with each mixture. These cotton balls were irradiated with a diode laser at 664 nm under the irradiation conditions described later, and then observed the emitted fluorescence at 672 nm using the microscopic system to determine whether the dose-dependent fluorescence intensity is grossly detectable.

Subjects

The study subjects were 47 consecutive patients who received the protocol-specified surgery after being diagnosed with glioma by preoperative diagnostic imaging by a single surgeon (JA)

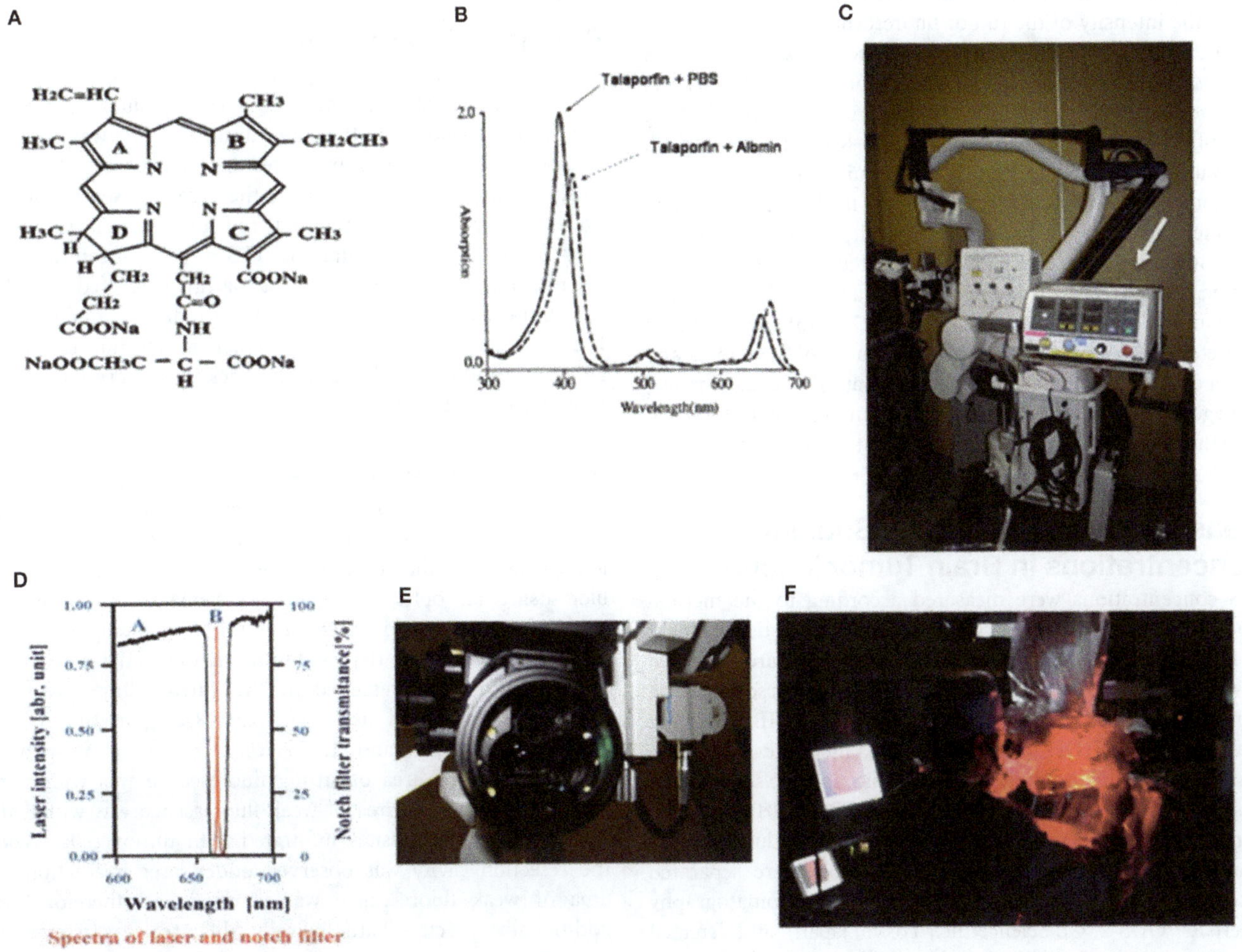

FIGURE 1 | (A) Chemical structure of talaporfin sodium (mono-L-aspartyl chlorine e6, NPe6). **(B)** Absorption spectrum of talaporfin sodium and change in absorption wavelength following conjugation with albumin (solid line: talaporfin sodium and phosphate buffer solution, dotted line: talaporfin sodium conjugated with albumin). Talaporfin sodium has absorption peaks in the Soret band (398 nm) and Q bands (502, 530, 620, and 654 nm) in pH 7.4 phosphate buffer solution (PBS). When it conjugates with albumin, its absorption band wavelength becomes ~10 nm longer (bathochromic shift). **(C)** MM80® surgical microscope (Mitaka Kohki Co., Ltd.) equipped with a compact diode laser (PD Laser®, Panasonic Health Care Ltd., arrow). **(D)** A very narrow notch filter (Nitto Optical Co. Ltd.) that can cut out light excited at 664 nm and can capture fluorescence emitted at 672 nm is mounted in a surgical microscope. **(E)** Six white LEDs (Nichia Corporation) are mounted as light sources in the applicator at the objective lens side of the microscope, in order to illuminate the brain surface during laser irradiation. **(F)** From the surgical microscope, the diode laser irradiates the surgical field.

from April 2005 to December 2008 at the Department of Neurosurgery, Tokyo Medical University. The final pathological diagnosis was glioma in 42 patients, newly diagnosed tumor in 24 patients, and recurrent tumor in 18 patients. The histological malignancy grade was Grade I in 1 patient, Grade II in 5 patients, Grade III in 8 patients and Grade IV in 28 patients. There were 5 patients whose final pathological diagnosis was not glioma after undergoing the protocol-specified surgery based on the diagnosis of glioma made by preoperative diagnostic imaging. The final pathological diagnosis in these patients was metastatic brain tumor in 2 patients (from lung cancer and mammary gland cancer), primary central nervous system lymphoma in 1 patient and meningioma in 2 patients. The institutional review board approved the participation of humans in research at Tokyo Medical University approved our fluorescence-guided intracranial tumor resection protocol, and all patients gave their informed consent before participating.

PDT and Intraoperative PD Procedures

TPS was administered as a bolus intravenously at a dose of 40 mg/m^2 in light-shielded conditions 24 h prior to surgery. Craniotomy was performed under illumination at ≤500 lux. First, the brain surface was observed under halogen light illumination. Then, the halogen light was turned off, and the brain surface was irradiated with a diode laser at 664 nm at a power density of 10 mW/cm^2, with a beam diameter of 40 mm and an irradiation area of 12.6 cm^2, to observe the presence or absence of tumor fluorescence. The illuminance of the white LEDs was adjusted as appropriate to check the difference in color tone from the brain surface. Every time tumor tissue was resected, the resected tissue was irradiated with a laser in order to check the intensity of the tumor fluorescence. The fluorescence intensity displayed on the monitor was grossly assessed in three grades: strong fluorescence (S), weak fluorescence (W), and no fluorescence (N). The tumor resection was performed using an optical navigation system (Brainlab K.K., Tokyo, Japan), as awake craniotomy and fluorescence-guided resection, under physiological monitoring. When reaching the limit for resection, the resection cavity was irradiated with a diode laser. When weak or strong fluorescence was grossly detected in the cavity, PDT was performed as reported previously (at a power density of 150 mW/cm^2 and an irradiation energy of 27 J/cm^2, with a beam diameter of 15 mm and an irradiation area of 1.8 cm^2), and the operation was ended. After the operation, the patient was managed in a shielded condition under illumination at $\leq$500 lux, until the result of the skin photosensitivity test turned to negative.

Measurement of Talaporfin Sodium Concentrations in Brain Tumor Tissue

TPS concentrations were measured according to the method reported by Yoshida et al. (21), using 5-mm cubic tissue blocks of 124 samples from 47 cases excised from each area assessed as strong, weak or no during the surgery. To the resected brain tumor tissue per 100 mg, 5 mL of a mixture of HEPES buffer solution and CH_3OH (1:9) was added, then the tissue was homogenized while cooling in ice for 1 min, and the supernatant was used as a measurement sample. The TPS and the internal standard, fluoranthene (Wako Pure Chemical Industries Ltd., Osaka, Japan), in each measurement sample were separated based on the principle of reverse phase liquid chromatography (Inertsil® ODS-2, GL Science Inc., Tokyo, Japan), and detected by a fluorescence detector. Based on each peak area obtained, the peak area ratio relative to fluoranthene was calculated and used the values as TPS concentrations. For patients in whom the concentration was measured at multiple sites in each area assessed as strong, weak or no fluorescence, the mean concentration was used for the evaluation.

Calculation of the Extent Of Resection

Based on MRI images obtained before surgical resection and within 3 days of the resection, the extent of resection was determined. For gadolinium-enhanced tumors, gadolinium-enhanced T1-weighted axial imaging was used. The sum of the products of perpendicular diameters (SPD) of the contrast-enhanced lesions was calculated. Then, the SPD of residual lesions on immediate postoperative imaging was determined, and the extent of resection was calculated. For non-gadolinium-enhanced tumors, the SPD of the areas of prolonged T2 on T2-weighted imaging was assessed to calculate the extent of resection.

Statistical Analysis

A significance test for TPS concentrations in each tissue was performed by Student's *t*-test, using SPSS analysis software (Advanced Statistics Version 17 by SPSS, Chicago, USA).

RESULTS

Phantom Experiment

From the cotton balls impregnated with mixtures of the TPS solutions at 3 concentrations and 10% BSA, red fluorescence with intensities dependent on the concentration of TPS was observed by laser irradiation. A clear fluorescence was observed in light shielded conditions. However, in the case of laser irradiation under halogen light illumination, red fluorescence was visible only from the tissue containing TPS at the concentration of 100 μg/mL, but fluorescence was hardly perceived at other concentrations. In the case of laser irradiation under white LED illumination, both the dose-dependent red fluorescence at all concentrations of TPS and the background are considered observable (**Figures 2A–C**).

Representative Cases

Case 10: A 56-year-old man had glioblastoma in the right parietal lobe, manifested by involuntary twitching at the left corner of the mouth. The tumor was resected en bloc using an optical navigation system under continuous somatosensory evoked potential monitoring. Being irradiated with a laser, resected tissues emitted strong red fluorescence, with weak red fluorescence in the surrounding area. The TPS concentration in tissue was 2.9538 μg/g in the area of strong fluorescence and 1.5765 μg/g in the area of weak fluorescence. The area of strong fluorescence was within the tumor bulk, and the area of weak fluorescence was within the surrounding brain tissues infiltrated with tumor cells. When the resection cavity was observed under laser irradiation, an area of weak fluorescence was detected and therefore was additionally resected. Pathologically, this area was assessed as a tumor infiltration area containing MIB-1 positive cells. A postoperative contrast-enhanced MRI revealed that the tumor was totally resected, and the additionally resected area was clearly identifiable (**Figures 3A–F**).

Case 18: A 41-year-old woman had glioblastoma in the left frontal lobe, manifested by mild motor aphasia and right hemiplegia. She underwent awake surgery, and laser irradiation was performed on the brain surface during the operation. By the laser irradiation, strong red fluorescence suggestive of a localized tumor was observed on the brain surface along with fluorescence from the blood vessels on the brain surface. When a laser was irradiated under white LEDs, a clear contrast was observed between the fluorescence and the surrounding brain surface. The tumor was resected en bloc and examined on the longitudinal cross-section. Strong ring-like red fluorescence was observed, which was similar to the ring-like enhancement surrounding the central necrosis on MRI images. Observation under LED illumination revealed a more detailed relationship with the surrounding brain tissue. The TPS concentration in tissue was 2.1861 μg/g in the strong fluorescence area, 0.9349 μg/g in the weak fluorescence area, and 0.4044 μg/g in the no fluorescence area in the periphery. A postoperative MRI confirmed that the contrast-enhanced lesion was totally resected (**Figures 4A–F**).

Case 2: A 30-year-old man had oligoastrocytoma in the left frontal lobe, manifested by a first episode of generalized tonic-clonic seizures. No obvious contrast enhancement was observed

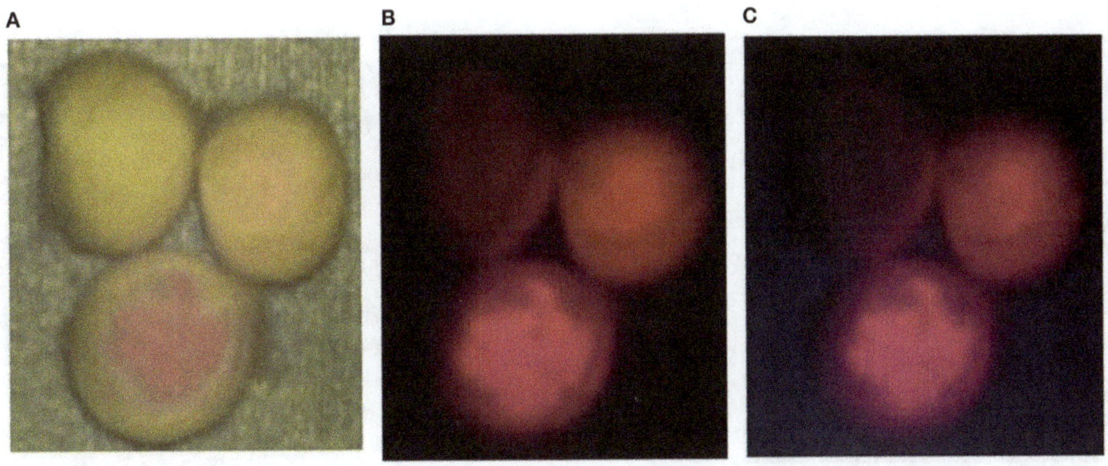

FIGURE 2 | Phantom experiment. **(A)** Talaporfin sodium (TPS) dissolved in 1 mL of physiological saline at 3 concentrations of 1, 10 and 100 μg/mL was mixed with 1 mL of 10% bovine serum albumin (BSA). Then, each mixture was dripped onto a cotton ball. First, when each cotton ball was irradiated with a laser under halogen light illumination of the surgical microscope, clear fluorescence was observed from the cotton ball impregnated with TPS at 100 μg/mL. **(B)** The halogen light illumination of the surgical microscope was turned off, and laser irradiation was performed. Differences in fluorescence intensity dependent on the TPS concentration were clearly identified. **(C)** When laser irradiation was performed while the halogen light was off and the 4 LED light sources were on, color tones of the non-woven fabric on the background were perceived, and differences in concentration among the cotton balls became more distinct.

on the preoperative contrast-enhanced MRI. When the resected tumor tissue was irradiated with a laser, weak red fluorescence was observed at the site where the tumor had been located. The TPS concentration in tissue in this area was 0.6914 μg/g. A postoperative MRI confirmed that the lesion of prolonged T2 was totally resected (**Figures 5A–D**).

Case 1: An 18-year-old man had pilocytic astrocytoma in the vermis cerebelli, manifested by sudden headache and nausea. A preoperative contrast-enhanced MRI showed an enhanced mural nodule. During the surgery, the cyst was opened and irradiated with a laser. As a result, nodular fluorescence, tending to be strong, appeared with weak fluorescence from the surrounding cystic wall. The TPS concentration in tissue was high, being 3.163 μg/g in the strong fluorescence area and 1.614 μg/g in the weak fluorescence area. A postoperative MRI confirmed that the lesion including the cystic wall was totally resected (**Figures 6A–D**).

Results of Intraoperative Observation of Fluorescence From Tumors

Fluorescence Positive Rate (Figure 7, Table 1 and Supplementary Table 1)

In glioma cases, 1 case of Grade I pilocytic astrocytoma showed strong fluorescence. In five Grade II cases, none showed strong fluorescence, but all showed weak fluorescence. In eight Grade III cases, all showed at least weak fluorescence, including 5 cases (62.5%) showing strong fluorescence. In 28 Grade IV cases, 22 cases (78.6%) showed strong fluorescence and 26 cases (92.9%) showed weak fluorescence; thus all showed fluorescence, as seen in Grade III cases. In the Grade IV cases, strong fluorescence was shown in 14 (93.3%) of 15 newly diagnosed cases and 8 (61.5%) of 13 recurrent cases. In the recurrent cases, some showed only weak fluorescence. In the other 5 cases, except for 1 case of metastatic brain tumor, 4 cases showed strong fluorescence.

Correlation Between Fluorescence Intensity and Tissue Concentration (Figure 8, Table 1 and Supplementary Table 1)

The TPS concentrations in tissue in the strong, weak and no fluorescence areas that were assessed grossly were 1.6184 ± 0.9661, 0.6708 ± 0.3765 and 0.1885 ± 0.1253 μg/g, respectively. There were significant differences in concentration between the strong and weak fluorescence areas and between the weak and no fluorescence areas ($P < 0.001$). In the glioma cases, 1 Grade I case showed strong fluorescence with a tissue concentration of 3.1628 μg/g, but all Grade II cases showed weak fluorescence. The tissue concentrations in strong fluorescence areas in Grade III and IV cases were 1.3751 ± 0.7480 and 1.4948 ± 0.7783 μg/g, respectively, showing no significant difference between the Grade III and IV cases ($P = 0.718$). In Grade IV cases, the mean tissue concentrations in strong, weak and no fluorescence areas were 1.4948, 0.6752, and 0.1655 μg/g, respectively, showing significant differences ($P < 0.001$) among the tissue concentrations in these areas. The tissue concentration in the strong fluorescence area in Grade IV cases was 1.5797 ± 0.9082 μg/g in newly diagnosed cases and 1.3589 ± 0.5239 μg/g in recurrent cases, showing no significant difference between the newly diagnosed and recurrent cases ($P = 0.493$). Also in the weak and no fluorescence areas, no significant differences were observed between the newly diagnosed and recurrent cases ($P = 0.821$ for weak fluorescence area and $P = 0.853$ for no fluorescence area). In non-glioma cases, the tissue concentration in the strong fluorescence area was 2.100 ± 1.528 μg/g, showing no significant difference from the result obtained for the strong fluorescence area in Grade IV cases ($P = 0.153$).

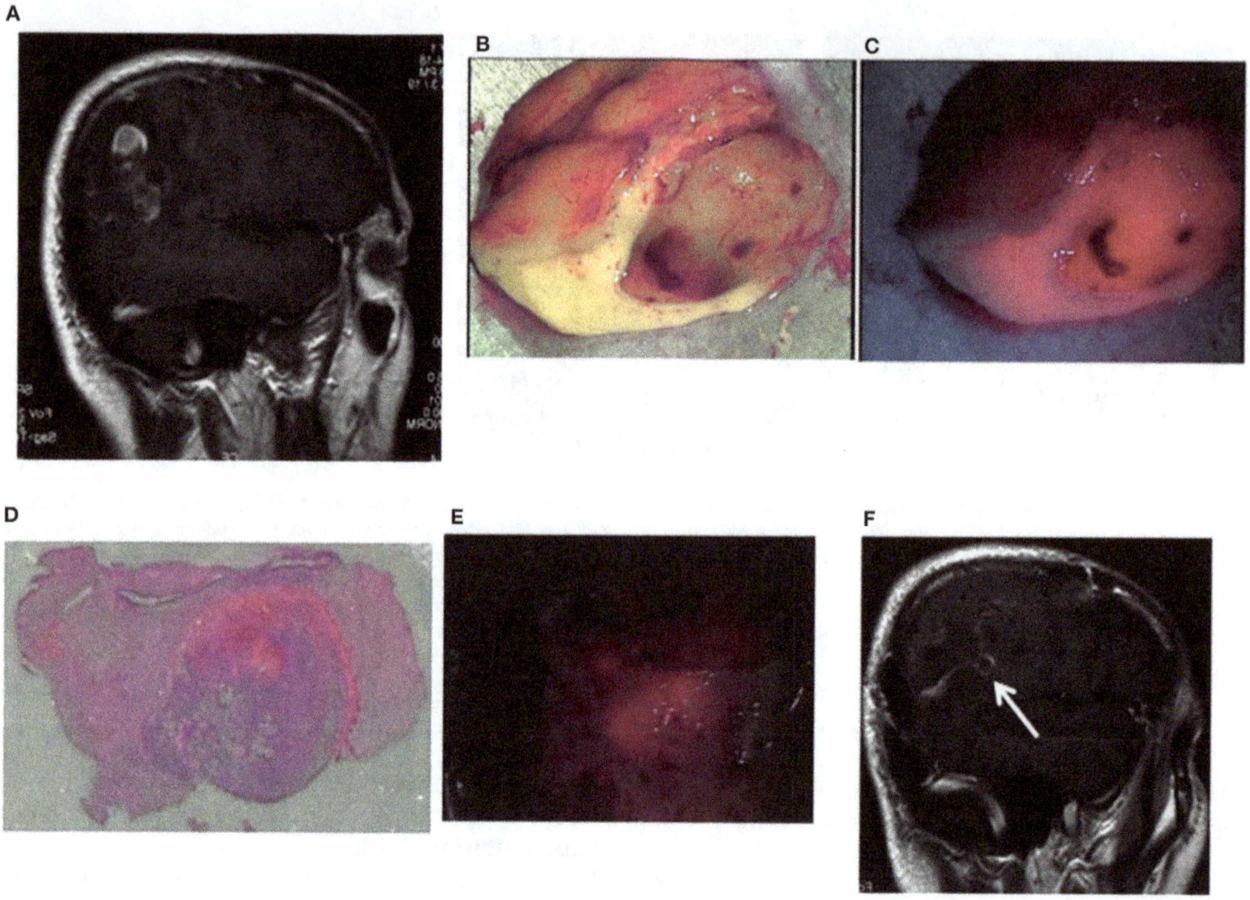

FIGURE 3 | Representative case 10. **(A)** A gadolinium-enhanced T1-weighted sagittal image. The image revealed an irregularly enhanced glioblastoma lesion in the right parietal lobe. **(B)** Brain tissues containing a tumor tissue were resected to the widest extent possible, using an optical navigation system while somatosensory-evoked monitoring was performed. Well-demarcated tumor tissue was observed in the subcortical white matter. **(C)** When laser irradiation was performed under LED illumination, strong fluorescence from the tumor bulk and weak fluorescence from the surrounding white matter were observed. **(D)** A postoperative histopathological image revealed the presence of tumor cells infiltrating from the strong fluorescence area into the weak fluorescence area (hematoxylin and eosin staining). **(E)** When a laser was irradiated to the white matter in the tumor resection cavity under LED illumination, weak fluorescence areas were found in the normal white matter. Therefore, the tissue resection was continued until the fluorescence disappeared. **(F)** The postoperative gadolinium-enhanced MRI confirmed the additionally resected areas (arrow) as well as the total resection of the enhanced lesion.

Extent of Resection (Supplementary Table 1)

By the FGR using TPS, total resection confirmed on imaging was achieved in 22 (52.3%) of 42 patients with gliomas. In most of the 24 newly diagnosed cases, a clear difference in fluorescence intensity was obtained, allowing the resection of not only strong fluorescence areas but also weak to no fluorescence areas. As a result, total resection was achieved in 16 cases (66.7%). Even in cases with residual lesions, the resection of 94 ± 4.3% (89–99%) of the tumor was achieved, according to an SPD analysis. On the other hand, in 18 recurrent cases, it was difficult to obtain a clear difference in fluorescence intensity. In the majority of these cases, weak fluorescence was blurrily spread, making it difficult to grossly determine the disappearance of the fluorescence. Consequently, total resection was achieved only in 6 cases (33.3%), which is an extremely low extent of resection. In cases showing residual lesions, the extent of resection was limited to 81.4 ± 8.9% (63−95%). Of course, when a tumor clearly infiltrates in the functional regions of the brain, it is difficult to resect the tumor even though fluorescence is detected, and PDT should be performed additionally. PDT was performed in 5 newly diagnosed cases and 11 recurrent cases. In most of these recurrent cases, PDT was added due to concern that there may be residual tumors because it was difficult to confirm the disappearance of fluorescence. In non-glioma cases, 1 case with atypical meningioma with repeated recurrences underwent PDT for the residual tumor because total resection had to be abandoned due to intracerebral infiltration of the tumor in the motor cortex, although fluorescence was identified. In this case, however, total resection of other tumor lesions was achieved.

DISCUSSION

In the surgery of glioma, which is characterized by invasive growth, the concept of "maximal safe resection" is important. Evidence for the fact that enhancement of the extent of surgical

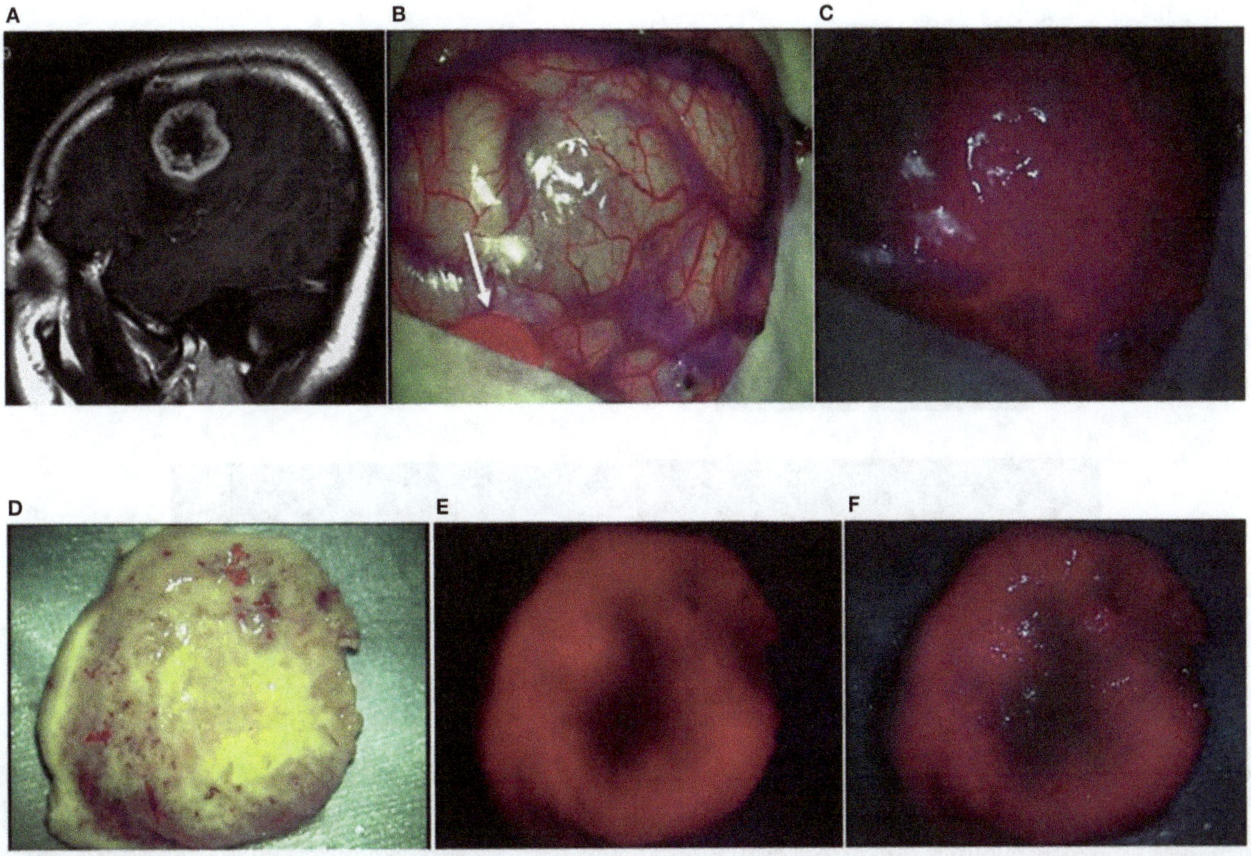

FIGURE 4 | Representative case 18. **(A)** A gadolinium-enhanced T1-weighted sagittal image revealed a ring-like enhanced glioblastoma in the left middle frontal gyrus. **(B)** An image of the brain surface under halogen light illumination showed marked swelling in the left middle frontal gyrus, but tumor tissue was not exposed (arrowed red circle: primary motor cortex). **(C)** In the fluorescence diagnosis under white LED illumination, strong fluorescence from the tumor was observed, and fluorescence from residual TPS in the surrounding blood vessels was identified simultaneously, facilitating the fluorescence-guided resection. **(D)** The tumor together with some surrounding brain tissue attached to the tumor was resected en bloc. The median section observed under halogen light illumination revealed the presence of a light brownish tumor tissue in a doughnut shape. **(E)** Laser irradiation revealed strong fluorescence almost surrounding the central necrotic lesion, clearly identifying the contrast-enhanced lesion on preoperative MRI. **(F)** In the fluorescence diagnosis under white LED illumination, the difference in fluorescence intensity between the strong fluorescence areas and the necrotic lesion or the surrounding brain tissue became more distinct.

resection leads to improved prognosis of malignant gliomas has been accumulating, and there have been a series of discussions regarding how to achieve total resection of gadolinium-enhanced lesions on MRI images and, at the same time, how to protect neurological functions (22–24). FGR using dyes, such as fluorescein and 5-ALA, has been widely accepted as an intraoperative real-time navigation method that visualizes tumor bulk, and many studies on the efficacy of FGR have been reported (25–27). A representative study among these is a randomized controlled trial (RCT) of FGR with 5-ALA, led by Stummer et al. in which FGR has been demonstrated to improve the extent of resection, resulting in significant prolongation of PFS in patients who underwent FGR. Therefore, this methodology has been accepted in many countries (9, 11, 12). However, FGR with 5-ALA alone failed to prolong overall survival (OS). In other words, the results indicate that the total resection of gadolinium-enhanced lesions by FGR only does not prolong OS (10).

A scheme proposed by Wilson for the extent of tumor cell infiltration shows that curative resection cannot be achieved by glioma surgery, as well as that resection of not only contrast-enhanced lesions on imaging but also the surrounding tissue infiltrated by tumor cells can contribute to reducing the residual tumor cells (28). In recent years, a supra-total resection, i.e., an extended resection of high signal-intensity areas on FLAIR images in tissue surrounding the tumor to the extent that the neurological function is not deteriorated, has been reported to prolong OS (29, 30). Therefore, in malignant glioma surgery, in addition to total resection of gadolinium-enhanced lesions using FGR under proper monitoring of neurological functions, the surrounding tissue infiltrated by tumor cells should be resected to the extent possible up to the boundary of the functional regions of the brain (29, 30). For cases where tumor cells have infiltrated in the functional region of the brain, we consider it significant to perform PDT, which is capable of specifically destroying tumor cells (18, 19). In that sense, the TPS we used this time is a PS

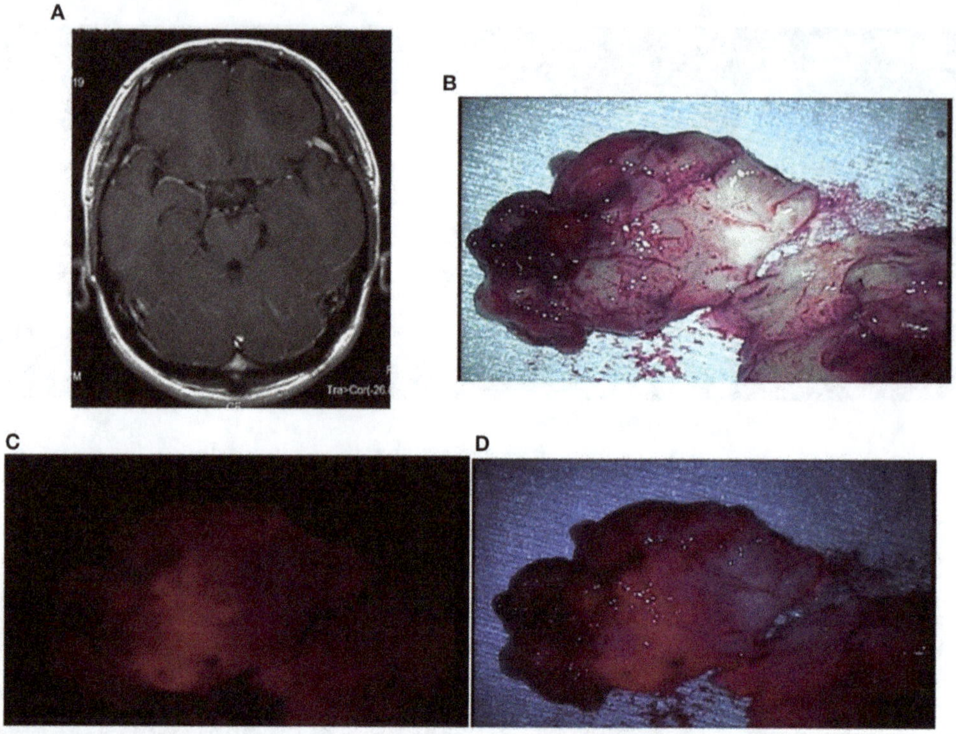

FIGURE 5 | Representative case 2. **(A)** A gadolinium-enhanced T1-weighted axial image showed a slightly enhanced tumor in the left frontal lobe. **(B)** The tumor bulk was resected en bloc. The median section observed under halogen light illumination revealed the presence of a yellowish-gray gelatinous tumor in the cortex. **(C)** By laser irradiation, weak fluorescence from the cortex was detected, and the white matter tended to emit further weaker fluorescence. **(D)** Observed under white LED illumination, the fluorescence from the cortex was enhanced, making the gradation of fluorescence intensity between the cortex and the white matter more distinct.

that can be used in two ways, not only for PD but also for PDT. Thus, TPS is a tool allowing us to carry out the best approach for malignant glioma. In fact, clinical studies of PDT using TPS have reported PFS of 12 months and OS of 24.8 months in patients with newly diagnosed glioblastoma, showing a clear therapeutic add-on effect to the standard treatment, and this method has been rapidly spreading in Japan (19).

In this article, we report that intraoperative PD using TPS and an excitation diode laser can identify gadolinium-enhanced lesions and non-gadolinium-enhanced lesions infiltrated by tumor cells, based on differences in fluorescence intensity, in glioma cases. In particular, a positive correlation was observed between the histological malignancy grade and the fluorescence positive rate or the fluorescence intensity. In particular, in Grade IV cases, strong fluorescence was observed in 93.3% of newly diagnosed cases and 61.5% of recurrent cases, and there were no cases without fluorescence. In recurrent cases, the fluorescence intensity tended to be weaker than that observed in newly diagnosed cases. The reason for this might be associated with the use of radiotherapy in these cases. Even in cases of lower grade gliomas, in which the detection of fluorescence with the use of 5-ALA is difficult, weak fluorescence was observed, although the number of cases was limited. These results suggest the usefulness of FGR using TPS in all glioma surgeries. Very strong fluorescence was observed in 1 case of pilocytic astrocytoma. In addition, strong fluorescence was observed also in cases of malignant lymphoma, metastases and malignant meningioma. These results suggest that FGR using TPS can be performed for tumors enhanced by gadolinium on MRI, regardless of histological type.

Tsurubuchi et al. (31) examined the intracerebral distribution of 5-ALA and TPS, using a glioma rat model, and reported that the lesion-to-normal brain ratio (L/N ratio) in the tumor bulk was 7.78 ± 4.61 at 2 h after administration of 5-ALA and 23.1 ± 11.9 at 12 h after administration of TPS, with the fluorescence intensity being approximately 10-fold stronger with TPS than with 5-ALA (31). On the other hand, both drugs elicited fluorescence even in vasogenic edema in a cold injury model for brain edema. With 5-ALA, the time to peak fluorescence after administration in edema was delayed compared with that in tumor. On the other hand, with TPS, the time to peak fluorescence was 2 h after administration in peritumoral edema and 12 h after administration in tumor tissue. This time course of the fluorescence intensity perfectly reflects the mechanism of TPS uptake by tumor cells, which is considered as follows: TPS, a water-soluble drug, is conjugated with albumin immediately after intravenous injection, and the conjugate circulates in the bloodstream. After leaking from tumor blood vessels due to the disruption of the blood brain barrier (BBB), the conjugate is taken up by tumor cells, mediated by SLC46A1, a heme carrier

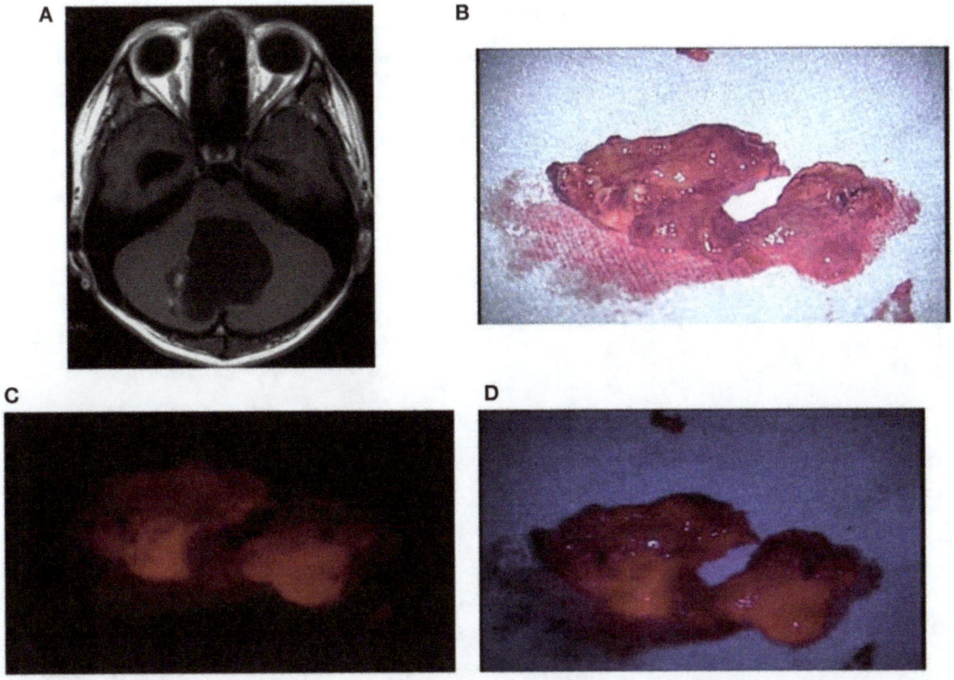

FIGURE 6 | Representative case 1. **(A)** A gadolinium-enhanced T1-weighted axial image showed a cystic tumor with a mural nodule in the vermis cerebelli, in which the nodule was slightly enhanced. **(B)** The resected nodule was rich in blood vessels, exhibiting red color also under halogen light illumination. **(C)** By laser irradiation, strong fluorescence from the nodule was observed. **(D)** Under white LED illumination, strong fluorescence emitted from the entire nodule was clearly observed.

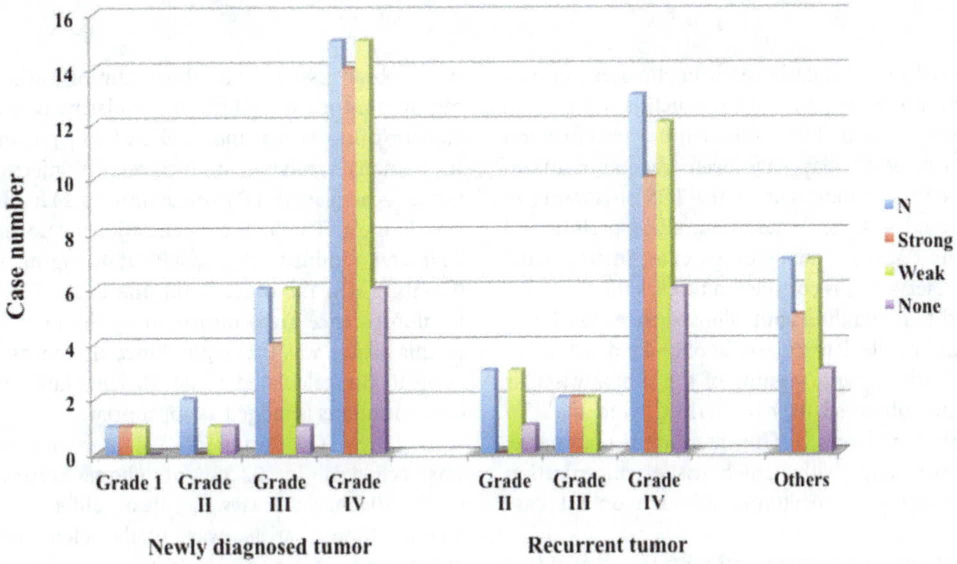

FIGURE 7 | Fluorescence positive rate of newly diagnosed glioma, recurrent glioma and other tumors. In Grade IV, 92.9% of newly diagnosed cases and 61.5% of recurrent cases emitted strong fluorescence.

protein 1, and other factors, and accumulates into the tumor cells due to the enhanced permeability and retention (EPR) effect (31, 32). Comparing the distribution of fluorescence intensity in resected tissues with the images in the clinical cases presented this time, it was confirmed that the gadolinium-enhanced lesions on MRI exhibited strong fluorescence, with high TPS concentrations in these tissues, suggesting that these findings reflect the TPS uptake by tumor cells. In addition, the findings highly suggest that the weak fluorescence in non-enhanced areas is derived from not only the TPS taken up by infiltrating tumor cells but

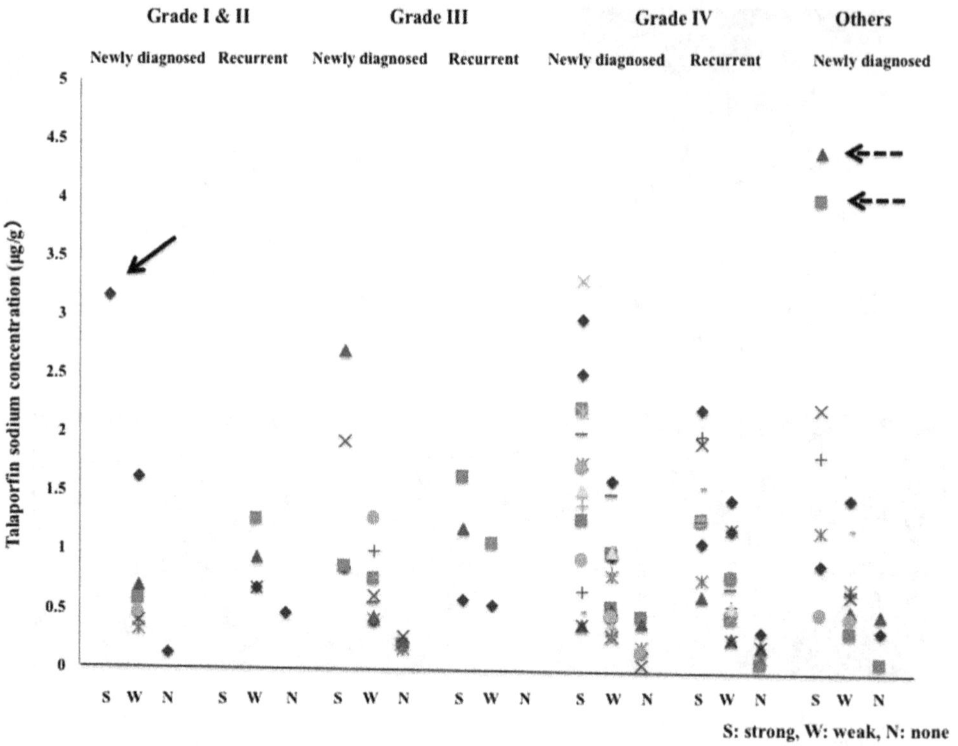

FIGURE 8 | The tissue concentrations of talaporfin sodium in the strong fluorescence (S), weak fluorescence (W) and no fluorescence (N) areas in newly diagnosed cases and recurrent cases with Grade I to IV gliomas and other tumors. Arrow: Pilocytic astrocytoma, Dotted arrow: Primary central nervous system lymphoma.

also the TPS diffused extracellularly. Also in the areas grossly assessed as showing no fluorescence, TPS, which is not present in normal brain tissue, was detected although its concentration was low. The TPS detected may have been trace amounts of TPS diffused outside the tumor cells or the TPS circulating in normal cerebral blood vessels. In addition, since peritumoral brain edema is found also in low-grade gliomas, in which the BBB is generally preserved, it is considered that, as the first step, TPS diffused into the edema fluid emits fluorescence after being taken up by the tumor cells. Particularly in oligodendrogliomas, which is associated with a large volume of the tumor vascular bed, the fluorescence observed may be derived from the TPS present in the tumor blood vessels. This inference is reasonable, because strong fluorescence with a high tissue concentration was observed in pilocytic astrocytoma, although only 1 case was examined.

The finding that the fluorescence intensity was dependent on the histological malignancy grade of glioma cells suggests that the fluorescence intensity of TPS reflects the tumor cell density, proliferative capacity or vascular bed volume, as seen in the studies of 5-ALA (33). Therefore, it is essential to examine the relationship of the fluorescene intensity of TPS with histopathological images in terms of these factors (34).

According to the drug information of TPS, the $t_{1/2\alpha}$ and $t_{1/2\beta}$ of TPS are 14.6 ± 2.96 and 138 ± 21.4 h, respectively (35). Experiments in rats revealed that the TPS concentration in cerebral tissue 24 h after administration of TPS at 40 mg/m^2 was one forty-fifth of the plasma concentration (4.56 ± 0.65 μg/g in plasma and 0.09 ± 0.01 μg/g in cerebral tissue). In humans receiving an intravenous injection of TPS at 40 mg/m^2, the plasma TPS concentration 24 h after administration was 11 μg/g. The TPS concentration in normal cerebral tissue 24 h after administration of TPS at 40 mg/m^2 is calculated to be 0.24 μg/g. On the other hand, the mean TPS concentration in no fluorescence areas measured by the methodology presented in this article was 0.21 μg/g. Since this measured value is very close to the calculated value, this method for measuring TPS concentrations is judged as appropriate.

By the FGR using TPS, total resection on imaging was achieved in 52.3% of glioma cases. Particularly in newly diagnosed cases, a clear difference in fluorescence among tumor areas was easily identified also under a microscope. As a result, total resection was achieved in 66.7% of the cases, and PDT was properly performed for tumors infiltrating in the functional regions in the brain. On the other hand, in the majority of recurrent cases, weak fluorescence appeared blurrily, and even though the resection was continued, the fluorescence persisted. The resection was extended to the boundary of the functional regions in the brain and then PDT was implemented in many cases. The reasons for this may include tumor vascular changes due to radiotherapy and

TABLE 1 | Pathological diagnosis and fluorescence positive rate, tissue TPS concentrations, extent of resection and number of patients who underwent PDT.

	N	Fluorescence			Concentration (μg/g)			Resection		PDT
		Strong	**Weak**	**None**	**Strong**	**Weak**	**None**	**N of GTR**	**EOR**	***N***
Newly diagnosed tumor	24									
Grade I	1	1	1	0	3.163	1.614		1	100%	0
Grade II	2	0	2	1		0.489 ± 0.145	0.123	1	95% (95–100)	0
Grade III	6	3	6	3	1.573 ± 0.901	0.608 ± 0.304	0.2	3	98% (90–100)	1
Grade IV	15	14	15	6	1.580 ± 0.908	0.675 ± 0.413	0.193 ± 0.156	11	98% (89–100)	4
Recurrent tumor	18									
Grade I	0									
Grade II	3	0	3	1		0.878 ± 0.276	0.46	1	92% (80–100)	1
Grade III	2	2	2	0	1.112 ± 0.529	0.776 ± 0.375		0	88% (80–95)	1
Grade IV	13	8	11	6	1.347 ± 0.524	0.656 ± 0.381	0.132 ± 0.156	5	88% (63–100)	9
Others										
Meta	2	1	2	1	0.851	0.520 ± 0.097		2	100%	0
PCNSL	1	1	1		4.166 ± 0.294	0.647		1	100%	0
MGM	1	1	1	1	1.657 ± 0.735	0.8382 ± 0.807	0.279	1	100%	0
Atypical MGM	1	1	1	1	1.103 ± 0.957	0.720 ± 0.390	0.424	0	75%	1

N, number; Meta, metastatic brain tumor; PCNSL, primary central nervous system lymphoma; MGM, meningioma; GTR, gross total removal; EOR, extent of resection; PDT, photodynamic therapy.

decreased proliferative capacity of recurrent tumors. In fact, TPS concentrations in tumors tended to be lower in recurrent cases than in newly diagnosed cases, although there was no significant difference. This issue also needs to be studied in future.

Yoshida et al. reported 0.36- to 5.69-fold higher TPS concentrations in cancer tissue than in normal tissue, measured 4 h after the administration of TPS at 40 mg/m^2 in 16 patients with early head and neck cancer (21). In addition, they stated, from their experience with PDT performed in these cases, that the TPS concentration in the irradiation target tissue needed to be at least 1 μg/g in order to demonstrate the efficacy of PDT (21). In the present study, the mean TPS concentration in tumor tissue 24 h after the administration of TPS in glioblastoma cases was 1.580 μg/g in strong fluorescence areas and 0.672 μg/g in weak fluorescence areas. The tissue TPS concentration in strong fluorescence areas was 7.52-fold higher than that in normal brain tissue. Although there are differences in the time after the administration of TPS to observation as well as in the PDT implementation conditions, these findings suggest that PDT may not have clinical significance in some cases because, unless the target tissue emits at least weak fluorescence, reactions to PDT are unlikely to occur. This needs to be kept in mind when considering the implementation of PDT after FGR in malignant glioma cases in the future.

There are several limitations to acknowledge in this study. First, since this case group was enrolled only for a certain period of time, it can not deny that there was a limit in the number of cases. In particular, as TPS is a photosensitizer that is used for PDT, which is generally only performed on patients who are suspected of having a malignant brain tumor on preoperative neuroimaging, there is little data on the use of TPS in brain tumors except glioma. Second, there was lack of investigation of relationship between histopathological findings and fluorescence intensity or TPS concentration. Such analysis is the focus of our ongoing study.

CONCLUSION

We examined the fluorescence emission from malignant brain tumors, using TPS, a second-generation photosensitizer, and an excitation laser specific to it, and demonstrated that TPS is applicable to FGR. In glioma cases, the fluorescence intensity and the TPS concentration in tumor tissue have been found to be correlated with the histological malignancy grade, and, particularly in newly diagnosed patients, have been suggested to contribute to improving the extent of resection. We will further investigate the relationship between histopathological images of brain tumors and the fluorescence intensity or tissue TPS concentration, in order to verify the usefulness of FGR using TPS in malignant brain tumor surgery.

AUTHOR CONTRIBUTIONS

MK and AM supervised the project. JA, SF, and MI developed the concept and the design of the study. JA and SF designed and made the experimental set up for data acquisition. JA, SF, and MI carried out patient care, surgery, and sample acquisition. JA performed data collection. JA, SF, MI, AM, and MK analyzed and interpreted the data. JA drafted the manuscript. SF and MK critically revised the manuscript. AM was contributed to the review of the manuscript and answer to the reviewer's comment. All authors have approved the final manuscript.

ACKNOWLEDGMENTS

The authors are indebted to Associate Professor Edward F. Barroga and Akiko Popiel Helena, Department of International Medical Communications of Tokyo Medical University, for their review of the manuscript. The authors also thank Panasonic HealthCare Co. Ltd., Japan, Mitaka Kohki Co. Ltd., Japan and Meiji Seika Pharma Co. Ltd., Japan for supplies of equipments and drugs.

REFERENCES

1. Perria C, Capuzzo T, Cavagnaro G, Datti R, Francaviglia N, Rivano C, et al. First attempts at the photodynamic treatment of human gliomas. *J Neurosurg Sci.* (1980) 24:119–29.
2. Kaye AH, Morstyn G, Appuzo MJ. Photoradiation therapy and its potential in the management of neurological tumors. *J Neurosurg.* (1988) 69:1–14. doi: 10.3171/jns.1988.69.1.0001
3. Stylli SS, Kaye AH, MacGregor L, Howes M, Rajendra P. Photodynamic therapy of high grade glioma- long term survival. *J Clin Neurosci.* (2005) 12:389–98. doi: 10.1016/j.jocn.2005.01.006
4. Muller PJ, Wilson BC. Photodynamic therapy of brain tumor- a work in progress. *Laser Surg Med.* (2006) 38: 384–89. doi: 10.1002/lsm.20338
5. Eljamel MS. Brain photodiagnosis (PD), fluorescence guided resection (FGR) and photodynamic therapy (PDT): past, present and future. *Photodiagnosis Photodyn Ther.* (2008) 5:29–35. doi: 10.1016/j.pdpdt.2008.01.006
6. Nelson JS, Liaw LH, Orenstein A, Berns MW. Mechanism of tumor destruction following photodynamic therapy with hematoporphyrin derivative, chlorine, and phthalocyanine. *J Natl Cancer Inst.* (1988) 80:1599–605. doi: 10.1093/jnci/80.20.1599
7. Castano AP, Demidova TN, Hamblin MR. Mechanism in photodynamic therapy: part one – photosensitizers, photochemistry and cellular localization. *Photodiagnosis Photodyn Ther.* (2004) 1:279–93. doi: 10.1016/S1572-1000(05)00007-4
8. Stummer W, Stocker S, Wagner S, Stepp H, Fritsch C, Goetz C, et al. Intraoperative detection of malignant gliomas by 5-aminolevulinic acid-induced prophyrin fluorescence. *Neurosurgery.* (1988) 42:518–26.
9. Stummer W, Novotny A, Stepp H, Goetz C, Bise K, Reulen HJ. Fluorescence-guided resection of glioblastoma multiforme by using 5-aminolevulinic acid-induced porphyrins: a prospective study in 52 consecutive patients. *J Neurosurg.* (2000) 93:1003–13. doi: 10.3171/jns.2000.93.6.1003
10. Stummer W, Pichlmeier U, Meinel T, Wiestler OD, Zanella F, Reulen HJ. Fluorescence-guided surgery with 5-aminolevulinic acid for resection of malignant glioma: a randomised controlled multicentre phase III trial. *Lancet Oncol.* (2006) 7:392–401. doi: 10.1016/S1470-2045(06)70665-9
11. Widhalm G, Wolfsberger S, Minchev G, Woeher A, Krssak M, Czech T, et al. 5-Aminolevulinic acid is a promising marker for detection of anaplastic foci in diffusely infiltrating gliomas with non-significant contrast enhancement. *Cancer.* (2010) 116:1545–52. doi: 10.1002/cncr.24903
12. Valdes PA, Leblond F, Kim A, Harris BT, Wilson BC, Fan X, et al. Quantitative fluorescence in intracranial tumor: implications for ALA-induced PpIX as an intraoperative biomarker. *J Neurosurg.* (2011) 115:11–17. doi: 10.3171/2011.2.JNS101451
13. Kennedy JC, Pottier RH. Endogeneous protoporphyrin IX, a clinically useful photosensitizer for photodynamic therapy. *J Photochem Photobiol B.* (1992) 14:275–92. doi: 10.1016/1011-1344(92)85108-7
14. Roberts DW, Valdes PA, Harris BT, Fontaine KM, Hartov A, Fan X, et al. Coregistered fluorescence-enhanced tumor resection of malignant glioma: relationship between δ-amino-levulinic acid-induced protoporphyrin IX fluorescence, magnetic resonance imaging enhancement, and neuropathological parameters. *J Neurosurg.* (2011) 114:595–603. doi: 10.3171/2010.2.JNS091322
15. Tsutsumi M, Miki Y, Akimoto J, Haraoka J, Aizawa K, Hirano M, et al. Photodynamic therapy with talaporfin sodium induces dose-dependent apoptotic cell death in human glioma cell lines. *Photodiagnosis Photodyn Ther.* (2013) 10:103–10. doi: 10.1016/j.pdpdt.2012.08.002
16. Matsumura H, Akimoto J, Haraoka J, Aizawa K. Uptake and retention of the mono-L-asparthyl chlorine e6 in experimental glioma. *Lasers Med Sci.* (2008) 23:237–45. doi: 10.1007/s10103-007-0469-3
17. Namatame H, Akimoto J, Matsumura H, Haraoka J, Aizawa K. Photodynamic therapy of C6-implanted glioma cells in the rat brain employing second-generation photosensitizer Talaporfin sodium. *Photodiagnosis Photodyn Ther.* (2008) 5:198–209. doi: 10.1016/j.pdpdt.2008.08.001
18. Akimoto J, Haraoka J, Aizawa K. Preliminary clinical report of safety and efficacy of photodynamic therapy using Talaporfin sodium for malignant gliomas. *Photodiagnosis Photodyn Ther.* (2012) 9:91–99. doi: 10.1016/j.pdpdt.2012.01.001
19. Muragaki Y, Akimoto J, Maruyama T, Iseki H, Ikuta S, Nitta M, et al. Phase II clinical study on intraoperative photodynamic therapy with talaporfin sodium and semiconductor laser in patients with malignant brain tumors. *J Neurosurg.* (2013) 119:845–52. doi: 10.3171/2013.7.JNS13415
20. Usuda J, Tsutsui H, Honda H, Ichinose S, Ishizumi T, Hirata T, et al. (2007) Photodynamic therapy for lung cancers based on novel photodynamic diagnosis using talaporfin sodium (NPe6) and autofluorescence bronchoscopy. *Lung Cancer.* 58:317–23. doi: 10.1016/j.lungcan.2007.06.026
21. Yoshida T, Tokashiki R, Ito H, Shimizu A, Nakamura K, Hiramatsu H, et al. Therapeutic effects of a new photosensitizer for photodynamic therapy of early head and neck cancer in relation to tissue concentration. *Auris Nasus Larynx.* (2008) 35:545–51. doi: 10.1016/j.anl.2007.10.008
22. Sanai N, Polley MY, McDermott MW, Parsa AT, Berger MS. An extent of resection threshold for newly diagnosed glioblastomas. *J Neurosurg.* (2011) 115:3–8. doi: 10.3171/2011.2.JNS10998
23. Chen L, Mao Y. Gross total resection plays a leading role in survival of patients with glioblastoma multiforme. *World Neurosurg.* (2014) 82:105–7. doi: 10.1016/j.wneu.2014.04.074
24. Grabowski MM, Recinos PF, Nowacki AS, Schroeder JL, Angelov L, Barnett GH, et al. Residual tumor volume versus extent of resection: predictors of survival after surgery of glioblastoma. *J Neurosurg.* (2014) 121:1115–23. doi: 10.3171/2014.7.JNS132449
25. Schwake M, Stummer W, Suero Molina EJ, Wolfeer J. Simultaneous fluorescein sodium and 5-ALA in fluorescence-guided glioma surgery. *Acta Neurochir.* (2015) 157:877–79. doi: 10.1007/s00701-015-2401-0
26. Liu JTC, Meza D, Sanai N. Trends in fluorescence image-guided surgery for gliomas. *Neurosurgery.* (2014) 75:61–71. doi: 10.1227/NEU.0000000000000344
27. Zimmermann A, Ritsch-Marte M, Kostron H. mTHPC-mediated photodynamic diagnosis of malignant brain tumors. *Photochem Photobiol.* (2001) 74:611–16. doi: 10.1562/0031-8655(2001)074<0611:MMPDOM>2.0.CO;2
28. Wilson CB. Glioblastoma: the past, the present, and the future. *Clin Neurosurg.* (1992) 38:32–48.
29. Yordanova YN, Moritz SG, Duffau H. Awake surgery for WHO II gliomas within "noneloquent" areas in the left dominant hemisphere: toward a "supratotal" resection. *J Neurosurg.* (2011) 115:232–39. doi: 10.3171/2011.3.JNS101333

30. Li YM, Suki D, Hess K, Sawaya R. The influence of maximum safe resection of glioblastoma on survival in 1229 patients: can we do better than gross-total resection? *J Neurosurg.* (2016) 124:977–988. doi: 10.3171/2015.5.JNS142087
31. Tsurubuchi T, Zoboronok A, Yamamoto T, Nakai K, Yoshida F, Shirakawa M, et al. The optimization of fluorescence imaging of brain tumor tissue differentiated from brain edema- *In vivo* kinetic study of 5-aminolevulinic acid and talaporfin sodium. *Photodiagnosis Photodyn Ther.* (2009) 6:19–27. doi: 10.1016/j.pdpdt.2009.03.005
32. Takada T, Tamura M, Yamamoto T, Matsui H, Matsumura A. Selective accumulation of hematoporphyrin deriveative in glioma through proton-coupled folate transporter SLC46A1. *J Clin Biochem Nutr.* (2014) 54:26–30. doi: 10.3164/jcbn.13-87
33. Stummer W, Tonn JC, Goetz C, Ullrich W, Stepp H, Bink A, et al. 5-Aminolevulinic acid-derived tumor fluorescence: the diagnostic accuracy of visible fluorescence qualities as corroborated by spectrum and histology and postoperative imaging. *Neurosurgery.* (2014) 74:310–9. doi: 10.1227/NEU.0000000000000267
34. Mitra S, Foster TH. *In vivo* confocal fluorescence imaging of the intratumor distribution of the photosensitizer mono-L-aspartylchlorin-e6. *Neoplasia.* (2008) 10:429–38. doi: 10.1593/neo.08104
35. Kessel D. Pharmacokinetics of N-asparthyl chlorin e6 in cancer patients. *J Photochem Photobiol B.* (1997) 39:81–3. doi: 10.1016/S1011-1344(96)00009-7

7

Progress in Confocal Laser Endomicroscopy for Neurosurgery and Technical Nuances for Brain Tumor Imaging with Fluorescein

Evgenii Belykh[1,2], Eric J. Miller[1], Alessandro Carotenuto[1], Arpan A. Patel[1], Claudio Cavallo[1], Nikolay L. Martirosyan[1], Debbie R. Healey[3], Vadim A. Byvaltsev[2], Adrienne C. Scheck[3†], Michael T. Lawton[1], Jennifer M. Eschbacher[4], Peter Nakaji[1] and Mark C. Preul[1]*

[1] Department of Neurosurgery, Barrow Neurological Institute, St. Joseph's Hospital and Medical Center, Phoenix, AZ, United States, [2] Department of Neurosurgery, Irkutsk State Medical University, Irkutsk, Russia, [3] Department of Neuro-Oncology Research, Barrow Neurological Institute, St. Joseph's Hospital and Medical Center, Phoenix, AZ, United States, [4] Department of Neuropathology, Barrow Neurological Institute, St. Joseph's Hospital and Medical Center, Phoenix, AZ, United States

***Correspondence:**
Mark C. Preul
neuropub@barrowneuro.org

†Present Address:
Adrienne C. Scheck, Institute of Molecular Medicine, Phoenix Children's Research Institute, Phoenix Children's Hospital, Phoenix, AZ, United States

Background: Previous studies showed that confocal laser endomicroscopy (CLE) images of brain tumors acquired by a first-generation (Gen1) CLE system using fluorescein sodium (FNa) contrast yielded a diagnostic accuracy similar to frozen surgical sections and histologic analysis. We investigated performance improvements of a second-generation (Gen2) CLE system designed specifically for neurosurgical use.

Methods: Rodent glioma models were used for *in vivo* and rapid *ex vivo* CLE imaging. FNa and 5-aminolevulinic acid were used as contrast agents. Gen1 and Gen2 CLE images were compared to distinguish cytoarchitectural features of tumor mass and margin and surrounding and normal brain regions. We assessed imaging parameters (gain, laser power, brightness, scanning speed, imaging depth, and Z-stack [3D image acquisition]) and evaluated optimal values for better neurosurgical imaging performance with Gen2.

Results: Efficacy of Gen1 and Gen2 was similar in identifying normal brain tissue, vasculature, and tumor cells in masses or at margins. Gen2 had smaller field of view, but higher image resolution, and sharper, clearer images. Other advantages of the Gen2 were auto-brightness correction, user interface, image metadata handling, and image transfer. CLE imaging with FNa allowed identification of nuclear and cytoplasmic contours in tumor cells. Injection of higher dosages of FNa (20 and 40 mg/kg vs. 0.1–8 mg/kg) resulted in better image clarity and structural identification. When used with 5-aminolevulinic acid, CLE was not able to detect individual glioma cells labeled with protoporphyrin IX, but overall fluorescence intensity was higher ($p < 0.01$) than in the normal hemisphere. Gen2 Z-stack imaging allowed a unique 3D image volume presentation through the focal depth.

Conclusion: Compared with Gen1, advantages of Gen2 CLE included a more responsive and intuitive user interface, collection of metadata with each image, automatic

Z-stack imaging, sharper images, and a sterile sheath. Shortcomings of Gen2 were a slightly slower maximal imaging speed and smaller field of view. Optimal Gen2 imaging parameters to visualize brain tumor cytoarchitecture with FNa as a fluorescent contrast were defined to aid further neurosurgical clinical *in vivo* and rapid *ex vivo* use. Further validation of the Gen2 CLE for microscopic visualization and diagnosis of brain tumors is ongoing.

Keywords: 5-ALA, brain tumor, confocal, endomicroscopy, fluorescein, fluorescence, glioma, imaging

INTRODUCTION

Intraoperative diagnosis in neurosurgery has traditionally relied on frozen and formalin-fixed, paraffin-embedded section analysis of biopsied tissue samples. Although this technique is considered to be the "gold standard" for establishing a histopathologic diagnosis, it entails a number of significant limitations. These limitations include the time required for transferring, processing, and interpreting the tissue (1); the presence of artifacts and sampling errors (1–3); as well as the differences present when comparing frozen and permanent sections that may lead to misdiagnosis (1, 4). Rapid intraoperative diagnosis has become possible with refinement and miniaturization of the research-type confocal laser scanning microscope into a handheld confocal laser endomicroscopy (CLE) system (5, 6). Combined with appropriate fluorescent stains or labels, CLE provides an imaging technique for real-time intraoperative *in vivo* visualization of histopathologic features of suspected tumor and healthy tissues.

Previous studies using a CLE system originally designed for nonneurosurgical use (e.g., gastrointestinal luminal examination) showed that a blinded review of CLE imaging of brain gliomas and meningiomas by a neuropathologist yielded an accuracy rate of 92.9%, similar to those previously reported with frozen-section analysis (4, 7–9). In terms of analysis of tumor margins, CLE has not yet been thoroughly investigated in human brain tumors; however, in experimental animals, CLE was able to visualize border regions of glioma (10, 11). In humans, CLE was shown to increase accuracy of delineation of margins in early gastric cancer (12). CLE may be used as a diagnostic tool, but it also has the potential to aid in optimizing surgical resection of brain tumors, including maximal safe tumor resection, which is a strategy that would be expected to have a positive impact on long-term neurosurgical patient survival, especially among patients with invasive malignant tumors (10, 13–18).

Various CLE devices have been developed; the proximal scanning fiber optic CLE (19, 20) and distal scanning CLE (1) systems are the most advanced in terms of potential for becoming adopted into wide clinical use (21). Importantly, each CLE system has different pre-set, mostly unchangeable, imaging parameters that may result in unique and different diagnostic performance; therefore, meticulous independent assessment of each microscope system is required. We previously evaluated the diagnostic performance and other application parameters of a handheld scanning CLE system (Optiscan Pty., Ltd., Mulgrave, Australia), referred to in this report as the first-generation (Gen1) device and designed for gastrointestinal use. This system has recently served as the imaging platform for development of a second-generation (Gen2) CLE system specifically aimed at neurosurgery.

The Gen2 CLE device was designed to function specifically for intraoperative application in neurosurgery and to integrate with the robotic operating microscope visualization platform for neurosurgery (22). The goals for this device in neurosurgery are ultimately to increase the positive yield of biopsies and to serve as a tool to microscopically explore, in portable and rapid fashion, for tumor cells beyond the obvious margin of infiltrating tumors, such as cells in and around the surgical resection bed, or to define suspected tumor invasion within eloquent cortex. Previous studies regarding *in vivo* investigation of distal scanning CLE in human and animal model brain tumors were conducted using the Gen1 device, which had several performance characteristics that limited its use in neurosurgery. These included lack of a sterile attachment cover sheath for the imaging probe, a different design and function of the handheld probe that was not optimal for the neurosurgeon's usual hand position, and nonoptimal imaging processing and display (1, 7, 10, 23–25). Therefore, this study was designed to assess performance of the Gen2 CLE system, assess differences in image quality or diagnostic accuracy of the Gen1 and Gen2 systems, and provide additional information on the probe conformation, and optimal handling practices that were designed to produce high-quality confocal intraoperative images for neurosurgery on-the-fly.

Gen1 and Gen2 functionalities were compared using fluorescein sodium (FNa), the primary fluorophore with which they were designed to work, and with 5-aminolevulinic acid (5-ALA)-induced protoporphyrin IX (PpIX) fluorescence. Although the fluorescence signal from PpIX is not within the optimal detection range for these CLE systems, 5-ALA is also of interest in brain tumor surgery, especially for use in invasive gliomas, and our preliminary studies suggested that the PpIX signal may be faintly detected with the CLE systems. This study aimed to expand on the current literature related to CLE for brain tumor imaging, including further investigating the relationship between FNa dosage and image quality, the ability to differentiate cellular structures with CLE and FNa, and the

Abbreviations: 5-ALA, 5-aminolevulinic acid; AF, acriflavine; AO, acridine orange; CLE, confocal laser endomicroscopy; DAPI, 4′6-diamidino-2-phenylindole; FNa, fluorescein sodium; FOV, field of view; Gen1, first generation; Gen2, second generation; H&E, hematoxylin and eosin; LSM, laser scanning microscopy; PpIX, protoporphyrin.

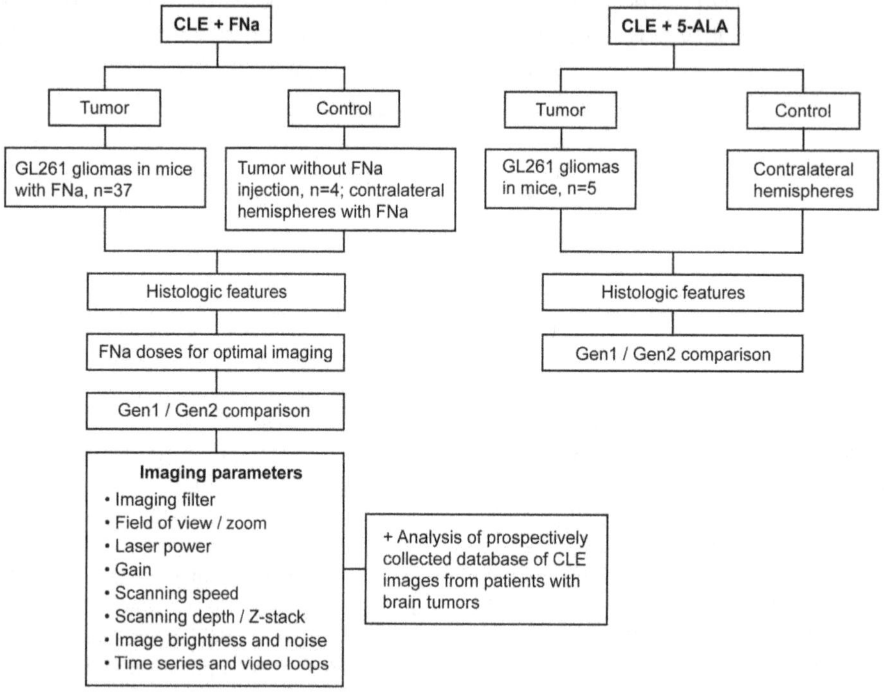

FIGURE 1 | Study design flowchart. CLE, confocal laser endomicroscope; FNa, fluorescein sodium; Gen1, generation 1; Gen2, generation 2; 5-ALA, 5-aminolevulinic acid. Used with permission from Barrow Neurological Institute, Phoenix, Arizona.

utility of both generations of CLE with 5-ALA for the detection of tumor tissue.

METHODS

Ethics Approval

All animal investigations were performed according to the guidelines outlined by the National Institutes of Health *Guide for the Care and Use of Laboratory Animals* and with approval from the Institutional Animal Care and Use Committee of the Barrow Neurological Institute and St. Joseph's Hospital and Medical Center, Phoenix, Arizona. Animals were maintained under approved veterinary care in the vivarium of St. Joseph's Hospital and Medical Center.

Patient tissues used for this project were acquired from a prospective ongoing brain tumor clinical study. Patients with preoperative diagnoses of brain masses requiring surgical removal and for whom the decision was to use the assistance of fluorescence surgical guidance with FNa were prospectively enrolled. Extra biopsies from tumor tissue that would have to be safely removed during the normal course of the surgery were used. De-identified samples were placed on a wet telfa and submitted for immediate *ex vivo* CLE analysis. The same samples were then sent for routine histologic processing and review by a neuropathologist. All patients gave voluntary informed consent as a part of a study protocol approved by the Institutional Review Board of the Barrow Neurological Institute, St. Joseph's Hospital and Medical Center, Phoenix, Arizona. A flowchart describing the study protocol is presented in **Figure 1**.

Mouse Glioma Model

Ten-week-old female B6(Cg)-Tyr^{c-2J}/J mice (albino variant C57BL/6J, The Jackson Laboratory, Bar Harbor, ME) weighing 20 g (mean) were anesthetized and placed in a small-animal stereotactic head frame. Glioma models were created according to the previously described protocol (26). Briefly, 2 μL of GL261-luc tumor cells (1.45×10^7 cells/mL; Division of Cancer Treatment and Diagnosis, National Cancer Institute, Bethesda, MD) were infused 2 mm lateral and 2 mm posterior to bregma at a depth of 2.5 mm from the brain surface through a bur hole at the targeted brain location after the syringe needle was withdrawn 0.5 mm to a total depth of 2 mm below the surface of the brain to create a 0.5 mm pocket for the cells. The 2-μL cell suspension was infused using a controllable microinjector (0.67 μL/min × 3 min with the needle in place for 2 min afterward) (10).

A week prior to surgery, the mice were injected with 15 μg/kg of luciferin (PerkinElmer, Waltham, MA), anesthetized using isoflurane in a 37°C chamber, and glioma growth was confirmed using bioluminescence detection in the IVIS Spectrum *in vivo* imaging system (PerkinElmer). Bioluminescence images were examined and quantified in Living Image 4.3 software (PerkinElmer) (26).

Drug Administration

CLE imaging was performed within the first 2 h after FNa injection. We used escalating dosages of FNa: 0.1 ($n = 4$), 1 ($n = 7$), 2 ($n = 2$), 5 ($n = 7$), 8 ($n = 5$), 20 ($n = 6$), and 40 ($n = 6$) mg/kg. These doses approximate the doses of FNa that can be used in humans, as we have previously used 5 mg/kg IV in clinical study. The 5-ALA (Clinical grade, NIOPIK, Moscow, Russia) was injected intraperitoneally 2 h before surgery at a dose of 5 mg dissolved in 200 μL of normal saline ($n = 5$). Chosen dosages are similar to those previously used in comparable animal studies with 5-ALA (27–29) and FNa (10, 30–32) and are similar to or higher than those used in humans to compensate for differences in metabolism.

Intraoperative CLE Imaging

After confirmation of tumor growth and size, on average 21 days after implantation, the mice underwent craniectomy. The animals were anesthetized, and their oxygen supply and body temperature were maintained throughout the procedure. An operating microscope (Pentero 900, Carl Zeiss AG, Oberkochen, Germany) was used to visualize the exposed surfaces of both cerebral hemispheres. Brain tumors were identified macroscopically in the right hemisphere of all mice, and the CLE scanning was performed. After imaging was performed, the anesthetized animals were euthanized according to protocol guidelines. Brains were extracted, sliced fresh coronally (1 mm in thickness) through the center of the tumor in a mouse brain slicer matrix (ZIVIC Instruments, Pittsburgh, PA), and imaged rapidly *ex vivo* with CLE again.

Gen1 (Optiscan 5.1, Carl Zeiss AG) and Gen2 CLE (Convivo, Carl Zeiss AG) were compared in terms of intraoperative fluorescence visualization using either FNa ($n = 37$), 5-ALA ($n = 5$), or no dye injection ($n = 4$ control). This comparison was completed initially using the Gen1 CLE in a designated area. Once adequate images were acquired, the Gen2 CLE was used to take further images at the same area. All scanning was performed *in vivo* and then *ex vivo* within the 2-h interval alternating Gen1 and Gen2 confocal microscopes targeting multiple regions of interest. Further testing included evaluation of Gen2 imaging with different available filters (green bandpass or green longpass and red longpass) and with various gain, laser intensity, brightness, acquisition speed, and zoom settings controlling for image quality and noise levels. In 2 animals, topical acridine orange was used for nuclear staining as described elsewhere (10).

Operating Microscopy Fluorescence Imaging

Gross FNa and protoporphyrin IX fluorescence in the brain was assessed with the operating microscopes equipped with the Yellow 560 and Blue 400 filters, respectively (Pentero 900 and Kinevo 900, Carl Zeiss AG).

Benchtop Confocal Laser Microscopy

The benchtop laser scanning microscopy (LSM) imaging (LSM 710 DUO, Carl Zeiss AG) was performed with a C-Apochromat 40×/1.20 W Korr M27 objective. Sliced fresh brain samples were imaged on 35-mm glass-bottom Petri dishes (MatTek, Ashland, MA). For PpIX visualization, the excitation and detection wavelengths used were 405 and 635–750 nm, respectively. Additionally, topical staining was performed with acridine orange (AO), acriflavine (AF), Hoechst 33342 (ThermoFisher Scientific, Waltham, MA), and 4′6-diamidino-2-phenylindole (DAPI). The excitation wavelength was 488 nm for AO, AF, or FNa, and 405 nm for DAPI and Hoechst; and the detection wavelength was 493–625 nm for AO, AF, or FNa, and 410–585 nm for DAPI and Hoechst. Examples of imaging modalities are shown in **Supplemental Figure 1**.

Image Assessment and Statistical Analysis

Imaging analysis and cell and nuclei size measurements were performed in FIJI software (open source software) (33). Statistical analysis was completed in Excel (Microsoft, Redmond, WA). Quality of CLE imaging was scored independently by 5 respondents trained in interpreting CLE images as bad (1), average (2), good (3), or excellent (4), based on the ability to visualize characteristic GL261 tumor histologic characteristics and patterns. Grading was performed based on the assessment of the best confocal images from each animal. Student *t*-test, Mann-Whitney U test, and Kruskal-Wallis analysis of variance (ANOVA) with significance set at $p < 0.05$ were used to establish whether differences were statistically significant, and the Spearman *R*-value was used to assess correlations.

RESULTS

Assessment of CLE Imaging Parameters

To produce clear images, several parameters were controlled in both systems: gain, brightness level, laser power, scanning speed, imaging depth, and Z-stack thickness (Gen2 only). Because many imaging parameters were similar between Gen1 and Gen2 CLE, salient results are presented of observations for Gen2, and are specifically mentioned when differences were observed with Gen1. Gen2 imaging parameters are summarized in **Table 1**.

Field of View

The field of view (FOV) of the Gen2 (475 × 267 μm, 1980 pixels/line) was half the size of the Gen1 image (475 × 475 μm, 1080 pixels/line). Gen2 images were essentially twice the resolution. Gen2 images appear sharper, but upon magnification, they have a grainier appearance compared with Gen1 images. This graininess is due to the raw image TIFF format of Gen2 images, compared to compressed and smoothing JPG formatting of Gen1 images.

Gain

Specimens with grossly average fluorescence brightness produced clear CLE images on Gen2 gain setting of 2,400 (**Table 1**). When the brain tumor appeared grossly intensely bright yellow, lowering the gain allowed imaging with a CLE brightness level within a 20–60% range, which produced optimal quality images without oversaturated pixels and with low noise. However, in specimens with low gross fluorescence intensity, the quality and resolution of CLE images did not improve regardless of the changes in imaging parameters. The increased level of black noise with an increase of brightness level and laser power only lowered image quality in dark images.

Scanning Speed

Scanning speed was critically important for time series imaging. Comparison of imaging speed recorded for both generations of

TABLE 1 | Confocal laser endomicroscopy (CLE) imaging parameters.

Parameter	Gen1	Gen2	Comment
Laser wavelength	488 nm	488 nm	Always the same
Laser power	Range: 0–1,000 μm	Range: 0–100%	Percentages correlate to the actual laser power. Fifty percent results in ~500 μm laser power; 10%, 100 μm. TIFF image metadata records actual laser power in microwatts, which may be used for further analysis
Depth	Displayed only relative value showing the arrow position on the horizontal scale; not recorded	Range: −50 to 200 μm; also displayed as relative value on the vertical scale	Knowledge of depth position is crucial for understanding of imaging location and adjustment of depth on the fly for optimal image quality. Awareness of depth helps to avoid low-quality images by not imaging too deep into a tissue. The axial imaging resolution is <4.5 μm
Brightness	Range: 0–100%	Range: 0–100%	The brightness is the built-in adjustable proprietary setting parameter used during CLE imaging. Unlike the gain and laser power, the brightness could be adjusted during the imaging. Knowledge of brightness is important to assess the true brightness of the fluorescent staining
Gain	Options: low, normal, high, max	Range: 1,800–3,000	Gain is an important parameter to consider, as it influences the image brightness. We mostly used the system with gain at the midlevel (normal or 2,400). We found it useful to increase or reduce the gain for imaging of very bright and dark fluorescent samples respectively
Speed (resolution)	Options: 1024 × 1024 μm 475 × 475 μm	Options: 1,080 540 270 135	Numbers represent the number of horizontal lines that the laser travels during image acquisition. Acquisition speed 1,080 results in a 1,920 × 1,080 pixel scan at <0.5 μm axial resolution; speed 540 results in a 1,920 × 540 pixel scan, etc. Scan area–aspect ratio is kept the same as 16 × 9. Most images are taken in the "high-image quality low-speed" mode (1,080). Higher speeds (270 and 135) are rarely used and do not produce diagnostic-quality images. Higher speed might be adjusted for an initial search of an optimal imaging position to quickly verify the presence of fluorescence. At the settings window, the user can select two speeds that would be rapidly available to choose from on the primary screen
Zoom	Constant; changes not available	Options: 1× 1.4× 2×	Zoom is usually set at 1× giving a FOV size of 475 × 267 μm (width/height). This FOV size is 2× less compared to Gen1 system; however, with FNa Gen2 provides subjectively similar appearing images to Gen1. We almost never use 2× zoom with FNa, as we feel that a larger field of view is favorable for imaging with FNa. However, 1.4× and 2× zoom are useful with other fluorophores like acridine orange or acriflavine, which bind to the cellular structures and therefore result in more contrasted images
Filter	Options: Green fluoro (505–585 nm) Green-red fluoro (505–750 nm)	Options: Gray filter Green bandpass Green longpass Red filter	Our experience with FNa is that the green longpass filter provides overall brighter images than the green bandpass filter. The red bandpass filter may be unnecessary for the work with FNa. We were not able to detect reliable PpIX (peak emission~630 nm) signal with red or green longpass filters, which we believe is mostly due to the absence of an appropriate excitation laser source (405 nm for PpIX)
Z-stack	Not available	Start position offset, range: −50 to +47 μm End position offset, range: −47 to +50 μm Step size, range: 3–20 μm	We find that for most cases +10 μm and −15 μm offsets (total depth 25 μm) with the minimally possible (3 μm) Z-step are the most optimal for 3-dimensional reconstruction of the Z-stack
Time stamp	Not available on the image	2017-04-14_12-39-20-34	Time stamp is critical for matching individual CLE images with the time on microscope and navigation in order to track the optical biopsy location

FOV, field of view; FNa, fluorescein sodium; Gen1, first generation; Gen2, second generation; PpIX, protoporphyrin; TIFF, tagged image file format.

CLEs is presented in **Supplemental Table 1**. Scanning speed of Gen1 was 0.8 s per frame for a 1,024 × 512-pixel image and 1.2 s per frame for a 1,024 × 1,024-pixel image. The scanning speed for Gen2 ranged from 1.3 s per frame for the highest quality imaging to 0.27 s per frame for the lowest quality imaging. Despite the difference in scanning speed, all images were recorded and stored as 1,920 × 1,080-pixel red, green, blue (RGB) TIFF files.

Scanning Depth

Optimal imaging depth with FNa was within the first few microns in depth from the surface of the imaged tissue. The CLE Z-stack function (Gen2 only) resulted in a series of images, the first of which was a central image from the current position on the Z axis. A series of images were acquired starting from the surface and ending at the deepest position, with the Z-step image thickness selection to be between 3 and 20 μm. The interval of the scanning depth could be chosen by selecting two offset positions. The maximal range was obtained at the offsets from −47 to +50, which resulted in a 97-μm thick Z-stack. The number of images per Z-stack was limited by the size of the Z-step (3 μm minimum), which for the 97-μm Z-stack resulted in 35 images. Higher ranges are not practically necessary, so the

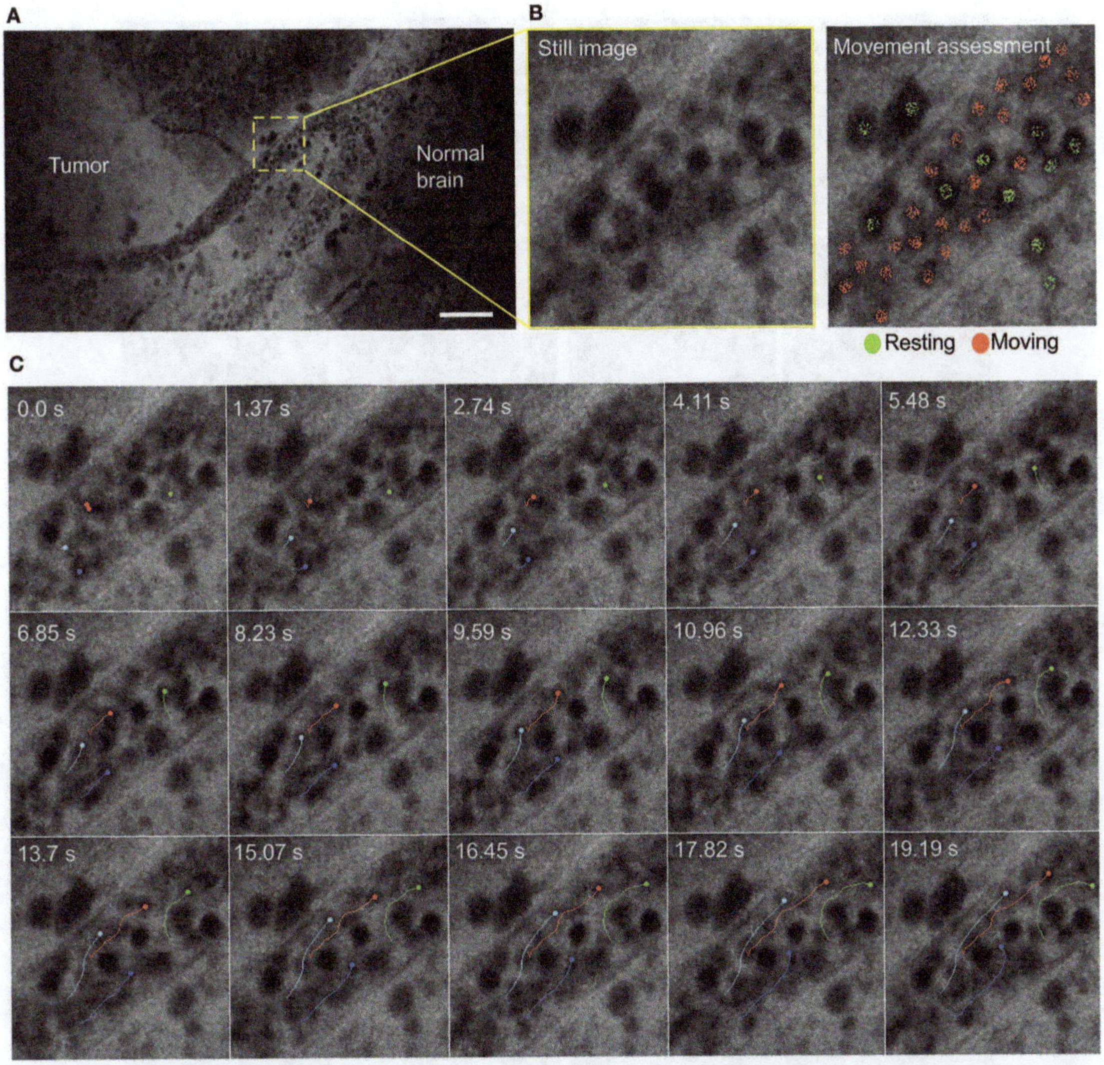

FIGURE 2 | Time series imaging to differentiate stationary and mobile cells using a Gen2 confocal laser endomicroscope. **(A)** Single frame from time-lapse image. **(B)** Enlarged view of the vessel (left) and same image with moving cells labeled red and stationary cells labeled green (right). **(C)** Tracking of the selected cells shows intravascular movement of individual blood cells. Particle tracking performed in FIJI. Scale bar is 50 μm. Used with permission from Barrow Neurological Institute, Phoenix, Arizona.

available CLE Z-stack range is sufficient for use in human brain tissue. Previous experiments have shown that the maximal depth of brain tumor tissue (using FNa) for interrogation through Z-stack imaging is 36 μm in animal and 28 μm in human brain tissue (34).

Probe movements during image capturing produced similar artifacts in both Gen1 and Gen2 CLEs. Although free-hand probe positioning yielded informative images, remaining in a steady position for an optimal Z-stack was difficult for image series acquisition. A semiflexible surgical probe holder was used to decrease movement artifacts.

Time Series and Video Loops

Time series imaging (in both Gen1 and Gen2) allowed observation of blood cell movements inside and outside the vessels (**Figure 2**). Tumor cell movements seen with tissue squeezing under the CLE lens were also noted during *in vivo* imaging, which is not possible on fixed tissues. In contrast to the static hematoxylin and eosin (H&E) slide, *in vivo* CLE revealed histologic features of the living tumor cells and their behavior. In animal gliomas, many tumor cells were actually moving independently, squeezing and pushing each other, captivated by the stream of oozing blood. Such tumor cells were flowing independent of the tumor core, especially when they were at the border of the brain slice. When imaged *in vivo*, GL261 glioma cells were actually not tightly connected to one another, as they appear on H&E slides, although they grow as relatively solid tumors. CLE imaging revealed pericellular spaces that were filled with FNa, which were not previously visualized well on H&E stained slides.

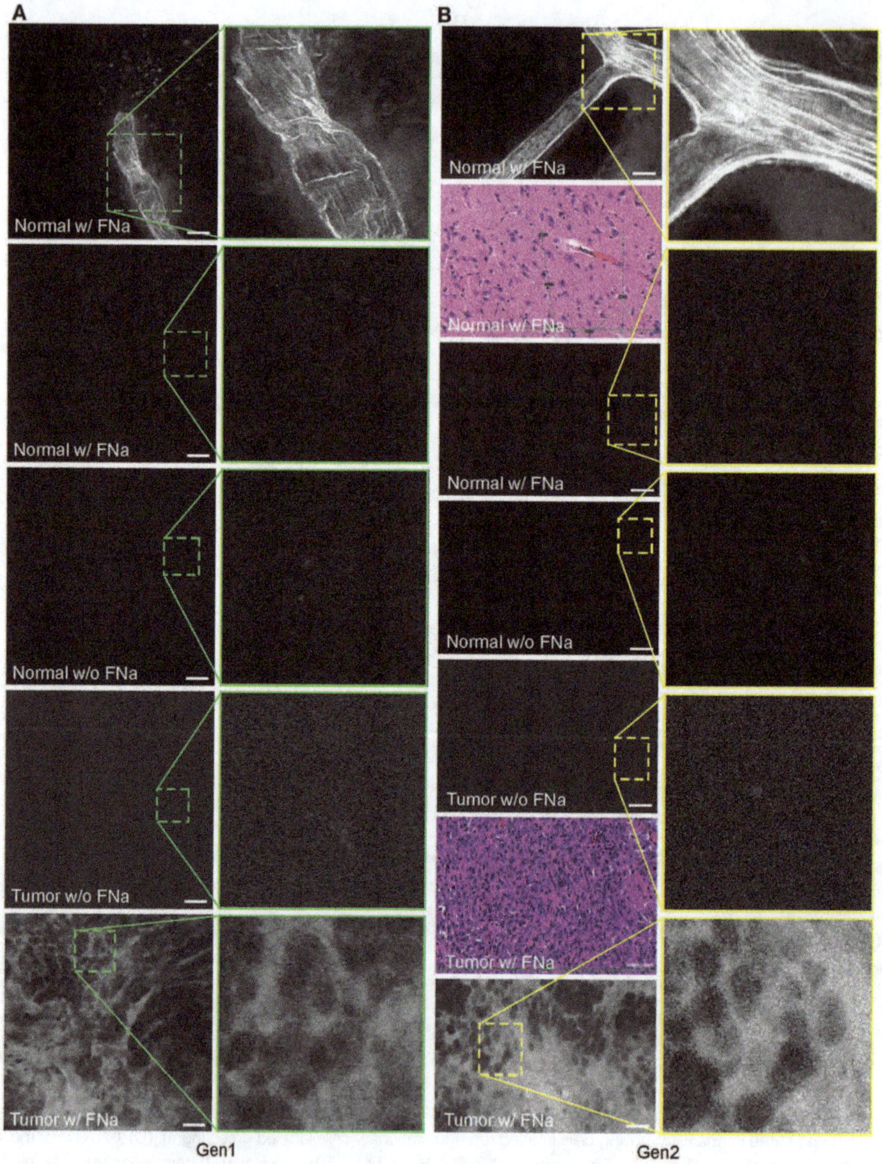

FIGURE 3 | Confocal laser endomicroscopy (CLE) images of normal mouse brain, GL261 brain glioma, visualized with and without fluorescein sodium (FNa), using **(A)** generation 1 (Gen1) and **(B)** generation 2 (Gen2) CLE. Brain vasculature, brain parenchyma, and tumor staining patterns were observed with similar quality between Gen1 and Gen2 systems. The insets show similarly magnified views from Gen1 and Gen2 systems. Additional hematoxylin and eosin (H&E) images are provided from the regions of interest of normal brain and glioma areas scanned with Gen1 and Gen2 CLE. Scale bars are 50 μm. Used with permission from Barrow Neurological Institute, Phoenix, Arizona.

Histologic Features During CLE Imaging With FNa (Gen1 and Gen2)

In no case was the tumor location uncertain based on CLE images after successful intravenous FNa injection. When imaging normal brain without tumor using CLE, FNa could be seen inside blood vessels, and occasionally leaking from vessels because of damage from surgery. Red blood cells could be visualized in these vessels as dark moving objects. No FNa was seen in other areas of the normal brain, other than intravascularly, except for sparse autofluorescent cells. Ultimately, the area of the brain away from the vessels appeared similar to the brain when FNa had not been injected, with both generally lacking fluorescence, except for rare autofluorescent cells and with limited fluorescence (**Figure 3**). After FNa injection, tumor cells were seen as nonfluorescent cells on a highlighted fluorescent background.

Abnormal tumor vasculature was seen in several tumor biopsy spots (**Supplemental Figure 2**). A gradient of FNa in the tumor was observed on images and may suggest proximity to the tumor vessels (**Supplemental Figure 3**).

Average nuclei sizes measured on AO-stained tumor images (11.9 ± 2.5 μm) were not different (p = 0.10) from those measured on FNa-contrasted CLE brain tumor images (11.6

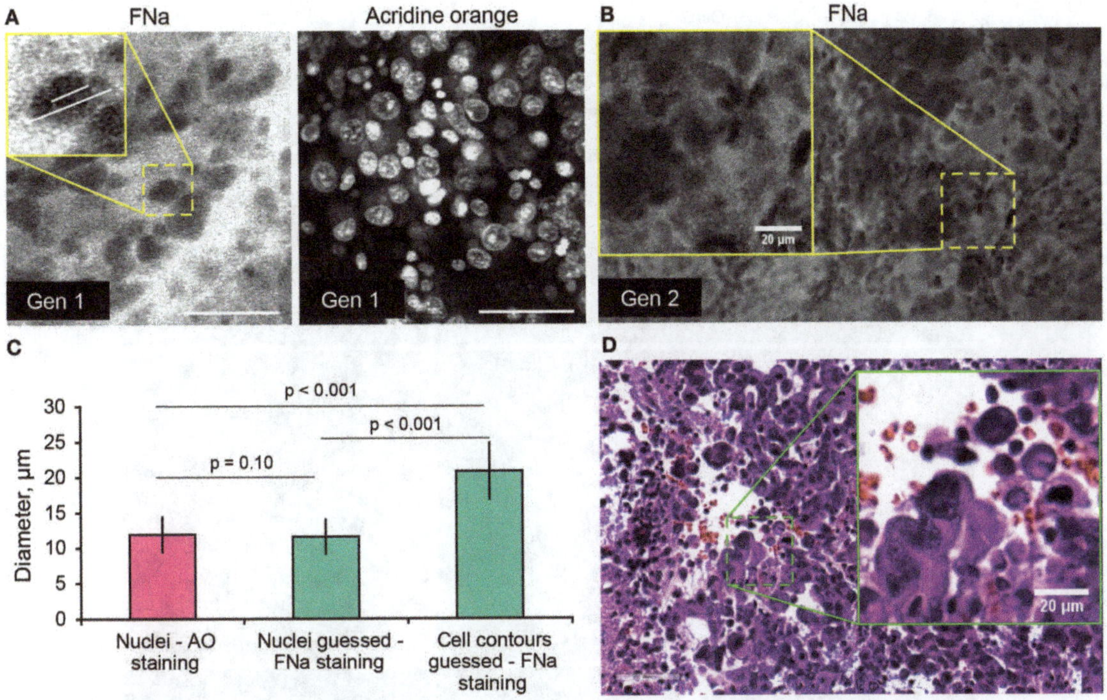

FIGURE 4 | (A,B) Comparison of the tumor cellular features visible on confocal laser endomicroscopy images with fluorescein sodium (FNa) and acridine orange (AO). AO staining of the same specimen shows true nuclei size. Gradient of FNa distribution delineates cell contours with bright gray, while cell nuclei may be visible in some of the cells in a darker gray. **(C)** Comparison of the nuclei size measured on the images with AO staining to the nuclei size measured on the images with the FNa staining ($n = 106$ cells measured with AO stain; $n = 53$ nuclei and $n = 52$ cell diameters were measured with FNa stain). The average nucleus size determined on the FNa images was similar to the true average nucleus size based on the AO staining. Generation (Gen) 2 CLE image **(B)** shows anisocytosis, similar to **(D)** histologic findings. Scale bar in **(A)** is 50 µm. Used with permission from Barrow Neurological Institute, Phoenix, Arizona.

± 2.5 µm), suggesting validity of identification of nuclei on the FNa-based confocal images. The average nuclei size was significantly smaller ($p < 0.01$) than the cell sizes (20.8 ± 3.9 µm) (**Figure 4**). Benchtop confocal LSM of fresh samples stained with FNa (*in vivo*, intravenous) and Hoechst (rapid *ex vivo*, topical live cell nuclear stain) showed images similar to CLE grayscale images and provided additional confirmation regarding the dimensions of nuclei and cells observed with CLE (**Figure 5**).

The tumor margin was visible in the GL261 model with both CLEs. The tumor border region appeared as a nonuniform delineation between the area with low FNa signal that did not contain atypical cellular features (normal brain) and an area with high FNa signal containing silhouettes of the abnormal tumor cells (**Figure 6**). Benchtop confocal microscopy of samples stained with FNa *in vivo* and rapidly counterstained *ex vivo* with Hoechst suggested that FNa signal "followed" invasions of the tumor cells in the normal brain. It confirmed that many small cell contours visible with FNa are actually anuclear red blood cells. A gradient of FNa distribution from the tumor into the normal brain was also visible with the higher FOV confocal microscopy.

When normal brain tissue was injured, leaking FNa signal was visible. Brain regions of injury without tumor could be differentiated from regions of brain with tumor on CLE images by small and nonvariable red blood cells being present, rather than large, numerous, and variable tumor cells (32).

FNa Doses for Optimal CLE Imaging

Different concentrations of intravenous FNa as a contrast for CLE imaging yielded variations in image appearance. Bolus injections of higher concentrations of FNa resulted in brighter images of tumors with less noise, and an overall increase in the fraction of diagnostic frames, compared to lower FNa concentrations ($R = 0.5$, $p < 0.05$) (**Figure 7**). The best working dosages were 20 and 40 mg/kg and are in accordance with previous publications [100 mg/kg (11); 8 mg/kg (24); 7.7 mg/kg (30)]. Based on our experience, imaging closer to the time of FNa injection produced images with greater contrast and overall higher quality compared with images obtained longer after the injection.

Histologic Features During CLE Imaging With 5-ALA (Gen1 and Gen2)

Neither Gen1 nor Gen2 CLE was reliably able to detect PpIX fluorescence in experimental tumors after 5-ALA administration. At the same time, Pentero 900 imaging with a dedicated Blue 400 filter showed very bright red PpIX fluorescence with all tumor masses. Gen2 CLE detected some signal in several tumor areas; however, this signal was not consistent in different locations imaged over the tumor area. Most imaging of the tumor showed dark images without visible signal. In all 5 animals interrogated with both Gen1 and Gen2, reliable histologic features of tumor or normal brain were not discernible with PpIX fluorescence.

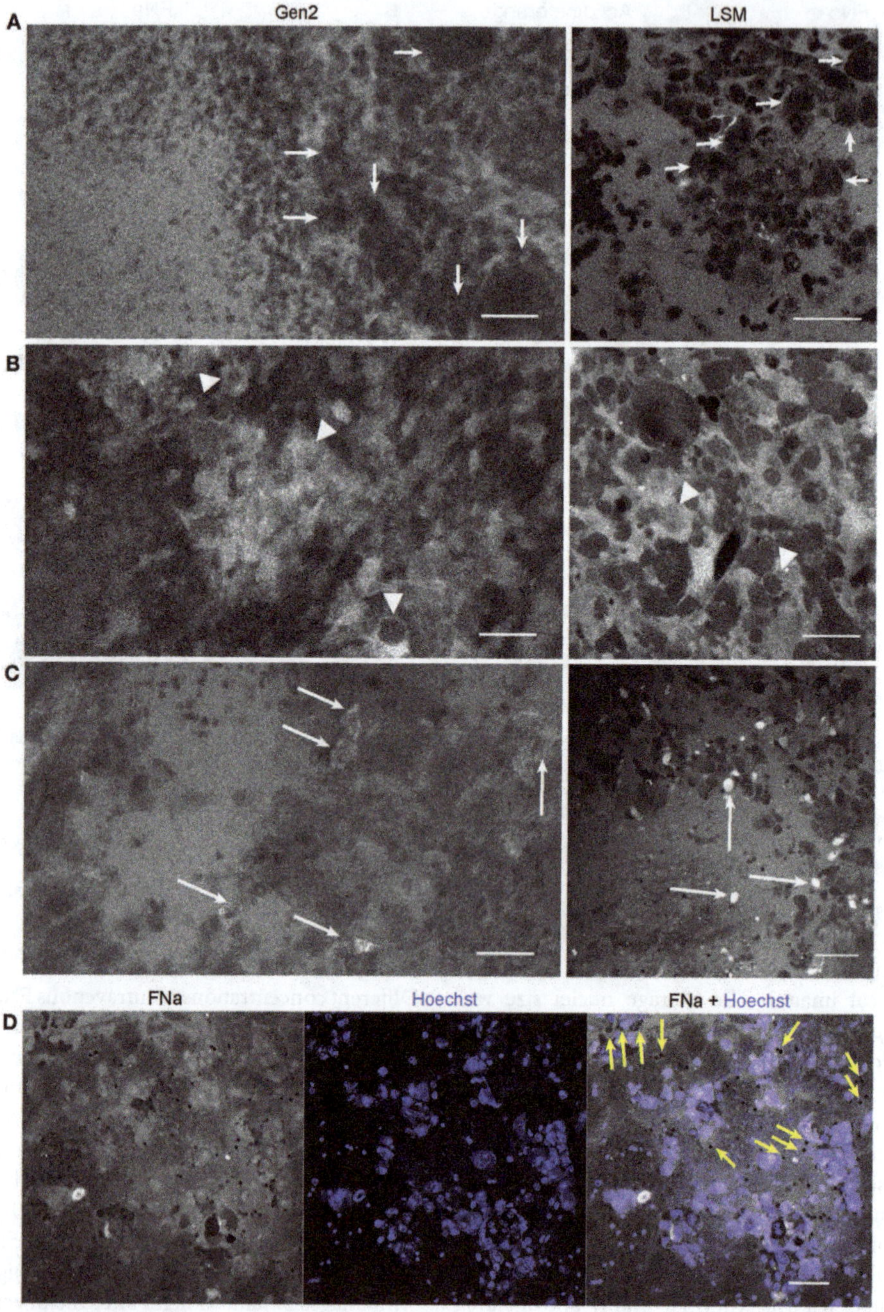

FIGURE 5 | Confocal laser endomicroscopy (CLE) patterns of GL261 glioma core. *In vivo* Gen2 CLE and rapid *ex vivo* laser scanning microscopy (LSM) images show higher fluorescein sodium (FNa) signal in the tumor area and visible contours of the tumor cells. Overall tissue architecture presents similarly in CLE and LSM images. **(A)** Most often tumor cells appeared darker than the background (arrows), while in some areas **(B,C)** tumor cells absorbed FNa and appeared bright. **(D)** Red blood cells, which were not stained by the Hoechst dye, are visible on a bright FNa background (yellow arrows). Scale bars are 50 μm. Used with permission from Barrow Neurological Institute, Phoenix, Arizona.

However, sparse fluorescent spots were observed in normal brain and tumor in experimental animals and were likely autofluorescence (35). When the overall image intensities of normal brain and tumor areas, acquired with similar parameters, were compared, they differed significantly ($p < 0.01$) (**Figure 8**).

Influence of Imaging Parameters on the Image Quality (Gen2 System)

Imaging Filter

Imaging using green bandpass or green longpass filters was compared on both systems to visualize FNa in mouse glioma

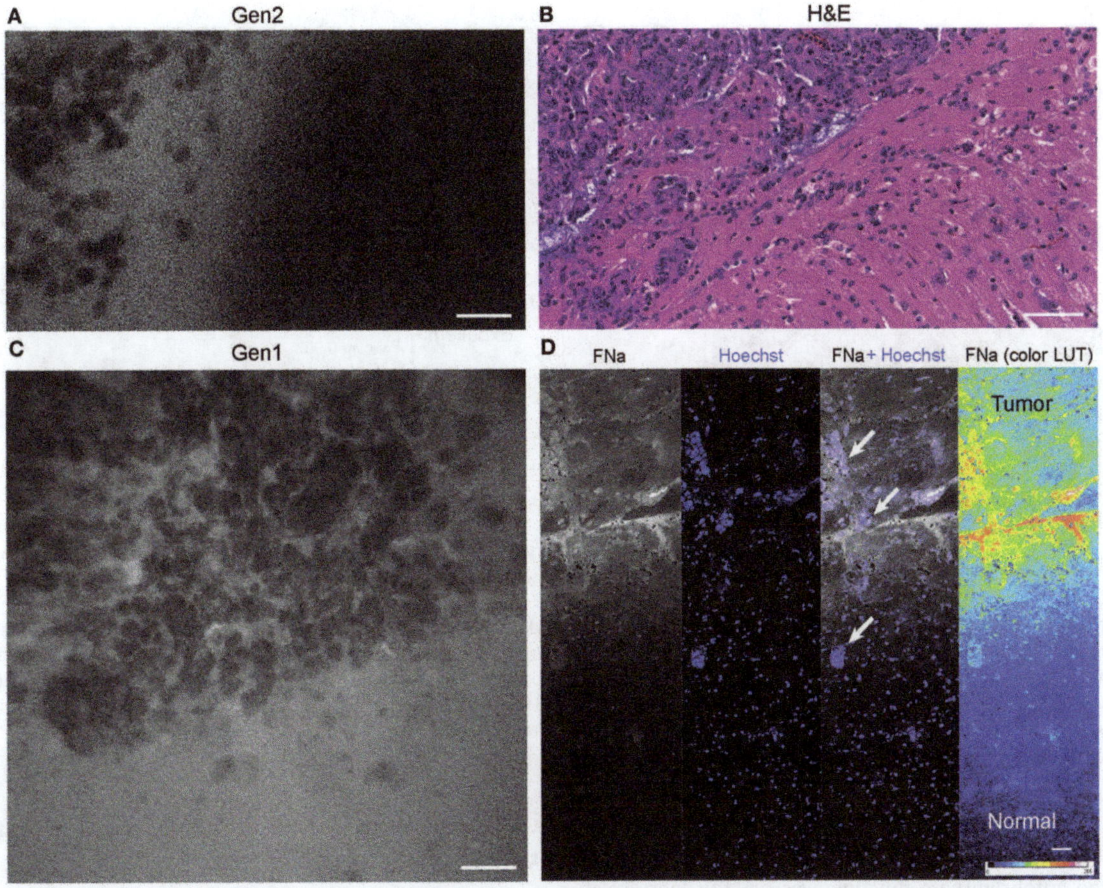

FIGURE 6 | Tumor border 1 h after intravenous fluorescein sodium (FNa) injection. **(A)** Generation 2 (Gen2) and **(C)** generation 1 (Gen1) confocal laser endomicroscopy images show a similar cellular architecture pattern of the GL261 glioma border region. **(B)** Hematoxylin and eosin (H&E) image of the tumor border from a matched sample. **(D)** Larger field of view *ex vivo* benchtop confocal image shows gradient of fluorescein diffusion from the tumor to the normal brain. Arrows indicate invading tumor cell groups. LUT, look-up table. Scale bars are 50 μm. Used with permission from Barrow Neurological Institute, Phoenix, Arizona.

models. Images acquired with the longpass filter appeared brighter. At the same time, quantitative analysis showed that the bandpass filter resulted in significantly better-contrasted images (**Figure 9**). With autobrightness function on, some Gen2 images (using FNa or AO as a contrast) appeared subjectively dark. However, adjusting the brightness during post-processing resulted in significantly better-contrasted images than when using the longpass filter. The red longpass filter was not useful for FNa imaging; however, scant cells and structures emitted light in the red spectrum within normal brain and tumor areas.

Detector Gain

When FNa was used, images were acquired mainly with a gain at the mid-position (2,400). Very bright fluorescent specimens (10–40 mg/kg FNa) required gain adjustments on only rare occasions, as control was usually possible for oversaturated pixels and image quality by lowering the laser power and brightness (**Figure 10**).

Laser Power

For FNa imaging, the laser power was usually at 50% (500 μm). In locations that produced dark images (low FNa or bleached areas), increasing the laser intensity improved image quality and brightness to some extent, but further increases in laser power did not result in quality improvement. The functioning of laser power control was not different between Gen1 and Gen2 systems. Overall, grossly bright fluorescent samples resulted in excellent contrast and quality at 50% laser power and gain position in the midpoint range (2,400) (**Figure 11**).

Image Brightness and Noise

The autobrightness function auto-adjusts the brightness of the image on the fly during continuous imaging based on the brightness histogram of the precedent image, independently from the gain and laser power settings. With one exception, the autobrightness function of the Gen2 was advantageous for rapid image and optimal brightness display, contrasting with the Gen1 that lacked this function and required frequent manual adjustments. The exception occurred when the image had abnormally bright artifacts. In such situations, the autobrightness function decreased the overall image brightness, with the FNa signal in the tumor interstitium becoming low and barely detectable—this was observed both qualitatively in real time and

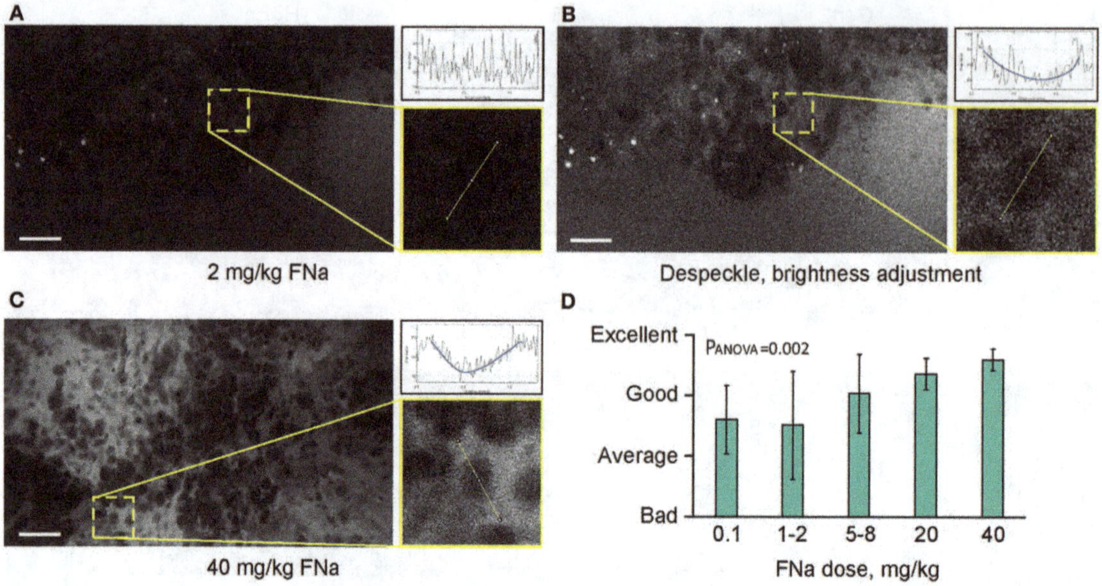

FIGURE 7 | Higher concentrations of fluorescein sodium (FNa) produces images with less noise on a generation 2 confocal laser endomicroscope. Images acquired with a low dose of FNa **(A)** could be post-processed to improve brightness **(B)**, so they appear similar to higher FNa dose images **(C)**. Comparison of the enlarged regions in **(A–C)** shows that cell contours are distinguished on all images; however, noise level [diagrams in **(A–C)**] is less with a higher FNa concentration. **(D)** Subjective grading of overall CLE imaging quality is presented as a mean of all grades from 5 independent raters. The image quality is significantly better with higher FNa dosages ($P_{ANOVA} = 0.002$). Scale bars are 50 μm. Used with permission from Barrow Neurological Institute, Phoenix, Arizona.

quantitatively during post-processing. In such situations, manual brightness setup was used to obtain better overall image quality.

When the autobrightness function was on, the increase in gain resulted in a proportional decrease in automatic brightness level. Brightness values can be indicative of noise level. Brightness levels below 80% were the most optimal with less black noise, compared to a brightness level of 80% and above. The brightness values were maintained below 80% to keep the noise levels low (**Figure 12**).

Background noise levels were further studied to assess the effects of Gen2 imaging parameters on image quality. Imaging of normal brain with various manually set brightness levels revealed that mean image intensity and standard deviation of the individual pixels had a positive correlation with brightness level (**Figure 13**). At a brightness of 91%, laser power of 50% (505 μm), speed of 1080 pixels (~1.26 seconds per frame), and gain of 2400, the average pixel intensity from a normal brain (black color) was 53.5 arbitrary units, corresponding to about 20% saturation of the 8-bit image.

Image Acquisition Speed

Most images were acquired at a speed setting of 1080 pixels (~1.26 seconds per frame), which resulted in the best image quality (**Table 1**). Faster scanning at speeds of 135 pixels (~0.26 seconds per frame) and 270 pixels (~0.4 seconds per frame) were useful for rapid scanning of large areas to determine the presence or absence of an FNa signal or for blood flow imaging (**Figure 14**). Some gross tumor tissue structures were visible at speeds of 135 and 270 but appeared overly pixelated on the CLE display. Image quality and contrast were significantly better at 1080 pixels (~1.26 seconds per frame), especially in areas with small vessels contrasted with FNa or when using nuclear stains (AO, AF).

DISCUSSION

The Gen2 CLE system is compatible with the specific demands of neurosurgical use. With the disposable sterile sheath that includes a coverslip, the Gen2 CLE can now be safely used on the human brain during surgery without the need for a complex sterilization procedure after surgery, as was the case with the Gen1 system (**Supplemental Figure 4**). The ergonomics of the probe conformation are such that it resembles a curved, lightweight neurosurgical suction device that will lie comfortably in the hand, grasped by the first few fingers, in a fashion that allows smooth, stabilized movement as a neurosurgeon is used to for surgical instruments. In this study, we performed a preclinical investigation of the Gen2 CLE and characterized its operation, capabilities, and limitations, and compared its performance to the Gen1 CLE system.

Image Quality Comparison (Gen1 vs. Gen2)

Imaging Parameters (Gen1 and Gen2)

Multiple imaging parameters can be adjusted in both Gen1 and Gen2 systems making them flexible and capable of detecting a single-channel fluorescent signal over a broad range of intensity values. Gen2 is more adjustable, as it allows for changing most parameters rapidly during scanning, while with the Gen1, the user is required to create a new imaging session using the operating software interface to change the gain or filter. Another

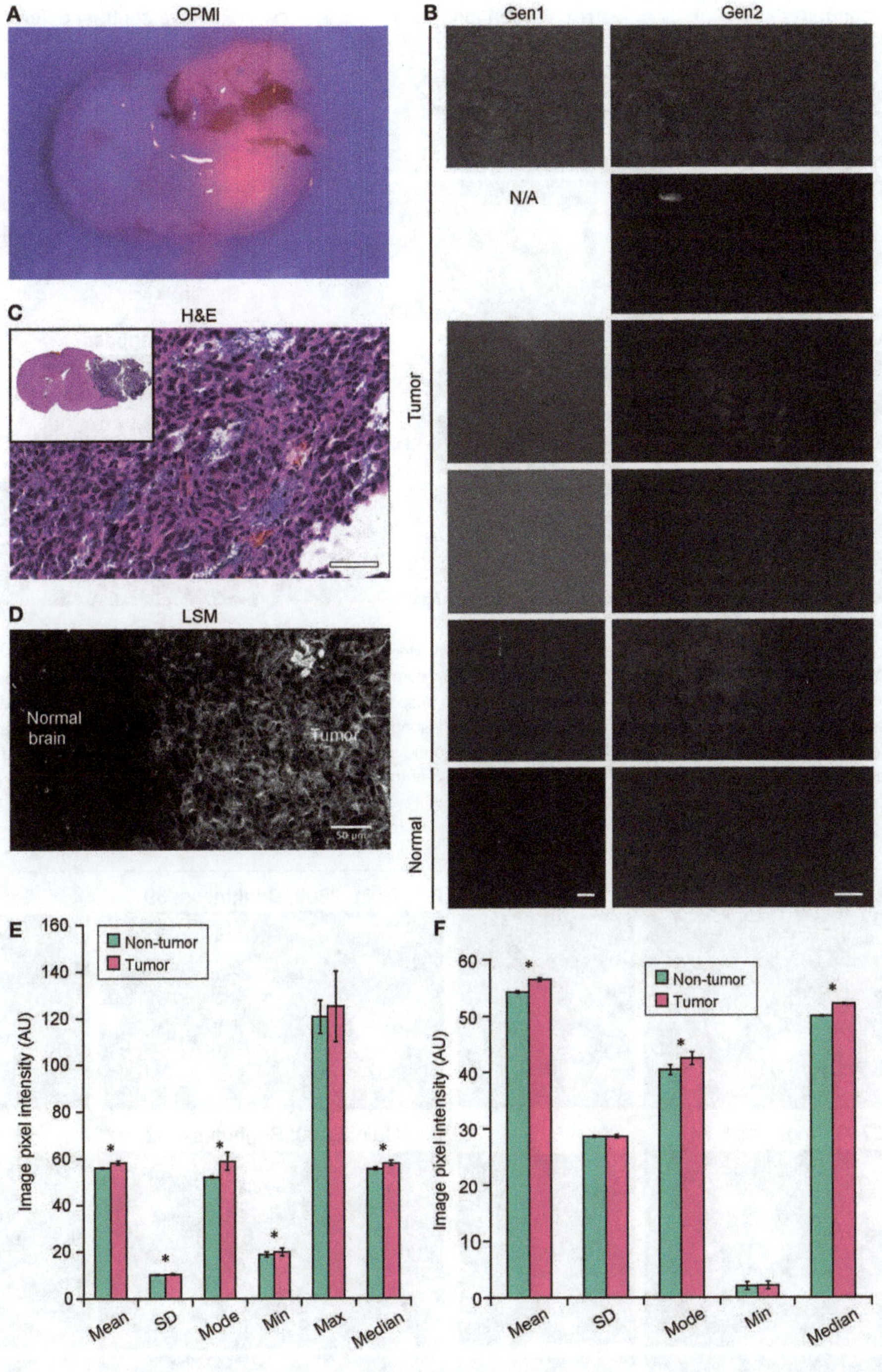

FIGURE 8 | Confocal laser endomicroscopy (CLE) imaging of GL261 glioma with 5-aminolevulenic acid (5-ALA). **(A)** Representative image of a coronal brain slice with a tumor viewed through the Pentero 900 operative microscope in Blue 400 mode shows bright red fluorescence from the tumor. **(B)** The best representative generation 1 (Gen1) and generation 2 (Gen2) CLE images of tumor (rows are 5 separate animals) and normal brain 2 h after intraperitoneal 5-ALA administration. Normal brain shows no fluorescent signal in any of the cases. Fluorescent signal from tumor is very low, visible from only a few areas, and is not consistent across the biopsy locations and across the animals imaged. **(C)** Hematoxylin and eosin (H&E) coronal slice of the brain with a tumor shows hypercellular tumor in the areas from which CLE imaging was performed. **(D)** Laser scanning microscopy (LSM) image at the tumor margin shows the protoporphyrin signal localized to tumor cell cytoplasm. The image displayed in gray scale and size is similar to Gen2 CLE. (Image acquired with 40× 1.2 W objective; 405 nm excitation; 598–740 nm detection range.) **(E)** Gen1 CLE imaging of GL261 gliomas and contralateral normal brain as a control with 5-ALA. Quantification of the images ($n = 54$ control; $n = 59$ tumor images from 5 animals) showed minimal but significant difference in the overall pixel intensities of the images taken from the tumor vs. normal brain. Groups were compared using Student *t*-tests; an asterisk indicates $p < 0.01$. **(F)** Quantification of the Gen2 CLE images ($n = 5$ control; $n = 4$ tumor) showed minimal but significant differences in the overall pixel intensities of the selected best images taken from the tumor and normal brain. Groups were compared using Student *t*-tests; an asterisk indicates $p < 0.01$. Selected images were acquired with similar CLE settings. Scale bars are 50 μm. AU, arbitrary unit. Used with permission from Barrow Neurological Institute, Phoenix, Arizona.

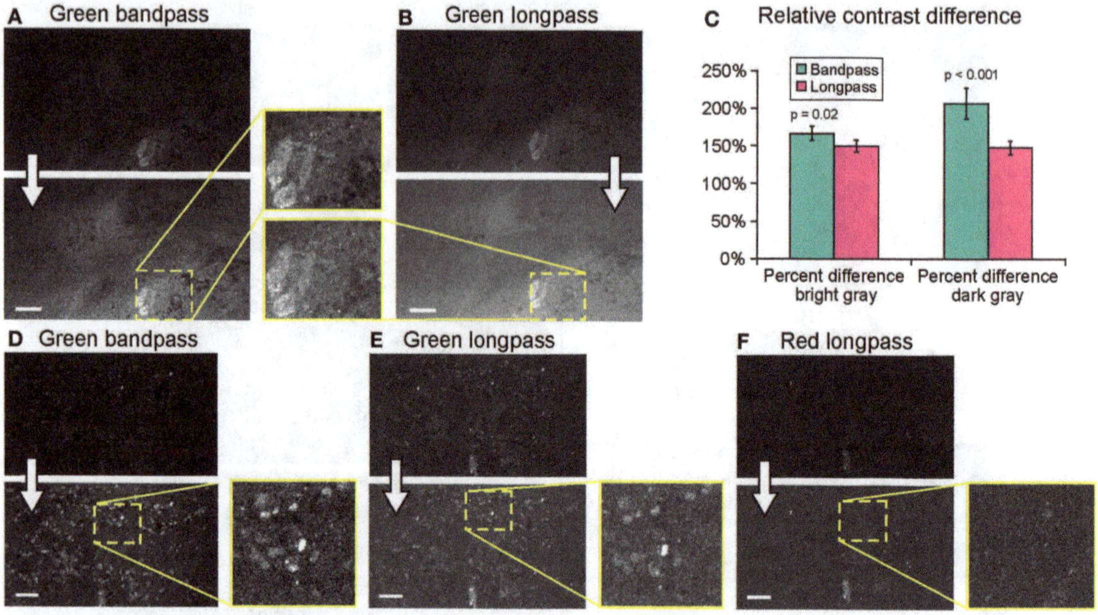

FIGURE 9 | Generation 2 confocal laser endomicroscope (CLE) imaging with various filters. Comparison of the CLE images taken from the same regions of interest with green bandpass **(A,D)**, green longpass **(B,E)**, and red **(F)** optical filters. Human glioma samples (patients were injected with FNa intraoperatively) were used for analysis and illustration. Thick arrows signify post-processing in FIJI, which includes despeckling and maximum brightness adjustment. **(C)** Matching regions of interest (ROI) were selected in FIJI to compare contrast between various structures in longpass and bandpass filters. ROIs were manually drawn over the brightest structures ($n = 5$), over the surrounding gray background ($n = 3$), and on the dark round structures ($n = 5$). Paired Student t-tests were used for comparison. **(D–F)** Green bandpass **(D)**, green longpass **(E)**, and red longpass **(F)** filter images obtained at the same location. Scale bars are 50 μm. Used with permission from Barrow Neurological Institute, Phoenix, Arizona.

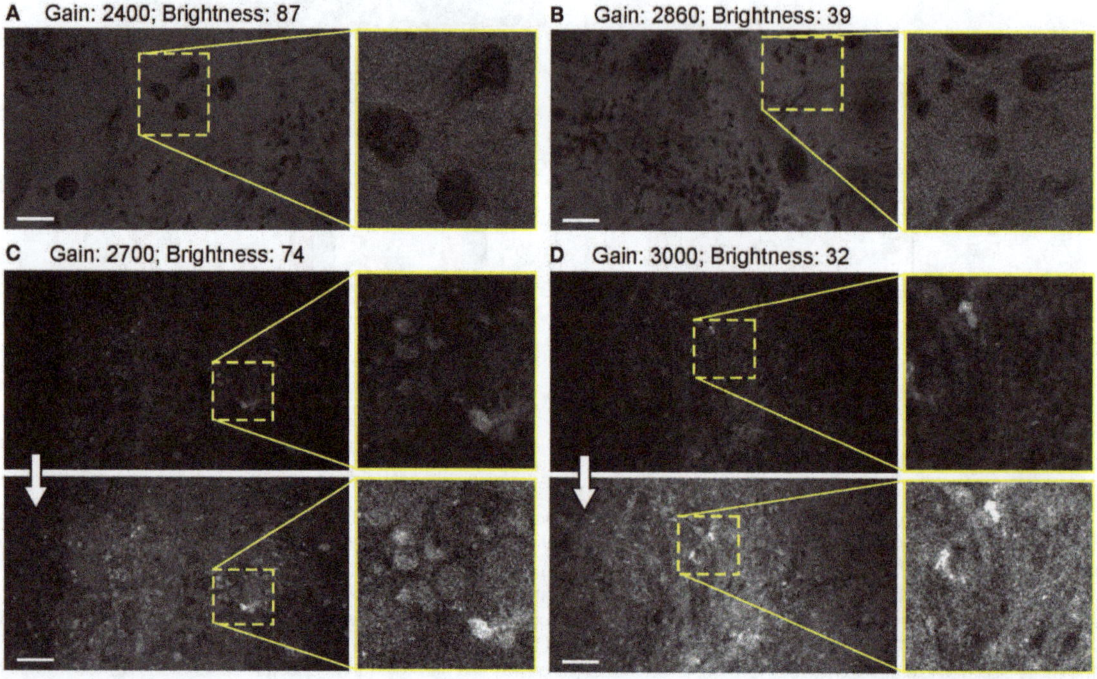

FIGURE 10 | Balanced generation 2 (Gen2) confocal laser endomicroscope (CLE) images with different gain results in comparable image quality. **(A–D)** Comparison of the CLE images taken with various gain setup. Human meningioma **(A,B)** and glioblastoma **(C,D)** samples scanned *ex vivo* 2 h after fluorescein sodium (2-mg/kg) injection are used for analysis and illustration. Increase in the gain requires reciprocal adjustments in the brightness. Overall, the resulting images have comparable quality. **(A,B)** are visualized from one patient, while **(C,D)** are visualized from a different patient. Thick arrows signify post-processing in FIJI, which includes despeckling and maximum brightness adjustment. Scale bars are 50 μm. Used with permission from Barrow Neurological Institute, Phoenix, Arizona.

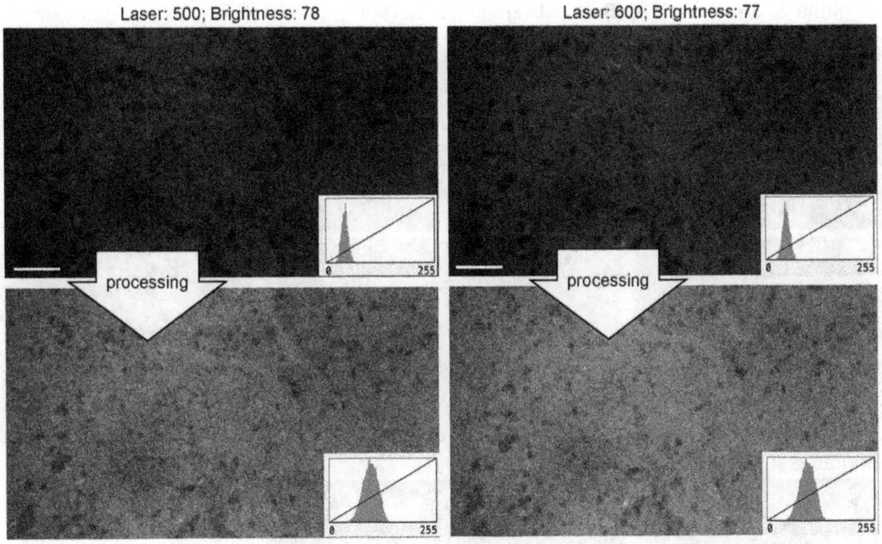

FIGURE 11 | Generation 2 confocal laser endomicroscope images taken at different laser intensity values. A human meningioma sample is used for analysis and illustration. Brightness was kept at a similar level during image acquisition. Increase in the laser intensity from 500 μm (upper left) to 600 μm (upper right) leads to a brighter overall image. Further increase in laser power does not improve contrast. Thick arrows signify post-processing in FIJI, which includes despeckling and maximum brightness adjustment. There are no subjective differences in images after post-processing (lower row). Scale bars are 50 μm. Used with permission from Barrow Neurological Institute, Phoenix, Arizona.

convenient advantage is that, unlike the Gen1, the Gen2 imaging parameters are recorded as part of the file properties. Having access to these parameters is important for quantitative analysis and comparison among various images, especially to evaluate fluorophore signal intensity in the image, which correlates with the concentration of the fluorophore in the sample. For FNa-guided optical biopsy in brain tumors, such information may be used to assess the degree of blood-brain barrier disruption, to eliminate imaging artifacts, to identify potential causes of suboptimal images, or to improve images in post-processing.

Still Images (Gen1 and Gen2)

While continuous imaging occurs at a chosen speed in both CLE systems, the recording options are different. Both systems have the option to record a single still image and time series, while the Gen2 can also automatically record Z-stacks. Still image recordings were used when the sample quality was perfect and when there was no concern about having only a few selected imaging frames recorded while interrogating the tissue. However, in most cases, continuous recording was preferred and advantageous, which is discussed later. Finding the exact same position again is nearly impossible with a CLE system due to the minute dimensions on the order of fractions of a millimeter (475 × 475 μm for Gen1; 475 × 267 μm for Gen2), contact probe design, and pliable nature of unfixed brain tissue. Thus, there was always a concern about not being able to return the CLE to the previous imaging plane. Therefore, still recordings were used less frequently than Z-stacks or time series. Incorporation and registration of the probe into an image-guided surgery navigation system would allow improvement in reassessing tissue imaging location.

Z-Stack Function (Gen2 Only)

A Z-stack is a series of images taken in rapid succession at different depths and a constant position (34). The "Z-step" is the depth distance between images and is a novel feature for handheld CLE imaging with the Gen2 CLE system. The range of the Z-stack can be set by the user, and the Z-step is a constant 3 μm, resulting in 2–35 images per stack. At least several slices (maximum 10–13) from the Z-stack were acquired at optimal Z positions that were in focus, usable, and diagnostic (36). Informative images from a Z-stack can be easily processed into video loops or semitransparent volumetric images for detailed assessment and further interpretation.

It is also worth mentioning that the size of objects becomes larger when they are imaged out of focus and deeper within the tissue. This could potentially make small red blood cells look larger than they are, thus imposing a minor potential for misdiagnosing small cells as tumor cells.

Time Series Recording and Video Loops (Gen1 and Gen2)

Time series (or "cine"-series) recordings were used extensively for post-processing and creation of video loops. Continuous nonstop recording during Gen1 or Gen2 CLE interrogation of the sample was helpful compared with "on-demand" snapshot recording because with the latter technique, some locations were bleached out before the image was recorded. Gradual photobleaching was observed, but with practice, minimizing the scan time avoided this problem. We did not investigate whether laser interrogation results in tissue damage. Although tissue damage is unlikely, we are conducting an ongoing investigation of the potential phototoxicity of CLE scanning. Additionally, minute tissue shifts

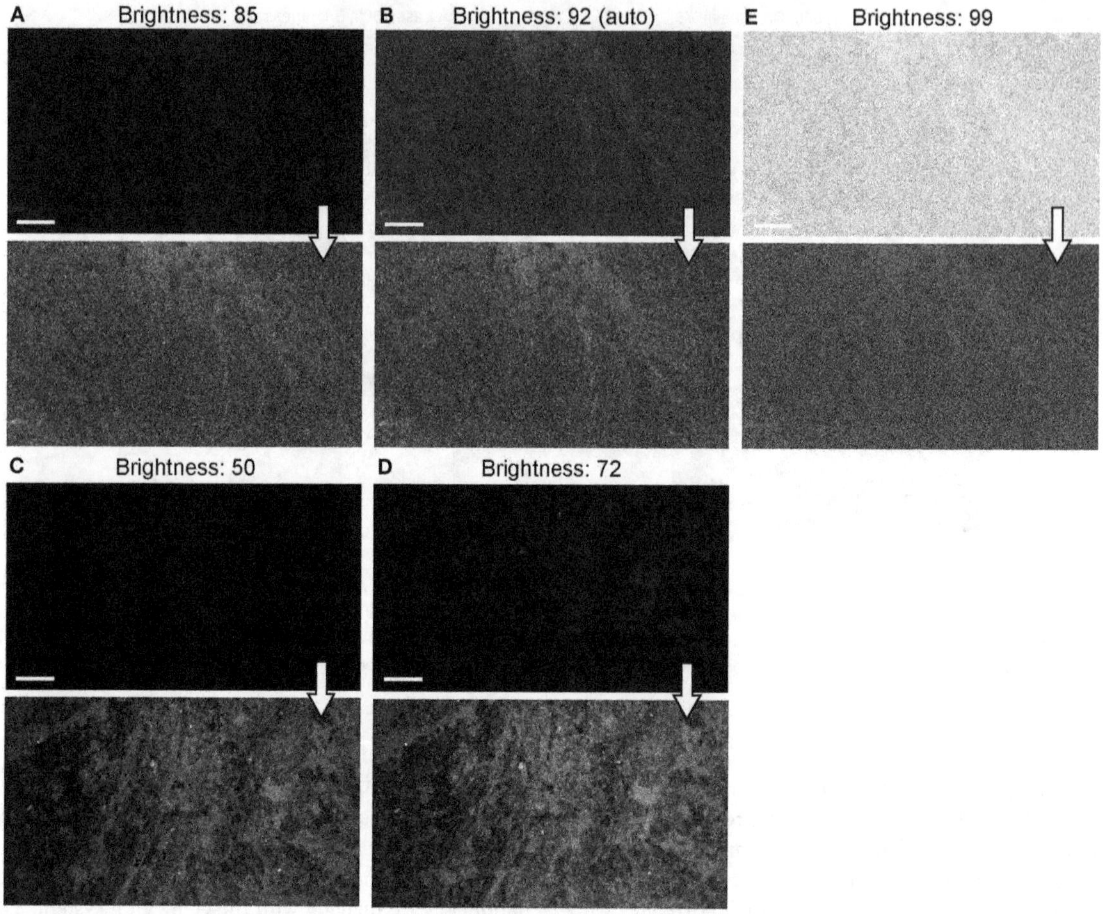

FIGURE 12 | Generation 2 confocal laser endomicroscope (CLE) images taken with different brightness setup. **(A–E)** Comparison of the CLE images taken with various brightness settings. The same fields of view of meningioma **(A–C)** and low-grade glioma **(D,E)** human samples are used for analysis and illustration. Brightness is in the automatic position for **(B)**; in all other figures, brightness is set manually. Increase in brightness higher than automatic position does not increase image quality quantitatively **(C)**. Thick arrows signify post-processing in FIJI, which includes despeckling and maximum brightness adjustment, except for **(C)** in which brightness is decreased with post-processing. Scale bars are 50 μm. Used with permission from Barrow Neurological Institute, Phoenix, Arizona.

changed the observed image before taking a picture, and the probe often could not be returned to the desired location because of the pliable nature of unfixed brain tissue. Z-position, brightness, and laser power can be adjusted during the time series imaging to record optimal quality images.

Notably, time series imaging revealed a "movement" feature of the tissue and supplemented visual information gained from still images. This feature is useful in several aspects for tissue histologic characteristics and CLE image interpretation. Primarily, differentiation of freely moving red blood cells from other moving or stationary cells becomes much easier and thus fosters the diagnostic accuracy of image and tissue interpretation. Additionally, it becomes easier to differentiate real signal from noise. By viewing time series, differentiation is possible between what is meaningful and what is merely stochastic noise. Such judgment is usually difficult on still images because of the nature of FNa. FNa is a nonspecific dye that is not bound to any structure, but rather provides a bright background (i.e., a silhouetted appearance) on which to observe, contrast, and differentiate structures. Noise is an inherent limitation of FNa. *In vivo* CLE demonstrated dynamics of the glioma environment for the first time, something that is not possible in fixed brain tissue.

It should also be noted that CLE allowed for *in vivo* tracking of blood flow in vessels. Tracking of individual blood cells is not always possible because of fast movements that require high-speed scanning confocal imaging systems, such as spinning disk confocal microscopes (37–39).

Histologic Pictures Visualized by CLE With FNa (Gen1 and Gen2)

The use of FNa with both distal scanning CLE systems was effective to visualize brain vasculature, red blood cells, silhouettes of neoplastic cells, nuclear and cell dimensions, GL261 glioma border, and brain injury. FNa aided detection of normal and tumor vessels and did not significantly highlight normal brain tissue. Cell nuclei and cytoplasm may be distinguished in some of the cells by a gradient of FNa penetration through

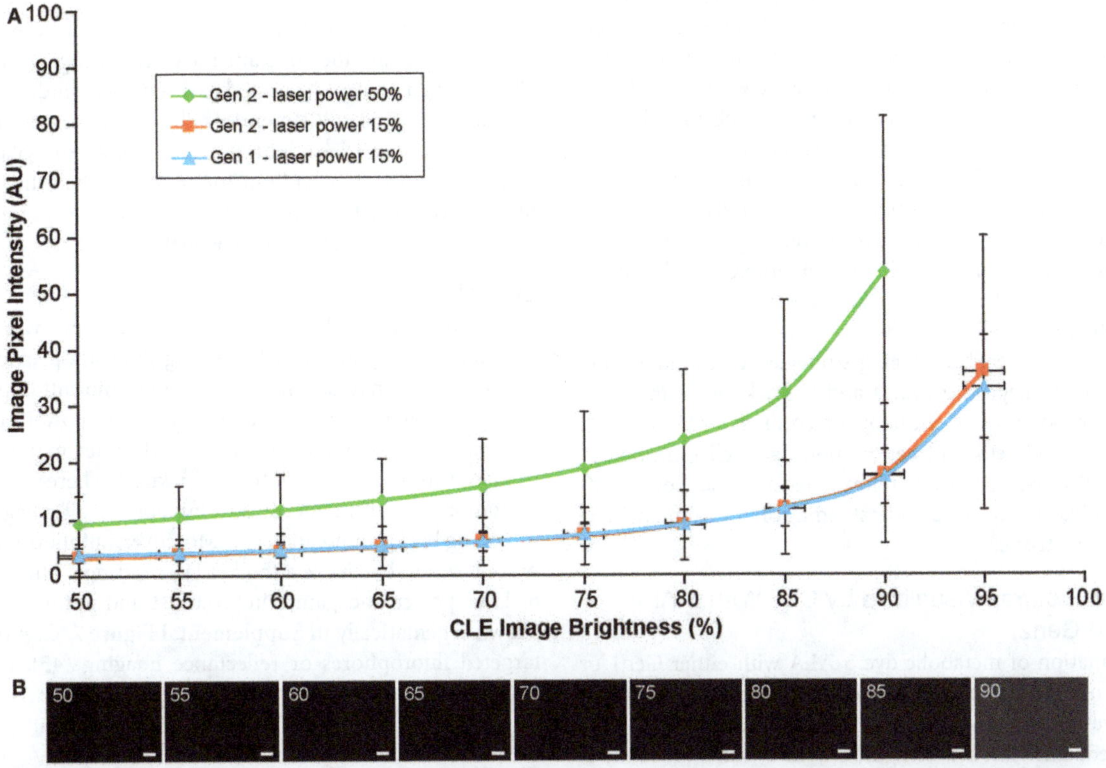

FIGURE 13 | Image brightness and background noise level with the generation 1 (Gen1) and generation 2 (Gen2) confocal laser endomicroscope (CLE). Image brightness and background noise level depend on the laser power and image brightness set up of the CLE. **(A)** Graph showing observed image intensity in arbitrary units (AU) (y axis) at the various brightness positions, while imaging normal brain area. This value represents "black" noise. Brightness setting above 80% results in a significant increase of black noise, which may decrease image quality. Therefore, when imaging, one should aim at getting a picture at a brightness level below 80%. **(B)** Unprocessed Gen 2 CLE images taken at various indicated brightness levels (%) that are set manually. Scale bars are 50 µm. Used with permission from Barrow Neurological Institute, Phoenix, Arizona.

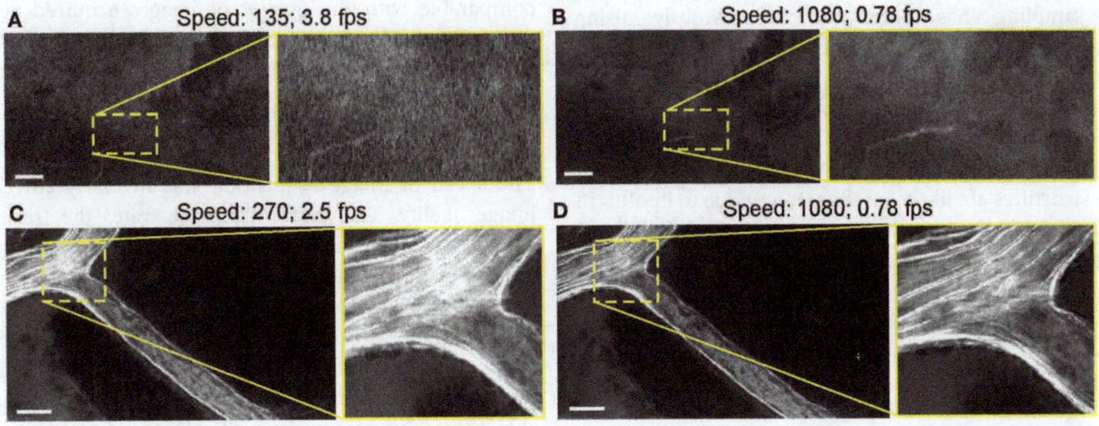

FIGURE 14 | Generation 2 confocal laser endomicroscope (CLE) images taken at different speeds. Comparison of CLE images taken with 3 various acquisition speed settings: **(A)** 135, **(B,D)** 1,080, and **(C)** 270. Images acquired at an intermediate speed setting **(C)** of 270 (calculated mean 2.5 frames per second) are of average quality and are able to resolve more structural details than images taken at the faster speed of 135 **(A)**. Significant improvement in image quality at the slower speed of 1,080 **(B,D)** is mostly apparent in the areas with high contrast, such as small vessels when fluorescein sodium is used. When viewed as smaller pictures, the differences are less pronounced. However, on a large high-definition display, the image quality at different speeds differs substantially. Scale bars are 50 µm. Used with permission from Barrow Neurological Institute, Phoenix, Arizona.

different biological membranes (**Supplemental Figure 5**). FNa extravasation due to injury can be differentiated from the FNa diffusion in the tumor using characteristic histologic patterns on CLE (32). It is worth noting that individual fluorescent cells were frequently observed in both tumor and normal brain (**Supplemental Figure 6**). This phenomenon had various patterns and was observed more frequently with increased imaging time after FNa injection. Singular and multiple cells were observed that took up FNa on the cut surface of the tumors. Even though such images did not represent a characteristic CLE image of the tumor, they were helpful to assess the cell morphology, tissue architecture, and cytoplasm-to-nucleus ratio. The reason for such FNa uptake by some cells is still unknown because tumor cells do not show FNa uptake *in vitro* (30). However, it might be due to cell membrane disruption caused by injury, as such findings were seen mostly in *ex vivo* samples. Additionally, large singular cells that took up FNa seen in the tumor may be macrophages.

When considering FNa imaging strategies, continuous cine-like time series image recordings and Z-stacks were the most useful and productive. Continuous recordings were used to identify red blood cells and better appreciate cell morphology based on cell movement while reformatted volume views of Z-stacks provided an improved understanding of the 3-dimensional structure of the tissue.

Histologic Pictures Visualized by CLE With 5-ALA (Gen1 and Gen2)

The combination of metabolic dye 5-ALA with either Gen1 or Gen2 was not a reliable method for identification of tumor in our observations, as characteristic histologic features could not be identified. The laser wavelength of both systems (488 nm) is not optimally tuned for excitation of PpIX, and CLE images did not show specific information. CLE images did not reproduce findings when LSM with the appropriate excitation laser was used to image PpIX in the same mouse glioma model (40).

While it was possible to differentiate glioma from normal brain tissue by comparing overall average image intensity, this charcteristic was not deemed useful. Similar "fluorescence intensity" sampling has been shown previously using spectrophotometric methods (41–43). Of note, sparse fluorescent "spots" seen using the Gen2 CLE with 5-ALA were consistent with the previous intraoperative observations of patients with brain tumors with the Gen1 CLE, although the exact identification of these PpIX fluorescent signals is not confirmed (25). These structures are likely autofluorescent due to lipofuscin (35). Imaging of histologic patterns created by 5-ALA-induced PpIX in brain tumors remains limited to benchtop confocal microscopes, or hand-held fluorescence microscopes specifically designed for PpIX excitation and detection, such as a dual axis confocal microscope (44) or a scanning fiber endoscope system (40).

CLE Parameters for Best Image Quality With FNa (Gen2 Only)

Filter

The first parameter to consider during CLE imaging is the filter. Between the two types of green filters (i.e., the longpass filter and bandpass filter), the longpass filter produced brighter images. Although images with such longpass filters may look more pleasing, they include nonspecific light from the background that attenuates FNa-induced contrast. Ultimately, the bandpass filter produced images with higher contrast and was preferable for obtaining better quality and interpretable images.

Gain

Unlike in the benchtop confocal microscope, where the gain is fine-tuned during the constant image capturing, with the Gen2 CLE the gain control is located in a separate window and is not available for rapid adjustments on the fly. However, adjustments of brightness and laser power were enough to obtain quality images in most cases without the need to adjust the gain. Only in a few very bright or very dim specimens was there a need to adjust the gain for optimal image quality.

Laser Power

Laser power at mid-range (50% or 500 μm) was generally optimal for imaging, with increasing intensity providing some improvements in image quality. Lack of significant improvement in image quality with increasing laser power is mainly explained by the nature of FNa, which, after extravasation, is diffused through almost all tissue thickness. Therefore, increased excitation results in increased emission in all image regions, including background and cells. Moreover, autofluorescence and noise begin to be visible at higher laser settings. This association of laser power and gain with contrast and autofluorescence is shown schematically in **Supplemental Figure 7**. Compared with targeted fluorophores or reflectance imaging (45), imaging of FNa is always associated with higher levels of noise.

Brightness

The brightness is the built-in adjustable proprietary setting parameter used during CLE imaging. It has a range of settings from 0 to 100% and, unlike the gain and laser power settings, could be adjusted during the imaging. Brightness was a primary setting of both CLE systems. Autobrightness is a new Gen2 function that saved time and made imaging process faster. Images acquired in autobrightness mode had good quality, comparable with the quality of images acquired at manually set brightness levels. Additionally, an optimal brightness level, or even pseudocoloring, can be applied later during post-processing (34).

Speed

The speed of image acquisition was inversely correlated with image quality. This relationship illustrates the tradeoff of the convenience of using high-speed imaging to locate informative structures quickly within a large area with little detail versus taking more time to look at higher resolution images in greater detail. For areas of high contrast, such as intact vessels with FNa within the normal brain, or pronounced hypercellular tumor areas with bright FNa nearby, high-speed imaging was able to resolve structures well. However, in most cases, fast scanning was not able to resolve red blood cells and fine cellular details.

Zoom

Although the FOV of Gen2 images is about half the size of Gen1 images, it was sufficient to obtain similar image interpretation for corresponding histological structures. Subjective image quality appraisal between the systems is dependent on the display size. The Gen2 is capable of increasing optical zoom by a factor of two, but this results in a corresponding decrease in FOV size, which is not particularly helpful for the identification of cell or tissue architecture using FNa imaging. However, a zoom function might be advantageous for dyes such as AO or AF (**Supplemental Figure 8**). Unlike benchtop confocal scanning microscope systems, where zoom can be adjusted in real time (45, 46), handheld CLE systems are limited to a preset zoom because of limitations in miniature design and construction.

Because of the inherent cellular composition of different tumor types, including cellular and regional tissue architectural heterogeneity, CLE system functionality may benefit the surgeon or pathologist by use of a lower resolution and larger FOV image assessment. This situation would allow a closer match to the lower power magnification of a conventional pathology microscope, which would allow the surgeon a larger FOV for scanning the tissue surface (40). However, the portability and capability to move the CLE probe compensate for the smaller FOV, along with Z-stack functionality. Combining multiple small FOV frames together using mosaicking computational algorithms has been shown to yield a larger reconstructed FOV (47).

Different Concentrations and Timing of FNa Administration

FNa doses in animals are higher than human doses used in brain tumor surgery either with epifluorescence guidance using the operating microscope with a dedicated filter [2–20 mg/kg (48)] or previously used with CLE [5 mg/kg (1)], which most likely is due to faster metabolism of such fluorophores in rodents. CLE imaging likely requires similar or higher, but not lower, dosages than epifluorescent imaging to obtain informative images. CLE imaging was performed within a period of 5 min to 2 h after FNa injection. This timing was chosen to approximate the duration of tumor surgery in humans and complements the previous data on the biodistribution of FNa in a rodent model (30). Overall, the shorter time periods produced a higher number of diagnostic frames, while imaging at longer time periods produced less contrasted images, which corresponds to the findings by Folaron et al. (31).

Limitations

The current study was performed using a mouse GL261 glioma model. Histologic patterns and the feasibility of FNa imaging with CLE in other experimental tumor models were not addressed in this project. However, clinical experience (1, 7) and the available literature indicate the general feasibility of such an approach for intraoperative brain tumor imaging. The limitations that have not been addressed in this discussion include the need for the development of remote access to the system by another surgeon or neuropathologist or the ability to push images out to cellular devices for rapid assessment or consultation. In addition, the number of images acquired during a case can be very high—in the thousands—and the number of images with artifact caused by motion or other distortions causing them to be unusable is high. Thus, image stabilization control and associated software built into system would be beneficial for quick informative image selection, identification, review, and optimization (49–51).

CONCLUSIONS

Functionality and parameters were assessed for a CLE system (Gen2) designed specifically to perform to the demands and progress of neurosurgery to potentially assist in managing invasive brain tumors in a preclinical setting. Experimental brain tumor models (*in vivo*) and human tumor samples (*ex vivo*) were employed to discern and describe optimal imaging parameters for microscopic histologic visualization with a clinical-grade CLE system and intravenous FNa as a contrast fluorophore. Visualized histologic patterns and pixel intensity values were of comparable quality on Gen1 and Gen2 systems, if not improved with the Gen2 system. The Gen2 had a limitation of a smaller FOV, while having higher resolution, clearer images, and a more responsive user interface, including an autobrightness function and volumetric Z-stack image acquisition that enrich diagnostic possibilities and imaging functionality.

Such portable CLE systems are designed ultimately for *in vivo* use. CLE systems cannot replace the extensive functionality of benchtop confocal scanning microscopes, and they are not designed to accomplish such tasks. CLE systems depend on their specificity, rapid applicability, and portability; their functions, ergonomics, and employment depend on the demands of the surgical or diagnostic specialty. Additionally, the properties of the emitted and detected light range and concomitant fluorophores have a critical impact on use and efficacy.

The CLE provides the neurosurgeon with real-time intraoperative image resolution at the cellular level that is the critical basis of the potential for cell-precision surgery (although neurosurgical instrumentation does not yet provide for precision maneuvers at the cellular level). Although CLE has been used routinely in other medical and surgical specialties, such as for gastrointestinal diagnosis, neurosurgery is in its infancy with respect to CLE use. CLE technology does appear to be responding to the demands of neurosurgeons and neuropathologists for practical introduction into the operating room as an aid in surgery for invasive brain tumors after nearly a decade of developmental exploration and testing.

Concepts for CLE use that must be considered are those that will make the system meaningful in a surgical setting. CLE usefulness to neurosurgery must be proven by being shown to provide a measurable ability to discriminate and guide removal of tumor invasion, thereby extending or optimizing the resection. As much as CLE may provide precise information on where to biopsy or remove tissue, it may be just as crucially used to inform the neurosurgeon where to stop the resection. Further clinical investigation of the diagnostic value of the Gen2 CLE system in fluorescence-guided brain tumor surgery is ongoing.

ETHICS STATEMENT

All patients gave voluntary informed consent as a part of a study protocol approved by the Institutional Review Board of the Barrow Neurological Institute, St. Joseph's Hospital and Medical Center, Phoenix, Arizona.

AUTHOR CONTRIBUTIONS

EB, PN, and MP conception and design. EB, EM, AC, AP, and CC acquisition of data, experiments. EB, EM, NM, VB, JE, PN, and MP analysis and interpretation of data. MP, DH, and AS resources, animal model development. MP, PN, and ML supervision. EB, EM, and CC drafting the article. EB, AC, AP, DH, NM, VB, AS, ML, JE, PN, and MP revising article critically for important intellectual content. All authors final approval of the manuscript.

Foundation. This project received materials support from Carl Zeiss AG, Oberkochen, Germany. EB received scholarship support SP-2240.2018.4.

ACKNOWLEDGMENTS

The authors thank the staff of Neuroscience Publications at Barrow Neurological Institute for assistance with manuscript preparation.

REFERENCES

1. Martirosyan NL, Eschbacher JM, Kalani MY, Turner JD, Belykh E, Spetzler RF, et al. Prospective evaluation of the utility of intraoperative confocal laser endomicroscopy in patients with brain neoplasms using fluorescein sodium: experience with 74 cases. *Neurosurg Focus.* (2016) 40:E11. doi: 10.3171/2016.1.FOCUS15559
2. Ackerman LV, Ramirez GA. The indications for and limitations of frozen section diagnosis; a review of 1269 consecutive frozen section diagnoses. *Br J Surg.* (1959) 46:336–50.
3. Novis DA, Zarbo RJ. Interinstitutional comparison of frozen section turnaround time. A College of American Pathologists Q-Probes study of 32868 frozen sections in 700 hospitals. *Arch Pathol Lab Med.* (1997) 121:559–67.
4. Plesec TP, Prayson RA. Frozen section discrepancy in the evaluation of central nervous system tumors. *Arch Pathol Lab Med.* (2007) 131:1532–40. doi: 10.1043/1543-2165(2007)131[1532:FSDITE]2.0.CO;2
5. Osman H, Georges J, Elsahy D, Hattab EM, Yocom S, Cohen-Gadol AA. *In vivo* microscopy in neurosurgical oncology. *World Neurosurg.* (2018) 115:110–27. doi: 10.1016/j.wneu.2018.03.218
6. Belykh E, Martirosyan NL, Yagmurlu K, Miller EJ, Eschbacher JM, Izadyyazdanabadi M, et al. Intraoperative fluorescence imaging for personalized brain tumor resection: current state and future directions. *Front Surg.* (2016) 3:55. doi: 10.3389/fsurg.2016.00055
7. Eschbacher J, Martirosyan NL, Nakaji P, Sanai N, Preul MC, Smith KA, et al. *In vivo* intraoperative confocal microscopy for real-time histopathological imaging of brain tumors. *J Neurosurg.* (2012) 116:854–60. doi: 10.3171/2011.12.JNS11696
8. Roessler K, Dietrich W, Kitz K. High diagnostic accuracy of cytologic smears of central nervous system tumors. A 15-year experience based on 4,172 patients. *Acta cytologica.* (2002) 46:667–74. doi: 10.1159/000326973
9. Rao S, Rajkumar A, Ehtesham MD, Duvuru P. Challenges in neurosurgical intraoperative consultation. *Neurology India.* (2009) 57:464–8. doi: 10.4103/0028-3886.55598
10. Martirosyan NL, Georges J, Eschbacher JM, Cavalcanti DD, Elhadi AM, Abdelwahab MG, et al. Potential application of a handheld confocal endomicroscope imaging system using a variety of fluorophores in experimental gliomas and normal brain. *Neurosurg Focus.* (2014) 36:E16. doi: 10.3171/2013.11.FOCUS13486
11. Foersch S, Heimann A, Ayyad A, Spoden GA, Florin L, Mpoukouvalas K, et al. Confocal laser endomicroscopy for diagnosis and histomorphologic imaging of brain tumors *in vivo*. *PLoS ONE.* (2012) 7:e41760. doi: 10.1371/journal.pone.0041760
12. Park JC, Park Y, Kim HK, Jo JH, Park CH, Kim EH, et al. Probe-based confocal laser endomicroscopy in the margin delineation of early gastric cancer for endoscopic submucosal dissection. *J Gastroenterol Hepatol.* (2017) 32:1046–54. doi: 10.1111/jgh.13635
13. Ammirati M, Vick N, Liao YL, Ciric I, Mikhael M. Effect of the extent of surgical resection on survival and quality of life in patients with supratentorial glioblastomas and anaplastic astrocytomas. *Neurosurgery.* (1987) 21:201–6.
14. Devaux BC, O'Fallon JR, Kelly PJ. Resection, biopsy, and survival in malignant glial neoplasms. A retrospective study of clinical parameters, therapy, and outcome. *J Neurosurg.* (1993) 78:767–75.
15. Lacroix M, Abi-Said D, Fourney DR, Gokaslan ZL, Shi W, DeMonte F, et al. A multivariate analysis of 416 patients with glioblastoma multiforme: prognosis, extent of resection, and survival. *J Neurosurg.* (2001) 95:190–8. doi: 10.3171/jns.2001.95.2.0190
16. Nitta T, Sato K. Prognostic implications of the extent of surgical resection in patients with intracranial malignant gliomas. *Cancer.* (1995) 75:2727–31.
17. Rostomily RC, Spence AM, Duong D, McCormick K, Bland M, Berger MS. Multimodality management of recurrent adult malignant gliomas: results of a phase II multiagent chemotherapy study and analysis of cytoreductive surgery. *Neurosurgery.* (1994) 35:378–88; discussion: 88.
18. Wood JR, Green SB, Shapiro WR. The prognostic importance of tumor size in malignant gliomas: a computed tomographic scan study by the Brain Tumor Cooperative Group. *J Clin Oncol.* (1988) 6:338–43.
19. Pavlov V, Meyronet D, Meyer-Bisch V, Armoiry X, Pikul B, Dumot C, et al. Intraoperative probe-based confocal laser endomicroscopy in surgery and stereotactic biopsy of low-grade and high-grade gliomas: a feasibility study in humans. *Neurosurgery.* (2016) 79:604–12. doi: 10.1227/NEU.0000000000001365
20. Charalampaki P, Javed M, Daali S, Heiroth HJ, Igressa A, Weber F. Confocal laser endomicroscopy for real-time histomorphological diagnosis: our clinical experience with 150 brain and spinal tumor cases. *Neurosurgery.* (2015) 62(Suppl. 1):171–6. doi: 10.1227/NEU.0000000000000805
21. Belykh E, Cavallo C, Gandhi S, Zhao X, Veljanoski D, Izady Yazdanabadi M, et al. Utilization of intraoperative confocal laser endomicroscopy in brain tumor surgery. *J Neurosurg Sci.* (2018) 62:704–17. doi: 10.23736/S0390-5616.18.04553-8
22. Belykh EG, Zhao X, Cavallo C, Bohl MA, Yagmurlu K, Aklinski JL, et al. Laboratory evaluation of a robotic operative microscope - visualization platform for neurosurgery. *Cureus.* (2018)10:e3072. doi: 10.7759/cureus.3072.
23. Fenton KE, Martirosyan NL, Abdelwahab MG, Coons SW, Preul MC, Scheck AC. *In vivo* visualization of GL261-luc2 mouse glioma cells by use of Alexa Fluor-labeled TRP-2 antibodies. *Neurosurg Focus.* (2014) 36:E12. doi: 10.3171/2013.12.FOCUS13488
24. Sankar T, Delaney PM, Ryan RW, Eschbacher J, Abdelwahab M, Nakaji P, et al. Miniaturized handheld confocal microscopy for neurosurgery: results in an experimental glioblastoma model. *Neurosurgery.* (2010) 66:410–7; discussion: 7–8. doi: 10.1227/01.NEU.0000365772.66324.6F
25. Sanai N, Snyder LA, Honea NJ, Coons SW, Eschbacher JM, Smith KA, et al. Intraoperative confocal microscopy in the visualization of 5-aminolevulinic acid fluorescence in low-grade gliomas. *J Neurosurg.* (2011) 115:740–8. doi: 10.3171/2011.6.JNS11252
26. Abdelwahab MG, Sankar T, Preul MC, Scheck AC. Intracranial implantation with subsequent 3D *in vivo* bioluminescent imaging of murine gliomas. *J Vis Exp.* (2011) 57:e3403. doi: 10.3791/3403
27. Swanson KI, Clark PA, Zhang RR, Kandela IK, Farhoud M, Weichert JP, et al. Fluorescent cancer-selective alkylphosphocholine analogs for intraoperative glioma detection. *Neurosurgery.* (2015) 76:115–23; discussion: 23–4. doi: 10.1227/NEU.0000000000000622
28. Cho HR, Kim DH, Kim D, Doble P, Bishop D, Hare D, et al. Malignant glioma: MR imaging by using 5-aminolevulinic acid in an animal model. *Radiology* (2014) 272:720–30. doi: 10.1148/radiol.14131459
29. Fisher CJ, Niu C, Foltz W, Chen Y, Sidorova-Darmos E, Eubanks JH, et al. ALA-PpIX mediated photodynamic therapy of malignant gliomas augmented by hypothermia. *PLoS ONE.* (2017) 12:e0181654. doi: 10.1371/journal.pone.0181654
30. Diaz RJ, Dios RR, Hattab EM, Burrell K, Rakopoulos P, Sabha N, et al. Study of the biodistribution of fluorescein in glioma-infiltrated mouse brain and histopathological correlation of intraoperative findings in high-grade

gliomas resected under fluorescein fluorescence guidance. *J Neurosurg.* (2015) 122:1360–9. doi: 10.3171/2015.2.JNS132507

31. Folaron M, Strawbridge R, Samkoe KS, Filan C, Roberts DW, Davis SC. Elucidating the kinetics of sodium fluorescein for fluorescence-guided surgery of glioma. *J Neurosurg.* (2018) 1–11. doi: 10.3171/2018.4.JNS172644
32. Belykh E, Miller EJ, Patel AA, Yazdanabadi MI, Martirosyan NL, Yagmurlu K, et al. Diagnostic accuracy of a confocal laser endomicroscope for *in vivo* differentiation between normal injured and tumor tissue during fluorescein-guided glioma resection: laboratory investigation. *World Neurosurg.* (2018) 115:e337–48. doi: 10.1016/j.wneu.2018.04.048
33. Schindelin J, Arganda-Carreras I, Frise E, Kaynig V, Longair M, Pietzsch T, et al. Fiji: an open-source platform for biological-image analysis. *Nat Methods* (2012) 9:676–82. doi: 10.1038/nmeth.2019
34. Belykh E, Patel AA, Miller EJ, Bozkurt B, Yağmurlu K, Woolf EC, et al. Probe-based three-dimensional confocal laser endomicroscopy of brain tumors: technical note. *Cancer Manage Res.* (2018) 10:3109–23. doi: 10.2147/cmar.s165980.
35. Croce AC, Bottiroli G. Autofluorescence spectroscopy and imaging: a tool for biomedical research and diagnosis. *Eur J Histochem.* (2014) 58:2461. doi: 10.4081/ejh.2014.2461
36. Belykh E, Patel AA, Miller EJ, Bozkurt B, Yagmurlu K, Woolf EC, et al. Probe-based three-dimensional confocal laser endomicroscopy of brain tumors: technical note. *Cancer Manag Res.* (2018) 10:3109–23. doi: 10.2147/CMAR.S165980
37. Goetz M, Thomas S, Heimann A, Delaney P, Schneider C, Relle M, et al. Dynamic *in vivo* imaging of microvasculature and perfusion by miniaturized confocal laser microscopy. *Eur Surg Res.* (2008) 41:290–7. doi: 10.1159/000148242
38. Norman MU, Hulliger S, Colarusso P, Kubes P. Multichannel fluorescence spinning disk microscopy reveals early endogenous CD4 T cell recruitment in contact sensitivity via complement. *J Immunol.* (2008) 180:510–21. doi: 10.4049/jimmunol.180.1.510
39. Belykh E, Cavallo C, Zhao X, Lawton MT, Nakaji P, Preul MC. 312 Intraoperative imaging of cerebral vasculature and blood flow using confocal laser endomicroscopy: new perspectives in precise real-time brain fluorescence microimaging. *Neurosurgery.* (2018) 65(Suppl. 1):126–7. doi: 10.1093/neuros/nyy303.312
40. Belykh E, Miller EJ, Hu D, Martirosyan NL, Woolf EC, Scheck AC, et al. Scanning fiber endoscope improves detection of 5-aminolevulinic acid-induced protoporphyrin IX fluorescence at the boundary of infiltrative glioma. *World Neurosurg.* (2018) 113:e51–69. doi: 10.1016/j.wneu.2018.01.151
41. Potapov AA, Goryaynov SA, Okhlopkov VA, Shishkina LV, Loschenov VB, Savelieva TA, et al. Laser biospectroscopy and 5-ALA fluorescence navigation as a helpful tool in the meningioma resection. *Neurosurg Rev.* (2016) 39:437–47. doi: 10.1007/s10143-015-0697-0
42. Potapov AA, Goriainov SA, Loshchenov VB, Savel'eva TA, Gavrilov AG, Okhlopkov VA, et al. [Intraoperative combined spectroscopy (optical biopsy) of cerebral gliomas]. *Zh Vopr Neirokhir Im N N Burdenko.* (2013) 77:3–10.
43. Stummer W, Tonn JC, Goetz C, Ullrich W, Stepp H, Bink A, et al. 5-Aminolevulinic acid-derived tumor fluorescence: the diagnostic accuracy of visible fluorescence qualities as corroborated by spectrometry and histology and postoperative imaging. *Neurosurgery.* (2014) 74:310–9; discussion: 9–20. doi: 10.1227/NEU.0000000000000267
44. Wei L, Chen Y, Yin C, Borwege S, Sanai N, Liu JTC. Optical-sectioning microscopy of protoporphyrin IX fluorescence in human gliomas: standardization and quantitative comparison with histology. *J Biomed Opt.* (2017) 22:46005. doi: 10.1117/1.JBO.22.4.046005
45. Martirosyan NL, Georges J, Eschbacher JM, Belykh E, Carotenuto A, Spetzler RF, et al. Confocal scanning microscopy provides rapid, detailed intraoperative histological assessment of brain neoplasms: experience with 106 cases. *Clin Neurol Neurosurg.* (2018) 169:21–8. doi: 10.1016/j.clineuro.2018.03.015
46. Eschbacher JM, Georges JF, Belykh E, Yazdanabadi MI, Martirosyan NL, Szeto E, et al. Immediate label-free *ex vivo* evaluation of human brain tumor biopsies with confocal reflectance microscopy. *J Neuropathol Exp Neurol.* (2017) 76:1008–22. doi: 10.1093/jnen/nlx089
47. Becker V, Vercauteren T, von Weyhern CH, Prinz C, Schmid RM, Meining A. High-resolution miniprobe-based confocal microscopy in combination with video mosaicing (with video). *Gastrointest Endosc.* (2007) 66:1001–7. doi: 10.1016/j.gie.2007.04.015
48. Schebesch KM, Brawanski A, Hohenberger C, Hohne J. Fluorescein sodium-guided surgery of malignant brain tumors: history, current concepts, and future project. *Turk Neurosurg.* (2016) 26:185–94. doi: 10.5137/1019-5149.JTN.16952-16.0
49. Kamen A, Sun S, Wan S, Kluckner S, Chen T, Gigler AM, et al. Automatic tissue differentiation based on confocal endomicroscopic images for intraoperative guidance in neurosurgery. *Biomed Res Int.* (2016) 2016:6183218. doi: 10.1155/2016/6183218
50. Izadyyazdanabadi M, Belykh E, Mooney MA, Eschbacher JM, Nakaji P, Yang Y, et al. Prospects for theranostics in neurosurgical imaging: empowering confocal laser endomicroscopy diagnostics via deep learning. *Front Oncol.* (2018) 8:240. doi: 10.3389/fonc.2018.00240
51. Izadyyazdanabadi M, Belykh E, Cavallo C, Zhao X, Gandhi S, Moreira LB, et al. Weakly-supervised learning-based feature localization for confocal laser endomicroscopy glioma images. In: Frangi A, Schnabel J, Davatzikos C, Alberola-López C, Fichtinger G, editors. *Medical Image Computing and Computer Assisted Intervention – MICCAI 2018, MICCAI 2018. Lecture Notes in Computer Science.* Vol 11071. Springer: Cham. (2018) p. 300–8. doi: 10.1007/978-3-030-00934-2_34

8

The Use of Spectroscopy Handheld Tools in Brain Tumor Surgery

Nikita Lakomkin [1,2] *and Constantinos G. Hadjipanayis* [1,2*]

[1] *Department of Neurosurgery, Mount Sinai Health System, Icahn School of Medicine at Mount Sinai, New York, NY, United States,* [2] *Department of Neurosurgery, Mount Sinai Health System, Icahn School of Medicine, New York, NY, United States*

Correspondence:
Constantinos G. Hadjipanayis
constantinos.hadjipanayis@mountsinai.org

The fundamental principle in the operative treatment of brain tumors involves achieving maximal safe resection in order to improve postoperative outcomes. At present, challenges in visualizing microscopic disease and residual tumor remain an impediment to complete tumor removal. Spectroscopic tools have the theoretical advantage of accurate tissue identification, coupled with the potential for manual intraoperative adjustments to improve visualization of remaining tumor tissue that would otherwise be difficult to detect. The current evidence and techniques for handheld spectroscopic tools in surgical neuro-oncology are explored here.

Keywords: handheld technologies, gliomas, fluorescence-guided surgery, brain tumors, 5-ALA = 5-aminolevulinic acid, Raman spectroscopy

INTRODUCTION

The fundamental goal in the surgical treatment of brain tumors is achieving the greatest possible extent of resection while minimizing injury to surrounding pathways present in the adjacent brain. Indeed, numerous studies in the literature have demonstrated that the proportion of tumor removed is significantly associated with key postoperative outcome metrics, including overall survival (OS) and progression-free survival (PFS) (1–3). Despite this, however, complete tumor resection remains challenging due to the presence of microscopic disease and infiltrative tumor tissue that is difficult to visually differentiate from the surrounding brain. As such, numerous tools have been developed, for both pre- and intra-operative use [e.g., neuronavigation and intraoperative MRI (iMRI)], in order to assist in the identification and removal of neoplastic tissue (4). More sophisticated MRI techniques, such as whole brain magnetic resonance spectroscopic imaging (MRSI), has allowed for more precise visualization of tumor than would otherwise be possible with standard MRI (5). Multiple studies have highlighted the fact that microscopic involvement of high-grade gliomas (HGGs) extends well-beyond the contrast-enhancing lesion visible on T2-weighted MRI (5, 6). Other techniques, such as neurosurgical virtual reality and simulation have facilitated preoperative visualization and planning (7). Although these instruments have demonstrated utility, intraoperative retraction and tumor resection often result in brain shift, making it challenging to assess the extent of resection in real time. Also, non-specific enhancement after iMRI may be confused with residual tumor. Fluorescence-guided surgery using 5-aminolevulinic acid (5-ALA) has been a crucial addition to the neurosurgeon's toolkit, allowing for direct fluorescence visualization of HGGs using wide-field surgical microscopy (8). However, the infiltrative margin of HGGs and World Health Organization (WHO) grade II low grade gliomas (LGGs) have remained challenging to visualize, since sufficient levels of fluorescence often cannot be detected using traditionally employed visualization technologies (9). Handheld tools were developed as an adjunct to intraoperative resection, under the premise that real-time use and the ability to adjust the angle of the instrument could facilitate detection of remaining tumor at the time of surgery. Among the most studied techniques has been the use of handheld Raman spectroscopy in the identification of cancer cells during surgery. Other devices aimed at improving visualization in fluorescence guidance surgery have recently been developed. The purpose of this review is to examine the technique and evidence for the utility of handheld spectroscopy tools in neuro-oncologic surgery.

TECHNIQUE

Raman Spectroscopic Probes

Handheld Raman spectroscopic probes harness the traditionally employed Raman spectroscopic technique described decades ago (10). Monochromatic light from a laser is used to shine on an object of interest, resulting in a change in vibrational energy states, which can be detected as electromagnetic radiation that is filtered through a monochromator (11). This results in a molecular fingerprint that can be subsequently harnessed to differentiate various tissue types (12). Neoplastic cells, for instance, have a molecular composition that is distinct from normal brain parenchyma and thus allows for their identification during surgery (13, 14). Glioblastoma (GBM) has been shown to exhibit a decreased lipid band and an increased protein band, while cholesterol bands were found to be absent in metastatic brain lesions (15). One specific advantage of this technique is that water molecules do not interfere with the Raman scattering, thereby increasing its utility in surgical applications. In the operating room, the laser/collection cones, lens, and filter can be combined into a hand-held probe that is then connected to a camera and spectrometer device. This probe can be used intraoperatively during resection in order to both identify tumor cells outside of contrast-enhancing areas on anatomic MRI as well as residual tumor following debulking and resection (16). Unlike the MRI neuronavigation, virtual reality, and other imaging techniques, the handheld probe allows the surgeon to make intraoperative adjustments in terms of positioning and angles following changes in the relative location of anatomic structures during surgery.

5-ALA Fluorescence Visualization

5-ALA is an oral pro-drug and the preoperative administration of this agent results in the accumulation of the fluorescent metabolite protoporphyrin IX in neoplastic lesions, which can be visualized during surgery (17, 18). This is accomplished via excitation of protoporphyrin IX-rich tissue with blue 440 nanometer wavelength light, resulting in the emission of a violet-colored signal (19). Improved visualization of tumors consequently allows for a greater extent of resection than would otherwise be possible under white light. Numerous randomized, controlled trials have demonstrated a benefit to patient survival using this agent, resulting in it gaining recent FDA approval for the treatment of suspected HGGs in the United States (20–22).

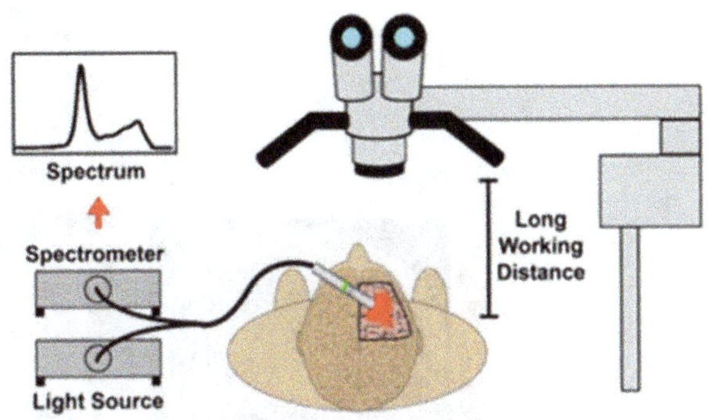

FIGURE 1 | A schematic depicting the intraoperative use of a handheld spectroscopic probe in order to quantify relative protoporphyrin IX levels in various tissues [With permission from Kairdolf et al. (25)].

Despite this, however, the evidence for its utility in the treatment of LGGs is less robust, due to the difficulty in achieving adequate fluorescent signal using wide-field microscopic illumination from a long working distance (9, 23). In addition, visualization of the infiltrative tumor margin becomes more difficult with fluorescence due to the lower number of tumor cells residing away from the tumor bulk. Handheld probes offer distinct advantages in visualizing these tumors, due to both the ability to place the instrument in close proximity to the tissue, as well as potentially generate a precise, quantitative measurement of protoporphyrin IX concentrations (24, 25). These techniques involve utilizing a handheld probe coupled to spectrometer that can be manipulated within the intraoperative field (**Figure 1**) (25, 26).

EVIDENCE

Raman Spectroscopy

Basic Science

An array of *ex-vivo* and animal model studies have demonstrated the value of handheld Raman spectroscopy in differentiating tumor from normal brain tissue. Ji et al. examined the ability of Raman microscopy to discriminate tumor samples from 22 biopsy specimens, and found that Raman spectroscopy detected tumor infiltration in near-perfect agreement with hematoxylin and eosin (H&E) staining (27). The authors concluded that the sensitivity and specificity of the technique was 97.5 and 98.5%, respectively. Similarly, Kalkanis et al. utilized a training set and subsequent validation series in order to employ Raman spectroscopy in distinguishing GBM from gray matter and necrosis. The authors reported 99.6 and 97.8% accuracy in the training and validation cohorts, respectively (28). An *in-vitro* study by Aguiar et al. revealed a sensitivity of 97.4% and a specificity of 100% in the diagnosis of GBM, medulloblastoma, and meningioma (29).

Other studies have revolved around the identification of important biomarkers that could be employed in distinguishing various tumor types. For instance, Zhou et al. demonstrated the utility of Raman spectroscopy in differentiating malignant tissue

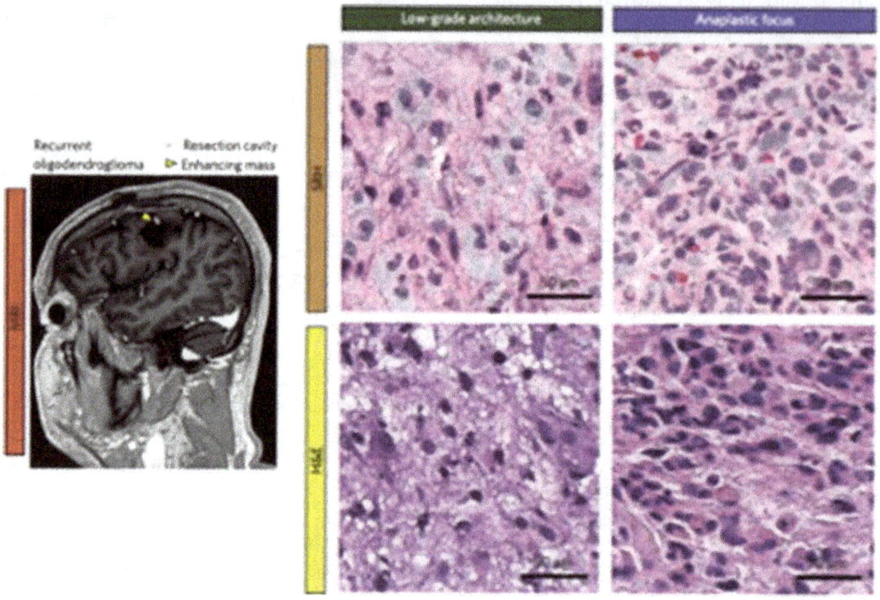

FIGURE 2 | Depiction of Raman-stimulated histology slides alongside traditional haematoxylin and eosin for a patient with a history of recurrent oligodendroglioma [With permission from Orringer et al. (31)].

in 87 samples, revealing the presence of peaks corresponding to lactic acid and ATP in certain tumor tissues when compared to controls (30). These initiatives have been harnessed by investigations focused on their clinical application. Orringer et al. leveraged portable Raman spectroscopy to not only create virtual H&E-stained slides, but to create an algorithm that predicts brain tumor subtypes with 90% accuracy (31). A side-by-side comparison of images generated via Raman-stimulated histology and traditional haematoxylin and eosin staining is depicted in **Figure 2**. These techniques have already been replicated in the pediatric population, where Hollon et al. created a Raman spectroscopic-based algorithm that had near-perfect histologic concordance and could differentiate low and high-grade tumors with 100% accuracy (32). These findings demonstrate the substantial potential of algorithm-driven, handheld spectroscopy tools in providing valuable real-time data that could alter clinical management.

Clinical Studies

Comparatively few studies have examined the feasibility and utility of handheld Raman spectroscopy using real-time, *in-vivo* experimental design. Jermyn et al. employed a handheld probe in 17 patients with grade 2-4 gliomas and compared imaging findings with obtained biopsy specimens (33). The authors concluded that intraoperative Raman imaging facilitated the detection of cancer cells with an accuracy of 92%, compared to 73% using bright microscopy and MRI. The sensitivity and specificity in the differentiation of neoplasia from normal brain parenchyma were 93 and 91%, respectively. Desroches et al. developed a handheld Raman spectroscopy system and demonstrated its preliminary use in a swine brain biopsy model, followed by a human validation study involving 19 grade 2-4 glioma patients. The authors concluded that the handheld spectroscopy was able to detect malignancy during surgery with a sensitivity and specificity of 80 and 90%, respectively (34). Characteristics of selected studies on the role of Raman in diagnosing different types of brain tumors are presented in **Table 1**.

Future Multimodal Techniques

Much of the recent literature on Raman spectroscopy in neurosurgical oncology revolves around the coupling of this technique to other, novel modalities in order to facilitate visualization. For instance, Neuschmelting et al. examined a combined approach of surface-enhanced Raman scattering and multispectral optoacoustic tomography in the detection of GBM cells in mouse brains. The authors reported that this new model exhibited a highly sensitive surface detection of infiltrating GBMs and could be transferrable to other animal models and potentially human trials (35). Meanwhile, Karabeber et al. demonstrated that the use of surface-enhanced Raman nanoparticles in the guidance of mouse GBM resection resulted in greater removal of residual tumor when compared to the use of white light alone (36). Jermyn et al. employed a combined, multimodal spectroscopic technique that incorporated fluorescence spectroscopy, diffuse reflectance spectroscopy, and Raman spectroscopy. The authors described high rates of accuracy, sensitivity, and specificity in differentiating brain, lung, colon, and skin malignancies *in situ* (37).

Visualization in Fluorescence-Guided Surgeries

Basic Science

Numerous laboratory investigations have examined the feasibility and efficacy of handheld probes in detecting protoporphyrin IX. Kim et al. used a handheld, fiberoptic

TABLE 1 | Characteristics of selected studies reporting on the utility of Raman spectroscopy in tumor.

References	Journal	Number of samples	Tumor histology	Relevant outcome metric	Rate	Notes
CLINICAL AND BASIC SCIENCE STUDIES						
Ji et al. (27)	Sci Transl Med	22	Gliomas (both LGG and HGG)	Tumor infiltration (compared to H&E)	Sensitivity = 97.5% Specificity = 98.5%	–
Kalkanis et al. (28)	J Neurooncol	40	GBM	Differentiation of GBM from gray matter and necrosis	99.6 and 97.8% accuracy in training and validation cohorts, respectively	Utilized a training set with subsequent validation series
Aguiar et al. (29)	Photomed Laser Surg	172	GBM, medulloblastoma, meningioma	Diagnosis of tumor types	Sensitivity = 97.4% Specificity = 100%	–
Orringer et al. (31)	Nat Biomed Eng	30	Gliomas (both LGG and HGG) + meningioma, lymphoma, medulloblastoma, and metastases	Prediction of brain tumor subtypes (compared to H&E)	>92% accuracy	–
Hollon et al. (32)	Cancer Res	25	All tumor types	Prediction of brain tumor subtypes (compared to H&E)	92–96% accuracy	Pediatric brain tumor patients
Jermyn et al. (33)	Sci Transl Med	161	Gliomas (WHO grades II-IV)	Detection of malignancy (vs. bright microscopy and MRI)	Sensitivity = 93% Specificity = 91%	*In-vivo* experimental design
Desroches et al. (34)	Sci Rep	280	Gliomas (WHO grades II-IV)	Detection of malignancy (compared to H&E)	Sensitivity = 80% Specificity = 90%	Authors used handheld probe in swine brain biopsy model first, followed by human validation study

GBM, Glioblastoma multiforme; HGG, High grade glioma; LGG, Low grade glioma; MRI, Magnetic resonance imaging; WHO, World Health Organization.

probe in order to quantify the fluorescence signal in *ex vivo* mouse brain tumors (38). They subsequently validated their technique using an *in vivo* rabbit brain tumor surgery model and were able to accurately differentiate tumor tissue from normal brain parenchyma. Cornelius et al. employed this same tool in order to examine its ability to differentiate different tumor types in humans (39). The authors concluded that the probe was a very sensitive tool in detecting 5-ALA-based fluorescence among 17 tumor biopsies, including differentiating between GBM and meningioma samples with the same precision as a laboratory spectrometer. Kairdolf et al. employed a low-cost hand-held spectroscopic instrument in order to compare the sensitivity of the handheld device with traditional surgical microscopes (25). They found that the handheld tool was, at a minimum, 3 times more sensitive and demonstrated strong specificity in differentiating tumor cells from normal brain tissue.

Clinical Studies

These handheld visualization devices have also been studied to assess their use and efficacy in the operating room. Haj-Hosseini et al. employed a handheld spectroscopic tool in order to make intraoperative measurements of white, gray, and known tumor tissue from patients undergoing GBM resection under 5-ALA fluorescence (26). The authors demonstrated the feasibility of this probe to accurately detect protoporphyrin IX fluorescence at the tumor margins *in vivo*. Richter et al. performed a study to directly compare the sensitivity of a hand-held fluorescence probe with fluorescence-guided microscopy in 16 patients undergoing resection of HGGs using 5-ALA. The authors highlighted that they were able to not only successfully integrate the tool into the operative routine, but that the handheld probe was superior to the microscope in sensitivity and detected additional tumor foci after the initial debulking using fluorescence-guided microscopy (40). The intraoperative use of the hand-held fluorescence probe is highlighted in **Figure 3**. These techniques have also been studied in other tumor types. Valdes et al. used a handheld probe tip in the intraoperative resection of low-grade gliomas, meningiomas, metastatic tumors, and GBM in order to compare quantitative fluorescence spectra across tumor types (41). They concluded that there was a significant difference in the quantitative measurements of protoporphyrin IX concentrations for all tumor groups when compared to normal brain tissue, as well as high sensitivity when compared to conventional fluorescence measurements.

DISCUSSION

Tumor Identification Using Raman Probes

Overall, the use of handheld Raman spectroscopic imaging as an adjunct to neurosurgical resection is a promising development in brain tumor treatment and has been corroborated in a variety of clinical and basic science literature. The unique spectra allow for the differentiation of various tissue types. Numerous investigations have identified key biomarkers that can be employed to not only discriminate between tumor and normal parenchyma, but between various tumor types for both intra- and extra-axial lesions. Zhou et al., for instance, reported a detailed

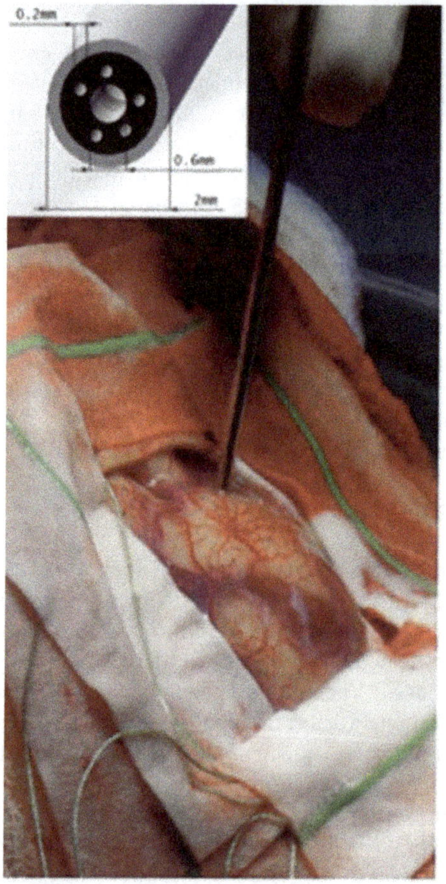

FIGURE 3 | Intraoperative placement of the hand-held fluorescent probe on the cortical surface [With permission from Richter et al. (40)].

analysis of Raman spectra for an array of tumors, including GBM, acoustic neuroma, pituitary adenoma, and meningioma (42). This is turn has been used in several studies to create predictive algorithms with the capability to correctly predict histologic subtype with >90% accuracy (31, 32). The strong predictive capacity of this modality makes it useful in both the diagnosis and subsequent operative treatment of brain tumors.

Intraoperative Advantages

Although numerous other modalities facilitate improved preoperative visualization of tumor, handheld spectroscopic tools offer the advantage of not only strong discriminatory capacity based on molecular footprint, but the ability to make physical adjustments intraoperatively. Unlike other visualization techniques, including intraoperative MRI, handheld probes can be angled away in order to inspect portions of the resection cavity that may not otherwise be visible. This may facilitate the identification of Raman-positive foci and removal of additional tumor. Karabeber et al. performed a study involving the surgical resection of GBM in mice, comparing resection with light microscopy, Raman microscopy, and hand-held Raman scanning (36). The authors demonstrated that the hand-held device was associated with a greater extent of resection, and noted several instances where the hand-held tool detected foci that were missed using microscopy, including the presence of tumor within the right lateral ventricle. This increased flexibility of hand-held devices offers the theoretical advantage of a potential combined therapy, where intraoperative Raman identification may be used alongside 5-ALA fluorescence-guided resection or conventional microscopic imaging. Although the application of 5-ALA has been shown to alter the Raman spectra of bladder tissues, this interference may be improved via fluorescence-subtraction algorithms, making a dual approach potentially viable *in-vivo* (43). Further studies are needed to explore the utility of combined modalities in the resection of brain tumors.

5-ALA Visualization

Other handheld tools have been developed in order to facilitate both visualization and quantification of protoporphyrin IX concentrations for patients undergoing tumor resection with 5-ALA. While the detection of fluorescence using traditional wide-field microscopy has been challenging for LGGs and other tumor types, handheld probes offer several advantages that can improve the utility of 5-ALA for these tumors. First, the ability to place these probes in close proximity to the tissue helps ameliorate the light scatter and suboptimal angle between traditionally employed microscopes and the resection bed (9). Second, the tools can be equipped with spectroscopic instrumentation that allows for the quantification of metabolite concentration, rather than relying on the subjective intraoperative assessment of visualized fluorescent signal (23). These advantages have been demonstrated in numerous studies highlighting the feasibility and efficacy of handheld probes *in vivo*. The ability to directly quantify fluorescence measurements in LGGs, meningiomas, and metastatic lesions, as well as the ability to intraoperatively distinguish them from brain parenchyma may increase the role of 5-ALA for these tumor types in the near future (41).

Clinical Relevance

There is substantial literature reporting the relationship between the extent of resection and subsequent postoperative outcomes in patients with brain tumors (1–3). Identification of microscopic disease and residual tumor remains the primary challenge in neuro-oncology. As such, all tools that facilitate the intraoperative visualization of lesions have the potential to provide clinical benefit to patients. Despite this, however, there is a dearth of literature examining the relationship between the use of spectroscopic handheld tools and improved postoperative clinical endpoints. Additional studies are needed to examine the association between intraoperative Raman spectroscopy, protoporphyrin IX quantification tools, extent of resection, and OS/PFS.

CONCLUSIONS

There is significant evidence demonstrating the utility of Raman spectroscopic imaging in identifying areas of malignancy in both human and animal specimens. Several studies have highlighted the use of concomitant algorithms in accurately diagnosing histologic tumor subtype and the feasibility of using handheld spectroscopy tools in the operative setting. In addition, numerous studies have demonstrated the efficacy of handheld probes in the operative quantification of protoporphyrin IX levels for patients undergoing 5-ALA fluorescence-guided resection. Further studies exploring the relationship between *in-vivo* spectroscopic use, extent of resection, and postoperative survival are needed to better assess the impact of these tools on patient outcomes.

AUTHOR CONTRIBUTIONS

All authors listed have made a substantial, direct and intellectual contribution to the work, and approved it for publication.

REFERENCES

1. Brown TJ, Brennan MC, Li M, Church EW, Brandmeir NJ, Rakszawski KL, et al. Association of the extent of resection with survival in glioblastoma: a systematic review and meta-analysis. *JAMA Oncol.* (2016) 2:1460–9. doi: 10.1001/jamaoncol.2016.1373
2. Xia L, Fang C, Chen G, Sun C. Relationship between the extent of resection and the survival of patients with low-grade gliomas: a systematic review and meta-analysis. *BMC Cancer.* (2018) 18:48. doi: 10.1186/s12885-017-3909-x
3. Kuhnt D, Becker A, Ganslandt O, Bauer M, Buchfelder M, Nimsky C. Correlation of the extent of tumor volume resection and patient survival in surgery of glioblastoma multiforme with high-field intraoperative MRI guidance. *Neuro Oncol.* (2011) 13:1339–48. doi: 10.1093/neuonc/nor133
4. Schulder M, Carmel PW. Intraoperative magnetic resonance imaging: impact on brain tumor surgery. *Cancer Control J Moffitt Cancer Cent.* (2003) 10:115–24. doi: 10.1177/107327480301000203
5. Cordova JS, Shu HK, Liang Z, Gurbani SS, Cooper LA, Holder CA, et al. Whole-brain spectroscopic MRI biomarkers identify infiltrating margins in glioblastoma patients. *Neuro Oncol.* (2016) 18:1180–9. doi: 10.1093/neuonc/now036
6. Cordova JS, Gurbani SS, Olson JJ, Liang Z, Cooper LA, Shu HG, et al. A systematic pipeline for the objective comparison of whole-brain spectroscopic MRI with histology in biopsy specimens from grade III glioma. *Tomogr Ann Arbor Mich.* (2016) 2:106–16. doi: 10.18383/j.tom.2016.00136
7. Chan S, Conti F, Salisbury K, Blevins NH. Virtual reality simulation in neurosurgery: technologies and evolution. *Neurosurgery.* (2013) 72 (Suppl 1):154–64. doi: 10.1227/NEU.0b013e3182750d26
8. Hadjipanayis CG, Widhalm G, Stummer W. What is the surgical benefit of utilizing 5-ALA for fluorescence-guided surgery of malignant gliomas? *Neurosurgery.* (2015) 77:663–73. doi: 10.1227/NEU.0000000000000929
9. Wei L, Roberts DW, Sanai N, Liu JTC. Visualization technologies for 5-ALA-based fluorescence-guided surgeries. *J Neurooncol.* (2018) 141:495–505. doi: 10.1007/s11060-018-03077-9
10. Raman CV. Part II.—The Raman effect. Investigation of molecular structure by light scattering. *Trans Faraday Soc.* (1929) 25:781–92. doi: 10.1039/TF9292500781
11. Downes A, Elfick A. Raman spectroscopy and related techniques in biomedicine. *Sensors.* (2010) 10:1871–89. doi: 10.3390/s100301871
12. Tu Q, Chang C. Diagnostic applications of Raman spectroscopy. *Nanomed Nanotechnol Biol Med.* (2012) 8:545–58. doi: 10.1016/j.nano.2011.09.013
13. Wills H, Kast R, Stewart C, Rabah R, Pandya A, Poulik J, et al.Raman spectroscopy detects and distinguishes neuroblastoma and related tissues in fresh and (banked) frozen specimens. *J Pediatr Surg.* (2009) 44:386–91. doi: 10.1016/j.jpedsurg.2008.10.095
14. Depciuch J, Kaznowska E, Zawlik I, Wojnarowska R, Cholewa M, Heraud P, et al. Application of Raman spectroscopy and infrared spectroscopy in the identification of breast cancer. *Appl Spectrosc.* (2016) 70:251–63. doi: 10.1177/0003702815620127
15. Uckermann O, Galli R, Meinhardt M, Steiner G, Schackert G, Kirsch M. Path-15. optical analysis of human brain tumors by raman spectroscopy. *Neuro Oncol.* (2017) 19(Suppl 6):vi173–vi173. doi: 10.1093/neuonc/nox168.706
16. Jermyn M, Desroches J, Mercier J, St-Arnaud K, Guiot MC, Leblond F, et al. Raman spectroscopy detects distant invasive brain cancer cells centimeters beyond MRI capability in humans. *Biomed Opt Express.* (2016) 7:5129–37. doi: 10.1364/BOE.7.005129
17. Tonn J-C, Stummer W. Fluorescence-guided resection of malignant gliomas using 5-aminolevulinic acid: practical use, risks, and pitfalls. *Clin Neurosurg.* (2008) 55:20–26. Available online at: https://pdfs.semanticscholar.org/29de/0409643ebcdcc768ade61f30ca33d1296026.pdf
18. Lakomkin N, Hadjipanayis CG. Fluorescence-guided surgery for high-grade gliomas. *J Surg Oncol.* (2018) 118:356–61. doi: 10.1002/jso.25154
19. Ferraro N, Barbarite E, Albert TR, Berchmans E, Shah AH, Bregy A, et al. The role of 5-aminolevulinic acid in brain tumor surgery: a systematic review. *Neurosurg Rev.* (2016) 39:545–55. doi: 10.1007/s10143-015-0695-2
20. Stummer W, Pichlmeier U, Meinel T, Wiestler OD, Zanella F, Reulen HJ, et al. Fluorescence-guided surgery with 5-aminolevulinic acid for resection of malignant glioma: a randomised controlled multicentre phase III trial. *Lancet Oncol.* (2006) 7:392–401. doi: 10.1016/S1470-2045(06)70665-9
21. Stummer W, Tonn JC, Mehdorn HM, Nestler U, Franz K, Goetz C, et al. Counterbalancing risks and gains from extended resections in malignant glioma surgery: a supplemental analysis from the randomized 5-aminolevulinic acid glioma resection study. Clinical article. *J Neurosurg.* (2011) 114:613–23. doi: 10.3171/2010.3.JNS097
22. Díez Valle R, Tejada Solis S, Idoate Gastearena MA, García de Eulate R, Domínguez Echávarri P, Aristu Mendiroz J. Surgery guided by 5-aminolevulinic fluorescence in glioblastoma: volumetric analysis of extent of resection in single-center experience. *J Neurooncol.* (2011) 102:105–13. doi: 10.1007/s11060-010-0296-4
23. Belykh E, Martirosyan NL, Yagmurlu K, Miller EJ, Eschbacher JM, Izadyyazdanabadi M, et al. Intraoperative fluorescence imaging for personalized brain tumor resection: current state and future directions. *Front Surg.* (2016) 3:55. doi: 10.3389/fsurg.2016.00055
24. Stummer W, Tonn JC, Goetz C, Ullrich W, Stepp H, Bink A, et al. 5-Aminolevulinic acid-derived tumor fluorescence: the diagnostic accuracy of visible fluorescence qualities as corroborated by spectrometry and histology and postoperative imaging. *Neurosurgery.* (2014) 74:310–9; discussion 319–20. doi: 10.1227/NEU.0000000000000267
25. Kairdolf BA, Bouras A, Kaluzova M, Sharma AK, Wang MD, Hadjipanayis CG, et al. Intraoperative spectroscopy with ultrahigh sensitivity for image-guided surgery of malignant brain tumors. *Anal Chem.* (2016) 88:858–67. doi: 10.1021/acs.analchem.5b03453
26. Haj-Hosseini N, Richter J, Andersson-Engels S, Wårdell K. Optical touch pointer for fluorescence guided glioblastoma resection using 5-aminolevulinic acid. *Lasers Surg Med.* (2010) 42:9–14. doi: 10.1002/lsm.20868
27. Ji M, Lewis S, Camelo-Piragua S, Ramkissoon SH, Snuderl M, Venneti S, et al. Detection of human brain tumor infiltration with quantitative stimulated Raman scattering microscopy. *Sci Transl Med.* (2015) 7:309ra163. doi: 10.1126/scitranslmed.aab0195
28. Kalkanis SN, Kast RE, Rosenblum ML, Mikkelsen T, Yurgelevic SM, Nelson KM, et al. Raman spectroscopy to distinguish grey matter, necrosis, and glioblastoma multiforme in frozen tissue sections. *J Neurooncol.* (2014) 116:477–85. doi: 10.1007/s11060-013-1326-9
29. Aguiar RP, Silveira L, Falcão ET, Pacheco MTT, Zângaro RA, Pasqualucci CA. Discriminating neoplastic and normal brain tissues *in vitro* through Raman spectroscopy: a principal components analysis classification model. *Photomed Laser Surg.* (2013) 31:595–604. doi: 10.1089/pho.2012.3460
30. Zhou Y, Liu C, Wu B, Zhang C, Yu X, Cheng G, et al. Invited article: molecular biomarkers characterization for human brain glioma grading using

visible resonance Raman spectroscopy. *APL Photonics*. (2018) 3:120802. doi: 10.1063/1.5036637
31. Orringer DA, Pandian B, Niknafs YS, Hollon TC, Boyle J, Lewis S, et al. Rapid intraoperative histology of unprocessed surgical specimens via fibre-laser-based stimulated Raman scattering microscopy. *Nat Biomed Eng*. (2017) 1:0027. doi: 10.1038/s41551-016-0027
32. Hollon TC, Lewis S, Pandian B, Niknafs YS, Garrard MR, Garton H, et al. Rapid intraoperative diagnosis of pediatric brain tumors using stimulated raman histology. *Cancer Res*. (2018) 78:278–89. doi: 10.1158/0008-5472.CAN-17-1974
33. Jermyn M, Mok K, Mercier J, Desroches J, Pichette J, Saint-Arnaud K, et al. Intraoperative brain cancer detection with Raman spectroscopy in humans. *Sci Transl Med*. (2015) 7:274ra19. doi: 10.1126/scitranslmed.aaa2384
34. Desroches J, Jermyn M, Pinto M, Picot F, Tremblay MA, Obaid S, et al. A new method using Raman spectroscopy for *in vivo* targeted brain cancer tissue biopsy. *Sci Rep*. (2018) 8:1792. doi: 10.1038/s41598-018-20233-3
35. Neuschmelting V, Harmsen S, Beziere N, Lockau H, Hsu HT, Huang R, et al. Dual-modality surface-enhanced resonance raman scattering and multispectral optoacoustic tomography nanoparticle approach for brain tumor delineation. *Small*. (2018) 14:e1800740. doi: 10.1002/smll.201800740
36. Karabeber H, Huang R, Iacono P, Samii JM, Pitter K, Holland EC, et al. Guiding brain tumor resection using surface-enhanced raman scattering nanoparticles and a hand-held raman scanner. *ACS Nano*. (2014) 8:9755–66. doi: 10.1021/nn503948b
37. Jermyn M, Mercier J, Aubertin K, Desroches J, Urmey K, Karamchandiani J, et al. Highly accurate detection of cancer *in situ* with intraoperative, label-free, multimodal optical spectroscopy. *Cancer Res*. (2017) 77:3942–50. doi: 10.1158/0008-5472.CAN-17-0668
38. Kim A, Khurana M, Moriyama Y, Wilson BC. Quantification of *in vivo* fluorescence decoupled from the effects of tissue optical properties using fiber-optic spectroscopy measurements. *J Biomed Opt*. (2010) 15:067006. doi: 10.1117/1.3523616
39. Cornelius JF, Placke JM, Knipps J, Fischer I, Kamp M, Steiger HJ. Minispectrometer with handheld probe for 5-ALA based fluorescence-guided surgery of brain tumors: preliminary study for clinical applications. *Photodiagn Photodyn Ther*. (2017) 17:147–53. doi: 10.1016/j.pdpdt.2016.12.007
40. Richter JCO, Haj-Hosseini N, Hallbeck M, Wårdell K. Combination of hand-held probe and microscopy for fluorescence guided surgery in the brain tumor marginal zone. *Photodiagn Photodyn Ther*. (2017) 18:185–92. doi: 10.1016/j.pdpdt.2017.01.188
41. Valdés PA, Leblond F, Kim A, Harris BT, Wilson BC, Fan X, et al. Quantitative fluorescence in intracranial tumor: implications for ALA-induced PpIX as an intraoperative biomarker. *J Neurosurg*. (2011) 115:11. doi: 10.3171/2011.2.JNS101451
42. Zhou Y, Liu CH, Sun Y, Pu Y, Boydston-White S, Liu Y, et al. Human brain cancer studied by resonance Raman spectroscopy. *J Biomed Opt*. (2012) 17:116021. doi: 10.1117/1.JBO.17.11.116021
43. Grimbergen MCM, van Swol CFP, van Moorselaar RJA, Uff J, Mahadevan-Jansen A, Stone N. Raman spectroscopy of bladder tissue in the presence of 5-aminolevulinic acid. *J Photochem Photobiol B*. (2009) 95:170–6. doi: 10.1016/j.jphotobiol.2009.03.002

9

Fluorescence Diagnosis in Neurooncology: Retrospective Analysis of 653 Cases

Sergey A. Goryaynov[1], Vladimir A. Okhlopkov[1], Denis A. Golbin[1], Konstantin A. Chernyshov[2], Dmitrij V. Svistov[3], Boris V. Martynov[3], Alexandr V. Kim[4], Vadim A. Byvaltsev[5,6], Galina V. Pavlova[7], Artem Batalov[1], Nikolay A. Konovalov[1], Petr V. Zelenkov[1], Victor B. Loschenov[8,9] and Alexandr A. Potapov[1]*

[1] N. N. Burdenko National Medical Research Center of Neurosurgery of the Ministry of Health of the Russian Federation, Moscow, Russia, [2] I. M. Sechenov First Moscow State Medical University of the Ministry of Health of the Russian Federation, Moscow, Russia, [3] S. M. Kirov Military Medical Academy of the Ministry of Defense of the Russian Federation, St-Petersburg, Russia, [4] V. A. Almazov Federal North-West Medical Research Centre of the Ministry of Health of the Russian Federation, St-Petersburg, Russia, [5] Laboratory of Neurosurgery, Irkutsk Scientific Center of Surgery and Traumatology, Irkutsk, Russia, [6] Department of Neurosurgery, Irkutsk State Medical University, Irkutsk, Russia, [7] Institute of Gene Biology, Russian Academy of Science, Moscow, Russia, [8] Prokhorov General Physics Institute of the Russian Academy of Science, Moscow, Russia, [9] National Research Nuclear University MEPhI, Moscow, Russia

Correspondence:
Sergey A. Goryaynov
sgoraynov@nsi.ru

Objective: This study is to analyze fluorescence sensitivity in the diagnosis of brain and spinal cord tumors.

Material and methods: The authors conducted a multicenter retrospective analysis of data on 653 cases in 641 patients: 553 of them had brain tumors and 88 spinal cord tumors. Brain tumor resection was performed in 523 patients, of whom 484 were adults and 39 children. The analyzed series was presented by 320 gliomas, 101 meningiomas, and 72 metastases. A stereotactic biopsy was performed in 20 patients and endoscopic surgery in 10 patients. In all cases, 20 mg/kg of 5–Aminolaevulinic acid was administered orally 2-h before surgery. All surgical interventions were performed with a microscope BLUE 400 to visualize fluorescence, while endoscopic surgery—with an endoscope equipped with a fluorescent module. Fluorescence spectroscopy was conducted in 20 cases of stereotactic biopsies and in 88 cases of spinal cord tumors.

Results: Among adult brain tumors operated by microsurgical techniques, meningiomas showed the highest 5-ALA fluorescence sensitivity 94% (n = 95/101), brain metastases 84.7% (n = 61/72), low-grade gliomas 46.4% (n = 26/56), and high-grade gliomas 90.2% (n = 238/264). In children the highest 5-ALA visible fluorescence was observed in anaplastic astrocytomas 100% (n = 4/4) and in anaplastic ependymomas 100% (n = 4/4); in low-grade gliomas it made up 31.8% (n = 7/22). As for the spinal cord tumors in adults, the highest sensitivity was demonstrated by glioblastomas 100% (n = 4/4) and by meningiomas 100% (n = 4/4); Fluorescence was not found in gemangioblastomas (n = 0/6) and neurinomas (n = 0/4). Fluorescence intensity reached 60% (n = 6/10) in endoscopic surgery and 90% (n = 18/20) in stereotactic biopsy.

Conclusion: 5-ALA fluorescence diagnosis proved to be most sensitive in surgery of HGG and meningioma (90.2 and 94.1%, respectively). Sensitivity in surgery of intracranial metastases and spinal cord tumors was slightly lower (84.7 and 63.6%, correspondingly). The lowest fluorescence sensitivity was marked in pediatric tumors and LGG (50 and 46.4%, correspondingly). Fluorescence diagnosis can also be used in transnasal endoscopic surgery of skull base tumors and in stereotactic biopsy.

Keywords: fluorescence diagnosis, 5-Aminolevulinic acid (ALA), glioma, meningioma, neurooncology

INTRODUCTION

In late 90-ies first data on the potential use of 5-ALA in surgery of malignant gliomas have appeared (1, 2). Recently, use of 5-ALA has become more popular for other classes of brain and spinal cord tumors like meningioma (3–7), metastasis (8–11), neurocytoma (12), ependymoma (13, 14), medulloblastoma (15), adenoma (16). Besides microneurosurgery, intraoperative FD has found its application in endoscopic (17–21) and stereotactic surgery (22, 23).

Our study was aimed at analyzing 5-ALA fluorescence sensitivity in patients with brain and spinal cord tumors using microsurgical, endoscopic techniques, along with stereotactic biopsy.

MATERIALS AND METHODS

Patients

The study enrolled 641 patients with brain and spinal cord tumors, operated within 2010–2017 in 3 clinical hospitals: N. N. Burdenko National Medical Research Center of Neurosurgery of the Ministry of Health of the Russian Federation, Moscow; S. M. Kirov Military Medical Academy of the Ministry of Defense of the Russian Federation, St-Petersburg; V. A. Almazov Federal North-West Medical Research Centre of the Ministry of Health of the Russian Federation, St-Petersburg. More data on patients are presented in **Table 1**. The written informed consent to the surgery and 5-ALA administration was obtained from all patients. The study was approved by the local ethics committee of the N. N. Burdenko National Medical Research Center of Neurosurgery.

Drugs and Equipment

Having got the informed consent and data on absence of any significant liver or kidney pathology, patients were administered 20 mg/kg of 5–Aminolevulinic acid ("Alasens," SSC "NIOPIK," Russian Federation) in 2-h before surgery. Contraindications for "Alasens" were: more than 3-or 4-time ALT, AST increase, porphyria, pregnancy, breastfeeding. In children, 5-ALA was ingested after obtaining the informed parents' consent and by the ethics committee approval. All operations were performed with OPMI Pentero (Carl Zeiss Meditec AG, Obrekochen, Germany) microscope equipped with a fluorescent 400-nm UV light and filters (BLUE 400). During stereotactic surgery MRI (magnetic resonance imaging) and PET (positron emission tomography) with methionine were performed to select the target area and to obtain histological samples.

Operations were performed using the stereotactic system "OREOL" ["Elektropribor," St-Petersburg; (24)]. All assessments were made on an optic-fiber fluorescence-reflectance multichannel ≪Skin-AGE≫ spectrometer (25). In patients with spinal cord tumors, laser spectroscopy was performed using LESA-01-BIOSPEK spectrum analyzer (laser electronic-spectral device, "Biospek" company, Moscow). The PpIX level between the tumor tissue and the intact brain was measured during spectroscopy.

For endoscopic procedures there was used an endoscope equipped with a fluorescence filter; in a number of cases, the combined video-recording system was applied, which was developed in the Laboratory of Laser biospectroscopy at the A. M. Prokhorov general physics institute of the Russian Academy of Sciences.

OUTCOMES OF 5-ALA USE IN SURGERY OF BRAIN AND SPINAL CORD TUMORS

5-ALA Fluorescence in Surgery of Brain Tumors in Adults (n = 493)

Visible fluorescence was marked in 90.2% (n = 238/264) of patients with WHO Grade III-IV gliomas and in 46.4% (n = 26/56) of patients with WHO Grade I-II gliomas. More data on patient distribution into subgroups by tumor histology are presented in **Table 1.** Positive fluorescence was marked in 96.2% (n = 75/78) of patients with WHO Grade I, in 85.7% (n = 18/21) of WHO Grade II, and in 100% (n = 2/2) of WHO Grade III meningiomas.

From two to four nodes were revealed in 17 of 63 patients with metastatic brain lesions; overall, 5-ALA fluorescence was measured in 72 tumor cases. Based on tumor location, it was positive in 84.7% (n = 61/72) of cases, namely: metastatic lung cancer was positive in 80.7% (n = 21/26), metastatic breast cancer in 90% (n = 18/20), others in 66.7% (n = 21/24).

5-ALA Fluorescence in Surgery of Brain and Spinal Cord Tumors in Children (n = 42)

In this subgroup 39 of 42 patients were operated (3 patients underwent repeated surgery). Anaplastic astrocytoma and anaplastic ependymoma demonstrated the maximal sensitivity, which made up 100% (n = 4/4), each; sensitivity in glioblastomas reached 80% (n = 4/5), and in low-grade gliomas, it averaged 31.8% (n = 7/22).

Abbreviations: 5-ALA, 5–Aminolevulinic acid; FD, Fluorescence diagnosis; HGG, High-grade gliomas (WHO Grades III-IV); LGG, Low-grade gliomas (WHO Grades I-II); PpIX, Protoporphyrin IX; PET, Positron Emission Tomography; PDD, Photodynamic diagnosis; STB, Stereotactic Biopsy.

TABLE 1 | Cases.

Object	5-ALA +	5-ALA -
Brain tumors, open resection ($n = 535$)		
Adults ($n = 493$)	420 (85.2%)	73 (14.8%)
Glioma ($n = 320$)	264 (82.5%)	56 (17.5%)
LGG ($n = 56$)	26 (46.4%)	30 (53.6%)
Pilloid astrocytoma	3 (100%)	0 (0%)
Diffuse astrocytoma	6 (25%)	18 (75%)
Gemistocytic astrocytoma	3 (100%)	0 (0%)
Ganglioastrocytoma	0 (0%)	1 (100%)
Non-infantile desmoplastic ganglioglioma	1 (100%)	0 (0%)
Oligoastrocytoma	8 (50%)	8 (50%)
Oligodendroglioma	3 (50%)	3 (50%)
Pleomorphic xanthoastrocytoma	2 (100%)	0 (0%)
HGG ($n = 264$)	238 (90.2%)	26 (9.8%)
Anaplastic astrocytoma	19 (65.5%)	10 (34.5%)
Anaplastic hemangiopericytoma	1 (100%)	0 (0%)
Anaplastic oligoastrocytoma	5 (71.4%)	2 (28.6%)
Anaplastic oligodendroglioma	4 (66.7%)	2 (33.3%)
Glioblastoma ($n = 211$)	203 (94%)	12 (6%)
Gliosarcoma	6 (100%)	0 (0%)
Meningioma ($n = 101$)	95 (94.1%)	6 (5.9%)
Grade I	75 (96.2%)	3 (3.8%)
Grade II	18 (85.7%)	3 (14.3%)
Grade III	2 (100%)	0 (0%)
Brain metastasis ($n = 72$)	61 (84.7%)	11 (15.3%)
Lungs cancer	21 (80.7%)	5 (19.3%)
Breast cancer	18 (90%)	2 (10%)
Other metastases	21 (66.7%)	3 (33.3%)
Pediatric ($n = 42$)	21 (50%)	21 (50%)
LGG ($n = 22$)	7 (31.8%)	15 (68.2%)
Disembrioplastic neuroepithelial tumor	0 (0%)	1 (100%)
Fibrillary protoplasmic astrocytoma	0 (0%)	2 (100%)
Pilocytic astrocytoma	0 (0%)	4 (100%)
Pilomixoid astrpcytoma	4 (57.1%)	3 (42.9%)
Oligoastrocytoma	1 (50%)	1 (50%)
Oligodendroglioma	0 (0%)	1 (100%)
Fibrillary astrocytoma	1 (50%)	1 (50%)
Ependymoma	1 (50%)	1 (50%)
Chorioid papilloma	0 (0%)	1 (100%)
HGG ($n = 20$)	14 (70%)	6 (30%)
Anaplastic astrocytoma	4 (100%)	0 (0%)
Anaplastic ependymoma	4 (100%)	0 (0%)
Glioblastoma	4 (80%)	1 (20%)
Medulloblastoma	1 (16.7%)	5 (83.3%)
Primitive neuroectodermal tumor	1 (100%)	0 (0%)
Brain tumor, Endoscopic surgery ($n = 10$)	6 (60%)	4 (40%)
Meningioma	3 (75%)	1 (25%)
Hordoma	1 (50%)	1 (50%)
Neurinoma	1 (100%)	0 (0%)
Inverted papilloma	1 (100%)	0 (0%)
Other tumors	0 (0%)	2 (100%)

(Continued)

TABLE 1 | Continued

Object	5-ALA +	5-ALA -
Brain tumors, open resection ($n = 535$)		
Brain tumor, stereotactic biopsy ($n = 20$)	18 (90%)	2 (10%)
Fibrillary protoplasmic astrocytoma	2 (66.7%)	1 (33.3)
Anaplastic astrocytoma	8 (100%)	0 (0%)
Glioblastoma	7 (100%)	0 (0%)
Other	1 (50%)	1 (50%)
Adults, spinal cord ($n = 88$)	56 (63.6%)	32 (36.4%)
Ependymoma	37 (72.5%)	14 (27.5%)
Astrocytoma	4 (33.3%)	8 (66.7%)
Glioblastoma	4 (100%)	0 (0%)
Gemangioblastoma	0 (0%)	6 (100%)
Meningioma	11 (100%)	0 (0%)
Neurinoma	0 (0%)	4 (100%)
Overall	**653**	

It is interesting to note, that medulloblastomas demonstrated "weak" fluorescence (16.7%, $n = 1/6$) despite their high grade of malignancy.

5-ALA Fluorescence in Endoscopic Neurosurgery ($n = 10$)

Ten operations have been performed: anterior cranial fossa tumor resection by a transnasal approach. By all that, fluorescence was marked in 75% ($n = 3/4$) of meningiomas, in 50% ($n = 1/2$) of chordomas, in 100% ($n = 1/1$) of neurinoma, and in 100% ($n = 1/1$) of inverted papilloma.

Fluorescence-Guided Stereotactic Biopsy of Brain Tumors ($n = 20$)

Stereotactic biopsy and stereotactic fluorescence biospectroscopy revealed positive tumor fluorescence in 90% ($n = 18/20$) of cases. Fluorescence spectroscopy was sensitive for detecting fibrillary-protoplasmatic astrocytomas in 66.7% ($n = 2/3$), anaplastic astrocytomas in 100% [($n = 8/8$), glioblastomas in 100% ($n = 7/7$)] of cases. The false-positive effect was marked in 5.6% ($n = 1/18$) of patients (reactive gliosis after earlier performed radiotherapy).

5-ALA Fluorescence in Surgery of Spinal Cord Tumors in Adults ($n = 88$)

Visible fluorescence was marked in 75% ($n = 33/44$) of intramedullary ependymomas, wherein, a strong PpIX fluorescence, revealed by laser spectroscopy, was observed in 100% ($n = 44/44$) of cases. Astrocytomas have been noted to fluoresce in 33.3% ($n = 4/12$) of cases, spectroscopy has demonstrated PpIX fluorescence in 50% ($n = 6/12$). The highest fluorescence sensitivity was marked in patients with glioblastoma (4/4) and meningioma (11/11). Fluorescence was visible in 57.1% ($n = 4/7$) of cauda equine ependymoma; PpIX fluorescence intensity, revealed by laser spectroscopy, was

($n = 7/7$) in all cases; negative PpIX fluorescence was observed in hemangioblastoma ($n = 0/6$) and neurinoma ($n = 0/4$).

DISCUSSION

At the end of 90-ies first data on the potential use of 5-ALA in neurosurgery appeared, with first publications being devoted to malignant gliomas (1, 22). Today, 5-ALA is applied in surgery of different types of brain and spinal cord tumors for both adults and children, including meningiomas (3–7, 26–28), metastasis (8–11), neurocytomas (12), ependymomas (13, 14), medulloblastomas (15).

Among the publications devoted to application of 5-ALA fluorescence in surgery of CNS tumors, Marbacher et al. (10) (n=458) reports the largest series of patients (10). In contrast to Marbacher et al. (10), our series ($n = 641$) enrolled patients with spinal cord tumors ($n = 88$), children ($n = 39$), and patients who underwent transnasal endoscopic surgery ($n = 10$). The novelty of our research is application of spectroscopy in cases of spinal cord tumors ($n = 88$) and stereotactic biopsy ($n = 20$).

We found it reasonable to combine data on intraoperative fluorescence sensitivity obtained in different tumors of the CNS. In our series, to visualize fluorescence in stereotactic biopsy and in spinal surgery, traditionally, besides microscope, the spectroscopic control is used.

Adults, Brain, Open Resection

High-Grade Gliomas

A number of papers have proved that use of fluorescence diagnosis in surgery of high-grade gliomas results in the increased rate of GTR (gross total resection) and the increased progression-free and overall survival time (29–32). Thus, use of fluorescence diagnosis in surgery of high-grade gliomas is an effective technique.

The results of 5-ALA application in adults with different types of brain tumors were highlighted in detail in our earlier publications (18, 18, 21, 26). In this study, fluorescence sensitivity in the treatment of high-grade gliomas was 90.2% ($n = 238/264$), which corresponded to findings of other authors (22, 32–34).

Low-Grade Gliomas

Whether it is reasonable to use 5-ALA in surgery of non-contrasting gliomas, is still undefined. On the one hand, it is evident knowledge that gross total resection results in the increased progression-free and overall survival time among patients with LGG (31). However, no research has proved that use of fluorescence in LGG results in the increased rate of GTR. For these reasons, there is a strong need for further studying and specifying this problem.

Widhalm et al. have reported that PpIX accumulates in anaplastic focus, where the tumor has higher grade areas of malignancy (Grade III) (23). According to our data, fluorescing focuses in LGG are areas with the Ki 67 index still not exceeding 5% (35). Medical publications provide contradictory opinions on fluorescence sensitivity in LGG, which varies from 7.7 to 40% (10, 36–38). In our group it made up 46.4% ($n = 26/56$), presumably due to comprising different types of gliomas; while the lowest sensitivity was observed in diffuse astrocytomas 25% ($n = 6/18$).

Metastases

In our series, 5-ALA-induced fluorescence for cerebral metastases was 84.7% ($n = 61/72$), which is slightly higher compared to other studies. Thus, according to Kamp and co-authors, fluorescence sensitivity for cerebral metastases varied from 52 to 81% (11). The absence of fluorescence in intracranial metastases indicated a significantly higher incidence of local tumor progression after surgery (11). It might be related to different surgeon's experience in using 5-ALA, which is particularly important when dealing with weak fluorescence intensity. The phenomenon of tumor bed, still fluorescing after metastatic node removal, is still hard to understand (clinical case, **Figure 1**).

Meningiomas

These data prove our previous research on 5-ALA sensitivity in intracranial meningioma surgery (39).

Children, Brain, Open Resection

As was earlier mentioned, use of fluorescence diagnosis in HGG in children results in the increased rate of GTR (gross total resection) and the increased progression-free and overall survival time (40, 41). New data on the clinical use of 5-ALA in children with some other types of brain tumors have been reported (15, 24, 41–43). Thus, fluorescence diagnosis is recommended for HGG. For other classes of tumors, its use is disputable (44).

In our series, fluorescence sensitivity in children with brain tumors was 50% ($n = 21/42$) (45), thus corresponding to other foreign authors' experience (24, 41, 43, 46). Fluorescence sensitivity depends on the tumor morphology and malignancy. According to Stummer et al. fluorescence sensitivity was noted to make up 15% ($n = 2/13$) for Grade I-II astrocytoma, and 85% ($n = 12/14$)—for glioblastoma. In our research, florescence sensitivity for low-grade gliomas was 31.8% ($n = 7/22$), for high-grade gliomas −70% ($n = 14/20$). Maximal sensitivity was revealed in anaplastic astrocytomas 100% ($n = 4/4$) and anaplastic ependymoma 100% ($n = 4/4$).

Still confusing is, that medulloblastomas in children show low fluorescence sensitivity. This high-grade class of tumors, however, reveals "weak" fluorescence (30). For instance, Beez et al. report fluorescence sensitivity reaching 25% ($n = 1/3$) (43). In our series, it made up 16.7% ($n = 1/6$) for medulloblastomas. As Zhang et al. reports, more complete resection rate with the following increased survival time was associated with positive fluorescence (44).

Adults, Spinal Cord

5-ALA fluorescence-assisted technology in adults has proved to be a good method of intraoperative neuroimaging (13, 14, 47–49). In our experience, fluorescence sensitivity for spinal cord tumors was 63.6% ($n = 56/88$), which was similar to other publications (13, 14, 48). Millesi et al. report fluorescence sensitivity to range from 0% ($n = 0/8$) in neurinomas to 100% ($n = 12/12$) in meningiomas (48), thus, also confiding with our

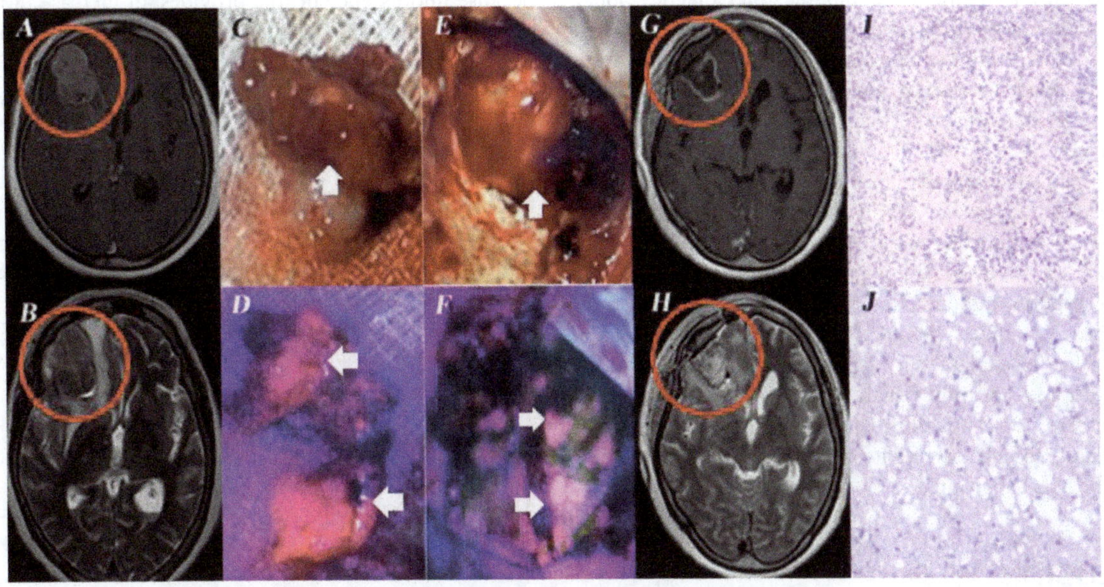

FIGURE 1 | Female, aged 60, admitted to the clinical center with complaints of headaches. In 2009 melanoma of the right lumbar region was removed, in 2017 she underwent resection of the superior lobe of the left lung. MRI of the brain revealed an intracerebral tumor in the right frontal lobe with perifocal edema **(A,B)**. Resection of the right frontal lobe tumor was performed under 5-ALA Fluorescence assistance. During surgery, bright fluorescence of the tumor node was marked **(C,D)**. Biopsy revealed melanoma metastasis **(I)**. immunohistochemical examination showed positive HMB45, MelA expression. After resection, the unchanged white matter of the frontal lobe was exposed in the tumor bed **(E)**. Visible tumor bed fluorescence was observed **(F)**. No tumor tissue was revealed by additional biopsy samples taken from the fluorescing region **(J)**. Postoperative MRI **(G,H)** demonstrated total tumor node resection. This case is interesting, first, by the fact that melanoma metastasis can fluorescence and second, that the resected tumor bed without tumor cells can also fluoresce. Informed consent has been obtained from the patient for the publication of data, including images.

data. Application of spectroscopy in our series allowed us to increase fluorescence sensitivity in astrocytomas (Grade II) from 33.3% (n = 4/12) to 50% (n = 6/12), and in ependymomas from 75% (n = 33/44) to 100% (n = 44/44), including cauda equine ependymoma, the sensitivity of which varied from 57.1% (n = 4/7) to 100% (7/7).

Endoscopic Surgery

The present-day microscope-assisted metabolic navigation possesses the insufficient quality of the fluorescence signal obtained during a deep and narrow approach. To solve this problem, a specific design of fluorescence endoscope has been adopted. 5-ALA fluorescence is known to be useful in visualizing the tumor tissue (18, 19, 50, 51), while fluorescence with indocyanine green (ICG)—for coloration of the vessels (52–55).

There are only a few medical publications devoted to endoscopic surgery with fluorescence assistance in neurooncology. Takeda et al. reported 2 cases of germinomas (56), in which 5-ALA fluorescence-guided endoscopic surgery was used. Cornelius et al. described the procedure of using 5-ALA endoscopic surgery in 2 patients with meningiomas (57). Our series included 10 patients with different skull base tumors; intraoperative fluorescence was visualized in 60% of cases. Alongside with this, meningiomas was visualized in 3 cases out of 4, chordoma in 1 case out of 2, neurinoma in 1 case of 1, inverted papilloma in 1 case of 1.

Patients who underwent microscopic 5-ALA fluorescence-assisted endoscopic surgery for brain tumors did not enter this series. These results were reported in our early publication in 2008 (18). We did not use 5-ALA fluorescence in transventricular endoscopic surgery of intraventricular tumors. Takeda et al. have earlier reported on that (56).

Stereotactic Biopsy

According to the world literature databank, STB proved to be not informative in 24% (58). There are three main methods neurosurgeons have for reduction the incidence of uninformative biopsies: a combination of MRI and PET is used for preoperative planning, biopsy in the operating room and the use 5-ALA fluorescence. A fluorescence-assisted stereotactic biopsy can be obtained in 2 ways: first, by measuring the concentration of PP IX in the tumor tissue along the stereotactic trajectory to the target using a spectral probe before extracting the biopsy (59). Second, by evaluating the tissue sample fluorescence using a neurosurgical microscope with a special fluorescence regimen, as described by Widhalm et al. (23). In the latter, specimens were put under fluorescence light of a surgical microscope to assess their fluorescence. Fluorescence sensitivity, according to Widhalm's report, was 100% for HGG and 0% for LGG. In addition, use of fluorescence was helpful in shortening the operation time and decreasing the average number of biopsies during surgery (60).

In our opinion, the combination of the stereotactic cannula and the spectral probe is easier and does not require an operative microscope with a fluorescence module. Stereotactic biopsy combined with fluorescence spectroscopy gives a chance when analyzing, to determine the zones of the highest concentration of PPIX and select the tumor site with the highest degree of anaplasia, thus increasing the diagnostic value of stereotactic biopsy as a technique (23, 61).

Fluorescence sensitivity in our series reached 90% ($n = 18/20$), thus corresponding to the world literature data. Marbacher et al. (10) reports fluorescence sensitivity of 88% ($n = 44/50$). Fluorescence sensitivity for a low-grade glioma, particularly for fibrillary protoplasmic glioma, was 66.7% (2/3), while in the study of Marbacher et al. it was 25% (3/12). In our experience, higher fluorescence can be explained by using stereotactic biopsy under spectroscopic, and not only visual, control. A small number of cases in our series does not allow us to perform the comparative analysis of fluorescence sensitivity for patients with low-grade glioma in the STB subgroup.

CONCLUSION

5-ALA fluorescence diagnosis proved to be most sensitive in surgery of HGG and meningioma (90.2 and 94.1%, respectively). Sensitivity in surgery of intracranial metastases and spinal cord tumors was slightly lower (84.7 and 63.6%, correspondingly). The lowest fluorescence sensitivity was marked in pediatric tumors and LGG (50 and 46.4%, correspondingly). Fluorescence diagnosis can also be used in transnasal endoscopic surgery of skull base tumors and in stereotactic biopsy.

LIMITATIONS

There are several limitations our work has. Firstly, we used brain tumor classification of the 2007 year (because it is a retrospective study). Secondly, it common knowledge that medulloblastomas (MB) are recommended to classify into subtypes, according to WHO classification, but our analysis was performed earlier than an official MB sub-type classification was generally accepted. In addition, MB sub-type classification is effective for a traditional classification of patients into moderate or high-grade risk groups and is important for further prognosis and choice of the differentiated treatment modality. In our opinion, the practical value of such a comparative analysis is not so important, because fluorescence degree provides an increase in the radical blastomatous tissue resection rate and not assessment of its molecular genetic features. Our group of MB patients is too small to claim any novelty. We just state that the data obtained can be helpful for a meta-analysis.

ETHICS STATEMENT

All procedures performed in studies involving human participants were in accordance with the ethical standards of the institutional and/or national research committee and with the 1964 Helsinki declaration and its later amendments or comparable ethical standards.

AUTHOR'S NOTE

AK is a corresponding member of RAS. AP is a full member of RAS.

AUTHOR CONTRIBUTIONS

SG and AP: research concept and design. VO, DG, DS, BM, AK, NK, PZ, AP, and AB: data collection and processing. KC: statistic support and writing text. VB, GP, and VL: editing. This work was supported by the ethical committee of Burdenko Neurosurgical Institute.

ACKNOWLEDGMENTS

We would like to acknowledge the help provided by our colleagues:

A. I. Kholyavin, N. P. Bechtereva Institute of the Human Brain, Russian Academy of Sciences, Saint Petersburg, Russia.

G. V. Papayan, I. P. Pavlov First St. Petersburg State Medical University, Ministry of Health of the Russian Federation, St. Petersburg, Russia.

D. S. Kim, Department of Pathomorphology, Burdenko NSI, Moscow.

I. N. Pronin, Full member of RAS, and A. I. Batalov, Burdenko NSI, Moscow.

Translation from Russian to English – N. A. Pestovskaya.

This work was partially supported by the Competitiveness Program of MEPhI.

REFERENCES

1. Stummer W, Novotny A, Stepp H, Goetz C, Bise K, Reulen HJ. Fluorescence-guided resection of glioblastoma multiforme utilizing 5-ALA-induced porphyrins: a prospective study in 52 consecutive patients. *J Neurosurg.* (2000) 93:1003–13. doi: 10.3171/jns.2000.93.6.1003
2. Stummer W, Goetz C, Stepp H, Stocker S, Reulen HJ. Intraoperative detection of malignant glioma by 5-ALA induced protoporphyrin IX fluorescence. *Clin Neurol Neurosurg.* (1997) 99:S93. doi: 10.1016/S0303-8467(97)81684-8
3. Coluccia D, Fandino J, Fujioka M, Cordovi S, Muroi C, Landolt H. Intraoperative 5-aminolevulinic-acid-induced fluorescence in meningiomas. *Acta Neurochir.* (2010) 152:1711–9. doi: 10.1007/s00701-010-0708-4
4. Foster N, Eljamel S. ALA-induced fluorescence image guided surgery of meningiomas: a meta-analyses. *Photodiagnosis Photodyn Ther.* (2016) 15:73–8. doi: 10.1016/j.pdpdt.2016.05.006
5. Cornelius J, Slotty P, Stoffels G, Galldiks N, Langen K, Steiger H. 5-Aminolevulinic acid and 18F-FET-PET as metabolic imaging tools for surgery of a recurrent skull base meningioma. *J Neurol Surg Part B Skull Base.* (2013) 74:211–6. doi: 10.1055/s-0033-1342918
6. Millesi M, Kiesel B, Mischkulnig M, Martínez-Moreno M, Wöhrer A, Wolfsberger S, et al. Analysis of the surgical benefits of 5-ALA–induced fluorescence in intracranial meningiomas: experience in 204 meningiomas. *Neurosurg.* (2016) 125:1408–19. doi: 10.3171/2015.12.JNS151513
7. Hefti M, Holenstein F, Albert I, Looser H, Luginbuehl V. Susceptibility to 5-aminolevulinic acid based photodynamic therapy in WHO I meningioma cells corresponds to ferrochelatase activity. *Photochem Photobiol.* (2011) 87:235–

41. doi: 10.1111/j.1751-1097.2010.00821.x

8. Utsuki S, Oka H, Sato S, Shimizu S, Suzuki S, Tanizaki Y, et al. Histological examination of false positive tissue resection using 5-aminolevulinic acid-induced fluorescence guidance. *Neurol Med Chir.* (2007) 47:210–3; discussion 213-4. doi: 10.2176/nmc.47.210
9. Belloch JP, Rovira V, Llácer JL, Riesgo PA, Cremades A. Fluorescence-guided surgery in high grade gliomas using an exoscope system. *Acta Neurochir.* (2014) 156:653–60. doi: 10.1007/s00701-013-1976-6
10. Marbacher S, Klinger E, Schwyzer L, Fischer I, Nevzati E, Diepers M, et al. Use of fluorescence to guide resection or biopsy of primary brain tumors and brain metastases. *Neurosurg Focus.* (2014) 36:E10. doi: 10.3171/2013.12.FOCUS13464
11. Kamp MA, Fischer I, Bühner J, Turowski B, Frederick Cornelius J, Steiger H-J, et al. 5-ALA fluorescence of cerebral metastases and its impact for the local-in-brain progression. *Oncotarget.* (2016) 7:66776–66789. doi: 10.18632/oncotarget.11488
12. Song SW, Kim Y-H, Park S-H, Park C-K. 5-Aminolevulinic acid fluorescence discriminates the histological grade of extraventricular neurocytoma. *Brain Tumor Res Treat.* (2013) 1:45. doi: 10.14791/btrt.2013.1.1.45
13. Eicker SO, Floeth FW, Kamp M, Steiger H-J, Hänggi D. The impact of fluorescence guidance on spinal intradural tumour surgery. *Eur Spine J.* (2013) 22:1394–401 doi: 10.1007/s00586-013-2657-0
14. Inoue T, Endo T, Nagamatsu K, Watanabe M, Tominaga T. 5-Aminolevulinic acid fluorescence-guided resection of intramedullary ependymoma. *Oper Neurosurg.* (2013) 72:ons159–68. doi: 10.1227/NEU.0b013e31827bc7a3
15. Skjøth-Rasmussen J, Bøgeskov L, Sehested A, Klausen C, Broholm H, Nysom K. The use of 5-ALA to assist complete removal of residual non-enhancing part of childhood medulloblastoma: a case report. *Child Nerv Syst.* (2015) 31:2173–7. doi: 10.1007/s00381-015-2762-y
16. Eljamel MS, Leese G, Moseley H. Intraoperative optical identification of pituitary adenomas. *J Neurooncol.* (2009) 92:417–21. doi: 10.1007/s11060-009-9820-9
17. Cho W-S, Kim JE, Kang H-S, Ha EJ, Jung M, Lee C, et al. Dual-channel endoscopic indocyanine green fluorescence angiography for clipping of cerebral aneurysms. *World Neurosurg.* (2017) 100:316–24. doi: 10.1016/j.wneu.2017.01.042
18. Potapov AA, Usachev DJ, Loshakov VA, Cherekaev VA, Kornienko VN, Pronin IN, et al. First experience in 5-ALA fluorescence-guided and endoscopically assisted microsurgery of brain tumors. *Med Laser Appl.* (2008) 23:202–8. doi: 10.1016/j.mla.2008.07.006
19. Ritz R, Feigl GC, Schuhmann MU, Ehrhardt A, Danz S, Noell S, et al. Use of 5-ALA fluorescence guided endoscopic biopsy of a deep-seated primary malignant brain tumor. *J Neurosurg.* (2011) 114:1410–3. doi: 10.3171/2010.11.JNS10250
20. Tsuzuki S, Aihara Y, Eguchi S, Amano K, Kawamata T, Okada Y. Application of indocyanine green (ICG) fluorescence for endoscopic biopsy of intraventricular tumors. *Child Nerv Syst.* (2014) 30:723–6. doi: 10.1007/s00381-013-2266-6
21. Belykh E, Miller EJ, Hu D, Martirosyan NL, Woolf EC, Scheck AC, et al. Scanning fiber endoscope improves detection of 5-aminolevulinic acid-induced protoporphyrin IX fluorescence at the boundary of infiltrative glioma. *World Neurosurg.* (2018) 113:e51–69. doi: 10.1016/j.wneu.2018.01.151
22. Stummer W, Pichlmeier U, Meinel T, Wiestler OD, Zanella F, Reulen H-J. Fluorescence-guided surgery with 5-aminolevulinic acid for resection of malignant glioma: a randomised controlled multicentre phase III trial. *Lancet Oncol.* (2006) 7:392–401. doi: 10.1016/S1470-2045(06)70665-9
23. Widhalm G, Minchev G, Woehrer A, Preusser M, Kiesel B, Furtner J, et al. Strong 5-aminolevulinic acid-induced fluorescence is a novel intraoperative marker for representative tissue samples in stereotactic brain tumor biopsies. *Neurosurg Rev.* (2012) 35:381–91. doi: 10.1007/s10143-012-0374-5
24. Stummer W, Rodrigues F, Schucht P, Preuss M, Wiewrodt D, Nestler U, et al. Predicting the "usefulness" of 5-ALA-derived tumor fluorescence for fluorescence-guided resections in pediatric brain tumors: a European survey. *Acta Neurochir.* (2014) 156:2315–24. doi: 10.1007/s00701-014-2234-2
25. Kang U, Papayan GV, Berezin VB, Petrischcv NN, Galagudza MM. Spectrometer for fluorescence-reflectance biomedical research. *Opt J.* (2013) 80:56–67. Available online at: https://yandex.ru/patents/doc/RU2539817C1_20150127
26. Potapov AA, Goryaynov SA, Danilov GV, Chelushkin DM, Okhlopkov VA, Shimanskiy VN, et al. Intraoperative fluorescence diagnostics in surgery of intracranial meningiomas: analysis of 101 cases. *Vopr neirokhirurgii Im NN Burdenko.* (2018) 82:17. doi: 10.17116/oftalma201882217-29
27. Belykh E, Martirosyan NL, Yagmurlu K, Miller EJ, Eschbacher JM, Izadyyazdanabadi M, et al. Intraoperative fluorescence imaging for personalized brain tumor resection: current state and future directions. *Front Surg.* (2016) 3:55. doi: 10.3389/fsurg.2016.00055
28. Belykh E, Miller EJ, Patel AA, Bozkurt B, Yagmurlu K, Robinson TR, et al. Optical characterization of neurosurgical operating microscopes: quantitative fluorescence and assessment of PpIX photobleaching. *Sci Rep.* (2018) 8:12543. doi: 10.1038/s41598-018-30247-6
29. Stummer W, Reulen H-J, Meinel T, Pichlmeier U, Schumacher W, Tonn J-C, et al. Extent of resection and survival in glioblastoma multiforme. *Neurosurgery.* (2008) 62:564–76. doi: 10.1227/01.neu.0000317304.31579.17
30. Aldave G, Tejada S, Pay E, Marigil M, Bejarano B, Idoate MA, et al. Prognostic value of residual fluorescent tissue in glioblastoma patients after gross total resection in 5-aminolevulinic acid-guided surgery. *Neurosurgery.* (2013) 72:915–21. doi: 10.1227/NEU.0b013e31828c3974
31. Schucht P, Beck J, Abu-Isa J, Andereggen L, Murek M, Seidel K, et al. Gross total resection rates in contemporary glioblastoma surgery: results of an institutional protocol combining 5-aminolevulinic acid intraoperative fluorescence imaging and brain mapping. *Neurosurgery.* (2012) 71:927–35. doi: 10.1227/NEU.0b013e31826d1e6b
32. Slotty PJ, Siantidis B, Beez T, Steiger HJ, Sabel M. The impact of improved treatment strategies on overall survival in glioblastoma patients. *Acta Neurochir.* (2013) 155:959–63. doi: 10.1007/s00701-013-1693-1
33. Díez Valle R, Slof J, Galván J, Arza C, Romariz C, Vidal C. Estudio observacional retrospectivo sobre la efectividad del ácido 5-aminolevulínico en la cirugía de los gliomas malignos en España (Estudio VISIONA). *Neurología.* (2014) 29:131–8. doi: 10.1016/j.nrl.2013.05.004
34. Chave-Cox DR, Corns MR, Sivakumar MG, Thomson MS. PP36. Improved glioblastoma survival following the introduction of a subspecialised surgical high grade brain tumour service. *Neuro Oncol.* (2017) 19 (Suppl. 1):i11. doi: 10.1093/neuonc/now293.036
35. Goryaynov SA, Widhalm G, Goldberg MF, Chelushkin D, Spallone A, Chernyshov KA, et al. The role of 5-ALA in low-grade gliomas and the influence of antiepileptic drugs on intraoperative fluorescence. *Front Oncol.* (2019) 9:423. doi: 10.3389/fonc.2019.00423
36. Widhalm G, Kiesel B, Woehrer A, Traub-Weidinger T, Preusser M, Marosi C, et al. 5-Aminolevulinic acid induced fluorescence is a powerful intraoperative marker for precise histopathological grading of gliomas with non-significant contrast-enhancement. *PLoS ONE.* (2013) 8:e76988. doi: 10.1371/journal.pone.0076988
37. Ewelt C, Floeth FW, Felsberg J, Steiger HJ, Sabel M, Langen K-J, et al. Finding the anaplastic focus in diffuse gliomas: the value of Gd-DTPA enhanced MRI, FET-PET, and intraoperative, ALA-derived tissue fluorescence. *Clin Neurol Neurosurg.* (2011) 113:541–7. doi: 10.1016/j.clineuro.2011.03.008
38. Jaber M, Wölfer J, Ewelt C, Holling M, Hasselblatt M, Niederstadt T, et al. The value of 5-aminolevulinic acid in low-grade gliomas and high-grade gliomas lacking glioblastoma imaging features. *Neurosurgery.* (2016) 78:401–11. doi: 10.1227/NEU.0000000000001020
39. Potapov AA, Goryaynov SA, Okhlopkov VA, Shishkina LV, Loschenov VB, Savelieva TA, et al. Laser biospectroscopy and 5-ALA fluorescence navigation as a helpful tool in the meningioma resection. *Neurosurg Rev.* (2016) 39:437–47. doi: 10.1007/s10143-015-0697-0
40. Kramm CM, Wagner S, Van Gool S, Schmid H, Sträter R, Gnekow A, et al. Improved survival after gross total resection of malignant gliomas in pediatric patients from the HIT-GBM studies. *Anticancer Res.* (2006) 26:3773–9.
41. Preuß M, Renner C, Krupp W, Christiansen H, Fischer L, Merkenschlager A, et al. The use of 5-aminolevulinic acid fluorescence guidance in resection of pediatric brain tumors. *Child Nerv Syst.* (2013) 29:1263–7. doi: 10.1007/s00381-013-2159-8
42. Bernal García LM, Cabezudo Artero JM, Royano Sánchez M, Marcelo Zamorano MB, López Macías M. Fluorescence-guided resection with 5-aminolevulinic acid of meningeal sarcoma in a

child. *Child Nerv Syst.* (2015) 31:1177–80. doi: 10.1007/s00381-015-2703-9
43. Beez T, Sarikaya-Seiwert S, Steiger H-J, Hänggi D. Fluorescence-guided surgery with 5-aminolevulinic acid for resection of brain tumors in children—a technical report. *Acta Neurochir.* (2014) 156:597–604. doi: 10.1007/s00701-014-1997-9
44. Zhang C, Boop FA, Ruge J. The use of 5-aminolevulinic acid in resection of pediatric brain tumors: a critical review. *J Neurooncol.* (2018) 141:567–763. doi: 10.1007/s11060-018-03004-y
45. Khachatryan WA, Kim AV, Samochernich KA, Tadevosian AR, Kazackaya EV, Don OA, et al. Experience with intraoperative fluorescence diagnosis in the surgical treatment of children with tumors of neuroepithelial brain. *Pediatr Neurosergery Neurol.* (2016) N2:37–51.
46. Kim AV, Khachatryan VA. Intraoperative fluorescence diagnosis using 5-aminolevulinic acid in surgical treatment of children with recurrent neuroepithelial tumors. *Zh Vopr Neirokhir Im N N Burdenko.* (2017) 81:51–7. doi: 10.17116/neiro201780751-57
47. De la Garza-Ramos R, Bydon M, Macki M, Huang J, Tamargo RJ, Bydon A. Fluorescent techniques in spine surgery. *Neurol Res.* (2014) 36:928–38. doi: 10.1179/1743132814Y.0000000340
48. Millesi M, Kiesel B, Woehrer A, Hainfellner JA, Novak K, Martínez-Moreno M, et al. Analysis of 5-aminolevulinic acid–induced fluorescence in 55 different spinal tumors. *Neurosurg Focus.* (2014) 36:E11. doi: 10.3171/2013.12.FOCUS13485
49. Rangel-Castilla L, Russin JJ, Zaidi HA, Martinez-del-Campo E, Park MS, Albuquerque FC, et al. Contemporary management of spinal AVFs and AVMs: lessons learned from 110 cases. *Neurosurg Focus.* (2014) 37:E14. doi: 10.3171/2014.7.FOCUS14236
50. Schwartz TH. Endoscopic-Assisted 5-Aminolevulinic Acid Imaging. World Neurosurg. (2014) 82:e117–8. doi: 10.1016/j.wneu.2013.07.110
51. Rapp M, Kamp M, Steiger H-J, Sabel M. Endoscopic-assisted visualization of 5-aminolevulinic acid–induced fluorescence in malignant glioma surgery: a technical note. *World Neurosurg.* (2014) 82:e277–9. doi: 10.1016/j.wneu.2013.07.002
52. Bruneau M, Appelboom G, Rynkowski M, Cutsem N, Mine B, Witte O. Endoscope-integrated ICG technology: first application during intracranial aneurysm surgery. *Neurosurg Rev.* (2012) 36:77–84. doi: 10.1007/s10143-012-0419-9
53. Mielke D, Malinova V, Rohde V. Comparison of intraoperative microscopic and endoscopic icg angiography in aneurysm surgery. *Neurosurgery.* (2014) 10:418–25. doi: 10.1227/NEU.0000000000000345
54. Hide T, Yano S, Kuratsu J. Indocyanine Green fluorescence endoscopy at endonasal transsphenoidal surgery for an intracavernous sinus dermoid cyst: case report. *Neurol Med Chir.* (2014) 54:999–1003. doi: 10.2176/nmc.cr.2014-0087
55. Hide T, Yano S, Shinojima N, Kuratsu J. Usefulness of the indocyanine green fluorescence endoscope in endonasal transsphenoidal surgery. *J Neurosurg.* (2015) 122:1185–92. doi: 10.3171/2014.9.JNS14599
56. Takeda J, Nonaka M, Li Y, Komori Y, Kamei T, Iwata R, et al. 5-ALA fluorescence-guided endoscopic surgery for mixed germ cell tumors. *J Neurooncol.* (2017) 134:119–24. doi: 10.1007/s11060-017-2494-9
57. Cornelius JF, Kamp MA, Tortora A, Knipps J, Krause-Molle Z, Beez T, et al. Surgery of small anterior skull base meningiomas by endoscopic 5-aminolevulinic acid fluorescence guidance: first clinical experience. *World Neurosurg.* (2018) 122:e890–5. doi: 10.1016/j.wneu.2018.10.171
58. Lu Y, Yeung C, Radmanesh A, Wiemann R, Black PM, Golby AJ. Comparative effectiveness of frame-based, frameless, and intraoperative magnetic resonance imaging-guided brain biopsy techniques. *World Neurosurg.* (2015) 83:261–8. doi: 10.1016/j.wneu.2014.07.043
59. Papayan GV, Martynov BV, Kholyavin AI, Nizkovolos VB, Svistov DV, Petrishchev NN, et al. Stereotactic fluorescence biospectroscopy in the diagnosis of brain glial neoplasms. *Top Issues Laser Med.* (2016) 2016:139–51. doi: 10.1093/neuros/nyy315
60. Millesi M, Kiesel B, Wöhrer A, Mercea PA, Bissolo M, Roetzer T, et al. Is intraoperative pathology needed if 5-aminolevulinic-acid-induced tissue fluorescence is found in stereotactic brain tumor biopsy? *Neurosurgery.* (2019) 2019:nyz086. doi: 10.1093/neuros/nyz086
61. Piquer J, Llácer JL, Rovira V, Riesgo P, Rodriguez R, Cremades A. Fluorescence-guided surgery and biopsy in gliomas with an exoscope system. *Biomed Res Int.* (2014) 2014:1–6. doi: 10.1155/2014/207974

10

Toward Quantitative Neurosurgical Guidance with High-Resolution Microscopy of 5-Aminolevulinic Acid-Induced Protoporphyrin IX

Linpeng Wei[1†], *Yoko Fujita*[2†], *Nader Sanai*[2] *and Jonathan T. C. Liu*[1,3*]

[1] Department of Mechanical Engineering, University of Washington, Seattle, WA, United States, [2] Department of Neurological Surgery, Barrow Neurological Institute, Phoenix, AZ, United States, [3] Department of Pathology, University of Washington School of Medicine, Seattle, WA, United States

***Correspondence:**
Jonathan T. C. Liu
jonliu@uw.edu

†Co-first authors

Low-power fluorescence microscopy of 5-ALA-induced PpIX has emerged as a valuable intraoperative imaging technology for improving the resection of malignant gliomas. However, current fluorescence imaging tools are not highly sensitive nor quantitative, which limits their effectiveness for optimizing operative decisions near the surgical margins of gliomas, in particular non-enhancing low-grade gliomas. Intraoperative high-resolution optical-sectioning microscopy can potentially serve as a valuable complement to low-power fluorescence microscopy by providing reproducible quantification of tumor parameters at the infiltrative margins of diffuse gliomas. In this forward-looking perspective article, we provide a brief discussion of recent technical advancements, pilot clinical studies, and our vision of the future adoption of handheld optical-sectioning microscopy at the final stages of glioma surgeries to enhance the extent of resection. We list a number of challenges for clinical acceptance, as well as potential strategies to overcome such obstacles for the surgical implementation of these *in vivo* microscopy techniques.

Keywords: fluorescence-guided surgery, handheld microscopy, 5-ALA, PpIX, gliomas, quantitative imaging

INTRODUCTION

Gliomas are the most common primary malignant brain tumors, with ~20,000 new cases each year in the United States (1). As the standard-of-care for all grades of gliomas, patients generally receive surgery as a first-line treatment. The goal of this "debulking" surgery is to maximize the extent of resection (EOR) while avoiding neurological damage. Mounting evidence suggests that more-extensive EOR is associated with increased overall survival and progression-free survival for both low- and high-grade gliomas patients (2–11). Unfortunately, optimal EOR is not achieved in many patients due to the lack of effective technologies to delineate tumor margins intraoperatively, with reported rates of gross-total resection (GTR) for high-grade gliomas (HGGs) ranging from 33 to 76% (12–19) and for low-grade gliomas (LGGs) ranging from 14 to 46% (7–9, 20, 21).

In recent years, numerous reports have detailed the benefits of using 5-aminolevulinic acid (5-ALA) for guiding HGG resections (22–38). In brief, 5-ALA is a non-fluorescent prodrug that is orally administered to patients several hours prior to surgery. 5-ALA is then intra-cellularly metabolized to form a fluorescent byproduct, protoporphyrin IX (PpIX), a heme-synthesis pathway substrate that accumulates preferentially in glioma cells due to metabolic dysregulation (39–43). In most cases, after 5-ALA administration, the bulk of a HGG tumor emits visible red fluorescence (~630 nm) when excited with blue (~405 nm) illumination, as viewed by the unassisted eye or with a wide-field fluorescence surgical microscope. A landmark phase III trial in Europe by Stummer et al. demonstrated that the use of this technique resulted in higher rates of GTR (65 vs. 36%) and 6-month progression-free survival (41 vs. 21.1%) compared to control patients (37). Intraoperative 5-ALA-induced fluorescence has since emerged as a valuable adjunct for HGG surgeries (22, 35–38), and has recently been approved by the US Food and Drug Administration (FDA) for neurosurgical guidance in 2017 (44).

In spite of its clear benefits, 5-ALA-based fluorescence-guided surgery (FGS) suffers from a number of shortcomings. First, it remains ineffective for guiding the resections of most LGGs and at the infiltrative margins of all diffuse gliomas (low- and high-grade) due to the fact that PpIX accumulation in these tissues is typically below the detection limit of conventional low-power wide-field surgical microscopes. Second, the visible fluorescence generated by PpIX is interpreted subjectively (45) and is difficult to quantify. This is because the visualized fluorescence is greatly affected by light-tissue interactions such as absorption and scattering, as well as detection parameters such as the angle and working distance of the microscope (46, 47). In light of these concerns, spectroscopy-based methods have been developed to provide a more accurate and reproducible measurement of the absolute concentration of PpIX expression in tissue, in which mathematical models are used to correct for the aforementioned confounding effects (22, 48–51). These quantitative detection methods should enable more-objective decision-making during tumor resection since the degree of PpIX accumulation has been shown to correlate with proliferative index, mitochondrial content, and other clinicopathologic metrics (22, 23, 40, 52, 53). However, while probe-based spectroscopy can provide improved sensitivity to detect weak PpIX fluorescence (i.e., in LGGs or at the tumor margins of all gliomas) in comparison to conventional wide-field surgical microscopy (54), spectroscopic approaches are typically limited to sampling localized points of tissue at low spatial resolution rather than generating an image over an extended field of view (FOV).

As a high-resolution, high-contrast imaging technique, handheld confocal microscopy has been explored as an alternative solution to guide the resection of both LGGs and HGGs. In 2011, a pilot study by Sanai et al. first demonstrated the feasibility of using a handheld *in vivo* confocal microscope to detect PpIX expression in LGGs (55), in which conventional wide-field surgical microscopy lacked the sensitivity to detect the PpIX fluorescence. Although the raw intensity of PpIX fluorescence, as previously mentioned, is subjective and cannot be reliably quantified, the spatial distribution (e.g., size, density, localization, etc.) of the signal can potentially serve as a reproducible tumor biomarker (56). Most recently, high-speed handheld confocal microscopy with video-mosaicking capabilities have also been developed and are continuing to be refined for 5-ALA-based FGS (57). In this perspective article, we outline a vision for a clinical workflow in which quantitative high-resolution microscopy is implemented to achieve optimal EOR for the ultimate benefit of patients suffering from LGGs and HGGs. We also describe key challenges to overcome and potential strategies to facilitate the clinical acceptance of these new technologies.

QUANTITATIVE PPIX VISUALIZATION WITH OPTICAL-SECTIONING MICROSCOPY

Optical-sectioning microscopy enables cross-sectional imaging of intact tissue at shallow depths (<0.5 mm deep) by removing the background "haze" due to out-of-focus and multiply-scattered photons. A technical description of various optical-sectioning approaches has been provided in previous review articles (58–61). In general, optical-sectioning microscopy provides the superior image contrast and spatial resolution that is necessary to detect the weak and sparse PpIX fluorescence generated by LGGs and at the infiltrative margins of all diffuse gliomas (55). An increasing number of studies have showcased the feasibility to examine PpIX expression in human gliomas at the microscopic level using optical-sectioning techniques (55, 56, 62, 63). Microscopic PpIX expression in gliomas is manifested as localized subcellular foci of fluorescence, a pattern that is consistent with our current biological understanding of subcellular PpIX generation by mitochondria (43). Quantification of microscopic PpIX expression based on a tabletop line-scanned dual-axis-confocal (LS-DAC) microscopy—a high-speed, high-contrast optical-sectioning technique—has been shown to agree with conventional fluorescence histology (56), suggesting that a miniature LS-DAC device could serve as a real-time non-invasive alternative to slide-based histopathology. As detailed in a recent review (47) and summarized in **Figure 1**, the main trade-off for high-resolution microscopy is a limited FOV that can lead to sampling bias in glioma tissues that are often spatially heterogeneous. To mitigate this problem, handheld confocal microscopy with video-mosaicking (i.e., stitching overlapping video frames to create an extended FOV over time using image processing algorithms) have been developed to sample a tissue region comparable in size to a physical biopsy specimen (several millimeters in scale) while maintaining high resolution and contrast (57, 64–68).

PROPOSED CLINICAL WORKFLOW

In the current clinical workflow for 5-ALA-based FGS, glioma margins are defined by pre-operative or intraoperative magnetic resonance imaging (MRI), as well as wide-field (low-power) surgical microscopy. However, since all gliomas are diffuse and ill-defined, the contrast-enhancing regions revealed by these wide-field imaging methods (e.g., Gd-enhancement for HGGs, T2-hyperintensity for LGGs, and macroscopic PpIX fluorescence for most HGGs) are not indicative of the actual extent of tumor infiltration. While frozen-section histopathology can confirm

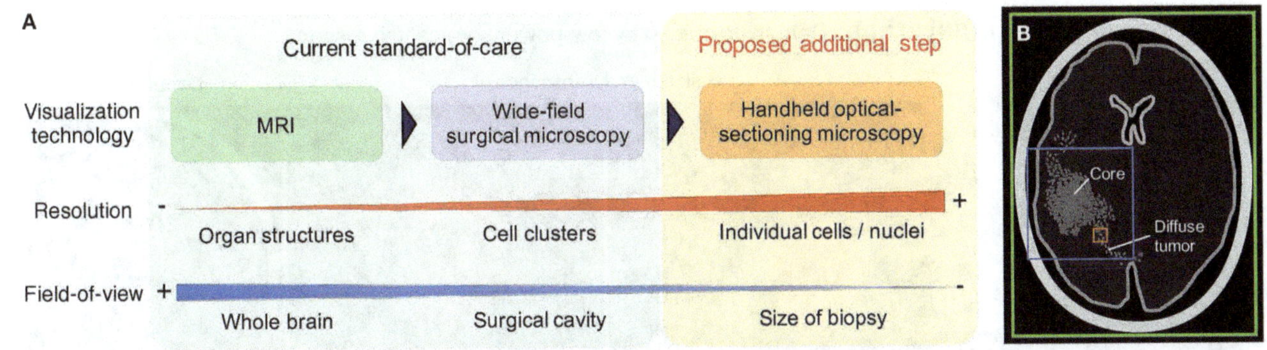

FIGURE 1 | Comparison of routine and emerging imaging techniques for neurosurgical guidance. **(A)** In the current standard-of-care, pre-operative MRI is used to assess the location and size of the bulk tumor, and wide-field surgical microscopy is used intraoperatively to guide debulking. Neither method provides sufficient spatial resolution or sensitivity to effectively visualize diffuse tumors at the surgical margins. Handheld optical-sectioning microscopy is an intraoperative imaging technique that provides superior resolution and sensitivity to detect infiltrating tumor cells at the margins, and can be potentially used to quantify tumor parameters at localized regions at the final stages of resection. **(B)** The colored boxes indicate the relative field-of-view (FOV) of the imaging modalities described. Larger FOVs are advantageous to mitigate sampling errors when imaging heterogeneous tissues, but typically require trade-offs in terms of resolution and sensitivity. Green: MRI. Blue: wide-field microscopy. Orange: optical-sectioning microscopy with mosaicking.

tissue status during the course of glioma resection, this strategy is invasive (requiring a physical biopsy) and time consuming. Our hypothesis, to be investigated in future prospective studies, is that when operating on gliomas adjacent to eloquent cortical and subcortical pathways, quantitative high-resolution microscopy can be used at the final stages of resection to interrogate tumor burden and other quantitative biomarkers at multiple suspicious sites in order to optimize the EOR (including beyond the radiographic margins) without jeopardizing functional pathways. As shown in **Figure 2**, a specific workflow for future clinical use is provided below:

(1) At the initial stages of the surgery, standard neurosurgical methods will be used for debulking the central portions of the tumor. As the neurosurgeon approaches the radiographic or functional boundaries of the tumor (indicated by anatomical/visual cues, MRI-based neuronavigation, intraoperative stimulation mapping, and 5-ALA-based FGS using wide-field surgical microscopy), regions adjacent to non-eloquent brain can be resected more aggressively to minimize residual tumor burden.

(2) At the final stages of surgery, ambiguous regions at critical locations (e.g., near eloquent brain) will be probed with high-resolution video-mosaicked microscopy of the exposed tissue surfaces, enabling a quantitative measure of microscopic PpIX expression that should ideally correlate with clinicopathologic metrics such as tumor burden and proliferative/mitotic index in order to guide operative decision-making. This provides a non-invasive and real-time alternative to intraoperative consultation with frozen-section histology. It should be noted that similar sterile probe-based microscopy/spectroscopy strategies have been implemented during neurosurgeries, as described in several reports (69–73).

(3) Conventional surgical tools (e.g., ultrasonic aspirator, suction catheters, etc.) will be used in an iterative process with intraoperative microscopy until optimal resection has been achieved. Ideally, neuronavigation would be used to track the spatial coordinates of all surgical devices (microscope, suction catheters, etc.) to ensure good co-registration between iterative rounds of imaging and resection.

CHALLENGES AND FUTURE STEPS

A number of translational milestones should ideally be achieved in order to bolster confidence in a high-resolution intraoperative imaging technique for adoption by surgeons. First, and perhaps the most critical step, is to establish a biological context and understanding of the pattern of sub-cellular PpIX expression that is visualized with an optical-sectioning microscope. Note that numerous studies have already shown that PpIX expression provides specific delineation of a variety of neoplasms under wide-field (low-resolution) imaging and spectroscopy (52, 74, 75), including a general correlation between PpIX concentrations and proliferative score as well as World Health Organization (WHO) histologic score (52). Preliminary studies [e.g., using high-resolution *in vivo* microscopy (55), or using fluorescent-activated cell sorting of dissociated human cells [unpublished data]] have also shown that PpIX expression at the cellular level is highly tumor-specific. However, larger-scale correlation studies are needed to improve our ability to interpret high-resolution images of PpIX in gliomas. For example, studies should ideally demonstrate a clear correlation between subcellular patterns of PpIX fluorescence and well-established clinicopathologic metrics such as tumor burden and proliferative/mitotic index (e.g., Ki-67 and pHH3 expression). Facilitated by the recent advancements in both imaging hardware [e.g., open-top light-sheet microscopy (63)] and artificial intelligence (e.g., deep-learning algorithms for classification and regression tasks), it should be possible to perform large correlative studies within a reasonable timeline. A second milestone, as mentioned previously, is to mitigate sampling bias due to tissue heterogeneity and to more-closely match the spatial precision of current surgical tools (typically several millimeters in scale). While it is technically challenging

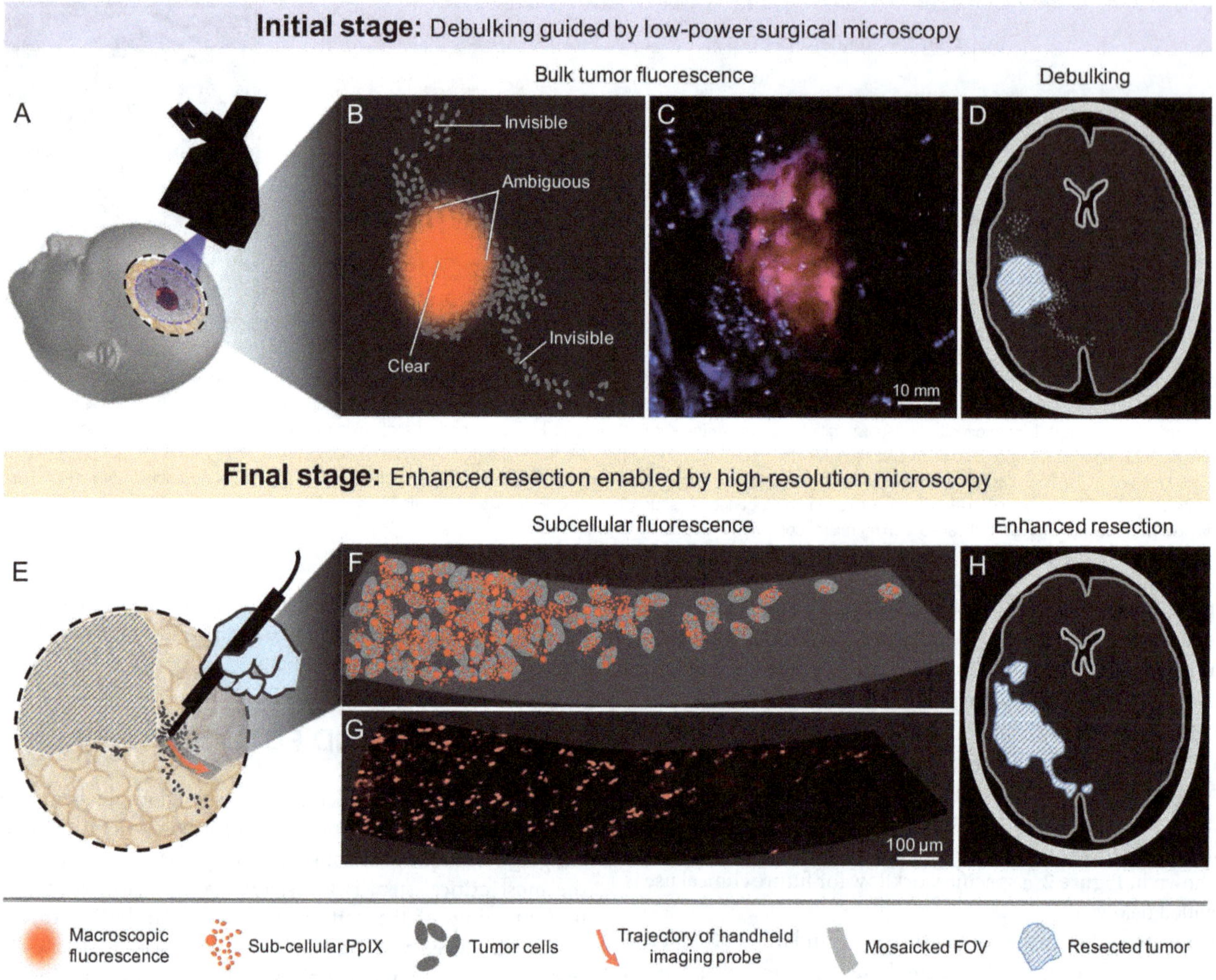

FIGURE 2 | Proposed clinical workflow of 5-ALA-based fluorescence-guided neurosurgery. **(A)** Conventional low-power fluorescence surgical microscopy provides a wide FOV that often covers the entire surgical cavity. **(B)** Macroscopic PpIX fluorescence is visible at the central portions of most HGGs, but not at the infiltrative margins. **(C)** Example low-power fluorescence microscopy image of PpIX expression from a bulk HGG region. The margins of the tumor are subjectively delineated and ambiguous. **(D)** Debulking guided by macroscopic PpIX fluorescence, resulting in residual tumor burden. **(E)** High-sensitivity probe-based optical-sectioning microscopy is used to examine localized regions near the surgical margins, providing a non-invasive alternative to intraoperative frozen section histopathology. **(F)** Visualization of subcellular PpIX fluorescence can potentially enable quantification of tumor parameters in order to guide surgical decisions at the final stages of resection. **(G)** Example image of microscopic PpIX fluorescence in a HGG biopsy using high-resolution optical-sectioning microscopy. **(H)** Optimal extent of resection is achieved after iterative tumor resection guided by video-mosaicked handheld optical-sectioning microscopy.

to engineer high-resolution microscopes with such large FOVs, robust computer vision algorithms have been developed and continue to be refined to stitch overlapping image frames together to create an extended FOV in real time while an imaging device is translated along the tissue surface (57, 64–68).

It bears repeating that the goal of optical-sectioning microscopy is NOT to image deeply, but rather to perform quantitative imaging near the exposed tissue surface, which requires the high contrast of an optical-sectioning device. However, in practice, the ability to image over a shallow range of depths (<150 microns) may be of practical value to identify an optimal depth where image quality and tissue integrity are maximized. Complementary imaging modalities for detecting PpIX fluorescence from deep subsurface tumors (76–78) are beyond the scope of this perspective paper. In terms of resolution, since current resection tools lack the spatial precision of a high-resolution microscope, the value of high-resolution imaging is not to enable cellular-scale resection, but to enable accurate quantification of PpIX, which in turn should correlate with relevant metrics of tumor burden/proliferation to guide surgical decisions. As with all innovative technologies, clinical validation is needed through well-powered and controlled studies. For example, "malignancy scores" based on quantitative PpIX microscopy should agree with traditional assessment methods such as histopathology and post-operative MRI, and should also be predictive of patient outcomes (e.g., recurrence). Note that for most glioma patients, adjuvant radiotherapy is a logical next-step following tumor resection. The development of technology that enables microscopic quantification of tumor burden and proliferation, and therefore identification of resection cavity regions with high-risk of tumor recurrence, could also inform postoperative radiotherapy planning and improve the efficacy of radiation-based strategies to control tumor progression.

In summary, the recent FDA approval of 5-ALA-based FGS and the advancement of fluorescence imaging technologies have provided a unique opportunity to improve glioma surgeries. We believe that handheld video-mosaicked optical-sectioning microscopy has an important role to play in improving the EOR for glioma surgeries through quantitative and reproducible delineation of the infiltrative margins of diffuse gliomas, for which current techniques fail to provide adequate guidance at the final most-critical stages of resection procedures. The successful translation of this technology will require collaborative efforts amongst multidisciplinary teams that include optical engineers, neurosurgeons, pathologists/biologists, computer scientists, industry partners, and regulatory/reimbursement stakeholders. Together with wide-field imaging techniques such as MRI and low-power surgical microscopy, we have provided a perspective that the use of intraoperative high-resolution microscopy within the surgical armamentarium should yield significant improvements in glioma patient outcomes.

AUTHOR CONTRIBUTIONS

All authors listed have made a substantial, direct and intellectual contribution to the work, and approved it for publication.

REFERENCES

1. Ostrom QT, Gittleman H, Liao P, Vecchione-Koval T, Wolinsky Y, Kruchko C, et al. CBTRUS Statistical report: primary brain and other central nervous system tumors diagnosed in the United States in 2010-2014. *Neuro Oncol.* (2017) 19(suppl_5):v1-v88. doi: 10.1093/neuonc/nox158
2. Hervey-Jumper SL, Berger MS. Evidence for improving outcome through extent of resection. *Neurosurg Clin N Am.* (2019) 30:85–93. doi: 10.1016/j.nec.2018.08.005
3. Lau D, Hervey-Jumper SL, Han SJ, Berger MS. Intraoperative perception and estimates on extent of resection during awake glioma surgery: overcoming the learning curve. *J Neurosurg.* (2018) 128:1410–8. doi: 10.3171/2017.1.JNS161811
4. Sharma M, Bellamkonda S, Mohapatra S, Meola A, Jia X, Mohammadi A, et al. Correlation between the residual tumor volume, extent of tumor resection, and O6-methylguanine DNA methyltransferase status in patients with glioblastoma. *World Neurosurg.* (2018) 116:e147-e61. doi: 10.1016/j.wneu.2018.04.134
5. Ahmadi R, Rezvan A, Dictus C, Christine D, Hartmann C, Christian H, et al. Long-term outcome and survival of surgically treated supratentorial low-grade glioma in adult patients. *Acta Neurochir.* (2009) 151:1359–65. doi: 10.1007/s00701-009-0435-x
6. Keles GE, Lamborn KR, Berger MS. Low-grade hemispheric gliomas in adults: a critical review of extent of resection as a factor influencing outcome. *J Neurosurg.* (2001) 95:735–45. doi: 10.3171/jns.2001.95.5.0735
7. McGirt MJ, Chaichana KL, Attenello FJ, Weingart JD, Than K, Burger PC, et al. Extent of surgical resection is independently associated with survival in patients with hemispheric infiltrating low-grade gliomas. *Neurosurgery.* (2008) 63:700–7- author reply 7-8. doi: 10.1227/01.NEU.0000325729.41085.73
8. Sanai N, Polley M-Y, Berger MS. Insular glioma resection: assessment of patient morbidity, survival, and tumor progression. *J Neurosurg.* (2010) 112:1–9. doi: 10.3171/2009.6.JNS0952
9. Smith JS, Chang EF, Lamborn KR, Chang SM, Prados MD, Cha S, et al. Role of extent of resection in the long-term outcome of low-grade hemispheric gliomas. *J Clin Oncol.* (2008) 26:1338–45. doi: 10.1200/JCO.2007.13.9337
10. Stummer W, van den Bent MJ, Westphal M. Cytoreductive surgery of glioblastoma as the key to successful adjuvant therapies: new arguments in an old discussion. *Acta Neurochir.* (2011) 153:1211–8. doi: 10.1007/s00701-011-1001-x
11. Stummer W, Reulen H-J, Meinel T, Pichlmeier U, Schumacher W, Tonn J-C, et al. Extent of resection and survival in glioblastoma multiforme: identification of and adjustment for bias. *Neurosurgery.* (2008) 62:564–76; discussion–76. doi: 10.1227/01.neu.0000317304.31579.17
12. DAmico RS, Englander ZK, Canoll P, Bruce JN. Extent of resection in glioma-a review of the cutting edge. *World Neurosurg.* (2017) 103:538–49. doi: 10.1016/j.wneu.2017.04.041
13. Hervey-Jumper SL, Berger MS. Maximizing safe resection of low- and high-grade glioma. *J Neurooncol.* (2016) 130:269–82. doi: 10.1007/s11060-016-2110-4
14. Sanai N, Berger MS. Operative techniques for gliomas and the value of extent of resection. *Neurother J Am Soc Exp NeuroTher.* (2009) 6:478–86. doi: 10.1016/j.nurt.2009.04.005
15. Brown PD, Maurer MJ, Rummans TA, Pollock BE, Ballman KV, Sloan JA, et al. A prospective study of quality of life in adults with newly diagnosed high-grade gliomas: the impact of the extent of resection on quality of life and survival. *Neurosurgery.* (2005) 57:495–504- discussion 495-504. doi: 10.1227/01.NEU.0000170562.25335.C7
16. Chaichana KL, Halthore AN, Parker SL, Olivi A, Weingart JD, Brem H, et al. Factors involved in maintaining prolonged functional independence following supratentorial glioblastoma resection. *J Neurosurg.* (2011) 114:604–12. doi: 10.3171/2010.4.JNS091340
17. Chaichana KL, Kosztowski T, Niranjan A, Olivi A, Weingart JD, Laterra J, et al. Prognostic significance of contrast-enhancing anaplastic astrocytomas in adults. *J Neurosurg.* (2010) 113:286–92. doi: 10.3171/2010.2.JNS091010
18. Stark AM, Nabavi A, Mehdorn HM, Blömer U. Glioblastoma multiforme-report of 267 cases treated at a single institution. *Surg Neurol.* (2005) 63:162–9-discussion 9. doi: 10.1016/j.surneu.2004.01.028
19. Ushio Y, Kochi M, Hamada J-i, Kai Y, Nakamura H. Effect of surgical removal on survival and quality of life in patients with supratentorial glioblastoma. *Neurol Med Chir.* (2005) 45:454–60- discussion 60-1. doi: 10.2176/nmc.45.454
20. Patel T, Bander ED, Venn RA, Powell T, Cederquist GY-M, Schaefer PM, et al. The role of extent of resection in IDH1 wild-type or mutant low-grade gliomas. *Neurosurgery.* (2018) 82:808–14. doi: 10.1093/neuros/nyx265
21. Wijnenga MMJ, French PJ, Dubbink HJ, Dinjens WNM, Atmodimedjo PN, Kros JM, et al. The impact of surgery in molecularly defined low-grade glioma: an integrated clinical, radiological, and molecular analysis. *Neuro-Oncology.* (2018) 20:103–12. doi: 10.1093/neuonc/nox176
22. Valdes PA, Leblond F, Kim A, Harris BT, Wilson BC, Fan XY, et al. Quantitative fluorescence in intracranial tumor: implications for ALA-induced PpIX as an intraoperative biomarker. *J Neurosurg.* (2011) 115:11–7. doi: 10.3171/2011.2.JNS101451
23. Stummer W, Tonn JC, Goetz C, Ullrich W, Stepp H, Bink A, et al. 5-Aminolevulinic acid-derived tumor fluorescence: the diagnostic accuracy of visible fluorescence qualities as corroborated by spectrometry and histology and postoperative imaging. *Neurosurgery.* (2014) 74:310–9; discussion 9-20. doi: 10.1227/NEU.0000000000000267
24. Stummer W, Novotny A, Stepp H, Goetz C, Bise K, Reulen HJ. Fluorescence-guided resection of glioblastoma multiforme by using 5-aminolevulinic acid-induced porphyrins: a prospective study in 52 consecutive patients. *J Neurosurg.* (2000) 93:1003–13. doi: 10.3171/jns.2000.93.6.1003
25. Panciani PP, Fontanella M, Schatlo B, Garbossa D, Agnoletti A, Ducati A, et al. Fluorescence and image guided resection in high grade glioma. *Clin Neurol Neurosurg.* (2012) 114:37–41. doi: 10.1016/j.clineuro.2011.09.001
26. Yamada S, Muragaki Y, Maruyama T, Komori T, Okada Y. Role of neurochemical navigation with 5-aminolevulinic acid during intraoperative

MRI-guided resection of intracranial malignant gliomas. *Clin Neurol Neurosurg.* (2015) 130:134–9. doi: 10.1016/j.clineuro.2015.01.005

27. Roberts DW, Valdes PA, Harris BT, Fontaine KM, Hartov A, Fan X, et al. Coregistered fluorescence-enhanced tumor resection of malignant glioma: relationships between delta-aminolevulinic acid-induced protoporphyrin IX fluorescence, magnetic resonance imaging enhancement, and neuropathological parameters. *J Neurosurg.* (2011) 114:595–603. doi: 10.3171/2010.2.JNS091322
28. Diez Valle R, Tejada Solis S, Idoate Gastearena MA, Garcia de Eulate R, Dominguez Echavarri P, Aristu Mendiroz J. Surgery guided by 5-aminolevulinic fluorescence in glioblastoma: volumetric analysis of extent of resection in single-center experience. *J Neurooncol.* (2011) 102:105–13. doi: 10.1007/s11060-010-0296-4
29. Hefti M, von Campe G, Moschopulos M, Siegner A, Looser H, Landolt H. 5-aminolevulinic acid induced protoporphyrin IX fluorescence in high-grade glioma surgery: a one-year experience at a single institutuion. *Swiss Med Wkly.* (2008) 138:180–5.
30. Acerbi F, Broggi M, Eoli M, Anghileri E, Cuppini L, Pollo B, et al. Fluorescein-guided surgery for grade IV gliomas with a dedicated filter on the surgical microscope: preliminary results in 12 cases. *Acta Neurochir.* (2013) 155:1277–86. doi: 10.1007/s00701-013-1734-9
31. Tsugu A, Ishizaka H, Mizokami Y, Osada T, Baba T, Yoshiyama M, et al. Impact of the combination of 5-aminolevulinic acid-induced fluorescence with intraoperative magnetic resonance imaging-guided surgery for glioma. *World Neurosurg.* (2011) 76:120–7. doi: 10.1016/j.wneu.2011.02.005
32. Hadjipanayis CG, Widhalm G, Stummer W. What is the surgical benefit of utilizing 5-aminolevulinic acid for fluorescence-guided surgery of malignant gliomas? *Neurosurgery.* (2015) 77:663–73. doi: 10.1227/NEU.0000000000000929
33. Rapp M, Kamp M, Steiger HJ, Sabel M. Endoscopic-assisted visualization of 5-aminolevulinic acid-induced fluorescence in malignant glioma surgery: a technical note. *World Neurosurg.* (2014) 82:E277–E9. doi: 10.1016/j.wneu.2013.07.002
34. Belloch JP, Rovira V, Llacer JL, Riesgo PA, Cremades A. Fluorescence-guided surgery in high grade gliomas using an exoscope system. *Acta Neurochir.* (2014) 156:653–60. doi: 10.1007/s00701-013-1976-6
35. Liao H, Noguchi M, Maruyama T, Muragaki Y, Kobayashi E, Iseki H, et al. An integrated diagnosis and therapeutic system using intra-operative 5-aminolevulinic-acid-induced fluorescence guided robotic laser ablation for precision neurosurgery. *Med Image Anal.* (2012) 16:754–66. doi: 10.1016/j.media.2010.11.004
36. Nabavi A, Thurm H, Zountsas B, Pietsch T, Lanfermann H, Pichlmeier U, et al. Five-aminolevulinic acid for fluorescence-guided resection of recurrent malignant gliomas: a phase ii study. *Neurosurgery.* (2009) 65:1070–6; discussion 6-7. doi: 10.1227/01.NEU.0000360128.03597.C7
37. Stummer W, Pichlmeier U, Meinel T, Wiestler OD, Zanella F, Reulen H-J, et al. Fluorescence-guided surgery with 5-aminolevulinic acid for resection of malignant glioma: a randomised controlled multicentre phase III trial. *Lancet Oncol.* (2006) 7:392–401. doi: 10.1016/S1470-2045(06)70665-9
38. Tonn J-C, Stummer W. Fluorescence-guided resection of malignant gliomas using 5-aminolevulinic acid: practical use, risks, and pitfalls. *Clin Neurosurg.* (2008) 55:20–6.
39. Duffner F, Ritz R, Freudenstein D, Weller M, Dietz K, Wessels J. Specific intensity imaging for glioblastoma and neural cell cultures with 5-aminolevulinic acid-derived protoporphyrin IX. *J Neurooncol.* (2005) 71:107–11. doi: 10.1007/s11060-004-9603-2
40. Gibbs SL, Chen B, O'Hara JA, Hoopes PJ, Hasan T, Pogue BW. Protoporphyrin IX level correlates with number of mitochondria, but increase in production correlates with tumor cell size. *Photochem Photobiol.* (2006) 82:1334–41. doi: 10.1562/2006-03-11-RA-843
41. Olivo M, Wilson BC. Mapping ALA-induced PPIX fluorescence in normal brain and brain tumour using confocal fluorescence microscopy. *Int J Oncol.* (2004) 25:37–45. doi: 10.3892/ijo.25.1.37
42. Stummer W, Stocker S, Novotny A, Heimann A, Sauer O, Kempski O, et al. *In vitro* and *in vivo* porphyrin accumulation by C6 glioma cells after exposure to 5-aminolevulinic acid. *J Photochem Photobiol B Biol.* (1998) 45:160–9. doi: 10.1016/S1011-1344(98)00176-6
43. Stepp H, Stummer W. 5-ALA in the management of malignant glioma. *Lasers Surg Med.* (2018) 50:399–419. doi: 10.1002/lsm.22933
44. Aminolevulinic acid hydrochloride, known as ALA HCl (Gleolan, NX Development Corp.) as an optical imaging agent indicated in patients with gliomas (2017).
45. Lau D, Hervey-Jumper SL, Chang S, Molinaro AM, McDermott MW, Phillips JJ, et al. A prospective Phase II clinical trial of 5-aminolevulinic acid to assess the correlation of intraoperative fluorescence intensity and degree of histologic cellularity during resection of high-grade gliomas. *J Neurosurg.* (2016) 124:1300–9. doi: 10.3171/2015.5.JNS1577
46. Valdes PA, Leblond F, Jacobs VL, Wilson BC, Paulsen KD, Roberts DW. Quantitative, spectrally-resolved intraoperative fluorescence imaging. *Sci Rep.* (2012) 2:798. doi: 10.1038/srep00798
47. Wei L, Roberts D, Sanai N, Liu JTC. Visualization technologies for 5-ALA-based fluorescence-guided surgeries. *J Neuro-Oncol.* (2019) 2019:9. doi: 10.1007/s11060-018-03077-9
48. Haj-Hosseini N, Richter J, Andersson-Engels S, Wardell K. Optical touch pointer for fluorescence guided glioblastoma resection using 5-aminolevulinic acid. *Lasers Surg Med.* (2010) 42:9–14. doi: 10.1002/lsm.20868
49. Kim A, Khurana M, Moriyama Y, Wilson BC. Quantification of in vivo fluorescence decoupled from the effects of tissue optical properties using fiber-optic spectroscopy measurements. *J Biomed Optics.* (2010) 15:6. doi: 10.1117/1.3523616
50. Ishihara R, Katayama Y, Watanabe T, Yoshino A, Fukushima T, Sakatani K. Quantitative spectroscopic analysis of 5-aminolevulinic acid-induced protoporphyrin IX fluorescence intensity in diffusely infiltrating astrocytomas. *Neurol Med Chir.* (2007) 47:53–7; discussion 7. doi: 10.2176/nmc.47.53
51. Utsuki S, Oka H, Sato S, Suzuki S, Shimizu S, Tanaka S, et al. Possibility of using laser spectroscopy for the intraoperative detection of nonfluorescing brain tumors and the boundaries of brain tumor infiltrates - Technical note. *J Neurosurg.* (2006) 104:618–20. doi: 10.3171/jns.2006.104.4.618
52. Valdes PA, Kim A, Brantsch M, Niu C, Moses ZB, Tosteson TD, et al. delta-aminolevulinic acid-induced protoporphyrin IX concentration correlates with histopathologic markers of malignancy in human gliomas: the need for quantitative fluorescence-guided resection to identify regions of increasing malignancy. *Neuro Oncol.* (2011) 13:846–56. doi: 10.1093/neuonc/nor086
53. Belykh E, Miller EJ, Hu D, Martirosyan NL, Woolf EC, Scheck AC, et al. Scanning fiber endoscope improves detection of 5-aminolevulinic acid-induced protoporphyrin IX fluorescence at the boundary of infiltrative glioma. *World Neurosurg.* (2018) 113:e51-e69. doi: 10.1016/j.wneu.2018.01.151
54. Valdes PA, Jacobs V, Harris BT, Wilson BC, Leblond F, Paulsen KD, et al. Quantitative fluorescence using 5-aminolevulinic acid-induced protoporphyrin IX biomarker as a surgical adjunct in low-grade glioma surgery. *J Neurosurg.* (2015) 123:771–80. doi: 10.3171/2014.12.JNS14391
55. Sanai N, Snyder LA, Honea NJ, Coons SW, Eschbacher JM, Smith KA, et al. Intraoperative confocal microscopy in the visualization of 5-aminolevulinic acid fluorescence in low-grade gliomas. *J Neurosurg.* (2011) 115:740–8. doi: 10.3171/2011.6.JNS11252
56. Wei L, Chen Y, Yin C, Borwege S, Sanai N, Liu JTC. Optical-sectioning microscopy of protoporphyrin IX fluorescence in human gliomas: standardization and quantitative comparison with histology. *J Biomed Opt.* (2017) 22:46005. doi: 10.1117/1.JBO.22.4.046005
57. Wei L, Yin C, Fujita Y, Sanai N, Liu JTC. Handheld line-scanned dual-axis confocal microscope with pistoned MEMS actuation for flat-field fluorescence imaging. *Opt Lett.* (2019) 44:671–4. doi: 10.1364/OL.44.000671
58. Conchello JA, Lichtman JW. Optical sectioning microscopy. *Nat Methods.* (2005) 2:920–31. doi: 10.1038/nmeth815
59. Helmchen F, Denk W. Deep tissue two-photon microscopy. *Nat Methods.* (2005) 2:932–40. doi: 10.1038/nmeth818
60. Huisken J, Stainier DY. Selective plane illumination microscopy techniques in developmental biology. *Development.* (2009) 136:1963–75. doi: 10.1242/dev.022426
61. Wei L, Yin C, Liu JTC. Dual-axis confocal microscopy for point-of-care pathology. *IEEE J Select Topics Quantum Electron.* (2019) 25:1–10. doi: 10.1109/JSTQE.2018.2854572

62. Meza D, Wang D, Wang Y, Borwege S, Sanai N, Liu JT. Comparing high-resolution microscopy techniques for potential intraoperative use in guiding low-grade glioma resections. *Lasers Surg Med.* (2015) 47:289–95. doi: 10.1002/lsm.22347
63. Glaser AK, Reder NP, Chen Y, McCarty EF, Yin C, Wei L, et al. Light-sheet microscopy for slide-free non-destructive pathology of large clinical specimens. *Nat Biomed Eng.* (2017) 1:0084. doi: 10.1038/s41551-017-0084
64. Vercauteren T, Perchant A, Pennec X, Ayache N. Mosaicing of confocal microscopic *in vivo* soft tissue video sequences. *Lect Notes Comput Sc.* (2005) 3749:753–60. doi: 10.1007/11566465_93
65. Vercauteren T, Perchant A, Malandain G, Pennec X, Ayache N. Robust mosaicing with correction of motion distortions and tissue deformations for *in vivo* fibered microscopy. *Med Image Anal.* (2006) 10:673–92. doi: 10.1016/j.media.2006.06.006
66. Loewke KE, Camarillo DB, Piyawattanametha W, Mandella MJ, Contag CH, Thrun S, et al. *In vivo* micro-image mosaicing. *IEEE T Bio-Med Eng.* (2011) 58:159–71. doi: 10.1109/TBME.2010.2085082
67. Kose K, Cordova M, Duffy M, Flores ES, Brooks DH, Rajadhyaksha M. Video-mosaicing of reflectance confocal images for examination of extended areas of skin *in vivo*. *Br J Dermatol.* (2014) 171:1239–41. doi: 10.1111/bjd.13050
68. Kose K, Gou M, Yelamos O, Cordova M, Rossi AM, Nehal KS, et al. Automated video-mosaicking approach for confocal microscopic imaging *in vivo*: an approach to address challenges in imaging living tissue and extend field of view. *Sci Rep.* (2017) 7:10759. doi: 10.1038/s41598-017-11072-9
69. Martirosyan NL, Eschbacher JM, Kalani MYS, Turner JD, Belykh E, Spetzler RF, et al. Prospective evaluation of the utility of intraoperative confocal laser endomicroscopy in patients with brain neoplasms using fluorescein sodium: experience with 74 cases. *Neurosurg Focus.* (2016) 40:3. doi: 10.3171/2016.1.FOCUS15559
70. Pavlov V, Meyronet D, Meyer-Bisch V, Armoiry X, Pikul B, Dumot C, et al. Intraoperative probe-based confocal laser endomicroscopy in surgery and stereotactic biopsy of low-grade and high-grade gliomas: a feasibility study in humans. *Neurosurgery.* (2016) 79:604–12. doi: 10.1227/NEU.0000000000001365
71. Belykh E, Cavallo C, Gandhi S, Zhao X, Veljanoski D, Izady Yazdanabadi M, et al. Utilization of intraoperative confocal laser endomicroscopy in brain tumor surgery. *J Neurosurg Sci.* (2018) 2018:8. doi: 10.23736/S0390-5616.18.04553-8
72. Sanai N, Eschbacher J, Hattendorf G, Coons SW, Preul MC, Smith KA, et al. Intraoperative confocal microscopy for brain tumors: a feasibility analysis in humans. *Neurosurgery.* (2011) 68(2 Suppl Operative):282–90; discussion 90. doi: 10.1227/NEU.0b013e318212464e
73. Eschbacher J, Martirosyan NL, Nakaji P, Sanai N, Preul MC, Smith KA, et al. *In vivo* intraoperative confocal microscopy for real-time histopathological imaging of brain tumors. *J Neurosurg.* (2012) 116:854–60. doi: 10.3171/2011.12.JNS11696
74. Yano H, Nakayama N, Ohe N, Miwa K, Shinoda J, Iwama T. Pathological analysis of the surgical margins of resected glioblastomas excised using photodynamic visualization with both 5-aminolevulinic acid and fluorescein sodium. *J Neurooncol.* (2017) 133:389–97. doi: 10.1007/s11060-017-2445-5
75. Yoneda T, Nonoguchi N, Ikeda N, Yagi R, Kawabata S, Furuse M, et al. Spectral radiance of protoporphyrin IX fluorescence and its histopathological implications in 5-aminolevulinic acid-guided surgery for glioblastoma. *Photomed Laser Surg.* (2018) 36:266–72. doi: 10.1089/pho.2017.4384
76. Konecky SD, Owen CM, Rice T, Valdes PA, Kolste K, Wilson BC, et al. Spatial frequency domain tomography of protoporphyrin IX fluorescence in preclinical glioma models. *J Biomed Opt.* (2012) 17:056008. doi: 10.1117/1.JBO.17.5.056008
77. Roberts DW, Olson JD, Evans LT, Kolste KK, Kanick SC, Fan X, et al. Red-light excitation of protoporphyrin IX fluorescence for subsurface tumor detection. *J Neurosurg.* (2018) 128:1690–7. doi: 10.3171/2017.1.JNS162061
78. Kolste KK, Kanick SC, Valdes PA, Jermyn M, Wilson BC, Roberts DW, et al. Macroscopic optical imaging technique for wide-field estimation of fluorescence depth in optically turbid media for application in brain tumor surgical guidance. *J Biomed Opt.* (2015) 20:26002. doi: 10.1117/1.JBO.20.2.026002

11

Fluorescein Application in Cranial and Spinal Tumors Enhancing at Preoperative MRI and Operated with a Dedicated Filter on the Surgical Microscope: Preliminary Results in 279 Patients Enrolled in the FLUOCERTUM Prospective Study

Jacopo Falco [1†], Claudio Cavallo [1,2†], Ignazio G. Vetrano [1], Camilla de Laurentis [1], Lampros Siozos [1], Marco Schiariti [1], Morgan Broggi [1], Paolo Ferroli [1] and Francesco Acerbi [1]*

[1] Department of Neurosurgery, Fondazione IRCCS Istituto Neurologico Carlo Besta, Milan, Italy, [2] Department of Neurosurgery, Barrow Neurological Institute, St. Joseph's Hospital and Medical Center, Phoenix, AZ, United States

***Correspondence:**
Francesco Acerbi
francesco.acerbi@istituto-besta.it

† These authors have contributed equally to this work

Objective: Sodium fluorescein, a green, water soluble dye, is used as neurosurgical fluorescent tracer thanks to its property to accumulate in cerebral regions of blood-brain barrier (BBB) disruption. The authors report the preliminary results of a prospective observational study regarding the use of fluorescein-guided technique for the resection of suspected malignant neoplasms of the central nervous system (CNS), contrast enhancing at preoperative magnetic resonance imaging (MRI), using a dedicated filter on the surgical microscope.

Methods: In March 2016 the authors started a prospective, observational trial to evaluate intraoperative fluorescence's characteristics of CNS tumors, the percentage of extent of resection thanks to fluorescein aid and side effects related to fluorescein administration. This report is based on a preliminary analysis of the results of first 279 enrolled patients. Fluorescein was intravenously injected after intubation or immediately at the entrance in the operating room for awake procedures; the tumor was removed using a dedicated filter on the surgical microscope in an inside-out fashion until all fluorescent tissue was removed, as considered feasible by the surgeon.

Results: The 279 patients finally enrolled in the trial, both firstly diagnosed and recurrent, were categorized according to WHO pathological classification and there were 212 neuroepithelial tumors, 25 brain metastases, 10 cerebral lymphomas, 7 hemangioblastomas, or hemangioendotheliomas and 25 other tumors and conditions. No adverse reaction related to the administration of fluorescein or to the combined use of fluorescein with other fluorophores was registered. Fluorescein accumulated in cerebral regions where the BBB was damaged, representing a significant surgical aid in most of the CNS tumors with contrast enhancement. In cases of complete removal of all fluorescent tissue, as intraoperatively judged by the surgeon, postoperative MRI revealed a gross total resection in 181/198 patients (91.4%).

Conclusions: Based on these preliminary results, fluorescein-guided surgery with a dedicated filter on the microscope is a safe and effective technique to improve visualization and resection of different CNS tumors and conditions, based on BBB alteration.

Keywords: biopsy, brain tumors, central nervous system, fluorescein, neuro-oncology, spinal tumors, YELLOW 560

INTRODUCTION

Even if Central Nervous System (CNS) tumors do not represent one of the most frequent kind of cancers, they are a major cause of cancer-related mortality and morbidity (1), with an annual incidence in the Western countries of 16.5 per 100.000 adults and of 2.4 new cases per 100.000 children per year. Surgery is the most important treatment in almost all aggressive brain tumors (2–4). The extent of resection (EOR) is a fundamental topic in neurosurgery; if feasible and safely achievable, the gross total resection (GTR) is the most important predictor of overall survival both in high-grade gliomas (HGG) and in metastases (2, 3, 5–9). Furthermore, GTR reduces the risk of recurrence of low-grade gliomas (LGG) or other benign tumors (10, 11). For solitary metastasis, surgical resection plus adjuvant radiotherapy, in form of whole brain radiotherapy or stereotactic radiosurgery, is considered the gold therapeutic standard (12–14); complete metastases resection associated to a favorable factor for prolonged survival. Also for other astrocytomas or rarer primary brain tumors, such as medulloblastomas or ependymomas, radical resection has been correlated to a better prognosis: regarding pilocytic astrocytoma (PA) and ependymomas, a complete resection can achieve local control improving the survival (15, 16).

This need for a radical tumor removal allowed the flourishing of many tools to better visualize the tumor tissue, improving the extent of resection, such as neuronavigation, intraoperative magnetic resonance imaging (MRI), and intraoperative ultrasounds with contrast-enhanced ultrasound (17–19). Among these, fluorophores have acquired an important role thanks to their ability to discriminate between pathological and normal tissue (20–22). Fluorescein is a green fluorescent synthetic organic compound which has countless medical applications (23–27). In form of fluorescein sodium salt (SF) it represents a water-soluble dye with a major blue excitation peak in the region of 460–500 nm and a major green emission peak in the region of 540 to 690 nm.

Although initially its use has been limited to ophthalmology, with historical and sporadic utilization in neurosurgery (28–30), since the introduction of a dedicated and integrated filter in the surgical microscope (YELLOW 560 -*Pentero 900* and *Kinevo; Carl Zeiss Meditec, Oberkochen, Germany*), SF applications in neurosurgery have increased exponentially (31–42). SF, differently to 5-aminolevulenic acid (5-ALA) which is a metabolic tracer (20), could be considered as a vascular fluorophore and its use as fluorescent tracer in neuro-oncological procedures relies on the property to accumulate in pathological areas of blood-brain barrier (BBB) disruption, as in gliomas, but also in other brain tumors, similar to the process of contrast enhancement (c.e.) on MRI.

In July 2015, based upon preliminary scientific results from different studies published in the international literature (34, 36, 37), including a prospective phase II trial from our group (32, 33, 38, 43–46) the Italian Medicine Agency (AIFA) has extended the indications for the utilization of fluorescein molecule (determination 905/2015, Gazette n.168, 22 July, 2015; http://www.gazzettaufficiale.it/atto/serie_generale/caricaDettaglioAtto/originario;jsessionid=izVcTOmnjOzfNRjjw56kAA__.ntc-as2-guri2b?atto.dataPubblicazioneGazzetta=2015-07-22&atto.codiceRedazionale=15A05620&elenco30giorni=false). According to this determination, the intravenous (i.v.) injection of SF as a neurosurgical tracer during oncological procedures for aggressive tumors of the CNS is approved and its cost are totally reimbursed by the Italian National Health System. Therefore, in March 2016, the authors started a new prospective observational study, called FLUOCERTUM (FLUOrescein in CERebral TUMors), regarding the use of SF as a fluorescent intra-operative tracer in patients with suspected aggressive tumors of the CNS. In this paper, we present the preliminary results of the first 279 patients enrolled in this study, until December 2018.

METHODS

Patients and Inclusion Criteria

The inclusion criteria were as follows: (1) patients of both genders, at any age; (2) patients with suspected aggressive lesions of the CNS, as suggested by preoperative MRI or computerized tomography (CT) with i.v. contrast agent administration. The exclusion criteria were: (1) impossibility to give consent due to cognitive deficits or language disorders; (2) known allergy to contrast agents or history of previous anaphylactic shocks;

Abbreviations: AA, anaplastic astrocytoma; AO, anaplastic oligodendroglioma; AIFA, agenzia italiana del farmaco (Italian Medicine Agency); BBB, blood brain barrier; c.e., contrast enhancement; CNS, central nervous system; CT, computerized tomography; EOR, extent of resection; FET, fluoro-ethyl-tyrosine; GBM, glioblastoma; GTR, gross total resection; HGG, high-grade glioma; ICG, indocyanine green; i.v., intravenous; LGG, low-grade glioma; MET, 11C-methionine; MRI, magnetic resonance imaging; PA, pilocytic astrocytoma; PET, positron emission tomography; PR, partial resection; SF, sodium fluorescein; STR, subtotal resection; 5-ALA, 5-aminolevulenic acid.

(3) known severe previous adverse reactions to SF; (4) acute myocardial infarction or stroke in the last 90 days; (5) severe renal failure; (6) severe hepatic failure; (7) severe heart failure; (8) women in their first trimester of pregnancy or lactation.

The study started in March 2016, when the first patient was enrolled. Written informed consent was obtained from all patients. The FLUOCERTUM study has been approved by the Ethical Committee of the Fondazione IRCCS Istituto Neurologico Carlo Besta.

Three hundred and twenty-eight patients were screened for participation in this prospective trial. Two patients were excluded from the analysis because they refused surgery, seventeen patients were excluded because SF was not intraoperatively injected, while fourteen patients were excluded because the specific YELLOW 560 filter of the microscope was not available or not working properly; finally, we excluded sixteen patients because surgery was performed under 5-ALA guidance but SF was administered only for confocal laser endomicroscopy evaluation. The final enrolment comprised 279 patients: 252 adult patients (145 male and 107 female) from 18 to 82 years (mean age 52.1 years) and 27 pediatric patients (14 male and 13 female) from 2 to 17 years (mean age 9.82 years).

Clinical and Radiological Management

As part of normal clinical practice at our Institution, preoperative assessment included physical and neurological examination, laboratory tests results, preoperative contrast-enhanced MRI or CT scans for neuronavigation, recording of concomitant medications (as steroids) and previous radiation therapies. In pre-operative MRI, patients were categorized based on pre-operative contrast enhancement characteristics and divided in cases with clear contrast enhancement and cases with only minimal/absent contrast enhancement. To evaluate the EOR, a volumetric MRI examination was performed for each patient within 72 h after surgery; in particular, to calculate the residual pathological volume, the hyperintense alterations in volumetric basal T1 acquisitions were subtracted from the volume of hyperintense tissue in post-contrast volumetric T1 images, to avoid the incidental inclusion of blood or blood product. The post-operative clinical evaluation included a standard neurological examination and exclusion of occurrence of any side effect related to fluorescein injection. In particular, according to AIFA determination, arterial blood pressure, heart rate, blood oxygen saturation, temperature, and skin color were monitored pre-operatively and three times per day during the first three post-operative days; plasmatic dosage of creatinine was controlled the first and third post-operative day. The follow-up considered in this trial ended at the completion of the immediate post-operative radiological examination and clinical observation, as in AIFA determination.

Surgical Protocol

Our surgical protocol of fluorescein-guided technique is the same used in the FLUOGLIO trial since 2012 and it has already been described in previous papers (32, 33, 38), and based on i.v. SF (*Monico SpA, Italy*) injection at standard dose of 5 mg/kg, by a central venous line, immediately upon completion of the induction of general anesthesia or anesthetic procedures in awake surgery. The surgery was performed with the aid of a surgical microscope equipped with an integrated fluorescent filter specific for fluorescein (*Pentero* or *Kinevo* microscopes, with YELLOW 560 filter; *Carl Zeiss Meditec, Oberkochen, Germany*). During resection, the microscope could be switched alternatively from fluorescent to white-light illumination; neuronavigation, intraoperative ultrasounds, and contrast-enhanced ultrasound or other tools could be used according to the surgeon's preference. In tumors located in eloquent areas, intraoperative neurophysiological monitoring was used. Tumors were removed in an inside-out fashion until all fluorescent tissue was removed, as considered feasible by the surgeon.

In cases where tumor vessels, or peritumoral arteries and veins needed to be intraoperatively evaluated, indocyanine green (ICG) video-angiography with FLOW 800 analysis (*Carl Zeiss Meditec, Oberkochen, Germany*) and, sometimes, ICG temporary clipping test were performed, as already reported (47–51).

Histological Analysis

Histopathological analysis was performed in each case; tumors were classified according to the 2016 WHO classification by the neuro-pathology group of our Institute, with no additional costs respect to clinical practice (52).

Statistical Analysis

The study population was classified about gender, age, histological subtype, tumor volume and location, and therefore evaluated with descriptive analysis. Fluorescence intensity was graded by the surgeon as intense/bright, inhomogeneous or homogeneous, moderate or slight/absent; surgeons were also asked to classify the use of SF per each procedure as helpful/useful, not essential, not helpful/useless to achieve surgical aims. The EOR was prospectively calculated as a percentage of tumor resection based on early contrast-enhanced postoperative MRI or CT imaging; according to the entity of resection, we distinguished five main categories: GTR (EOR 100%), sub-total resection (STR, with an EOR of 90–100%), partial resection (PR, 30–90%), open biopsy and frameless/stereotactic biopsy. Rate of removal was studied in the different histological subtypes and compared with ANOVA by Prism software.

RESULTS

All the 279 patients finally enrolled in the trial were classified and categorized as stated by the 2016 WHO central nervous system tumors classification; the results about intraoperative fluorescence characteristics, surgical utility and extent of resection, were then related to the different histotypes.

Briefly, there were 212 neuroepithelial tumors, 25 brain metastases, 10 cerebral lymphomas, 7 hemangioblastomas or hemangioendotheliomas and 25 other tumors and conditions in differential diagnosis or in which SF represented a surgical aid (**Tables 1, 2**).

TABLE 1 | Intraoperative fluorescence characteristics and utility, based on tumor histology, in the surgical group.

HISTOLOGIES		Number of patients	Intraoperative fluorescence	Extent of resection				Surgeon's opinion
				GTR (# - %)	Unexpected STR (no fluorescent residual tissue–not enhancing tumor) (# - %)	Expected STR (fluorescent residual tissue) (# - %)	PR (# - %)	
Tumors of neuroepithelial tissue	Diffuse astrocytic and oligodendro	143	- Heterogeneously intense (HGG) - Absent, only some spots (LGG)	104 (72.7)	13 (9.1)	19 (13.3)	7 (4.9)	- Helpful in HGG (132 cases) - Useless in LGG (11 cases)
	Ependymoma	14	Homogeneously intense	10 (71.5)	1 (7.1)	2 (14.3)	1 (7.1)	Helpful (14 cases)
	Glioneuronal	13	- Homogeneously intense - Slight/Absent (rosette-forming glioneuronal tumor)	9 (69.2)	1 (7.7)	3 (23.1)	0	- Helpful (9 cases) - Partial utility during surgery for drug-resistant epilepsy (3 cases) - Useless in rosette-forming glioneuronal tumor (1 case)
	PA and other astrocytic	18	- Heterogeneously intense (bright cystic fluid if present) - Homogeneously intense (SEGA)	10 (55.6)	2 (11.1)	5 (27.8)	1 (5.5)	Helpful (18 cases)
	Others (Embryonal, PPTID, ...)	8	Intense: - Heterogeneously (medulloblastoma, PPTID and angiocentric glioma) - Homogenously (choroid plexus papilloma)	7 (87.5)	0	0	1 (12.5)	- Helpful (7 cases) - Not essential in choroid plexus papilloma (1 case)
Cerebral metastases		25	Heterogeneously intense	24 (96)	0	1 (4)	0	- Helpful (20 cases) - Not essential in 3 skin melanoma metastases and in one hemorrhagic metastasis (4 cases) - Useless in 1 case (previous whole brain radiotherapy and radiosurgery)
Primary CNS lymphomas		4	Homogeneously intense	4 (100)	0	0	0	Helpful (4 cases)
Meningiomas		3	Homogeneously intense	3 (100)	0	0	0	Not essential (3 cases)
Cerebral hemangioblastomas and hemangioendothelioma		7	Moderate (Bright cystic fluid)	7 (100)	0	0	0	Not essential (7 cases)
Tumors of cranial and paraspinal nerves		7	Homogeneously intense	2 (28.6)	0	5 (71.4)	0	Not essential (7 cases)
Tumors of the sellar region		1	Homogeneously intense (motor oil liquid, not enhancing)	1 (100)	0	0	0	Helpful (1 case)
Tumors of soft tissue and bone (Nothocordal)		2	Heterogeneously fluorescent	0	0	2 (100)	0	Not essential (2 cases)

TABLE 2 | Intraoperative fluorescence characteristics and utility, based on histopathological results, in the biopsy group.

Histologies		Open biopsy			Needle biopsy		
		Number of procedures	**Intraoperative evaluation**	**Diagnostic accuracy**	**Number of procedures**	**Intraoperative evaluation**	**Diagnostic accuracy**
Tumors of neuroepithelial tissue	Diffuse astrocytic and oligodendro	4	Helpful to highlight the target of biopsy in multifocal presentation	100% (GBM)	10	Bright samples visualized under Y560 filter	70% (6 GBM, 1 AA) 1 choroid plexus 2 reactive gliosis
	Pilocytic astrocytoma	1	Helpful to highlight the fluorescent component in a diffuse spinal lesion	100% (PA)	0	/	/
	Pineal region	1	Helpful to obtain the specimen of the cystic wall	100% (Pineocytoma)	0	/	/
Primary CNS lymphomas		5	Helpful to highlight the target of biopsy in multifocal presentation	100% (B-cell NHL)	1	Bright samples visualized under Y560 filter	100% (B-cell Lymphoma)
Vasculitis processes		5	Helpful to highlight the target of biopsy in multifocal presentation	100% (4 Vasculitis and 1 Cerebral Amyloid Angiopathy)	1	Moderate fluorescence under Y560 filter	100% (Vasculitis)

Tumors of Neuroepithelial Tissue

Diffuse Astrocytic and Oligodendroglial Tumors

One-hundred fifty-seven patients underwent surgery, either for removal and for open or stereotactic biopsy. In 142 cases, the tumor presented inhomogeneous contrast-enhancement, with cystic-necrotic areas and solid components; only 15 selected cases of patients with minimal/absent contrast enhancement were scheduled for fluorescein-guided surgery in this subgroup of patients.

In the 142 cases presenting with intense and inhomogeneous contrast-enhancement, 128 underwent surgery for tumor removal and 14 underwent open (4 cases) or needle biopsy 10 (cases).

In the 128 cases submitted to tumor removal, the histological diagnosis was HGG in all cases. There were 78 primary and 35 recurrent glioblastoma (GBM), 4 newly diagnosed and 1 recurrent anaplastic astrocytoma (AA), 3 newly diagnosed and 5 recurrent anaplastic oligodendrogliomas (AO), 1 newly diagnosed and 1 recurrent NOS high-grade glioma. Intraoperatively (**Figure 1**), these tumors usually presented as brightly fluorescent, with a yellow-green signal clearly distinguishable by pinkish-appearing peritumoral parenchyma under Y560 filter (**Figures 1C,D**). Sometimes, in cases with a clear central necrotic core, this tissue showed a dark pinkish feature with scant fluorescein enhancement (**Figures 1C,D**). This heterogenous appearance was more pronounced in recurrent tumors, already submitted to radiotherapy, although previous fractionated radiation therapy did not determine substantial difference about fluorescence characteristics or usefulness upon surgical evaluation. Finally, in some cases a bright fluid component was reported which was the result of tumor central colliquation. In all these 128 cases, SF was considered helpful by the operating surgeon to help in distinguishing tumor from healthy tissue (100% of the cases). In 95 out of 128 cases (74.2%), fluorescent tissue was completely removed, and the post-operative MRI confirmed a gross-total resection. In 18 out of 128 cases (14.1%) residual fluorescent tissue was deliberately left at the end of surgery, due to the proximity to eloquent areas or the adherence to major brain vessels; in these cases, an expected subtotal resection was achieved at post-operative MRI. In 11 out of 128 cases (8.6%) fluorescent tissue was intraoperatively judged as completely removed, while postoperative MRI showed an unexpected subtotal resection. In 4 out of 128 cases (3.1%) a partial resection was achieved (**Table 1**).

SF was used also in 4 cases of multifocal lesions, to guide open biopsy to highlight the area of fluorescent tissue in the context of the tumor. In all of these cases (100%) SF was considered useful and the histological analysis was possible, with a diagnosis of GBM. Finally, in the 10 cases of needle biopsies, the samples were evaluated under the YELLOW 560 filter of the microscope and resulted to be fluorescent in all cases; however, diagnostic accuracy was confirmed in 7/10 (70%) with a histological diagnosis of GBM in 6 cases and AA in 1 case; in three cases histological analysis was not diagnostic (1 choroid plexus and 2 reactive gliosis) (**Table 2**).

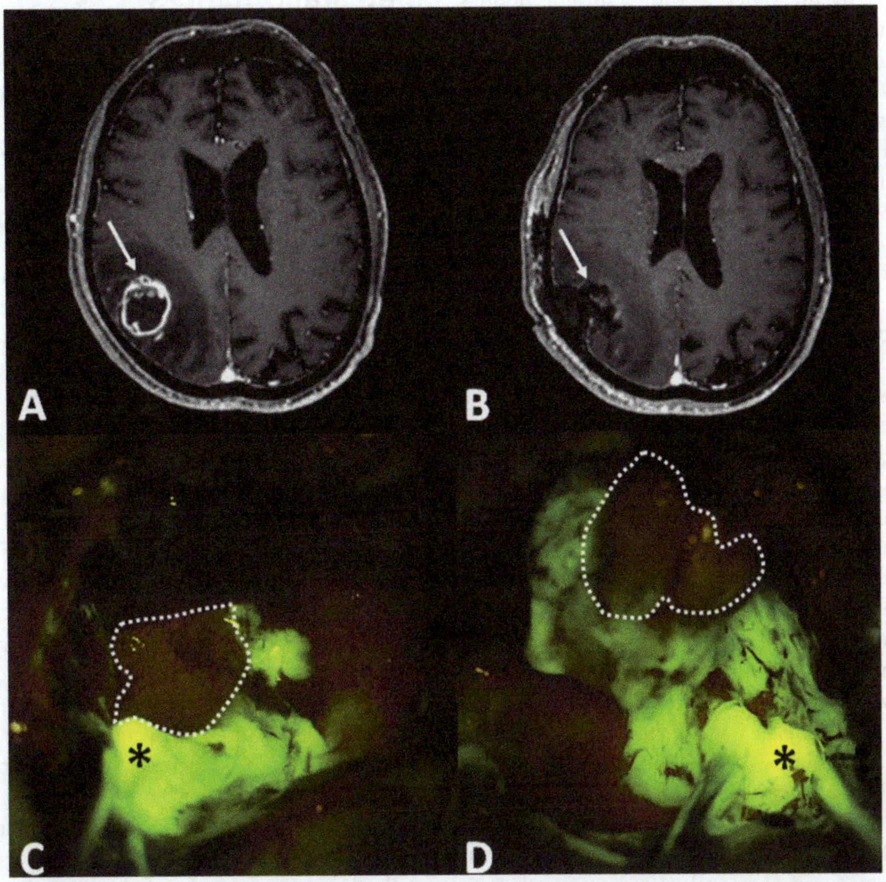

FIGURE 1 | (A) Preoperative post-contrast axial T1-weighted MRI scan showing a right parietal GBM (arrow), that was completely removed, as visible in post-operative T1 with contrast axial scan (**B**: in that case arrow is the surgical cavity). Intraoperative images, under Y560 filter **(C,D)**, depict bright yellow green signal (asterisk), in correspondence of nodular component, and dark pinkish feature in the necrotic core (dotted line).

Fifteen patients with minimal/absent contrast enhancement underwent tumor removal by fluorescein-guided technique. In 10 cases MRI showed a very extensive area of T2/FLAIR hyperintense signal abnormality, which suggested an aggressive behavior. In those cases, SF revealed in 6 out of 10 cases only minimal intralesional fluorescent spots. Therefore, SF was generally judged useless because no adjunctive information about residual tumor volume were provided compared to white light illumination. All that cases were histological grade II lesions (3 NOS grade II glioma, 3 diffuse astrocytomas and 4 oligodendrogliomas). Five patients presented with slight contrast enhancement at pre-operative MRI, and a positive 11C-methionine (MET) or fluoro-ethyl-tyrosine (FET) - Positron Emission Tomography (PET). In all cases, SF highlighted the pathological regions with higher metabolism, as suggested by PET findings, and it was judged useful in 4 patients, in which histopathological analysis revealed grade III lesions (AA in 3 cases and AO in 1 case). One patient affected by recurrent oligodendroglioma presented only few fluorescent spots, such as the MET positive regions, and SF was not judged useful during surgical removal (overall 80% of utility in the population of non-Gadolinium enhancing, but PET positive gliomas).

Other Neuroepithelial Tumors

Fourteen ependymomas, presenting with homogeneous and moderate enhancement at pre-operative MRI were submitted to fluorescein-guided resection. In all cases, the operating surgeon considered SF as a useful adjunct to better identify tumor-healthy tissues interface. GTR was achieved in 10 cases (71.4%); in one case (7.15%), despite the subjective surgical impression of complete fluorescent tissue removal, postoperative MRI showed tiny neoplastic remnants. In two ependymomas of the fourth ventricle (14.3%), there were small fluorescent residual spots due to extremely strong adherence to surrounding health parenchyma. Furthermore, a partial resection was performed in a very huge, recurrent posterior fossa ependymoma (7.15%), due to the significant bleeding (21.45% of expect subtotal or partial removal).

Thirteen neuronal and mixed neuronal-glial tumors were included in this series. Nine patients presented with enhancement (in 7 cases with a diffuse homogeneous enhancement whereas in the other 2 with a bright nodule associated with enhancing peripheral cyst), while four patients presented with minimal/absent enhancement or with an area of c.e. in the context of a larger not-enhancing tumor at pre-operative MRI. The surgeon found bright and homogeneously fluorescent tissue and SF was judged useful in 12 out of 13 cases, except for one case of a slight enhancing spinal rosette-forming glioneuronal tumor (92.3%). In 6 cases, all fluorescent tissue was removed whereas in 3 patients, small residual tumor was left due to the proximity to eloquent brain areas. Furthermore, in 3 patients scheduled for surgery due to drug-resistant epilepsy affected by supratentorial lesions, located in not-eloquent brain, SF was judged useful to identify the small, pathological nodule but the resection was supramaximal and extended to peritumoral gliosis and dysplastic parenchyma to achieve seizure control. Overall a GTR was achieved in 9 patients out of 12 cases (75%) when SF represented a surgical aid, whereas in 3 cases (25%) an expected STR was achieved (4, 53–56).

Pilocytic astrocytoma, pleomorphic xanthoastrocytoma and sub-ependymal giant cell astrocytoma, presented at pre-operative MRI with well-circumscribed margins, typically having both solid (predominant) and cystic components, with inhomogeneous contrast enhancement at pre-operative MRI. The fluorescein enhancement was typically intense in the vast majority of the solid portion of the neoplasia with characteristic bright fluorescent cystic fluid (**Figure 2**). GTR was achieved in 10 cases out of 19 patients scheduled for tumor removal (52.6%), in 2 cases a minimal residual volume was highlighted by postoperative MRI despite the intraoperative subjective evaluation of complete tumor removal (10.5%); in other 7 cases, the resection was subtotal with fluorescent residual spots to avoid neurological worsening (expected STR in 36.9%). In one case of spinal PA an open biopsy was performed: the most fluorescent component was removed for histological analysis which was diagnostic; the patient did not present any neurological sequelae.

For other neuroepithelial tumors (one choroid plexus papilloma, one recurrent angiocentric glioma and two medulloblastomas), all presenting with inhomogeneous contrast enhancement at pre-operative MRI, intraoperative fluorescein enhancement was intense and judged useful in all cases, even if in the case of choroid plexus papilloma, the tumor tissue was easily recognizable also under white light. SF represented an important surgical aid during pineal surgery, in two intermediate differentiation tumors of the pineal parenchyma, in one papillary pineal tumor and in one cerebellar metastasis of papillary pineal tumor. In these cases, preoperative MRI with Gadolinium showed an intense, inhomogeneous enhancement with cystic regions. Furthermore, SF was used in an open biopsy of a pineocytoma with a voluminous cystic component after its surgical fenestration; radiologically, it appeared as a voluminous cyst with peripheral enhancement. Despite histological differences, all those tumors had a strong and bright fluorescent enhancement and the Y560-guided surgery resulted really useful to identify pathological tissues, preserving normal brain parenchyma.

Metastatic Tumors

Overall 25 patients with cerebral metastasis had undergone fluorescence-guided surgery since 2016; 13 of them underwent previous radiotherapy/radiosurgical treatment. All lesions presented with typical inhomogeneous contrast enhancement at pre-operative MRI. About the primitive tumors, the majority of them were breast (8), lung (5) and colorectal (3) cancers; 3 seminomas, 3 melanomas and also ovarian, renal and thyroid (one case per each histotypes) were present too. GTR was achieved in 96% of patients (24/25); in the remaining one (4%), a right fronto-mesial metastasis enchasing the ipsilateral callosomarginal artery, the surgeon chose to leave lowercase fluorescent residual tissue around the encased artery.

Under YELLOW 560 visualization, metastases appeared intensively fluorescent, with large yellow areas corresponding to the Gadolinium enhancement spots (**Figure 3**). SF was considered really helpful to distinguish tumor or to identify the neoplastic nodules inside infiltrated parenchyma in 20 procedures (80%). In the 3 patients affected by melanoma (12%), visualization with Y560 filter was not essential in melanoma metastases, that showed a characteristic brown-bluish pigmentation; for the patient with a hemorrhagic metastasis (4%), the filter was activated only at the end of the procedure, to verify the absence of residual fluorescence. Finally, in one patient (4%) with a left frontal colorectal metastasis previously submitted to radiosurgery and whole brain radiotherapy, the lesion appeared strongly fluorescent, but this finding was considered not useful due to fluorescein enhancement of peritumoral parenchyma, secondary to radiation damages.

Furthermore, for 3 superficial metastases, after dural opening and YELLOW 560 activation, the surgeon identified an atypical and greater than usual meningeal fluorescence enhancement, in correspondence of the superficial part of the lesion: in these cases, the dura was sacrificed; the histopathological analysis identified leptomeningeal metastasis.

Primary Central Nervous System Lymphoma

Ten patients with radiological diagnosis of lymphoma were enrolled: in four of them, surgery was scheduled due to the spinal localization (two cases: one lumbar and one dorsal localization) or huge dimension of a single lesion in non-eloquent brain region (one left posterior temporal and one right parietal). Six patients had a multifocal presentation and were scheduled for open biopsy in five cases and for stereotactic biopsy of the deep, paraventricular, enhancing component in the remaining one; in every case, biopsies were judged diagnostic by the pathologist. Lymphomas, under YELLOW 560 filter visualization, appeared homogenously and brightly fluorescent: fluorescein guidance was always judged useful.

Cerebral Hemangioblastomas and Hemangioendotheliomas

Six patients with superficial hemangioblastomas and one patient with a left frontal recurrent epithelioid hemangioendothelioma were submitted to fluorescein-guided surgery; GTR was achieved

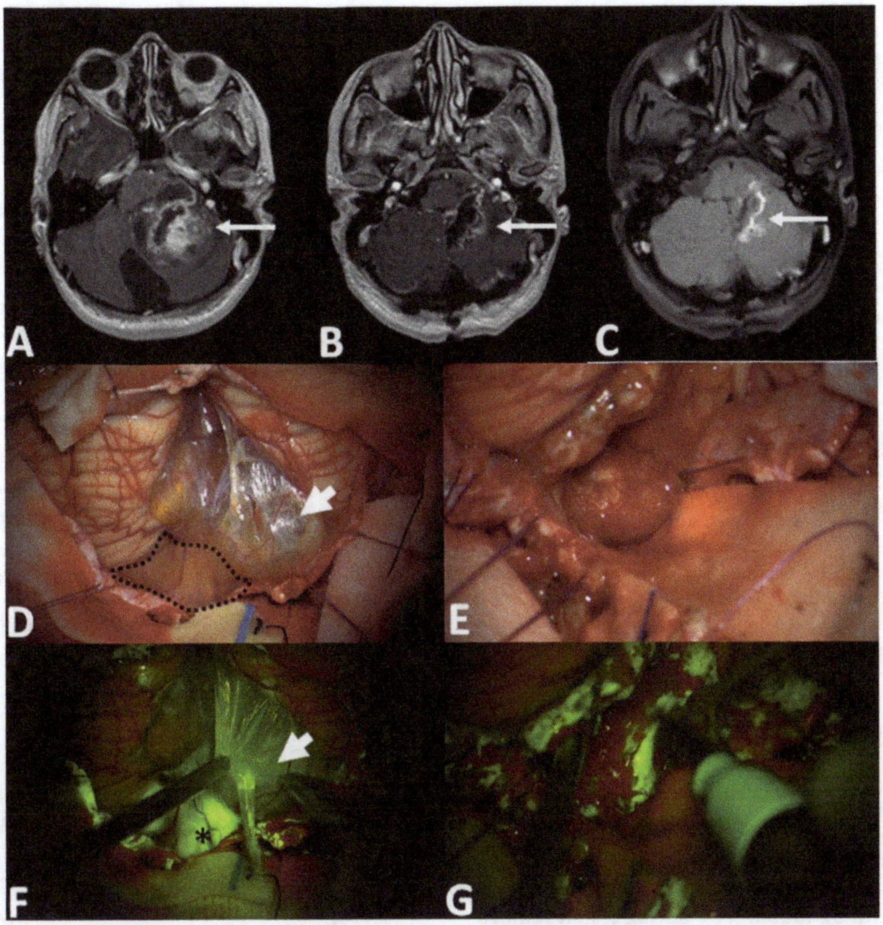

FIGURE 2 | Pre-operative T1 with contrast axial scan **(A)** shows a huge posterior fossa pilocytic astrocytoma (arrow) with a gross-total resection, as detectable by post-operative post-Gadolinium T1 MRI in **(B)**. The area of contrast-enhancement corresponds to the spontaneous hyperintense boundaries of surgical cavity **(C)**. After dural opening **(D,F)**, it is possible to appreciate a multilobulated cyst with a bright fluid (arrowhead in **D**, after its fenestration in **F**) and an inferior vermis nodular component (dotted line in **D**) with an intense fluorescein enhancement (asterisk in **F**). Intraoperative images, under white light **(E)** and Y560 filter **(G)**, during tumor removal with cavitron ultrasound aspirator, showing a bleeding, friable tissue with inhomogeneous fluorescein enhancement.

in all cases. Intraoperatively, the nodular component depicted a slight/moderate and homogenous fluorescence; the intra-cystic fluid, however, when present, appeared intensely fluorescent. Despite these findings, fluorescein was considered not essential because that tumor had a peculiar aspect with the typical orange nodule, that made them easily distinguishable from the surrounding structures. We may speculate that, for deep-seated tumors, SF could help to localize the pathological nodule.

Other Tumors and Conditions

Fluorescein was also used in five vestibular schwannomas, in two lumbar schwannomas and in two chordomas. Although all lesions presented with intense fluorescence, its use for not considered essential to remove the easily recognizable lesion, and because it was not possible to recognize not involved peritumoral cranial or spinal nerve.

SF was used in the only craniopharyngioma approached by craniotomy due to its large dimension and relapse despite the interferon therapy; in this case, the lesion showed an intense and homogeneous fluorescence under the YELLOW 560 filter. SF was considered useful by the surgeon, during the removal, in order to better identify the tumor capsule and to cleave it from the surrounding parenchyma.

SF was also used in three meningiomas: in everyone, it was considered not essential because the tumors were easily recognizable also under white light, even if all showed bright and homogeneous enhancement.

SF was incidentally used in a post-radiation cavernous malformation, located in the superior cerebellar vermis; intra-operatively, after the evacuation of an intra-parenchymal hematoma, the lesion showed an inhomogeneous fluorescence and SF was judged useful to achieve GTR, as confirmed by post-operative MRI, and to distinguish healthy cerebellar tissue.

In other five case, the radiological suspect of cerebral glioma was not confirmed during or after surgery (abscess, inflammatory pseudotumor, radionecrosis with residual pathological vessels of a previously-radiotreated arteriovenous malformation). The abscess appeared heterogeneously, intensely

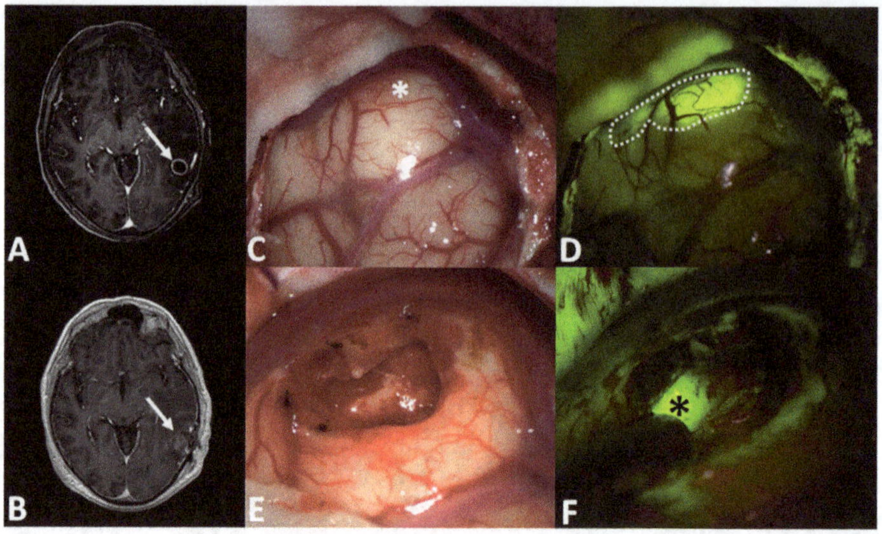

FIGURE 3 | (A,B) Pre- and post-operative post-contrast axial T1-weighted scans showing a left temporal metastasis from lung cancer, completely removed. After dural opening **(C)**, the Y560 filter **(D)** can highlight the superficial part of the metastasis, helping the surgeon in discriminating it from peritumoral brain parenchyma (dotted line in **D**), whereas under white light it is possible to appreciate a grayish, vanishing area (asterisk in **C**). During surgical resection **(E,F)**, fluorescein helps the surgeon to identify residual pathological tissue (black asterisks in **F**), not clearly visible under white light **(E)**.

fluorescent; it was intraoperatively recognized under white light, and, after an extemporaneous histopathological evaluation, the procedure was interrupted, and the material sent for bacteriological analysis. Inflammatory pseudotumor was characterized by a diffuse, moderate fluorescein enhancement which was judged useful by the surgeon during lesion removal. Finally, in the case of radionecrosis, the lesion showed a peripherical zone of strong fluorescein enhancement, with a good demarcation from health parenchyma: in this case, SF was judged not essential.

Six patients with a suspected diagnosis of vasculitis or inflammatory angiopathy, presenting with cerebral lesions at least partly enhancing at pre-operative MRI underwent fluorescein-guided open biopsy. In all cases, SF was helpful in recognizing the enhancing lesion under SF, obtaining a fluorescent sample to be analyzed. Fluorescein-guided biopsy was diagnostic in every case: histopathological analysis confirmed the diagnostic suspicion of cerebral vasculitis in five patient and cerebral amyloid angiopathy in the other one.

Reactions to Fluorescein, to Combined Use of SF With ICG or 5-ALA and Complications

No adverse drug reaction related to SF injection was reported in 309 patients; the only remarkable and visible effect was the transient yellowish staining of urine which disappeared in about 24 h. Moreover, no adverse neurosurgical or clinical event resulted from the combined use of two fluorophores (SF and 5-ALA, SF and ICG) during the same surgical procedure. Preoperative corticosteroid therapy did not affect fluorescence characteristics.

DISCUSSION

In our surgical series, the utilization of SF represented a useful adjunct in most of the CNS tumors presenting with some degree of contrast enhancement at preoperative neuroimaging scans.

During the last years SF has emerged as intraoperative tracer able to improve brain-tumor visualization, due to its non-specific, vascular mechanism of action related to the accumulation in brain regions with BBB disruption, as it happens with MRI contrast enhancement (34, 36, 38, 57). In fact, independently from their grading, the majority of CNS tumors, except for some grade I and II intra-axial histotypes, determine a BBB damage, thus they have a radiological presentation with contrast enhancement at MRI. Previous experiences had suggested that the use SF could be associated with a bright fluorescence of the tumor area in primary and recurrent HGG, in metastases, in lymphomas, and in spinal intramedullary lesions (34–36, 39). This was also associated with good results in term of extent of resection (39). However, there were in the literature significant variations in SF use, considering dosage and time of injections, in the studies published by different research groups (39).

As the reimbursement of SF as a fluorescent tracer in neuro-oncology has been approved by the Italian Drug Agency (AIFA) in July 2015 (determination 905/2015, Gazette n.168, 22 July, 2015), and based on our extensive experience with HGG (32, 33, 38), we decided to start a prospective observational study on the use of SF for the resection of aggressive tumors of the CNS, applying a standardized protocol, with a dosage of 5 mg/kg and an i.v. injection immediately after patient intubation or at the entrance in the OR for awake craniotomies (58).

As expected, the majority of the cases were HGG (51.6% of the total number of patients included in the study). Most of these patients underwent fluorescein-guided tumor resection based on a high suspect for a high-grade lesion based on pre-operative MRI. In all these cases, SF appeared extremely useful to improve the discrimination between tumor tissue and peritumoral brain parenchyma, with a positive impact in term of EOR, with a percentage of GTR in 74.2%. Coming from an unselected series of patients, these results seems to be extremely interesting, and in line with previous published studies (32, 33, 38, 39, 59).

A particular consideration regards instead the population of patients with gliomas with minimal/almost absent enhancement at preoperative MRI. In all that cases we noted that SF was useless due to the unpredictable, and usually focal fluorescence under the specific Y560 filter, except for the cases of patients with FET/MET-PET positive tumor, as suggested by Schebesch et al. (60). In our series of 5 patients with this characteristic, we could confirm a correlation between the positive PET areas and the fluorescein uptake by tumor tissue in all cases. This finding suggests a predictive ability of PET with amino acid tracers to detect areas with minimal BBB disruption, not shown by pre-operative MRI, which can be intra-operatively identified by using fluorescein-guided surgery. In that cases, SF enhancement could be related to the molecular property of SF which has a slightly lower molecular weight than Gadolinium. The intraoperative recognition of these positive PET areas could also be associated to a better diagnostic accuracy, as in 80% of our cases the final histological diagnosis was a grade III glioma.

Regarding brain metastasis, we could also confirm previous experiences (36), showing a very good tumor visualization in most of the cases with a percentage of GTR in 96% of the cases. Of notice, in 3 melanomas we did not find SF to be a useful adjunct, as the tumor was clearly visible under the microscope with white-light illumination.

We also found a good correspondence between pre-operative MRI enhancement and intraoperative fluorescence identification in in neuronal and mixed glioneuronal tumors, in other astrocytic tumors, in other types of neuroepithelial tumors and in lymphomas. SF was useful to identify pathological nodule, but also during surgery and at the end of resection, to verify the absence of residual tumor tissue. We administered fluorescein also in some cases of cranial and spinal schwannomas but, even if they showed an intense and homogeneous fluorescence, at the standard dosage fluorescein failed in distinguishing and identifying normal nerve fibers not related to the tumor. In addition, SF was considered not essential in hemangioblastomas that, despite the moderate but homogenous fluorescence both of nodular and fluid portions, present a peculiar and characteristic nodular component under white-light illumination, such to make not essential the use of fluorescein, at least with our protocol. On the contrary, we believe that a more appropriate application of fluorescein was proposed by Rey-Dios et al. (37) for these tumor subtypes. They reported the intravenous administration of fluorescein in bolus immediately before tumor resection to better visualize its vascular network, including arterial feeders, draining veins, and the nodule, as similarly reported by our group with ICG video-angiography (48, 49) (**Table 1**).

Two hundred and forty-five patients enrolled in the study were scheduled for surgery with a previous planning of macroscopic resection but keeping in mind the philosophy of maximal safe resection: in this series, we obtained a high percentage of GTR (181/245, 73.9%). Minimal residual tumor (lower than 10% of preoperative tumor volume) at postoperative MRI was expected in thirty-seven cases (15.1%), as it was involving eloquent areas or due to the adherences to major brain vessels or cranial nerves and was therefore independent from the use of fluorescein-guided technique. Conversely, in seventeen cases (6.9%), the residual tumor was an unexpected finding, based on the absence of clear residual intraoperative fluorescent tissue: this can be related, as for other fluorophores, to the fact that the residual tissue was not exposed during resection because hidden under the normal brain parenchyma. Finally, in the remaining ten cases (4.1%) the surgical resection was only partial due to the location in eloquent areas, or the significative encasement of major brain vessels or cranial nerves, especially for voluminous posterior fossa tumors (**Table 1**).

Twenty-eight patients were included in our protocol for fluorescein-guided biopsy. Regarding open biopsies, SF was used in four multifocal GBM, in five lymphomas and in five suspected vasculitis process/cerebral angiopathy with a cortico-subcortical component which was chosen as a target, in one pineocytoma with a voluminous cyst, after its surgical fenestration, and in one spinal PA, to identify the enhancing component for histopathological analysis. Regarding patients that underwent open biopsies, SF was always judged useful and, in every case, the tissue specimen was enough for an adequate histopathologic analysis. Regarding frameless/stereotactic biopsies, our series is limited to twelve patients, with a diagnostic accuracy of 75% (9/12): in particular, in two primitive multifocal gliomas, histopathological analysis revealed reactive gliosis despite the fluorescence of specimens, whereas in one recurrent thalamic glioma, the histology suggested choroidal plexus tissue, which can explain the SF enhancement of the samples, due to the absence of BBB, and physiological accumulation of SF in this cerebral area. In two of these patients, a fluorescein-guided diagnostic biopsy was repeated and was successful in obtaining a histological diagnosis (one AA and one oligodendroglioma). Although limited to 28 cases, these results seems to suggest, as already preliminarily shown in previous experiences (61), that SF could assist during biopsies of CNS lesions, for a correct identification of the best target for the histological diagnosis (**Table 2**).

Nobody, between patients of our series, presented fluorescein-related side effects or adverse reactions to SF administration, either singly or combined with other fluorophores. The only visible manifestation of intraoperative fluorescein administration is, as noted, the onset of transient yellowish stain of the urine, that rapidly disappear after 24–48 h : patients should be aware about this particular but totally harmless effect. We believe that the lack of any side effect, in particular any allergic reaction, was predominantly related to the low dosage used in this trial, thanks to the use of a dedicated filter into the microscope, that allowed a more accurate identification of fluorescent tissue, us suggested firstly by our group (27).

The main limitation of this study presented is represented by the lack of data about overall survival; in fact, the authors considered only a surrogate indicator which is the EOR, and by the lack of the direct comparison of surgery with and without SF aid due to ethical reasons. Furthermore, we did not make any comparison between the use of SF and other available fluorophores, like 5-aminolevulenic acid, that has been established as a surgical adjunct in surgery of HGG (20) and that has been reported as a possible advantage in selected cases of brain metastasis (62). Finally, the utility of SF in stereotactic/frameless biopsies is only descriptively considered without a proper statistical analysis, thus it is not able to establish a predictive value of SF. We have also to stress that, in most of the Countries, SF is still considered off label for neuro-oncological procedures. Thus, a widespread utilization of fluorescence-guided surgery will depend on the definitive approval by the competent authorities.

CONCLUSION

On the basis of its unspecific mechanism of action, the use of SF as fluorescent tracer in neuro-oncology should be considered in several applications. Indeed, as these preliminary results seem to suggest, the same unspecific mechanism may also be seen as its strength since SF can be used as an operative adjunct in every CNS tumor with some degree of BBB disruption as detectable by neuroradiological imaging after contrast medium administration, but also by PET with amino acids positivity. Further studies are required to clarify the field of application of SF in neuro-oncological procedures and definitively assess the value of this technique on improvement of the EOR and overall survival.

ETHICS STATEMENT

The FLUOCERTUM study has been approved by the Ethical Committee of the Fondazione IRCCS Istituto Neurologico Carlo Besta and written informed consent was obtained from all patients, in accordance with the Declaration of Helsinki.

AUTHOR CONTRIBUTIONS

JF, CC, and FA: study concept and design. JF, CC, IV, and FA: critical revision of the manuscript for intellectual content. All authors: acquisition of data, data analysis, and interpretation. PF and FA: study supervision.

REFERENCES

1. Ostrom QT, Gittleman H, Truitt G, Boscia A, Kruchko C, Barnholtz-Sloan JS. CBTRUS statistical report: primary brain and other central nervous system tumors diagnosed in the United States in 2011–2015. *Neuro Oncol.* (2018) 20:41–86. doi: 10.1093/neuonc/noy131
2. Lacroix M, Abi-Said D, Fourney DR, Gokaslan ZL, Shi W, DeMonte F, et al. A multivariate analysis of 416 patients with glioblastoma multiforme: prognosis, extent of resection, and survival. *J Neurosurg.* (2001) 95:190–8. doi: 10.3171/jns.2001.95.2.0190
3. Weller M, van den Bent M, Tonn JC, Stupp R, Preusser M, Cohen-Jonathan-Moyal E, et al. European Association for Neuro-Oncology (EANO) guideline on the diagnosis and treatment of adult astrocytic and oligodendroglial gliomas. *Lancet Oncol.* (2017) 18:e315–29. doi: 10.1016/S1470-2045(17)30194-8
4. Stone TJ, Rowell R, Jayasekera BAP, Cunningham MO, Jacques TS. Review: Molecular characteristics of long-term epilepsy-associated tumours (LEATs) and mechanisms for tumour-related epilepsy (TRE). *Neuropathol Appl Neurobiol.* (2018) 44:56–69. doi: 10.1111/nan.12459
5. Sanai N, Polley M-Y, McDermott MW, Parsa AT, Berger MS. An extent of resection threshold for newly diagnosed glioblastomas. *J Neurosurg.* (2011) 115:3–8. doi: 10.3171/2011.2.JNS10998
6. Li YM, Suki D, Hess K, Sawaya R. The influence of maximum safe resection of glioblastoma on survival in 1229 patients: can we do better than gross-total resection? *J Neurosurg.* (2016) 124:977–88. doi: 10.3171/2015.5.JNS142087
7. Grabowski MM, Recinos PF, Nowacki AS, Schroeder JL, Angelov L, Barnett GH, et al. Residual tumor volume versus extent of resection: predictors of survival after surgery for glioblastoma. *J Neurosurg.* (2014) 121:1115–23. doi: 10.3171/2014.7.JNS132449
8. Bloch O, Han SJ, Cha S, Sun MZ, Aghi MK, McDermott MW, et al. Impact of extent of resection for recurrent glioblastoma on overall survival. *J Neurosurg.* (2012) 117:1032–8. doi: 10.3171/2012.9.JNS12504
9. Brown TJ, Brennan MC, Li M, Church EW, Brandmeir NJ, Rakszawski KL, et al. Association of the extent of resection with survival in glioblastoma. *JAMA Oncol.* (2016) 2:1460. doi: 10.1001/jamaoncol.2016.1373
10. Aghi MK, Nahed BV, Sloan AE, Ryken TC, Kalkanis SN, Olson JJ. The role of surgery in the management of patients with diffuse low grade glioma. *J Neurooncol.* (2015) 125:503–30. doi: 10.1007/s11060-015-1867-1
11. Yang K, Nath S, Koziarz A, Badhiwala JH, Ghayur H, Sourour M, et al. Biopsy versus subtotal versus gross total resection in patients with low-grade glioma: a systematic review and meta-analysis. *World Neurosurg.* (2018) 120:e762–75. doi: 10.1016/j.wneu.2018.08.163
12. Tsao MN, Xu W, Wong RK, Lloyd N, Laperriere N, Sahgal A, et al. Whole brain radiotherapy for the treatment of newly diagnosed multiple brain metastases. *Cochrane Database Syst Rev.* (2018) 1:CD003869. doi: 10.1002/14651858.CD003869.pub4
13. Brown PD, Ballman KV, Cerhan JH, Anderson SK, Carrero XW, Whitton AC, et al. Postoperative stereotactic radiosurgery compared with whole brain radiotherapy for resected metastatic brain disease (NCCTG N107C/CEC·3): a multicentre, randomised, controlled, phase 3 trial. *Lancet Oncol.* (2017) 18:1049–60. doi: 10.1016/S1470-2045(17)30441-2
14. Mahajan A, Ahmed S, McAleer MF, Weinberg JS, Li J, Brown P, et al. Post-operative stereotactic radiosurgery versus observation for completely resected brain metastases: a single-centre, randomised, controlled, phase 3 trial. *Lancet Oncol.* (2017) 18:1040–8. doi: 10.1016/S1470-2045(17)30414-X
15. Vera-Bolanos E, Aldape K, Yuan Y, Wu J, Wani K, Necesito-Reyes MJ, et al. Clinical course and progression-free survival of adult intracranial and spinal ependymoma patients. *Neuro Oncol.* (2015) 17:440–7. doi: 10.1093/neuonc/nou162
16. Dodgshun AJ, Maixner WJ, Hansford JR, Sullivan MJ. Low rates of recurrence and slow progression of pediatric pilocytic astrocytoma after gross-total resection: justification for reducing surveillance imaging. *J Neurosurg Pediatr.* (2016) 17:569–72. doi: 10.3171/2015.9.PEDS15449
17. Jenkinson MD, Barone DG, Bryant A, Vale L, Bulbeck H, Lawrie TA, et al. Intraoperative imaging technology to maximise extent of resection for glioma. *Cochrane Database Syst Rev.* (2018) 1:CD012788. doi: 10.1002/14651858.CD012788.pub2
18. Senft C, Bink A, Franz K, Vatter H, Gasser T, Seifert V. Intraoperative MRI guidance and extent of resection in glioma surgery: a randomised, controlled trial. *Lancet Oncol.* (2011) 12:997–1003. doi: 10.1016/S1470-2045(11)70196-6

19. Prada F, Del Bene M, Rampini A, Mattei L, Casali C, Vetrano IG, et al. Intraoperative Strain Elastosonography in Brain Tumor Surgery. *Neurosurg.* (2018) 17:227–36. doi: 10.1093/ons/opy323
20. Stummer W, Pichlmeier U, Meinel T, Wiestler OD, Zanella F, Reulen HJ. Fluorescence-guided surgery with 5-aminolevulinic acid for resection of malignant glioma: a randomised controlled multicentre phase III trial. *Oncol.* (2006) 7:392–401. doi: 10.1016/s1470-2045(06)70665-9
21. Yano H, Nakayama N, Ohe N, Miwa K, Shinoda J, Iwama T. Pathological analysis of the surgical margins of resected glioblastomas excised using photodynamic visualization with both 5-aminolevulinic acid and fluorescein sodium. *J Neurooncol.* (2017) 133:389–97. doi: 10.1007/s11060-017-2445-5
22. Wei L, Roberts DW, Sanai N, Liu JTC. Visualization technologies for 5-ALA-based fluorescence-guided surgeries. *J Neurooncol.* (2019) 141:495–505. doi: 10.1007/s11060-018-03077-9
23. Copeman SM, Coke F, Gouldesbrough C. "Activated" (irradiated) fluorescein in the treatment of cancer. *Br Med J.* (1929) 2:233–42.
24. Siff LN, Hill AJ, Jallad K, Harnegie MP, Barber MD. Intraoperative evaluation of urinary tract injuries at the time of pelvic surgery. *Female Pelvic Med Reconstr Surg.* (2018). doi: 10.1097/SPV.0000000000000679. [Epub ahead of print].
25. O'goshi K, Serup J. Safety of sodium fluorescein for *in vivo* *Res Technol.* (2006) 12:155–61. doi: 10.1111/j.0909-752X.2006.00147.x
26. Hara T, Inami M, Hara T. Efficacy and safety of fluorescein angiography with orally administered sodium fluorescein. *Am J Ophthalmol* 126:560–4.
27. Keerl R, Weber RK, Draf W, Wienke A, Schaefer SD. Use of sodium fluorescein solution for detection of cerebrospinal fluid fistulas: an analysis of 420 administrations and reported complications in Europe and the United States. *Laryngoscope.* (2004) 114:266–72. doi: 10.1097/00005537-200402000-00016
28. Moore GE. Fluorescein as an agent in the differentiation of normal and malignant tissues. *Science.* (1947) 106:130–1. doi: 10.1126/science.106.2745.130-a
29. Moore GE, Hunter SW, Hubbard TB. Clinical and experimental studies of fluorescein dyes with special reference to their use for the diagnosis of central nervous system tumors. *Ann Surg.* (1949) 130:637–42.
30. Hubbard TB, Moore GE. The use of fluorescein dyes in the diagnosis of malignancy with special reference to tumors of the central nervous system. *J Natl Cancer Inst.* (1949) 10:303–14.
31. Kuroiwa T, Kajimoto Y, Ohta T. Development of a fluorescein operative microscope for use during malignant glioma surgery: a technical note and preliminary report. *Surg Neurol.* (1998) 50:41–8; discussion 48–9.
32. Acerbi F, Broggi M, Eoli M, Anghileri E, Cuppini L, Pollo B, et al. Fluorescein-guided surgery for grade IV gliomas with a dedicated filter on the surgical microscope: preliminary results in 12 cases. *Acta Neurochir.* (2013) 155:1277–86. doi: 10.1007/s00701-013-1734-9
33. Acerbi F, Broggi M, Eoli M, Anghileri E, Cavallo C, Boffano C, et al. Is fluorescein-guided technique able to help in resection of high-grade gliomas? *Neurosurg Focus.* (2014) 36:E5. doi: 10.3171/2013.11.FOCUS13487
34. Schebesch KM, Hoehne J, Hohenberger C, Acerbi F, Broggi M, Proescholdt M, et al. Fluorescein sodium-guided surgery in cerebral lymphoma. *Neurosurg.* (2015) 139:125–8. doi: 10.1016/j.clineuro.2015.09.015
35. Acerbi F, Cavallo C, Schebesch K-M, Akçakaya MO, de Laurentis C, Hamamcioglu MK, et al. Fluorescein-guided resection of intramedullary spinal cord tumors: results from a preliminary, multicentric, retrospective study. *World Neurosurg.* (2017) 108: 603–9. doi: 10.1016/j.wneu.2017.09.061
36. Höhne J, Hohenberger C, Proescholdt M, Riemenschneider MJ, Wendl C, Brawanski A, et al. Fluorescein sodium-guided resection *Clin Neurol* of cerebral metastases—an update. *Acta Neurochir.* (2017) 159:363–7. doi: 10.1007/s00701-016-3054-3
37. Rey-Dios R, Cohen-Gadol AA. Intraoperative fluorescence for resection of hemangioblastomas. *Acta Neurochir (Wien).* (2013) 155:1287–92. doi: 10.1007/s00701-013-1723-z
38. Acerbi F, Broggi M, Schebesch K-M, Höhne J, Cavallo C, De Laurentis C, et al. fluorescein-guided surgery for resection of high-grade gliomas: a multicentric prospective phase II study (FLUOGLIO). *Clin Cancer Res.* (2018) 24:52–61. doi: 10.1158/1078-0432.CCR-17-1184
39. Cavallo C, De Laurentis C, Vetrano IG, Falco J, Broggi M, Schiariti M, et al. The utilization of fluorescein in brain tumor surgery: a systematic review. *J Neurosurg Sci.* (2018) 62:690–703. doi: 10.23736/S0390-5616.18.04480-6
40. Neira JA, Ung TH, Sims JS, Malone HR, Chow DS, Samanamud JL, et al. Aggressive resection at the infiltrative margins of glioblastoma facilitated by intraoperative fluorescein guidance. *J Neurosurg.* (2017) 127:111–22. doi: 10.3171/2016.7.JNS16232
41. Rey-Dios R, Cohen-Gadol AA. Technical principles and neurosurgical applications of fluorescein fluorescence using a microscope-integrated fluorescence module. *Acta Neurochir (Wien).* (2013) 155(4):701-6. doi: 10.1007/s00701-013-1635-y
42. Acerbi F. Fluorescein assistance in neuro-oncological surgery: a trend of the moment or a real technical adjunt? *Clin Neurol Neurosurg.* (2016) 144:119–20. doi: 10.1016/j.clineuro.2016.03.011
43. da Silva CE, da Silva VD, da Silva JLB. Skull base meningiomas and cranial nerves contrast using sodium fluorescein: a new application of an old tool. *J Neurol Surg B Skull Base.* (2014) 75:255–60. doi: 10.1055/s-0034-1372466
44. Bohnstedt BN, Cohen-Gadol AA, Brain C, Lane B, Bohnstedt BN, Cohen-Gadol AA. A prospective comparative study of microscope-integrated intraoperative fluorescein and indocyanine videoangiography for clip ligation of complex cerebral aneurysms. *J Neurosurg.* (2015) 122:618–26. doi: 10.3171/2014.10.JNS132766
45. Li Y, Rey-Dios R, Roberts DW, Valdés PA, Cohen-Gadol AA. Intraoperative fluorescence-guided resection of high-grade gliomas: a comparison of the present techniques and evolution of future strategies. *World Neurosurg.* (2014) 82:175–85. doi: 10.1016/j.wneu.2013.06.014
46. Schebesch K-M, Proescholdt M, Höhne J, Hohenberger C, Hansen E, Riemenschneider MJ, et al. Sodium fluorescein-guided resection under the YELLOW 560 nm surgical microscope filter in malignant brain tumor surgery–a feasibility study. *Acta Neurochir (Wien).* (2013) 155:693–9. doi: 10.1007/s00701-013-1643-y
47. Ferroli P, Nakaji P, Acerbi F, Albanese E, Broggi G. Indocyanine green (ICG) temporary clipping test to assess collateral circulation before venous sacrifice. *World Neurosurg.* (2011) 75:122–5. doi: 10.1016/j.wneu.2010.09.011
48. Acerbi F, Vetrano IG, Sattin T, Falco J, de Laurentis C, Zattra CM, et al. Use of ICG videoangiography and FLOW 800 analysis to identify the patient-specific venous circulation and predict the effect of venous sacrifice: a retrospective study of 172 patients. *Neurosurg Focus.* (2018) 45:E7. doi: 10.3171/2018.4.FOCUS18120
49. Acerbi F, Vetrano IG, Sattin T, de Laurentis C, Bosio L, Rossini Z, et al. The role of indocyanine green videoangiography with FLOW 800 analysis for the surgical management of central nervous system tumors: an update. *Neurosurg Focus.* (2018) 44:E6. doi: 10.3171/2018.3.FOCUS1862
50. Acerbi F, Restelli F, Broggi M, Schiariti M, Ferroli P. Feasibility of simultaneous sodium fluorescein and indocyanine green injection in neurosurgical procedures. *Clin Neurol Neurosurg.* (2016) 146:123–9. doi: 10.1016/j.clineuro.2016.05.003
51. Ferroli P, Acerbi F, Tringali G, Albanese E, Broggi M, Franzini A, et al. Venous sacrifice in neurosurgery: new insights from venous indocyanine green videoangiography. *J Neurosurg.* (2011) 115:18–23. doi: 10.3171/2011.3.JNS10620
52. Louis DN, Perry A, Reifenberger G, von Deimling A, Figarella-Branger D, Cavenee WK, et al. The 2016 World Health Organization classification of tumors of the central nervous system: a summary. *Acta Neuropathol.* (2016) 131:803–20. doi: 10.1007/s00401-016-1545-1
53. Stone TJ, Keeley A, Virasami A, Harkness W, Tisdall M, Izquierdo Delgado E, et al. Comprehensive molecular characterisation of epilepsy-associated glioneuronal tumours. *Acta Neuropathol.* (2018) 135:115–29. doi: 10.1007/s00401-017-1773-z
54. Giulioni M, Marucci G, Pelliccia V, Gozzo F, Barba C, Didato G, et al. Epilepsy surgery of "low grade epilepsy associated neuroepithelial tumors": a retrospective nationwide Italian study. *Epilepsia.* (2017) 58:1832–41. doi: 10.1111/epi.13866
55. Englot DJ, Berger MS, Barbaro NM, Chang EF. Factors associated with seizure freedom in the surgical resection of glioneuronal tumors. *Epilepsia.* (2012) 53:51–7. doi: 10.1111/j.1528-1167.2011.03269.x
56. Zaghloul KA, Schramm J. Surgical management of glioneuronal tumors with drug-resistant epilepsy. *Acta Neurochir (Wien).* (2011) 153:1551–9. doi: 10.1007/s00701-011-1050-1
57. Diaz RJ, Dios RR, Hattab EM, Burrell K, Rakopoulos P, Sabha N, et al.

Study of the biodistribution of fluorescein in glioma-infiltrated mouse brain and histopathological correlation of intraoperative findings in high-grade gliomas resected under fluorescein fluorescence guidance. *J Neurosurg.* (2015) 122:1360–9. doi: 10.3171/2015.2.JNS132507

58. Acerbi F, Broggi M, Broggi G, Ferroli P. What is the best timing for fluorescein injection during surgical removal of high-grade gliomas? *Acta Neurochir (Wien).* (2015) 157:1377–8. doi: 10.1007/s00701-015-2455-z
59. Acerbi F, Cavallo C, Broggi M, Cordella R, Anghileri E, Eoli M, et al. Fluorescein-guided surgery for malignant gliomas: a review. *Neurosurg Rev.* (2014) 37:547–7. doi: 10.1007/s10143-014-0546-6
60. Schebesch K-M, Brawanski A, Doenitz C, Rosengarth K, Proescholdt M, Riemenschneider MJ, et al. Fluorescence-guidance in non-Gadolinium enhancing, but FET-PET positive gliomas. *Clin Neurol Neurosurg.* (2018) 172:177–82. doi: 10.1016/j.clineuro.2018.07.011
61. Rey-Dios R, Hattab EM, Cohen-Gadol AA. Use of intraoperative fluorescein sodium fluorescence to improve the accuracy of tissue diagnosis during stereotactic needle biopsy of high-grade gliomas. *Acta Neurochir (Wien)* (2014) 156:1071-5; discussion 1075. doi: 10.1007/s00701-014-2097-6
62. Ferraro N, Barbarite E, Albert TR, Berchmans E, Shah AH, Bregy A, et al. The role of 5-aminolevulinic acid in brain tumor surgery: a systematic review. *Neurosurg Rev.* (2016) 39:545–55. doi: 10.1007/s10143-015-0695-2

12

Quantitative Wide-Field Imaging Techniques for Fluorescence Guided Neurosurgery

Pablo A. Valdes[1], Parikshit Juvekar[1], Nathalie Y. R. Agar[1], Sylvain Gioux[2] and Alexandra J. Golby[1]*

[1] Department of Neurosurgery, Harvard Medical School, Brigham and Women's Hospital, Boston, MA, United States, [2] ICube Laboratory, University of Strasbourg, Télécom Physique Strasbourg, Alsace, France

***Correspondence:**
Pablo A. Valdes
pvaldesquevedo@bwh.harvard.edu

Fluorescence guided surgery (FGS) has fueled the development of novel technologies aimed at maximizing the utility of fluorescence imaging to help clinicians diagnose and in certain cases treat diseases across a breadth of disciplines such as dermatology, gynecology, oncology, ophthalmology, and neurosurgery. In neurosurgery, the goal of FGS technologies is to provide the neurosurgeon with additional information which can serve as a visual aid to better identify tumor tissue and associated margins. Yet, current clinical FGS technologies are qualitative in nature, limiting the ability to make accurate, reliable, and repeatable measurements. To this end, developments in fluorescence quantification are needed to overcome current limitations of FGS. Here we present an overview of the recent developments in quantitative fluorescence guidance technologies and conclude with the most recent developments aimed at wide-field quantitative fluorescence imaging approaches in neurosurgery.

Keywords: fluorescence-guided surgery, quantitative fluorescence imaging, protoporphyrin IX, tissue optical properties, brain tumors

INTRODUCTION

Fluorescence guided surgery (FGS) has fueled the development of novel technologies aimed at maximizing the utility of fluorescence imaging to help clinicians diagnose and in certain cases treat diseases across a breadth of disciplines such as dermatology, gynecology, oncology, ophthalmology, and neurosurgery. In neurosurgery, FGS has been applied in a variety of diseases including high grade gliomas where the largest experience exists, but also in other brain tumors including low-grade gliomas, meningiomas, lymphomas, and metastases. In addition to the use of FGS for brain tumors, neurosurgeon have used fluorescence for vascular imaging as well (1–11). The most common fluorophores, or fluorescent biomarkers in use include 5-aminolevulinic acid (5-ALA) induced protoporphyrin IX (PpIX), fluorescein sodium, methylene blue, and indocyanine green (ICG) (**Figures 1A–D**). There are also a variety of novel targeted fluorescent agents being tested in clinical trials (4, 9). FGS requires the development of novel agents with the ability to map the biological properties of interest (e.g., high specificity and sensitivity for tissue) as well as accompanying intraoperative instrumentation technologies for accurate, sensitive, specific, and objective assessment of the fluorescence emitted by these biomarkers.

Exciting developments in novel technologies for FGS to treat brain tumors include new wide-field fluorescence microscopes and hand-held devices. The goal of these technologies is to provide the neurosurgeon with additional information which can serve as a visual aid to better identify

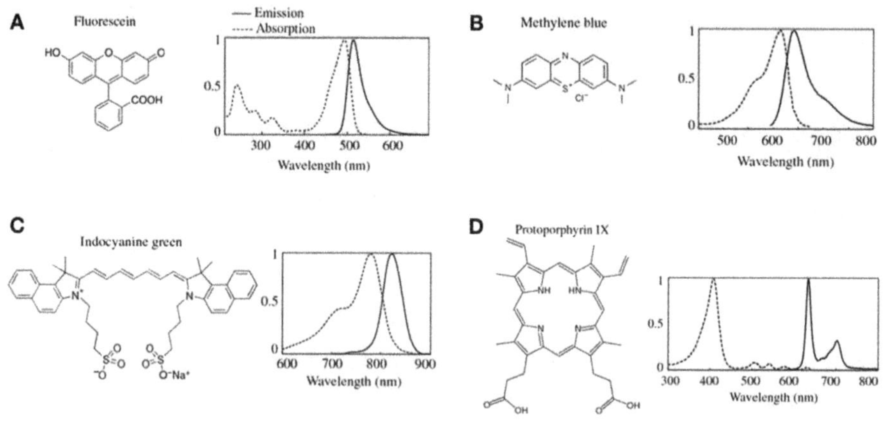

FIGURE 1 | Common fluorophores in clinical use. The chemical formulas and the associated excitation and emission spectra for the most common FDA approved fluorescence dyes are shown in **(A)** fluorescein, **(B)** methylene blue, **(C)** indocyanine green (ICG), and **(D)** protoporphryin IX (PpIX). Figure adapted with permission from DSouza et al. (12).

tumor tissue and associated margins. Beyond implementation of 5-ALA-PpIX across multiple different pathologies (e.g., gliomas, meningiomas, metastases, CNS lymphomas, spinal tumors), quantification of fluorescence in FGS opens a new avenue of research for novel technological development. Fluorescence quantification is needed to overcome current limitations of FGS which has been qualitative in nature, limiting the ability to make accurate, reliable and repeatable measurements. These limitations, in turn, impede consensus, standardization, and adoption of FGS in the field. To this end, various technologies, both pre-clinical and clinical, have been developed which are aimed at quantification and objective means of assessment of intraoperative fluorescence. Here we present an overview of the recent developments in quantitative fluorescence guidance technologies, with a focus on 5-ALA-PpIX, and conclude with the most recent developments aimed at wide-field quantitative fluorescence imaging approaches in neurosurgery.

FUNDAMENTAL CONCEPTS

State-of-the-art, clinically approved systems for FGS using PpIX provide surgeons with qualitative images of the "raw" fluorescence emissions as observed through the oculars of a surgical microscope modified for fluorescence imaging. During surgery, neurosurgeons can switch from conventional, white light illumination imaging mode to fluorescence light illumination mode to visualize either no visible fluorescence, or various graded, qualitative assessments of fluorescence intensities [e.g., in the case of fluorescein green-yellow (**Figure 1A**), or PpIX red-pink (**Figure 1D**)] from low to very bright fluorescence. Surgeons use these qualitative assessments of the fluorescence, herein called visible fluorescence imaging (vFI), to make clinical judgements. Neurosurgeons make qualitative assessments of the fluorescence visualized through the oculars, to ascertain the presence (or absence) of tumor (6, 7, 9, 11). PpIX emits in the 610–720 nm range when excited with 405 nm light to produce a red-pink fluorescence when visualized with state-of-the-art commercial surgical microscopes for FGS (3, 4, 11, 13) (**Figure 1D**). Numerous clinical studies have demonstrated a strong >90% positive predictive value of visible (e.g., bright pink fluorescence) PpIX vFI for predicting the presence tumor. As such, in areas with high or bright levels of visible fluorescence, the surgeon will make the judgement of the presence of tumor. Nevertheless, vFI assessments using state-of-the-art clinical microscopes during PpIX FGS have demonstrated a negative predictive value and sensitivity <50% in numerous studies (4, 11). Therefore, in areas with no visible fluorescence, the surgeon will make the judgement of no tumor present. Yet, given the high false negative rate of vFI PpIX there remains a high likelihood for the presence of residual tumor.

The low negative predictive value and sensitivity of vFI with 5-ALA-PpIX noted in glioma studies sheds light on important fundamental concepts in biomedical optics and on the limits of current state-of-the-art clinical technologies (4, 14, 15). It is well-known in biomedical optics, that multiple factors come into play with respect to *in vivo* fluorescence measurements during surgery or similar applications (3, 4, 14–16). Here, we will elaborate on some of the fundamental principles to consider in the implementation of fluorescence technologies during FGS, with a focus on further needs and developments in terms of quantification, or objective measures of the fluorescence intensity. We will describe the differences between visible fluorescence imaging (vFI) and the concept of quantitative fluorescence imaging (qFI). We will make use of fundamental ideas in biomedical optics to present the key factors to consider when developing quantitative FGS technologies. After building on the fundamental biophysics of tissue fluorescence measurements, we will describe current developments and applications of qFI in neurosurgery.

Tissue Optics

The measured fluorescence intensity, or fluorescence light that reaches the surgeon through the surgical oculars, or which reaches a detector (e.g., camera) and is displayed on a screen depends on multiple factors. These factors may be divided into instrumentation and intrinsic factors. Instrumentation factors include the specific camera properties (e.g., dark noise, pixel size, amplification, binning, etc.), light source excitation power, microscope optics (e.g., filters, mirrors, lenses), and set up (e.g., distance between excitation and tissue, distance between tissue and camera/oculars) (3, 14, 16). Here, we will not elaborate further on these components but acknowledge their significant role in our interpretation of the fluorescence and refer the reader to prior studies (12, 16–18). In the present review, we will focus on intrinsic factors impacting fluorescence, and how we can exploit understanding of these factors in developing quantitative fluorescence technologies.

Endogenous (Auto) Fluorescence

In the intraoperative setting, when tissues are interrogated for a fluorophore of interest (e.g., PpIX), two major intrinsic factors can impact the visualized or detected fluorescence: tissue autofluorescence (*AF*) and tissue optical properties—absorption (μ_a) and reduced scattering (μ_s'). Tissue ***AF*** results from endogenous fluorophores which make up cells and tissues (14). Multiple endogenous fluorophores varying by tissue composition include but are not limited to nicotinamide adenine dinucleotide (NADH), flavin adenine dinucleotide (FAD), aromatic amino acids (e.g., tryptophan), structural proteins (e.g., collagen, elastin), and degradation products (e.g., lipofuscin). These fluorophores have their excitation maxima in the range 200–400 nm and their emission maxima in the range 300–500 nm (14). As such, fluorescence imaging of tissues can have overlapping signal contributions from the fluorophore of interest (e.g., PpIX, fluorescein) and tissue ***AF***, which can lead to overestimation of fluorescence intensity from the fluorophore of interest. Thus, to properly quantify fluorescence, technologies require a means for spectral unmixing of tissue ***AF*** (and additional fluorophore contributions) from fluorescence due to the biomarker of interest such as PpIX, that make up the fluorescence measurements. For example, in the case of PpIX, photobleaching effects produce photoproducts (19–21), which can lead to inaccurate measurements of PpIX fluorescence given overlapping fluorescence emissions in the main PpIX emission peak. Other aspects to consider with fluorophores like fluorescence is fluorophore leakage from the vasculature, unlike PpIX which to the authors' knowledge, no large clinical study has noted leakage of intracellular PpIX contents as with fluorescein (4, 9, 22). Of note, current modified surgical microscopes for FGS provide surgeons with visualization of fluorescence emitted from tissues without any unmixing (e.g., subtraction) of tissue ***AF*** from the fluorescence produced by the fluorophore of interest (e.g., PpIX). These fluorescence measurements can then over or under estimate the actual fluorescence contribution from the fluorophore of interest, leading to inaccurate assessments of biomarker.

Tissue Optical Properties: Absorption and Scattering

The measured fluorescence intensity is significantly affected by tissue optical properties, which include the tissue absorption and reduced scattering at both the excitation ($\mu_{a(x)}$, $\mu_s'(x)$)

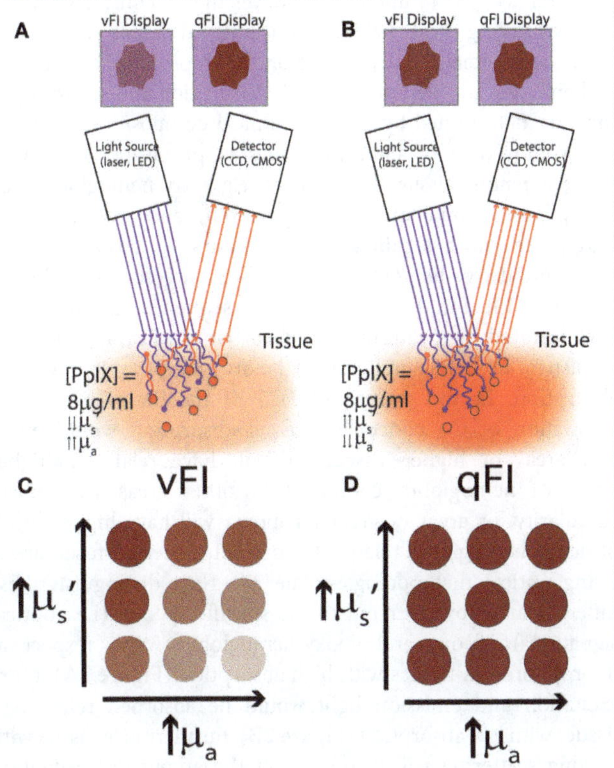

FIGURE 2 | Schematics of vFI and qFI for fluorescence guided surgery. **(A,B)** show schematics of an intraoperative FGS setup, which includes a light source for excitation light (e.g., lasers, light emitting diodes), and a detector to collect the fluorescence emissions (e.g., a CCD or CMOS camera). Tissues are illuminated with 405 nm violet light to excite the fluorophore, PpIX, which emits red to far red fluorescence in the 620–710 nm range. Excitation photons reach tissue and undergo multiple interactions with tissue including absorption and scattering of photons, with only a subset of excitation photons reaching the fluorophore, PpIX. Upon excitation, PpIX emits fluorescent photons which in turn travel through tissue undergoing multiple interactions including absorption and scattering, with only a subset of these fluorescent photons exiting tissue to reach the detector. In **(A)** less excitation photons reach PpIX and less fluorescent photons exit to reach the detector in tissues with high absorption and low reduced scattering. Meanwhile, in **(B)** more excitation photons reach PpIX and more fluorescent photons exit to reach the detector in tissues with low absorption and high reduced scattering, despite both **(A,B)** containing the same concentration and distribution of PpIX fluorophore. In **(A,B)** vFI shows highly different images of the surgical field of view (upper panel labeled vFI Display) despite equal PpIX concentrations, meanwhile, qFI shows equivalent images of the surgical field of view (upper panel labeled qFI Display) by correcting for intrinsic tissue factors including tissue optical properties. Schematics of tissue simulating phantoms containing the same concentration of PpIX but with different optical properties shown in **(C,D)**, with absorption increasing from left to right and reduced scattering increasing from bottom to top. **(C)** Shows images using vFI which either over- (top left corner) or under-estimates (bottom right corner) PpIX fluorescence with different tissue optical properties, meanwhile **(D)** shows images using qFI which performs accurate estimates of PpIX concentrations by correcting for tissue optical properties.

and emission wavelengths ($\mu_{a(m)}$, $\mu_s'(m)$). Tissue optical properties vary with wavelength. For example, hemoglobin has an μ_a (absorption) peak in the ultraviolet region ~10 times greater than its absorption in the red region of the visible spectrum (units cm^{-1}). Meanwhile, reduced scattering, μ_s', has a greater magnitude than absorption with a power law decrease as a function of wavelength. Thus, absorption and scattering will have significantly different effects on fluorescence imaging depending on the fluorophore's excitation and emission wavelengths (14, 15). Absorption and scattering in turn are determined by the biochemical composition of tissue. Absorption (μ_a) of light in tissues is primarily determined by endogenous tissue constituents, e.g., oxy-hemoglobin and deoxy-hemoglobin, melanin, myoglobin, and water. In the brain, the most significant contributors to absorption are oxy- and deoxy-hemoglobin with their largest absorption at <600 nm (9, 14, 23, 24). As a consequence, ultraviolet to near infrared light illuminated on to tissue will travel between ~100 µm to a few millimeters before complete loss due to absorption. In the context of FGS of the brain, a practical translation of the concept of tissue absorption would entail that areas of higher vascularity will have relatively higher levels of hemoglobin compared to other areas with lower vascularity, or areas of greater hypoxia will have higher levels of deoxy-hemoglobin relative to adjacent, better perfused areas. Using optical methodologies, one can then distinguish these different areas by referring to the specific spectra (i.e., optical signatures) of oxy and deoxy-hemoglobin. With respect to fluorophores, in tissues with high absorption (**Figure 2A**), more excitation and emission light would be absorbed relative to tissues with low absorption (**Figure 2B**). Furthermore, tissue with varying scattering will further affect the amount of excitation light that reaches fluorophores for excitation, and in turn, the number of photons which exit the tissue to reach the detector. This means that tissue with the same fluorophore concentration but different absorption and scattering will encounter less excitation light (i.e., fewer photons) reaching the fluorophore to enable excitation, and thus, less emission light would exit the tissue to reach the surgeon's oculars, or detector, leading to decreased detection of fluorescence intensity (4, 9, 14, 25).

Tissue scattering results from structural changes in tissues and is significant in the so called "therapeutic window" from 600 to 1,000 nm, where tissue absorption is small compared to scattering. Tissue scattering is determined by structures such as mitochondria, collagen fiber diameters, cell size and changes in the cell environment and its structures (14). For example, areas of higher cellularity and mitochondria content (e.g., cancerous tissue) will demonstrate different scattering than normal tissue. As such, tissue scattering can be indicative of pathophysiological changes and used as a means for optical contrast between tissues. Areas with higher scattering will allow more excitation light to travel through tissues, and furthermore, more emission light to exit tissues compared to areas with lower scattering (14). Current commercial systems for FGS in neurosurgery do not measure these optical properties or account for them in their fluorescence measurements.

Fluorescence Transport in Tissue

Intrinsic factors include the intrinsic properties of the fluorophore of interest (e.g., PpIX) and intrinsic tissue optical properties. The interplay of these factors determines the measured fluorescence intensity from tissue, ***F*** (i.e., the "raw fluorescence" intensity/number of photons measured by a detector or seen via the surgical oculars). Fluorophores possess their own intrinsic properties irrespective of the instrumentation used which include: concentration (**C**), quantum yield (***Q***), and extinction coefficient (***μ***); such that in the absence of any tissues (or in the setting of pure diluted fluorophore) the emitted (steady state) "raw fluorescence" intensity, ***F***, is linearly proportional to the concentration of fluorophore, **C** (Equation 1) (14, 15, 19, 20).

$$F = f = vFI = C * Q * \mu \qquad (1)$$

In the absence of tissues (or in the setting of pure diluted fluorophores) without the wavelength-dependent varying effects of tissue optical properties (μ_a, μ_s') and confounding/overlapping autofluorescence, ***AF***, from endogenous fluorophores, $\boldsymbol{E_f}$, the "raw" fluorescence intensity, ***F***, is equal to the quantitative fluorescence, ***f*** (Equation 1). In this ideal state, the fluorescence intensity seen by the surgeon, [i.e., the visible fluorescence (vFI)], is linearly proportional to the concentration of fluorophore in tissue (i.e., the brighter the fluorescence the higher the concentration independent of tissue variations). Nevertheless, in the operative setting, in which the surgeon visualizes different fluorescence intensities in tissue consisting of spatially varying levels of endogenous fluorophores (and in the case of PpIX, PpIX photoproducts), $\boldsymbol{E_f}$, and tissue optical properties, ***T***, the "raw" fluorescence intensity (e.g., vFI), is determined by a complex interaction of these factors (Equation 2) (14, 15, 17–21, 26–28).

$$F = f * E_f * T = C * Q * \mu * T \qquad (2)$$

During FGS of high-grade gliomas using PpIX as biomarker, the surgeon makes a qualitative assessment, i.e., vFI, of the "raw" fluorescence intensity and visually assessed what he/she sees as levels of red-pink fluorescence (no fluorescence, low fluorescence, high/bright fluorescence). The surgeon uses this information to infer the levels of tumor biomarker, i.e., PpIX, present. That is, tissues with high fluorescence implying high levels of PpIX, will be judged as containing tumor, and those without fluorescence, implying no PpIX, will likely be judged as not having tumor. Nevertheless, the "raw fluorescence" intensity, ***F***, as measured using vFI is determined by a variety of factors which include not only the PpIX concentration in tissue but also additional endogenous fluorophores, $\boldsymbol{E_f}$ (e.g., NAD, FADH, PpIX photoproducts) and tissue optical properties, ***T*** [absorption (μ_a) and scattering (μ_s')] that vary throughout every region of tissues in a wavelength-dependent manner (5, 8, 11, 14, 15, 17–21, 26–31). This is the critical shortcoming of FGS as currently practiced, because any assessment of the "raw fluorescence" intensity as currently practiced with vFI will be, at best, qualitative and approximate but always inaccurate regarding the true levels of fluorophore(s) present in tissue. "Raw" fluorescence intensity measurements are in reality an inaccurate estimate since it includes contributions from all these combined factors (fluorophore concentration, ***AF***, and tissue optical properties) (15). The raw fluorescence will always either over- or under-estimate the concentration of fluorescent biomarker, e.g., in glioma surgery under-estimation of fluorophore leads to the incorrect conclusion that the visualized tissue does not contain tumor biomarker, and can result in leaving significant residual tumor tissue unidentified and unresected, increasing the rate of recurrent disease and decreasing patient prognosis (7) (**Figure 2C**).

Inaccurate measurements of fluorescent biomarker levels in tissue has fueled the developing of tools and methods for measuring the quantitative fluorescence, *f*, in tissues, e.g., quantitative fluorescence imaging (qFI). Quantitative fluorescence measurements are accurate and true assessments of fluorophore(s) fluorescence decoupled from the distorting effects of tissue optical properties and endogenous fluorophores contributions (15). Thus, quantitative fluorescence measurements are linearly proportional to fluorophore concentrations in tissue and Equation (3)

$$\frac{F}{E_{f*}T} = f = C*Q*\mu \quad (3)$$

Quantitative fluorescence measurements could provide the surgeon a means for accurate assessment of fluorescent biomarker concentrations. The use of qFI would not have gross over- or under-estimation error in fluorophores levels as seen with vFI; and measurements across surgeons and institutions would be comparable given the objective scale of concentration levels (4, 11, 13, 15, 19, 22, 29, 30, 32–38) (**Figure 2D**).

Here we provided an overview of fundamental concepts in understanding the role of endogenous fluorescence, tissue optical properties, and fluorescence from fluorescent biomarkers currently used for FGS. These concepts provide a framework for understanding the need for quantitative fluorescence imaging (qFI) in neurosurgery. That is, current vFI technologies provide inaccurate assessments of the tissue fluorophore levels, and technological development should be geared toward creating technologies which are quantitative in their assessments of tissue fluorescence. To accomplish the goals of qFI, technologies require a means to correct for tissue optical properties and endogenous ***AF*** in the "raw" fluorescence data. In the next section, we provide an overview of the available technologies for wide-field quantitative fluorescence imaging (qFI) for fluorescence guided neurosurgery. We elaborate on precursors to qFI such as quantitative fluorescence spectroscopy, and subsequently describe technologies and clinical implementations of qFI in neurosurgery.

CLINICAL IMPLEMENTATION OF WIDE-FIELD QUANTITATIVE FLUORESCENCE GUIDED NEUROSURGERY

Quantitative Fluorescence Spectroscopy

To date, most clinical research implementing quantitative fluorescence assessments have used handheld spectroscopic probes (4, 9, 14, 23, 24). These probes consist of a fiber optic bundle for both light delivery and light collection with the tip of the probe held by the surgeon in contact with tissue. These probes are composed of light emitting diodes (LEDs) or laser sources to excite fluorophores and illuminate tissue, and spectrometers to collect the reflected light and/or emitted

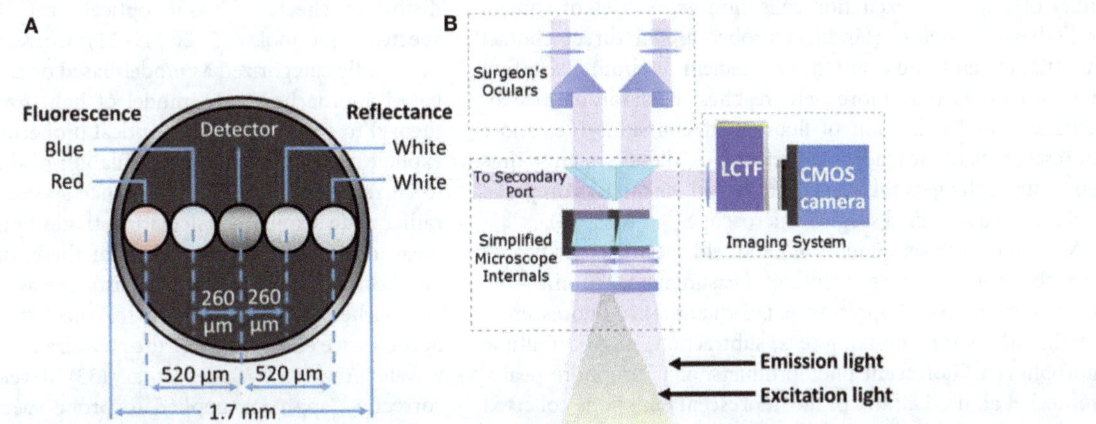

FIGURE 3 | Schematics of common quantitative probe and add-on modules for quantitative fluorescence. **(A)** Schematic of the distal contact end of a quantitative fluorescence probe with a linear arrangement of fibers for white light illumination, fluorescence excitation (violet-blue channel used for surface fluorescence, red channel not used in this study), and detector fiber. **(B)** Schematic of light path set up using a commercial surgical microscope modified for fluorescence imaging with corresponding white light illumination and excitation violet-blue light. A spectrally resolved add-on system connects to a free optical port for quantitative fluorescence imaging. Figure adapted with permission from Bravo et al. (38).

fluorescence in a wavelength-dependent manner (i.e., spectrally-resolved) (**Figure 3A**). A variety of spectroscopy systems have been used (4) in neurosurgery to collect fluorescence for tissue diagnostics and guidance, including probes used to collect the emitted fluorescence of endogenous (e.g., NADH, FADH), exogenously produced endogenous (e.g., PpIX), or exogenous (e.g., fluorescein) fluorophores in a wavelength dependent manner without correction for the distorting effects of tissue optical properties (5). Lin and colleagues detected *in vivo* tissue ***AF*** (i.e., without addition of exogenous fluorophores) as well as white light reflectance at 460 and 625 nm in 26 patients to distinguish normal tissue from tumor with a sensitivity and specificity of 100 and 76%, respectively. Similarly, the same group used the fluorescence peak at 500 nm as a means for identifying specific tissue pathology such as radiated tissue. In subsequent studies the authors developed discrimination algorithms with probe data to achieve sensitivities and specificities of up to 94% in distinguishing tumor from normal brain (39–44). A common theme with spectroscopy probes in neurosurgery is the use of the "raw" (i.e., arbitrary units of fluorescence) PpIX fluorescence intensity peak (5, 31, 45, 46). For example, a study by Stummer et al. (6) used a handheld spectroscopy probe to "quantify" the "raw" fluorescence at 635 nm for intraoperative diagnostic purposes. The authors used the "raw" fluorescence intensity peaks in a total of 33 patients with a receiver operating characteristic curve area under the curve of 88% using a threshold of 0.28 arbitrary units of fluorescence intensity with an associated specificity of 95% and sensitivity of 72%. This probe, like the majority in the neurosurgical literature, collect the "raw" emitted fluorescence from tissue fluorophores and the collected corresponding fluorescence spectra (i.e., wavelength dependent fluorescence light emissions). The collected "raw" fluorescence in these studies is equivalent to the "raw" fluorescence, ***F*** noted in Equation (2), which is a composite of multiple factors and thus, not truly "quantitative" measurements of the fluorescent biomarker. Nevertheless, these demonstrate the utility of improved excitation-collection geometries of contact probe-based systems. Handheld probes are in direct contact with tissue, and thus, are more efficient in both excitation of fluorophores (i.e., more light reaches the fluorophores for excitation) and collection of fluorescent emissions (i.e., more fluorescent light reaches the detector). These systems thus demonstrate the general trend of increased sensitivity compared to vFI using a modified surgical microscope (3, 14, 15, 23).

More recent developments of handheld spectroscopic probes with the aim of more accurate measurements of the true fluorophore-derived fluorescence, i.e., quantitative fluorescence, use algorithms for unmixing (e.g., subtraction) of ***AF***, multiple fluorophores, fluorescent photoproducts, or fluorophore peaks. Montcel et al. used a ratio of the fluorescent emissions collected via a handheld spectroscopic probe at 620 nm divided by the emissions at 634 nm. They corrected this ratio furthermore for tissue ***AF*** following correction of auto fluorescence as a means for more accurate spectroscopic detection (10). In similar fashion, Hosseini et al. used a spectroscopy system to "quantify" PpIX. In their work, they derived a "ratio number" for tissue diagnosis which was the ratio of the fluorescence intensity in arbitrary units at 635 nm minus the auto fluorescence at 635 nm. They then divided by the auto fluorescence at 510 nm to produce the "ratio number." The authors reported a higher "ratio number" in tumor compared to normal brain in a limited number of patients (47). In a subsequent study, they used the ratio of the raw fluorescence intensity at 630 over 600 nm for tissue diagnosis (48). These spectroscopy studies acknowledge the importance of different fluorescent contributions to the collected, "raw" fluorescence, ***F*** (Equation 2), and developed means to correct for them in their processing of fluorescence measurements. The different algorithms account for ***AF***, ***(Ef,*** Equation 2), or for PpIX associated photoproducts in their calculations of the PpIX specific fluorescence. PpIX is known to produce distinct photoproducts and to exist in distinct photochemical states with variation in their spectra depending on factors such as pH (10, 20). This is a significant advancement in spectroscopy probes which allows spectral unmixing of major component(s) in the "raw" fluorescence, ***F***, to arrive at a more quantitative, and accurate measurement of the "quantitative fluorescence," *f*, and fluorescent biomarker concentrations. Fluorophores exhibit different effects to continuous light excitation, which can lead to irreversible photodamage, or fluorescence quenching, and creation of photoproducts. PpIX is more prone to photobleaching effects than some modern fluorophores used in the basic sciences such as Alexa Fluor agents or quantum dots. In the case of PpIX, multiple photoproducts have been identified with fluorescence emissions which overlap with the main PpIX peak. As such, spectral unmixing is important in accounting for not just tissue autofluorescence, but also for these confounding photoproducts which may lead to inaccurate estimates of PpIX concentrations (4, 19–21). However, these systems do not correct for the non-linear, spatially dependent, and highly variable differences in tissue absorption and scattering, ***T*** (Equation 2), and thus cannot be accurately called "quantitative fluorescence."

Subsequent studies have used developing concepts in biomedical optics to apply correction techniques for the distorting effects of tissue optical properties with handheld spectroscopic tools (15, 26, 49–51). Correction techniques can be broadly categorized as model-based or empirical. The model-based approaches use a model of light transport (e.g., diffuse theory) to correct for tissue optical properties, usually requiring explicit measurement, and calculation of these properties prior to correcting the "raw" fluorescence spectra. Empirical models, rather than explicitly calculating tissue optical properties, will measure or calculate surrogates of these, for example, the use of reflectance measurements at distinct wavelengths. Ratiometric approaches, a common form of the latter, use ratios of the fluorescence emissions over the measured reflectance at specified wavelengths (15). Valdes et al. (33) developed a ratiometric correction approach applied to probe spectroscopy data. The authors collect the spectrally-resolved fluorescence from tissue. They then measure the reflectance near the excitation and main emission peaks; and use the calibrated reflectance correction factor to divide the "raw" fluorescence spectra to derive a "quantitative fluorescence" spectrum and quantitative PpIX concentrations (Equation 4). The "quantitative fluorescence" in this study performs well in phantoms and *in vivo* when correcting for absorption and scattering, by using the white light reflectance ratio as a surrogate for tissue optical properties effects (33) (Equation 4).

$$\frac{F}{R} = f, \tag{4}$$

Valdes et al. used the same quantitative probe with a model-based correction approach to calculate the quantitative fluorescence in tissues and thus, PpIX concentrations during brain tumor resections (19, 29, 35, 36). This approach used the white light reflectance to measure the reflected white light; and using a spatially resolved model of the diffuse reflectance explicitly calculate the tissue absorption and scattering. The tissue optical properties are used in a light transport model of the fluorescence to correct the "raw" fluorescence for the distorting effects of tissue optical properties and calculate the corrected, or quantitative fluorescence (and PpIX concentrations) at each interrogated site. This group used the probe on a variety of tumor pathologies including low- and high-grade gliomas, meningiomas, and metastases demonstrating improved detection of tumor compared to vFI using commercial systems. For example, the quantitative probe was able to detect significant amounts of PpIX in low grade gliomas which were not identified using vFI, and detection accuracies in low grade gliomas were similar to those using state-of-the-art vFI for high grade gliomas. Similar to the previous approaches which accounted for endogenous or other fluorophore contributions, the authors used a spectral unmixing algorithm to account for autofluorescence, PpIX photoproducts, and PpIX (4, 19–21). These latter two approaches describe the use of a spectroscopic handheld probe similar to the previously mentioned studies. The authors collected both spectrally resolved fluorescence and diffuse white light reflectance. Similar to previous studies, they accounted for additional fluorophore contributions other than PpIX such as the endogenous autofluorescence and PpIX photoproducts. A lesson learned from these later approaches is how they correct for tissue optical properties, either by a ratiometric, and empirical approach, or by means of a model-based, light transport approach. Correction for tissue optical properties in addition to additional fluorescence contributions, enabled the authors to explicitly calculate the quantitative fluorescence and as such, PpIX biomarker concentrations for tumor tissue identification.

Hand-held spectroscopy probes informed the community regarding important factors to consider when developing quantitative technologies and more importantly, the role these measurements might play in helping improve FGS with more accurate (and at times sensitive) measurements. The different probe implementations to date used methodologies to correct for endogenous ***AF***, for fluorophore photoproducts or distinct fluorescence states, the fluorophore of interest (e.g., PpIX), and for tissue optical properties. To accomplish these tasks, spectroscopy probes acquire spectrally-resolved data to analyze the fluorescence spectra in a wavelength dependent manner, and as such, enable such analyses of spectral-fitting. Furthermore, these studies used either surrogates of tissue optical properties in the case of ratiometric approaches, or explicitly measured them using models of light transport. These probes demonstrated improved accuracies for tumor detection across a broad range of pathologies, supporting the need for technologies that are not just more sensitive, but also which perform quantitative fluorescence measurements (4, 9, 14, 23).

Wide-Field Quantitative Fluorescence

Implementation of quantitative fluorescence systems for neurosurgical guidance is limited but included pre-clinical studies in phantoms and animals as well as clinical implementations of these novel imaging systems (3, 4, 15, 52). Yang et al. developed a multispectral fluorescence imaging system that measures fluorescence at multiple wavelengths. They tested this system during brain tumors surgeries using the agent Photofrin. This study used multi-wavelength excitation and emission light in a wide-field FGS imaging setup (53), unlike commercially available surgical microscopes which are single wavelength systems (e.g., a single bandpass for excitation and long pass filters), which limits their utility to one fluorophore at a time (3, 13). Further, as noted with the spectroscopy studies, this system is limited in its ability to correct and account for ***AF*** or additional fluorophore contributions as well as tissue optical properties on the collected fluorescence emissions. In 2011, Saager et al. (54) reported the development of a system capable of dual spatial frequency domain imaging (SFDI) and fluorescence imaging. This system performs patterned illumination at varying spatial frequencies and phases of the field of view (e.g., phantoms, animal brain) to recover the reflected light in a spectrally-resolved manner and calculate the tissue absorption and scattering at every pixel in the entire field of view (SFDI) (55). The authors were able to measure tissue optical properties to calculate a "correction map" and apply this for fluorescence correction and ultimately, quantification of PpIX concentrations. The authors validated their system in phantoms and ultimately applied to optical measurements of skin. Of note, although this study was not applied in neurosurgery or neurosurgical models, it is important because it lays the groundwork for future studies using explicit measurements of tissue optical properties for PpIX quantification. A more recent system (22) collects spectrally resolved white light reflectance and fluorescence emissions using an add-on module that adapts to a commercial surgical microscope (**Figure 3B**). This system collects multiple images at user-specified wavelengths in the visible range of the spectrum (e.g., 400–720 nm) enabling reconstruction of a full reflectance and fluorescence spectrum at each pixel in the image. The authors used an empiric ratiometric approach to correct for tissue optical properties by using a ratio of the "raw" fluorescence, ***F***, to the reflected white light, ***R***, to calculate the quantitative fluorescence in tissues and subsequently, using a calibration factor, calculated the true PpIX in tissues. This approach introduces important concepts in FGS. First, the authors developed a system for spectrally resolved detection of both the white light reflectance and emitted fluorescence, similar to the approach used in spectroscopy systems. Second, the authors use a fluorescence correction technique to derive the "quantitative fluorescence" in tissues. In this work, they used the reflected fluorescence as a surrogate for tissue optical properties. In the first iteration of their system, the authors used a low sensitivity, CCD camera that enabled detection levels down to ~100 ng/ml in tissue. Previous work from spectroscopic studies, noted that levels of PpIX in tumor tissues can be as low as 10 ng/ml. A subsequent system update by this team used a more sensitive scientific CMOS camera to improve both the lower threshold of detection and acquisition times by approximately one order of magnitude (19, 22). Jermyn et al developed a similar system for neurosurgical guidance using a more sensitive EMCCD camera (56). The authors noted detection levels down to 10 ng/ml of PpIX, significantly increased speeds for data collection, and improvement in overall system performance and quantification metrics compared to a CMOS based system (34). These latter studies used more sensitive, higher quality cameras, equivalent to those used for benchtop fluorescence microscopy studies, to implement into clinically compatible systems.

Xie et al. (1) developed a pre-clinical system that acquires spectrally resolved white light and fluorescence emissions, similar to Valdes et al. and Jermyn et al., and coupled it to a new algorithm for fluorescence correction. The authors developed an empirical algorithm for fluorescence correction. They correct the "raw" fluorescence by using a calibrated tissue reflectance. They calibrate their system to a known reflectance standard; and use a product of the reflectance at the excitation and emission wavelengths to subsequently correct the fluorescence spectrum. The authors tested the system in phantoms of varying absorption, scattering and PpIX concentrations to demonstrate reliable quantification <100 ng/ml with short acquisition times similar to those reported by prior studies. They noted excellent quantification ($r^2 = 0.94$) down to <100 ng/ml in phantoms, and furthermore, provided pilot data testing of this system in *ex vivo* glioblastoma samples, demonstrating the capabilities to detect PpIX concentrations of tumor infiltrated tissues in wide-field mode. This work presents an important advancement in qFI, by developing a novel algorithm to correct for the non-linear, and confounding effects of tissue optical properties on the measured "raw" fluorescence, further demonstrating the need for techniques to measure the quantitative fluorescence, and providing a detailed account and principles for system calibration

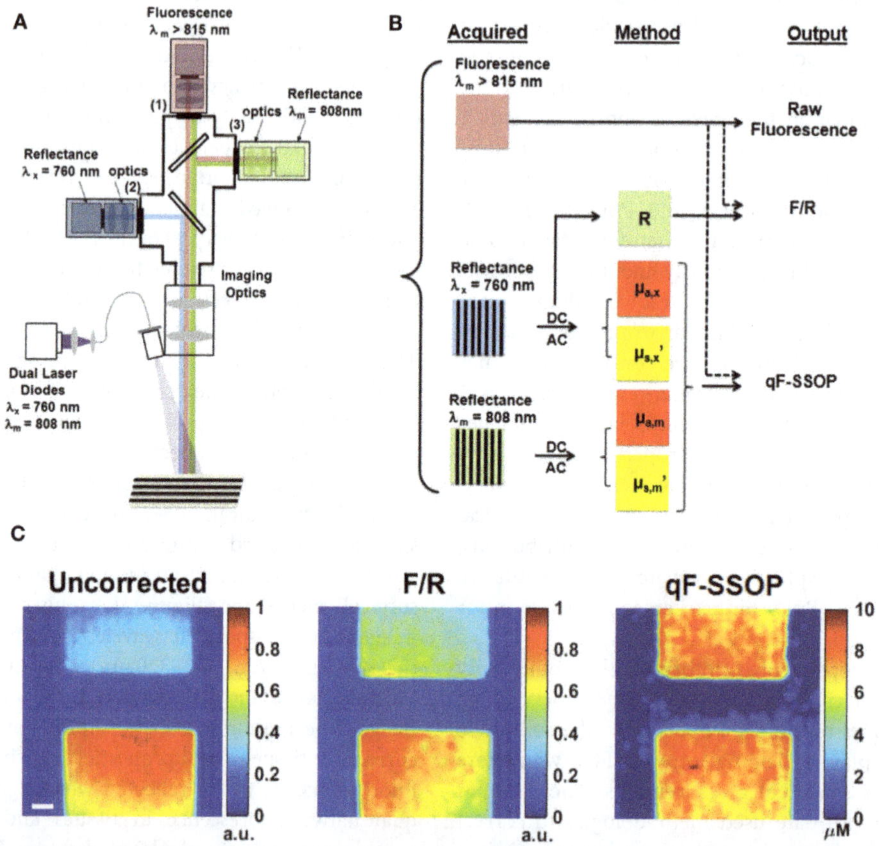

FIGURE 4 | Real time, quantitative fluorescence imaging system coupled with single snapshot optical properties imaging. **(A)** Schematics of a qFI system that performs simultaneous SSOP imaging and fluorescence detection by acquiring simultaneous reflectance and fluorescence imaging under SSOP mode. **(B)** Data processing scheme in which reflectance images are processed under SSOP conditions to estimate the absorption μ_a and reduced scattering μ_s'. **(C)** A light transport model is used to correct the raw fluorescence for the effects of tissue optical properties to calculate the quantitative fluorescence. Bottom panel shows one frame of a real-time dynamic video of tissue simulating phantoms displaying the raw fluorescence (uncorrected), the empirically corrected fluorescence (F/R), and the quantitative fluorescence using SSOP (qF-SSOP). Figure adapted with permission from Valdes et al. (37).

that inform the community when developing such quantitative fluorescence systems.

Sibai et al. (57) developed a bench top pre-clinical system capable of dual spatial frequency domain imaging (SFDI) and fluorescence imaging. This system performs patterned illumination at varying spatial frequencies and phases of the field of view (e.g., phantoms, animal brain) to recover the reflected light in a spectrally-resolved manner and calculate the tissue absorption and scattering at every pixel in the entire field of view (SFDI). In this study, each acquisition takes ~12 s followed by data processing. The optical properties are used to correct the collected fluorescence using a light transport model of the fluorescence; and reconstruct a qFI image of the full field of view. In this work, the authors validated their system in phantoms with varying optical properties and PpIX concentrations, and subsequently applied their system to a rodent model of glioma. They further validated their imaging results by comparison with the gold standard spectroscopy probe and *ex vivo,* tissue extraction homogenization technique demonstrating differences of μ_a and μ_s' of 14 and 19.4%, respectively and for PpIX of 10.5%. This work makes a significant advancement in quantitative fluorescence techniques in neurosurgery, by using a model-based approach for wide-field quantitative fluorescence imaging. The authors used a rigorous model-based approach for accurate estimates of tissue optical properties using a well-known SFDI technique (28). This is in contrast to the prior studies which use various calibration and empiric correction factors such as the raw reflectance as a surrogate for the tissue optical properties. After explicitly calculating the tissue optical properties across the full surgical field of view, these are integrated into a light transport model of the fluorescence to extract the quantitative fluorescence in tissue and thus, the quantitative PpIX concentrations.

Valdes et al. (37) developed a benchtop pre-clinical system to perform simultaneous single snapshot optical properties (SSOP) imaging and fluorescence imaging in wide field mode (**Figure 4A**). SSOP uses only one single frequency without the need for multiple phases during patterned illumination of tissue, unlike SFDI which uses multiple frequencies and phases to extract the tissue optical properties (28, 58, 59). SSOP enables fast, real time acquisition (milliseconds per acquisition) since it requires only one image to extract optical properties compared to at least 6 required for SFDI. The authors use SSOP imaging to estimate the tissue optical properties in phantoms of varying absorption, scattering and fluorophore concentrations to correct the "raw" fluorescence using a light transport model of the quantitative fluorescence (**Figure 4B**). They further demonstrate the ability to perform quantitative fluorescence imaging in video rate mode as a result of the high speed offered with SSOP imaging across the full field of view in a pixel-wide manner (**Figure 4C**). This work provides a further development in qFI methods by using a model-based approach to estimate tissue optical properties and correct the fluorescence for these effects. Furthermore, they implement this in a wide field of mode at video rate speeds. The ability to perform video rate imaging would

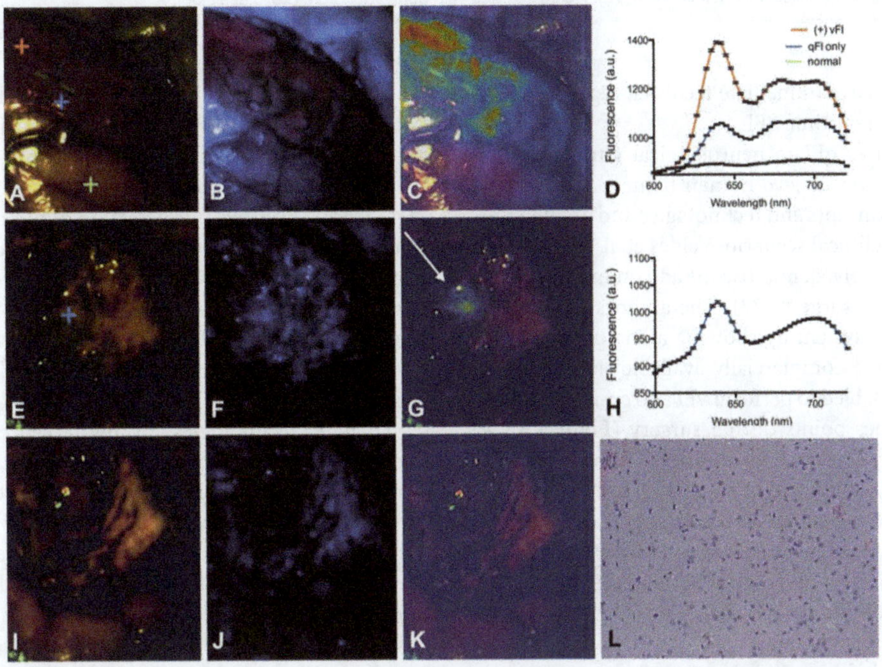

FIGURE 5 | Spectrally-resolved quantitative fluorescence imaging using a ratiometric approach during *in vivo* glioblastoma surgery. Intraoperative images under **(A,E,I)** conventional white light illumination, **(B,F,J)** blue light illumination for vFI using a commercial system, and **(C,G,K)** quantitative fluorescence images using a ratiometric approach at the beginning (top row), near the end (middle row), and at the end (bottom row) of surgery. Near the end of surgery, high levels of PpIX were found using qFI **(G)** but not using vFI **(C)** with histological corroboration of tumor **(L)**. Spectra at the beginning of surgery **(D)** show expected PpIX peaks and near the end of surgery **(H)** in the area of residual tumor **(G)**. Figure adapted with permission from Valdés et al. (22).

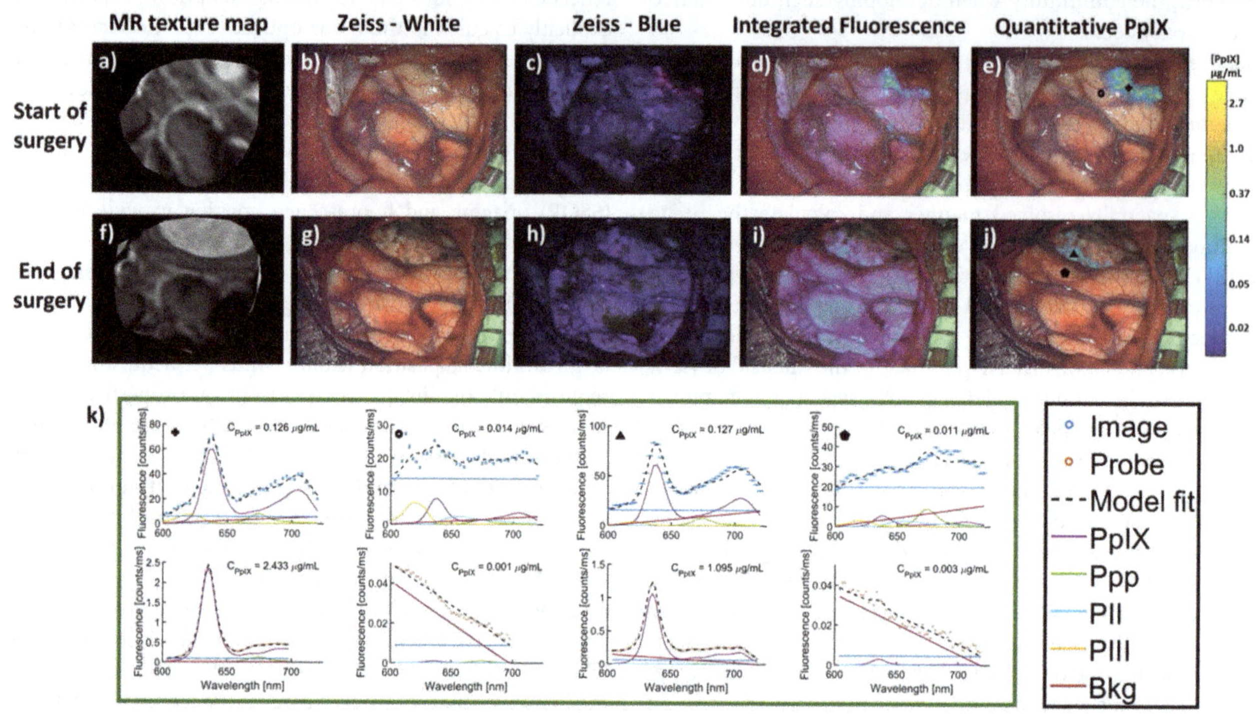

FIGURE 6 | MR images and intraoperative fluorescence using a filter corrected approach. Images were acquired at the start (top row) and end (bottom row) of surgery. **(a,f)**, MR images corresponding to the intraoperative **(b,g)** conventional white light images, **(c,h)** blue light vFI images using a commercial microscope system, **(d,i)** "raw" fluorescence intensity, or integrated fluorescence images, and **(e,j)** quantitative fluorescence images using a ratiometric and filter correction approach. **(k)** PpIX spectra using the qFI system (top row) and spectroscopic quantitative probe (bottom row) at multiple locations and timepoints during surgery [marked by corresponding symbols in images **(e,j)**]. PpIX concentration observed in the C_{PpIX} overlays. Ppp, Photoproduct I; PII, Photoproduct II; PIII, Photoproduct III; Bkg, Background; Offset, linear offset for background signal. Figure adapted with permission from Bravo et al. (38).

enable the surgeon to have immediate feedback regarding tissue in the field of view for real-time qFI.

The work above uses qFI in neurosurgical guidance in the pre-clinical setting, or on *ex vivo* human tissues. A few studies have used the above concepts and technologies and applied these in the intraoperative, clinical scenario. Valdes et al. subsequently used their spectrally-resolved, microscope add on module system in human glioblastoma surgery (22). The authors demonstrate the utility of their qFI system by showing a comparison of the images obtained using a commercially available state-of-the-art surgical microscope enabled to perform vFI and co-registered qFI images at various times points during surgery (**Figures 5A–D**, at the beginning of surgery; **Figures 5E–G**, near the end of surgery; **Figures 5I–K**, at the end of surgery). They demonstrate that the qFI system was able to detect tumor near the end of surgery in areas were vFI left residual tumor unidentified (i.e., vFI showed no visible fluorescence) (**Figure 5F**), but their qFI system was able to detect significant residual tumor (**Figures 5G,H**) which correlated with histopathology (**Figure 5L**). More recently, Bravo et al. (38) used this system *in vivo* to demonstrate the importance of spectral filtering of the fluorescence signals for more accurate PpIX quantification maps. The authors developed a metric called a "confidence ratio," which functions as a filter to remove regions of uncertainty from quantitative PpIX images; by removing those estimates that approach the detection limits of PpIX, the authors show their approach can decrease the rates of false positives (**Figure 6**). This work highlights the value of performing quantitative estimates of the fluorescence to significantly improve our detection of tumor tissue across tumor pathologies compared to the standard of care using commercially available vFI technologies, and the need for complex data processing to maximize qFI detection. Furthermore, this work highlights the importance of performing wide field quantitative detection compared to single small area detection provided by handheld probes.

To date, technologies for fluorescence quantification have used either handheld, contact probes, or wide field, non-contact imaging systems. Each system boasts of their own advantages and disadvantages. Handheld probes are in direct contact with tissue, which provides a geometry for more efficient (i.e., less loss of) light excitation and collection of reflectance and fluorescence emissions from tissue. Furthermore, these systems do not have to account for different distances as they have one distance between excitation and emission sources (since they are in contact with tissue), which simplifies models for fluorescence quantification. As such, these probes have a history of algorithms developed for rigorous model-based quantification, and in more recent developments, are able to

TABLE 1 | Comparative summary of wide-field imaging systems.

Group	Fluorophore	Technical Features and Advantages	Correction Method	Acquisition Time	Processing Time	Cost	Test population	Limitations
RESEARCH SYSTEMS								
Yang et al. (53)	Photofrin	Standalone Multispectral Fluorescence Imaging system—multiple (five band) excitation and emission wavelengths. Long working distance ~50 cm. Field of view ~ 3 cm diameter. Detector—CCD camera.	None	15 s	Real-time	~ $100,000	Phantoms. Human brain (*in vivo.*)	Inability to account and correct for ***AF, Ef***, additional fluorophore contributions and ***T***. Low concentration sensitivity (0.05 to 0.1 μg/g) and low depth sensitivity (0.5 mm.) Stand-alone system not integrated into surgical microscope. Results displayed on a personal computer.
Saager et al. (54)	5-ALA-PpIX	Standalone SFDI system—patterned illumination with varying spatial frequencies and phases of the field of view. Detector—CCD camera.	***T*** calculated as a "correction map" of the field of view using spatial frequency domain imaging	12 s	Not specified	Not specified	Phantoms. Human skin (*in vivo*).	Low concentration specificity (within 0.2 μg/ml of known concentration.) Longer acquisition times since 6 images are required to estimate ***T***. Not tested in human brains.
Valdes et al. (22)	5-ALA-PpIX Fluorescin	Integrated HIS (Hyperspectral Imaging System) for sequential spectrally resolved image acquisition in the range 400–720 nm at 10 nm intervals. Works as a portable, add-on module compatible with commercial surgical microscopes using the microscope optics and light source. Working distance ~30 cm. Field of view = 10 × 7.5 mm to 50 × 40 mm Allows reconstruction of the field of view with the full reflectance and fluorescence spectrum at each pixel as a 3D image cube. Detector—CCD camera (first iteration, concentration sensitivity ~100 ng/ml PpIX), sCMOS camera (second iteration, concentration sensitivity ~10 ng/ml PpIX.) System validated with phantoms, histopathology and comparison with commercial vFI systems.	Spectrally constrained dual-band normalization. Empiric ratiometric approach .	100 ms to 500 ms per wavelength. Up to 2–8 s per white light and fluorescence hyperspectral image capture.	Near real-time	~20,000–30,000	Phantoms. Rat brain (*in vivo*). Human brain (*in vivo*)	Penetration depth limited to a few hundred microns in depth. Quantification accuracy limited to > 40 ng/ml PpIX using the second generation sCMOS system compared to the gold standard optical probe of ~10 ng/ml PpIX. Empiric correction algorithm less accurate than model based correction approaches, unable to explicitly measure tissue optical properties and intrinsic tissue biomarkers other than PpIX
Jermyn et al. (56)	5-ALA-PpIX	Integrated HIS for sequential spectrally resolved image acquisition in the range 400–720 nm at 10 nm intervals. Works as a portable, add-on module compatible with commercial surgical microscopes using the microscope optics and light source. Working distance ~30 cm. Field of view ~ 20 cm X 20 cm. Allows reconstruction of the field of view with the full reflectance and fluorescence spectrum at each pixel as a 3D image cube . Detector—EMCCD camera (two orders of magnitude lower concentrations detected compared to CMOS, possibly comparable to the ~1 ng/ml detection limit of point probes) and sCMOS camera connected simultaneously for comparison.s	Spectrally constrained dual-band normalization. Empiric ratiometric approach .	5–100 ms. Up to 2 s per white light and fluorescence hyperspectral image capture.	Near real-time	~$50,000	Phantoms. Rat brain (*ex vivo*). Human brain (*ex vivo*)	Enhanced sensitivity of EMCCD detectors can be confounded to a greater degree by non-specific ***AF*** signals and ambient light. High cost of EMCCD detectors. Empiric correction algorithm less accurate than model based correction approaches, unable to explicitly measure tissue optical properties and intrinsic tissue biomarkers other than PpIX.

(Continued)

TABLE 1 | Continued

Group	Fluorophore	Technical Features and Advantages	Correction Method	Acquisition Time	Processing Time	Cost	Test population	Limitations
Xie et al. (1)	5-ALA-PpIX	Standalone system conceptually similar to those by Valdes et al and Jermyn et al. Detector—sCMOS camera. Concentration sensitivity ~ 10 ng/ml.	Empirical correction algorithm approach. Calibration to a known tissue reflectance standard and correction of F using a product of the R at excitation and emission wavelengths .	26 s	Not specified	Not specified	Phantoms. Human brain (*ex vivo*).	Penetration depth limited to a few hundred microns in depth. Long acquisition times due to data input/output latencies.
Sibai et al. (57)	5-ALA-PpIX	Standalone SFDI system (similar to Saager et al). Replaces previous approaches of ratiometric or semiratiometric correction in SFDI systems with a more rigorous light transport model. Allows reconstruction of the full-field of view representing qFI data post-correction. Field of view = 3 cm X 3 cm. Detector—CCD camera. System accuracy validated with spectroscopy probe (gold standard) and *ex vivo* homogenized extracted tissue. The method is also able to explicitly measure tissue optical properties and intrinsic tissue biomarkers unlike the systems by Valdes et al, Jermyn et al, and Xie et al.	Light transport model based approach using spatial frequency domain imaging.	36 s	Not specified	Not specified	Phantoms. Rat brains (post mortem in situ, *ex vivo*).	Benchtop preclinical system. Suboptimal results from *in vivo* rat brains (but these limitations may not translate to *in vivo* human experiments as the authors believe the rat glioma model to be the cause, rather than failure of the method or instrumentation). Less sensitive than spectroscopy probes by 2–4 times on account of spill-over or cross talk between image pixels and more tissue distortion and attenuation of weak fluorescence signals. Decreased concentration sensitivity and higher exposure times compared to systems with EMCCD detectors. Penetration depth limited to a few hundred microns in depth. Long acquisition times requiring 6 images to estimate T.
Valdes et al. (37)	5-ALA-PpIX	Standalone qF-SSOP system—single snapshot of optical properties. Able to perform real-time data acquisition since it requires a single image to estimate T (compared to the SFDI systems by Saager et al and Sibai et al which require multiple images).	Light transport model based approach using single snapshot of optical properties imaging	500 ms	21 ms	Not specified	Phantoms.	Benchtop preclinical system. System has not been validated against *ex vivo* or *in vivo* rodent or human brains.
Zeiss Surgical Microscope + Blue 400 module	5-ALA-PpIX	Commercial vFI system as an integrated add-on module for the Zeiss series of surgical microscopes. Real-time visualization of fluorescence through surgical oculars and projected unto a CCD camera.	No correction	Real-time	No processing	Quote requested	Humans (*in vivo*)	Requires purchase of expensive proprietary accessory. Qualitative, subjective information relayed to the surgeon without quantification. High rate of false negatives using PpIX.

(Continued)

TABLE 1 | Continued

Group	Fluorophore	Technical Features and Advantages	Correction Method	Acquisition Time	Processing Time	Cost	Test population	Limitations
COMMERCIAL SYSTEMS								
Leica Surgical Microscope + FL400 module	5-ALA-PpIX	Commercial vFI system as an integrated add-on module for the Leica series of surgical microscopes. Real-time visualization of fluorescence through surgical oculars and projected unto a CCD camera.	No correction	Real-time	No processing	Quote requested	Humans (*in vivo*)	Requires purchase of expensive proprietary accessory. Qualitative, subjective information relayed to the surgeon without quantification.

explicitly measure tissue optical properties and derive intrinsic biomarkers. These, in turn, are used in model-based approaches to correct the fluorescence emissions and quantify fluorophores. Despite the aforementioned advantages, handheld probes face a major disadvantage when it comes to wide-spread surgical implementation and intraoperative diagnostics. They require the surgeon to disrupt the surgical workflow to place the probe in direct contact with tissue, to then interrogate a small field of view (as small as 1 mm in diameter) for each acquisition (10, 14, 15, 19, 23, 31, 39, 43, 44, 47).

Wide-field, quantitative imaging systems allow the surgeons to view a larger area of interrogation up to multiple centimeters in diameter, including the full surgical field of view. This provides a more immediate, intuitive, and less disruptive view of tissue for intraoperative diagnostics. Nevertheless, current systems are limited in their ability to provide instantaneous, real-time quantification of this field of view. Another disadvantage involves a less efficient geometry for light excitation and emission given the ever-changing distances between light sources and the detector resulting from movement of the microscope and the imaging system. This, in turn, presents a challenge to accurate quantification, requiring more complex algorithms to account for these varying distances. Although, various pre-clinical systems (**Table 1**) have been developed that take advantage of model-based approaches for quantification (unlike systems using empiric algorithms), these have not been implemented in a seamless manner for immediate intraoperative surgical feedback. An important consideration with quantitative fluorescence is the need for calibration. Finally, spectroscopy and imaging systems require calibration against known standards of tissue optical properties and fluorophores to ensure accurate estimation of quantitative fluorescence intraoperatively (1, 4, 11, 15, 17, 22, 28, 34, 37, 38, 51, 53, 54, 56, 59). As such, reports on quantitative systems need to provide well-delineated calibration procedures to ensure translation of results between patients and institutions (18, 21, 28, 60).

CONCLUSION

The field of quantitative fluorescence in neurosurgery, with implementation of spectroscopic and wide-field systems is in its infancy. The majority of the literature on fluorescence imaging and its application to neurosurgical guidance in brain tumors uses vFI technologies (3). We have described limitations of vFI including subjectivity and inaccuracy of measurements, inter-observer dependence, and decreased sensitivity for residual disease. This work seeks to first introduce the reader to fundamental concepts in quantitative fluorescence, including concepts of autofluorescence, tissue optical properties and their effects on the fluorescence measurements, and fluorescence correction techniques (14, 15). Second, this study seeks to provide the reader with an overview of the major implementations of quantitative fluorescence in neurosurgery. Since the literature on quantitative fluorescence in neurosurgery is limited, we provide an overview of some of the preliminary studies seeking to arrive at quantitative assessments of the fluorescence in neurosurgery. We then highlight some lessons learned from each of these studies. Finally, we wish to inform the reader regarding the importance of quantitative fluorescence in neurosurgery both as a means for standardizing measurements across surgeons, but also, as a means for improved detection of residual disease.

The success of vFI has helped fuel technological developments including modified surgical microscopes for fluorescence imaging, exoscopes, and probe-based technologies such as spectroscopic, and confocal systems (3, 4). Furthermore, the success of vFI has subsequently led to development of quantitative fluorescence technologies discussed in this paper, as these technologies have highlighted the intrinsic limitations of vFI (subjectivity, inter-observer dependence, inaccurate measurements, decreased sensitivity for residual disease). Future developments in FGS require that these technologies provide seamless integration to the surgical workflow with fast acquisition times and ease of interpretation of the data to the surgeon. Technologies should provide means for improve visualization, calibration, and heads up display, to enable wide spread use across multiple centers. In summary, the use of qFI in neurosurgery is limited, but continued research and development will provide the neurosurgical community with more accurate technologies to ultimately improve patient outcomes.

AUTHOR CONTRIBUTIONS

All authors listed have made a substantial, direct and intellectual contribution to the work, and approved it for publication.

REFERENCES

1. Xie Y, Thom M, Ebner M, Wykes V, Desjardins A, Miserocchi A, et al. Wide-field spectrally resolved quantitative fluorescence imaging system: toward neurosurgical guidance in glioma resection. *J Biomed Opt.* (2017) 22:1–14. doi: 10.1117/1.JBO.22.11.116006
2. Whitson WJ, Valdes PA, Harris BT, Paulsen KD, Roberts DW. Confocal microscopy for the histological fluorescence pattern of a recurrent atypical meningioma: case report. *Neurosurgery.* (2011) 68:E1768–72; discussion E1772–3. doi: 10.1227/NEU.0b013e318217163c
3. Wei L, Roberts DW, Sanai N, Liu JTC. Visualization technologies for 5-ALA-based fluorescence-guided surgeries. *J Neurooncol.* (2018) 141:495–505. doi: 10.1007/s11060-018-03077-9
4. Valdés PA, Roberts DW, Lu FK, Golby A. Optical technologies for intraoperative neurosurgical guidance. *Neurosurg Focus.* (2016) 40:E8. doi: 10.3171/2015.12.FOCUS15550
5. Utsuki S, Oka H, Sato S, Suzuki S, Shimizu S, Tanaka S, et al. Possibility of using laser spectroscopy for the intraoperative detection of nonfluorescing brain tumors and the boundaries of brain tumor infiltrates. Technical note. *J Neurosurg.* (2006) 104:618–20. doi: 10.3171/jns.2006.104.4.618
6. Stummer W, Tonn JC, Goetz C, Ullrich W, Stepp H, Bink A, et al. 5-Aminolevulinic acid-derived tumor fluorescence: the diagnostic accuracy of visible fluorescence qualities as corroborated by spectrometry and histology and postoperative imaging. *Neurosurgery.* (2014) 74:310–9; discussion 319–20. doi: 10.1227/NEU.0000000000000267
7. Stummer W, Pichlmeier U, Meinel T, Wiestler OD, Zanella F, Reulen HJ, et al. Fluorescence-guided surgery with 5-aminolevulinic acid for resection of malignant glioma: a randomised controlled multicentre phase III trial. *Lancet Oncol.* (2006) 7:392–401. doi: 10.1016/S1470-2045(06)70665-9
8. Roberts DW, Valdés PA, Harris BT, Fontaine KM, Hartov A, Fan X, et al. Coregistered fluorescence-enhanced tumor resection of malignant glioma: relationships between delta-aminolevulinic acid-induced protoporphyrin IX fluorescence, magnetic resonance imaging enhancement, and neuropathological parameters. Clinical article. *J Neurosurg.* (2011) 114:595–603. doi: 10.3171/2010.2.JNS091322
9. Pogue BW, Gibbs-Strauss S, Valdés PA, Samkoe K, Roberts DW, Paulsen KD. Review of neurosurgical fluorescence imaging methodologies. *IEEE J Sel Top Quantum Electron.* (2010) 16:493–505. doi: 10.1109/JSTQE.2009.2034541
10. Montcel B, Mahieu-Williame L, Armoiry X, Meyronet D, Guyotat J. Two-peaked 5-ALA-induced PpIX fluorescence emission spectrum distinguishes glioblastomas from low grade gliomas and infiltrative component of glioblastomas. *Biomed Opt Express.* (2013) 4:548–58. doi: 10.1364/BOE.4.000548
11. Hadjipanayis CG, Widhalm G, Stummer W. What is the surgical benefit of utilizing 5-aminolevulinic acid for fluorescence-guided surgery of malignant gliomas? *Neurosurgery.* (2015) 77:663–73. doi: 10.1227/NEU.0000000000000929
12. DSouza AV, Lin H, Henderson ER, Samkoe KS, Pogue BW. Review of fluorescence guided surgery systems: identification of key performance capabilities beyond indocyanine green imaging. *J Biomed Opt.* (2016) 21:80901. doi: 10.1117/1.JBO.21.8.080901
13. Stummer W, Stepp H, Möller G, Ehrhardt A, Leonhard M, Reulen HJ. Technical principles for protoporphyrin-IX-fluorescence guided microsurgical resection of malignant glioma tissue. *Acta Neurochir.* (1998) 140:995–1000. doi: 10.1007/s007010050206
14. Richards-Kortum R, Sevick-Muraca E. Quantitative optical spectroscopy for tissue diagnosis. *Annu Rev Phys Chem.* (1996) 47:555–606. doi: 10.1146/annurev.physchem.47.1.555
15. Bradley RS, Thorniley MS. A review of attenuation correction techniques for tissue fluorescence. *J R Soc Interface.* (2006) 3:1–13. doi: 10.1098/rsif.2005.0066
16. Belykh E, Miller EJ, Patel AA, Bozkurt B, Yagmurlu K, Robinson TR, et al. Optical characterization of neurosurgical operating microscopes: quantitative fluorescence and assessment of PpIX photobleaching. *Sci Rep.* (2018) 8:12543. doi: 10.1038/s41598-018-30247-6
17. Gioux S, Choi HS, Frangioni JV. Image-guided surgery using invisible near-infrared light: fundamentals of clinical translation. *Mol Imaging.* (2010) 9:237–55. doi: 10.2310/7290.2010.00034
18. Pogue BW, Zhu TC, Ntziachristos V, Paulsen KD, Wilson BC, Pfefer J, et al. Fluorescence-guided surgery and intervention—An AAPM emerging technology blue paper. *Med Phys.* (2018) 45:2681–8. doi: 10.1002/mp.12909
19. Valdés PA, Leblond F, Kim A, Harris BT, Wilson BC, Fan X, et al. Quantitative fluorescence in intracranial tumor: implications for ALA-induced PpIX as an intraoperative biomarker. *J Neurosurg.* (2011) 115:11–7. doi: 10.3171/2011.2.JNS101451
20. Kim A, Khurana M, Moriyama Y, Wilson BC. Quantification of *in vivo* fluorescence decoupled from the effects of tissue optical properties using fiber-optic spectroscopy measurements. *J Biomed Opt.* (2010) 15:067006. doi: 10.1117/1.3523616
21. Gibbs SL. Near infrared fluorescence for image-guided surgery. *Quant Imaging Med Surg.* (2012) 2:177–87. doi: 10.3978/j.issn.2223-4292.2012.09.04
22. Valdés PA, Leblond F, Jacobs VL, Wilson BC, Paulsen KD, Roberts DW. Quantitative, spectrally-resolved intraoperative fluorescence imaging. *Sci Rep.* (2012) 2:798. doi: 10.1038/srep00798
23. Ramanujam N. Fluorescence spectroscopy of neoplastic and non-neoplastic tissues. *Neoplasia.* (2000) 2:89–117. doi: 10.1038/sj.neo.7900077
24. Sokolov K, Follen M, Richards-Kortum R. Optical spectroscopy for detection of neoplasia. *Curr Opin Chem Biol.* (2002) 6:651–8. doi: 10.1016/S1367-5931(02)00381-2
25. Boas DA, Franceschini MA. Haemoglobin oxygen saturation

as a biomarker: the problem and a solution. *Philos Trans A Math Phys Eng Sci.* (2011) 369:4407–24. doi: 10.1098/rsta.2011.0250

26. Müller MG, Georgakoudi I, Zhang Q, Wu J, Feld MS. Intrinsic fluorescence spectroscopy in turbid media: disentangling effects of scattering and absorption. *Appl Opt.* (2001) 40:4633–46. doi: 10.1364/AO.40.004633
27. Marois M, Bravo J, Davis SC, Kanick SC. Characterization and standardization of tissue-simulating protoporphyrin IX optical phantoms. *J Biomed Opt.* (2016) 21:35003. doi: 10.1117/1.JBO.21.3.035003
28. Angelo JP, Chen SJ, Ochoa M, Sunar U, Gioux S, Intes X. Review of structured light in diffuse optical imaging. *J Biomed Opt.* (2018) 24:1–20. doi: 10.1117/1.JBO.24.7.071602
29. Valdés PA, Kim A, Leblond F, Conde OM, Harris BT, Paulsen KD, et al. Combined fluorescence and reflectance spectroscopy for *in vivo* quantification of cancer biomarkers in low- and high-grade glioma surgery. *J Biomed Opt* (2011) 16:116007. doi: 10.1117/1.3646916
30. Valdés PA, Kim A, Brantsch M, Niu C, Moses ZB, Tosteson TD, et al. Delta-aminolevulinic acid-induced protoporphyrin IX concentration correlates with histopathologic markers of malignancy in human gliomas: the need for quantitative fluorescence-guided resection to identify regions of increasing malignancy. *Neuro Oncol.* (2011) 13:846–56. doi: 10.1093/neuonc/nor086
31. Ishihara R, Katayama Y, Watanabe T, Yoshino A, Fukushima T, Sakatani K. Quantitative spectroscopic analysis of 5-aminolevulinic acid-induced protoporphyrin IX fluorescence intensity in diffusely infiltrating astrocytomas. *Neurol Med Chir.* (2007) 47:53–7; discussion 57. doi: 10.2176/nmc.47.53
32. Valdes PA, Millesi M, Widhalm G, Roberts DW. 5-aminolevulinic acid induced protoporphyrin IX (ALA-PpIX) fluorescence guidance in meningioma surgery. *J Neurooncol.* (2019) 141:555–65. doi: 10.1007/s11060-018-03079-7
33. Valdés PA, Leblond F, Kim A, Wilson BC, Paulsen KD, Roberts DW. A spectrally constrained dual-band normalization technique for protoporphyrin IX quantification in fluorescence-guided surgery. *Opt Lett.* (2012) 37:1817–9. doi: 10.1364/OL.37.001817
34. Valdes PA, Jacobs VL, Wilson BC, Leblond F, Roberts DW, Paulsen KD. System and methods for wide-field quantitative fluorescence imaging during neurosurgery. *Opt Lett.* (2013) 38:2786–8. doi: 10.1364/OL.38.002786
35. Valdés PA, Jacobs V, Harris BT, Wilson BC, Leblond F, Paulsen KD, et al. Quantitative fluorescence using 5-aminolevulinic acid-induced protoporphyrin IX biomarker as a surgical adjunct in low-grade glioma surgery. *J Neurosurg.* (2015) 123:771–80. doi: 10.3171/2014.12.JNS14391
36. Valdes PA, Bekelis K, Harris BT, Wilson BC, Leblond F, Kim A, et al. 5-Aminolevulinic acid-induced protoporphyrin IX fluorescence in meningioma: qualitative and quantitative measurements *in vivo*. *Neurosurgery.* (2014) 10(Suppl. 1):74–82; discussion 82–3. doi: 10.1227/NEU.0000000000000117
37. Valdes PA, Angelo JP, Choi HS, Gioux S. qF-SSOP: real-time optical property corrected fluorescence imaging. *Biomed Opt Express.* (2017) 8:3597–605. doi: 10.1364/BOE.8.003597
38. Bravo JJ, Olson JD, Davis SC, Roberts DW, Paulsen KD, Kanick SC. Hyperspectral data processing improves PpIX contrast during fluorescence guided surgery of human brain tumors. *Sci Rep.* (2017) 7:9455. doi: 10.1038/s41598-017-09727-8
39. Lin WC, Mahadevan-Jansen A, Johnson MD, Weil RJ, Toms SA. *In vivo* optical spectroscopy detects radiation damage in brain tissue. *Neurosurgery.* (2005) 57:518–25; discussion 518–25. doi: 10.1227/01.NEU.0000170559.48166.AC
40. Toms SA, Lin WC, Weil RJ, Johnson MD, Jansen ED, Mahadevan-Jansen A. Intraoperative optical spectroscopy identifies infiltrating glioma margins with high sensitivity. *Neurosurgery.* (2007) 61(1 Suppl):327–35; discussion 335–6. doi: 10.1227/01.neu.0000279226.68751.21
41. Toms SA, Lin WC, Weil RJ, Johnson MD, Jansen ED, Mahadevan-Jansen A. Intraoperative optical spectroscopy identifies infiltrating glioma margins with high sensitivity. *Neurosurgery.* (2005) 57(4 Suppl):382–91; discussion 382–91. doi: 10.1227/01.NEU.000176855.39826.2D
42. Toms SA, Konrad PE, Lin WC, Weil RJ. Neuro-oncological applications of optical spectroscopy. *Technol Cancer Res Treat.* (2006) 5:231–8. doi: 10.1177/153303460600500306
43. Lin WC, Toms SA, Johnson M, Jansen ED, Mahadevan-Jansen A. *In vivo* brain tumor demarcation using optical spectroscopy. *Photochem Photobiol.* (2001) 73:396–402. doi: 10.1562/0031-8655(2001)0730396IVBTDU2.0.CO2
44. Lin WC, Sandberg DI, Bhatia S, Johnson M, Oh S, Ragheb J. Diffuse reflectance spectroscopy for *in vivo* pediatric brain tumor detection. *J Biomed Opt.* (2010) 15:061709. doi: 10.1117/1.3505012
45. Utsuki S, Oka H, Miyajima Y, Shimizu S, Suzuki S, Fujii K. Auditory alert system for fluorescence-guided resection of gliomas. *Neurol Med Chir.* (2008) 48:95–7; discussion 97–8. doi: 10.2176/nmc.48.95
46. Eljamel MS, Goodman C, Moseley H. ALA and Photofrin fluorescence-guided resection and repetitive PDT in glioblastoma multiforme: a single centre Phase III randomised controlled trial. *Lasers Med Sci.* (2008) 23:361–7. doi: 10.1007/s10103-007-0494-2
47. Haj-Hosseini N, Richter J, Andersson-Engels S, Wårdell K. Optical touch pointer for fluorescence guided glioblastoma resection using 5-aminolevulinic acid. *Lasers Surg Med.* (2010) 42:9–14. doi: 10.1002/lsm.20868
48. Black D, Hahn HK, Kikinis R, Wårdell K, Haj-Hosseini N. Auditory display for fluorescence-guided open brain tumor surgery. *Int J Comput Assist Radiol Surg.* (2018) 13:25–35. doi: 10.1007/s11548-017-1667-5
49. Diamond KR, Patterson MS, Farrell TJ. Quantification of fluorophore concentration in tissue-simulating media by fluorescence measurements with a single optical fiber. *Appl Opt.* (2003) 42:2436–42. doi: 10.1364/AO.42.002436
50. Wu J, Feld MS, Rava RP. Analytical model for extracting intrinsic fluorescence in turbid media. *Appl Opt.* (1993) 32:3585–95. doi: 10.1364/AO.32.003585
51. Weersink R, Patterson MS, Diamond K, Silver S, Padgett N. Noninvasive measurement of fluorophore concentration in turbid media with a simple fluorescence /reflectance ratio technique. *Appl Opt.* (2001) 40:6389–95. doi: 10.1364/AO.40.006389
52. Huang Z, Shi S, Qiu H, Li D, Zou J, Hu S. Fluorescence-guided resection of brain tumor: review of the significance of intraoperative quantification of protoporphyrin IX fluorescence. *Neurophotonics.* (2017) 4:011011. doi: 10.1117/1.NPh.4.1.011011
53. Yang VX, Muller PJ, Herman P, Wilson BC. A multispectral fluorescence imaging system: design and initial clinical tests in intra-operative Photofrin-photodynamic therapy of brain tumors. *Lasers Surg Med.* (2003) 32:224–32. doi: 10.1002/lsm.10131
54. Saager RB, Cuccia DJ, Saggese S, Kelly KM, Durkin AJ. Quantitative fluorescence imaging of protoporphyrin IX through determination of tissue optical properties in the spatial frequency domain. *J Biomed Opt.* (2011) 16:126013. doi: 10.1117/1.3665440
55. O'Sullivan TD, Cerussi AE, Cuccia DJ, Tromberg BJ. Diffuse optical imaging using spatially and temporally modulated light. *J Biomed Opt.* (2012) 17:071311. doi: 10.1117/1.JBO.17.7.071311
56. Jermyn M, Gosselin Y, Valdes PA, Sibai M, Kolste K, Mercier J, et al. Improved sensitivity to fluorescence for cancer detection in wide-field image-guided neurosurgery. *Biomed Opt Express.* (2015) 6:5063–74. doi: 10.1364/BOE.6.005063
57. Sibai M, Fisher C, Veilleux I, Elliott JT, Leblond F, Roberts DW, et al. Preclinical evaluation of spatial frequency domain-enabled wide-field quantitative imaging for enhanced glioma resection. *J Biomed Opt.* (2017) 22:76007. doi: 10.1117/1.JBO.22.7.076007
58. van de Giessen M, Angelo JP, Gioux S. Real-time, profile-corrected single snapshot imaging of optical properties. *Biomed Opt Express.* (2015) 6:4051–62. doi: 10.1364/BOE.6.004051
59. Vervandier J, Gioux S. Single snapshot imaging of optical properties. *Biomed Opt Express.* (2013) 4:2938–44. doi: 10.1364/BOE.4.002938
60. Hoogstins C, Burggraaf JJ, Koller M, Handgraaf H, Boogerd L, van Dam G, et al. Setting standards for reporting and quantification in fluorescence-guided surgery. *Mol Imaging Biol.* (2019) 21:11–18. doi: 10.1007/s11307-018-1220-0

13

Cross-Polarization Optical Coherence Tomography for Brain Tumor Imaging

Konstantin S. Yashin[1], Elena B. Kiseleva[2], Ekaterina V. Gubarkova[2], Alexander A. Moiseev[3], Sergey S. Kuznetsov[4], Pavel A. Shilyagin[3], Grigory V. Gelikonov[3], Igor A. Medyanik[1], Leonid Ya. Kravets[1], Alexander A. Potapov[5], Elena V. Zagaynova[6] and Natalia D. Gladkova[2]*

[1] Microneurosurgery Group, University Clinic, Privolzhsky Research Medical University, Nizhny Novgorod, Russia, [2] Laboratory of Optical Coherence Tomography, Research Institute of Experimental Oncology and Biomedical Technologies, Privolzhsky Research Medical University, Nizhny Novgorod, Russia, [3] Laboratory of High-Sensitivity Optical Measurements, Institute of Applied Physics, Russian Academy of Sciences, Nizhny Novgorod, Russia, [4] Department of Anatomical Pathology, Privolzhsky Research Medical University, Nizhny Novgorod, Russia, [5] Federal State Autonomous Institution "N.N. Burdenko National Scientific and Practical Center for Neurosurgery" of the Ministry of Healthcare of the Russian Federation, Moscow, Russia, [6] Research Institute of Experimental Oncology and Biomedical Technologies, Privolzhsky Research Medical University, Nizhny Novgorod, Russia

***Correspondence:**
Konstantin S. Yashin
jashinmed@gmail.com

This paper considers valuable visual assessment criteria for distinguishing between tumorous and non-tumorous tissues, intraoperatively, using cross-polarization OCT (CP OCT)—OCT with a functional extension, that enables detection of the polarization properties of the tissues in addition to their conventional light scattering.

Materials and Methods: The study was performed on 176 *ex vivo* human specimens obtained from 30 glioma patients. To measure the degree to which the typical parameters of CP OCT images can be matched to the actual histology, 100 images of tumors and white matter were selected for visual analysis to be undertaken by three "single-blinded" investigators. An evaluation of the inter-rater reliability between the investigators was performed. Application of the identified visual CP OCT criteria for intraoperative use was performed during brain tumor resection in 17 patients.

Results: The CP OCT image parameters that can typically be used for visual assessment were separated: (1) signal intensity; (2) homogeneity of intensity; (3) attenuation rate; (4) uniformity of attenuation. The degree of match between the CP OCT images and the histology of the specimens was significant for the parameters "signal intensity" in both polarizations, and "homogeneity of intensity" as well as the "uniformity of attenuation" in co-polarization. A test based on the identified criteria showed a diagnostic accuracy of 87–88%. Intraoperative *in vivo* CP OCT images of white matter and tumors have similar signals to *ex vivo* ones, whereas the cortex *in vivo* is characterized by indicative vertical striations arising from the "shadows" of the blood vessels; these are not seen in *ex vivo* images or in the case of tumor invasion.

Conclusion: Visual assessment of CP OCT images enables tumorous and non-tumorous tissues to be distinguished. The most powerful aspect of CP OCT images that can be used as a criterion for differentiation between tumorous tissue and white matter is the signal intensity. In distinguishing white matter from tumors the diagnostic accuracy using the identified visual CP OCT criteria was 87–88%. As the CP OCT data is easily associated with intraoperative neurophysiological and neuronavigation findings this can provide valuable complementary information for the neurosurgeon tumor resection.

Keywords: cross-polarization optical coherence tomography (CP OCT), malignant brain tumors, glioblastoma, intraoperative imaging, imaging assessment

INTRODUCTION

Optical coherence tomography (OCT) is a label-free, real-time imaging technique that allows three-dimensional images of biological tissues to be obtained at high resolution (around 2 μm). OCT is similar to ultrasonic imaging, in that both techniques detect reflected waves (light or acoustic). However, OCT uses a near-infrared light source (in the 700–1,300 nm wavelength range). OCT is a promising method for intraoperative guidance during the resection of glial tumors (astrocytomas) (1–3).

Recently, OCT has been proposed for intraoperative use in distinguishing tumorous and non-tumorous tissues using handled probes (4, 5) or microscope-integrated OCT systems (6, 7). OCT can provide differentiation between tumorous and non-tumorous tissues through both quantitative (4, 8) and qualitative (9, 10) assessment of the OCT signals. However, although visual assessment of the OCT data provided by clinically approved systems seems to be less sensitive when compared with the calculation of optical coefficients (which is not approved for clinical use), it is more user-friendly and intelligible. Meanwhile, for the intraoperative application of OCT it is necessary clearly to define the visual assessment criteria required for the OCT images in order to provide precise differentiation between glioma tissue and white matter.

Conventional, intensity-based OCT has demonstrated impressive results in detecting pathological changes in stratified tissues, such as those in the eye. However, the advanced visualization of structureless tissue types (brain, breast) needs novel contrast mechanisms such as can be achieved by using a so-called functional extension of OCT—polarization-sensitive (PS) OCT (11). PS OCT can detect the polarization state changes of the probing light in the tissue and, by means of this, generate tissue-specific contrast (11, 12). Based on the birefringence of the tissue structure, PS OCT provides better visualization of elongated structures and therefore provides advanced imaging of myelinated nerve fibers in nerves and the brain (13, 14), even showing the orientation of white matter tracts (15, 16). Cross-polarization OCT (CP OCT) is a variant of PS OCT that allows imaging of the initial polarization state changes both due to birefringence and cross-scattering in biological tissues (17, 18). In CP OCT two co-registered images are recorded: parallel (conventional OCT image or image in co-polarization) and orthogonal (image in cross-polarization) that detects tissue reflections with polarization state orthogonal to the incident one. Only orthogonally polarized backscattered light which is mutually coherent with the incident is contributing to the cross-polarized OCT image. The origin of such "coherent backscattering" includes random polarization during light propagation in the media, depolarization during the backscattering process, and "regular" polarization changes associated with propagation back and forth in birefringent media (19).

Some studies have demonstrated that tumorous tissue and white matter can be differentiated by visual assessment of such OCT images (8–10). This paper presents criteria based on the results of the CP OCT study of *ex vivo* specimens of human brain samples (20), compared with *in vivo* CP OCT images collected during brain tumor resections.

MATERIALS AND METHODS

This translational research was aimed to discover the CP OCT visual criteria for distinguishing timorous and non-tumorous tissue during surgical removal of a glioma. The study consists of two consecutive stages. During first part the *ex vivo* CP OCT analysis of brain human biopsy specimens matched to the actual histology was performed. Based on this data the visual criteria for distinguishing white matter and timorous tissue was discovered. The task of the second stage of the study was to develop the method of intraoperative using of the CP OCT and to confirm the discovered criteria during glioma removal.

Patients

Ex vivo Study on Human Brain Specimens

The *ex vivo* study was performed on material from human brain specimens that had been obtained during tumor resection from 30 patients with gliomas of differing degrees of malignancy: astrocytoma Grades I-II ($n = 8$), astrocytoma Grade III ($n = 7$), and glioblastoma Grade IV ($n = 15$) (**Figure 1A**). The tumor resections were performed taking into account eloquent brain areas and white matter tracts using a frameless navigation system with uploaded functional MRI data and intraoperative neurophysiological monitoring (also "awake" surgery). The surrounding tumor white matter in the peritumoral area that was routinely subjected to coagulation was accurately marked and removed. Samples were taken from different parts of each tumor.

The removed specimens were immediately placed in Petri dishes and closed to prevent dehydration. Tissues also were kept on ice until transfer to the imaging stage. Before OCT imaging, the tissue surface was cut to create a flat fresh surface of the sample. The CP OCT study of each sample was no longer than 30 min (including tissue preparation). In total, 176 samples of

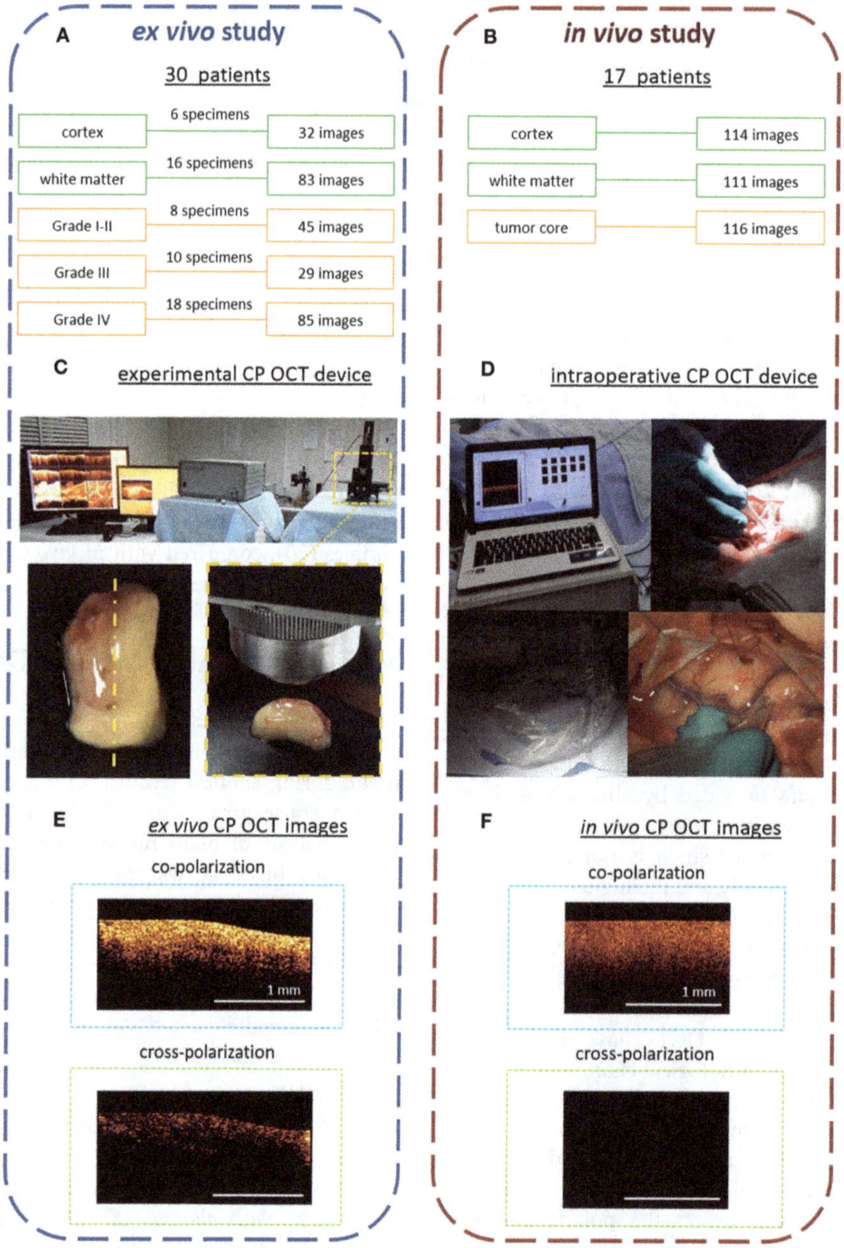

FIGURE 1 | Design of the *ex vivo* and *in vivo* CP OCT study: **(A)** the *ex vivo* study was performed on material from operative biopsies: 30 patients with gliomas of different grades of malignancy; in total 274 *ex vivo* images were analyzed; **(B)** the *in vivo* study was performed on 17 patients with different grades of malignant brain tumors; in total 341 *in vivo* images were analyzed; **(C)** working area for CP OCT scanning with the experimental CP OCT device and on-mount optical probe; specimen with schematic marking of the scanning area along the central line (yellow dotted line); **(D)** CP OCT device approved for clinical use, with a handled OCT probe in a sterile cover; **(F)** *in vivo*, and **(E)** *ex vivo* CP OCT images in co- and cross-polarizations. The signal in cross-polarized image is orthogonally polarized backscattered light, which is mutually coherent with the incident one and can appear if the tissue has anisotropic structures such as myelinated fibers.

different tissue types were studied and 274 *ex vivo* images were obtained. After surgery, any worsening in neurologic state of patients was not recorded.

Intraoperative Study

Here, *in vivo* CP OCT images were collected during tumor resections in 17 patients with different malignant brain tumors: astrocytoma Grades I-II ($n = 5$), astrocytoma Grade III ($n = 9$), glioblastoma Grade IV ($n = 2$), breast cancer metastasis ($n = 1$). During the tumor resections the *in vivo* OCT images were collected using an approved CP OCT device with a handled probe enclosed in a sterile cover. In total, 341 images of three areas of interest were analyzed: cortex—114, white matter—111, tumor core—116 (**Figure 1B**).

This study was carried out in accordance with the recommendations of the World Medical Association's

Declaration of Helsinki. The protocol was approved by the Ethical Committee of the Privolzhskiy Federal Research Medical Center of the Ministry of Health of the Russian Federation. All subjects gave written informed consent in accordance with the Declaration of Helsinki. All studies were performed in accordance with the relevant guidelines and regulations.

Cross-Polarization OCT Devices

The *ex vivo* studies were performed with an multimodal OCT device with cross-polarization detection developed by the Institute of Applied Physics of the Russian Academy of Sciences (Nizhny Novgorod, Russia) (21, 22). The device operates at a central wavelength of 1.3 μm providing axial and lateral resolutions, in air, of 10 and 15 μm, respectively. The probing beam uses circular polarization. The device has a scanning rate of 20,000 A-scans/s and performs 2D lateral scanning within a range of 2.4×2.4 mm^2 to obtain the 3D distribution of backscattered light in polarizations parallel and orthogonal to the polarization of the probing beam. Thus, the resulting CP OCT image includes an upper part—co-polarization image and a lower part—cross-polarization image. Scanning was performed in contactless mode (**Figure 1C**).

For *in vivo* study, time-domain "Polarization-sensitive optical coherence tomograph OCT-1300U" (BioMedTech LLC, Nizhny Novgorod, Russia) was used (**Figure 1D**). It is approved for clinical use (product license №FCP 2012/13479 from 30 May 2012) has the same characteristics of laser radiation as the experimental CP OCT device. However, its image data-processing system is not as effective, so the intensity of the intraoperative images in co- and cross-polarization is lower (~4 times) (**Figure 1F**) compared to those obtained using the experimental CP OCT device (**Figure 1E**).

Histological Study

After imaging the scanning area on the specimen was marked with histological ink, then the specimen was fixed in 10% formalin for 48 h and re-sectioned through the marked area, so that the plane of the histological sections coincided to en-face the CP OCT images. For the histological evaluation, hematoxylin and eosin staining was used. Two histopathologists independently evaluated the histological slides, with their diagnoses coinciding in 98% of cases.

Visual Assessment of CP OCT Images

Based on an initial analysis of the *ex vivo* CP OCT images of the white matter and tumors the parameters of the CP OCT signal for further analysis were selected. The differential criteria for CP OCT images must satisfy the following conditions:

- Simplicity and high speed of evaluation (the signal indicator(s) should be as simple as possible in use, and easy for the operating surgeon to remember);
- Be informative (reflect the histological morphology of the tissue);
- Have a high degree of inter-expert reliability (i.e., not resulting in significant disagreements in interpretation).

Visual assessment of the CP OCT images was performed using two special tests containing a training set and a proper test of 100 images (26 images of white matter and 74 images of tumorous tissue: Grade II−12, Grade III−22, Grade IV−40). The CP OCT images selected for these tests corresponded to specimens with typical histological structures of the tumor and white matter (cropped and damaged images, and images that, according to the histological samples contained large necrotic or hematoma areas were excluded). The first test, aimed at identifying the most useful CP OCT criteria, contained OCT images separately in co- and cross-polarization; the second test, aimed at determining the diagnostic accuracy of distinguishing tumor and white matter, contained OCT images separately in co- and cross-polarization, and simultaneously in both polarizations. Each test was performed by three "blinded" investigators.

In the first test, the visual assessment of the CP OCT image was performed on the basis of the following parameters (**Figure 2**) each with only two possible alternatives, which were selected to satisfy the condition of simplicity and high speed of evaluation (the indicator should be as simple as possible in use, and easy to remember by the operating surgeon):

(1) The signal intensity ("intense"/"non-intense")—the average level of the OCT signal throughout the image.
(2) The homogeneity of intensity ("homogeneous"/"heterogeneous")—the lack of variability of the brightness of the OCT signal.
(3) The attenuation rate ("high"/"low") as estimated by the penetration depth of the probing radiation;
(4) The uniformity of attenuation ("uniform"/"non-uniform")—the uniformity of the OCT signal attenuation along the inferior border of the structural OCT image.

The extent to which the parameters were "informative" was identified based on measuring the degree of association of each visual parameter with the results of the histology during visual assessment by the three "blinded" investigators, between whom the degree of inter-expert reliability was also identified.

The second test was also performed by three "blinded" investigators (neurosurgeons) and was based on the main and additional visual criteria identified during the first test. There were two possible answers: "tumor"/"white matter" (**Figure 3**). The inter-rater reliability between the investigators was also recorded.

Statistical Analysis

The statistical analysis was performed using Statistica 10.0, IBM SPSS Statistics 20. For evaluation of the association ratio of the coefficients Q (Yule) and φ (phi) were used, with a statistically significant value for $Q \geq 0.5$ and for $\varphi > 0.3$. The inter-rater reliability between investigators was registered using the Fleiss' kappa (κ) and Krippendorff's alpha (α) coefficients: $\kappa\ (\alpha) \geq 0.8$—perfect agreement; $0.7 \leq \kappa\ (\alpha) < 0.8$—substantial agreement; $\kappa\ (\alpha) < 0.7$—poor agreement. For the second test the diagnostic test parameters (sensitivity, specificity and accuracy) were calculated.

Intraoperative Application of the CP OCT

There was no histopathological evaluation of the *in vivo* CP OCT images, for error prevention and checking of complementarity between the OCT image and tissue type, the scanning being performed in areas with no doubt about their histology (white

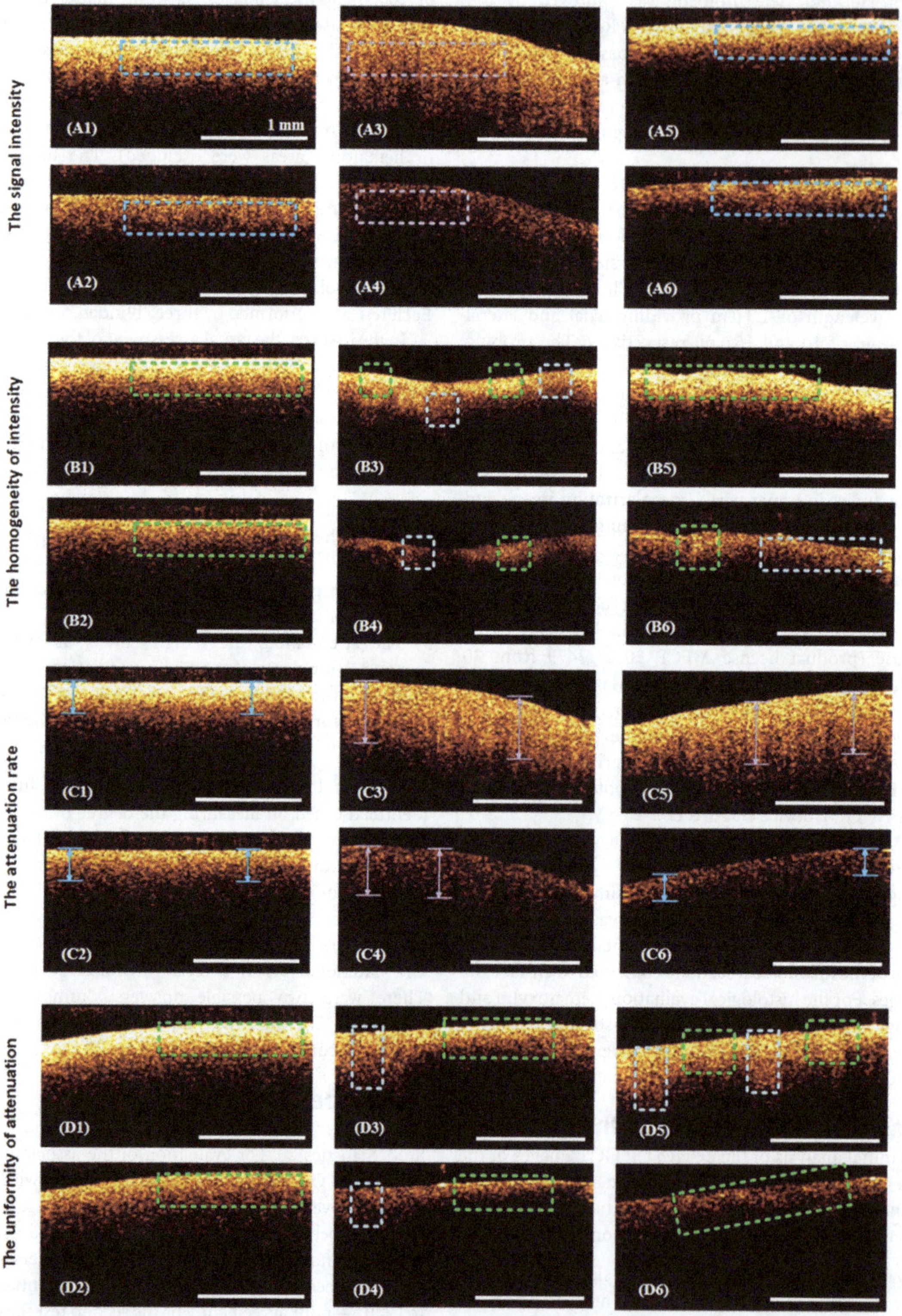

FIGURE 2 | Illustration from the training set of CP OCT images: **(A1–A6)**, **(B1–B6)**, **(C1–C6)**, **(D1–D6)** show examples of the assignment of certain characteristic to the CP OCT signal; **(A1–A6)**—intense signals are marked with blue rectangles, violet—a low-intensity signal; **(B1,B2)**—the regions of homogeneous signals are indicated by green rectangles; **(B3–B6)**—green areas and pale blue squares indicate areas of different intensities; **(C1–C6)**—blue arrows denote regions with high rates of signal attenuation, violet—with low signal attenuation rates; **(D1,D2,D6)**—the green rectangles indicate areas with uniform attenuation of the signal; **(D3–D5)**—rectangles of pale blue and green color indicate regions with different signal attenuation rates.

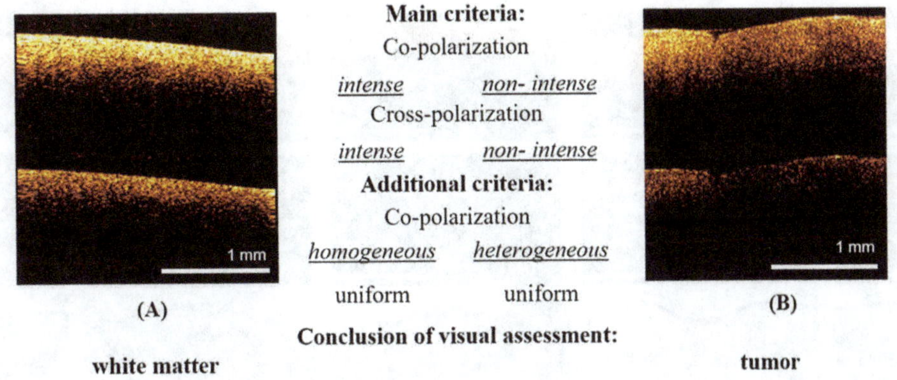

FIGURE 3 | Examples of images from the training set for the second test: **(A)**—white matter, **(B)**—tumor. The responder identifies tissue type using main criteria: white matter is characterized by high intense signal in co- and cross-polarization unlike low intensity signal of tumorous tissue. In the doubtful case, the additional criteria can be used.

matter and cortex far from the tumor mass, and of regions within the tumor core) using image guiding under a neuronavigation system and high magnification of surgical microscope. The *in vivo* CP OCT data were compared with the *ex vivo* set and also combined with surgical microscope view, the preoperative MRI and neuronavigation data, intraoperative neurophysiological and neuronavigation findings.

RESULTS

Ex vivo CP OCT Images of White Matter and Tumorous Tissue

The CP OCT signal of the *ex vivo* specimens is more intense and has a higher attenuation rate (in both the initial and orthogonal polarizations) than those obtained *in vivo*. However, previous comparative analysis of the optical properties of white matter and tumorous tissues has demonstrated that the CP OCT images obtained *ex vivo* show full qualitative similarity to the *in vivo* CP OCT images (23). For the cortex there are also structural differences between the *ex vivo* and *in vivo* images (23). In the *in vivo* studies, the CP OCT images show a specific vertical striation arising from "shadows" of the blood vessels located just under the tissue surface (**Figure 5A1**); this striation is practically invisible on the *ex vivo* images due to vasoconstriction.

White Matter

CP OCY analysis of *ex vivo* specimens showed that the white matter on the CP OCT images in co- and cross-polarizations (**Figures 4A2,B2**) presented by a narrow stripe of high intensity OCT signal. Histologically, the white matter is represented by a regular and dense arrangement of myelinated fibers (**Figure 4C1**) and therefore is characterized by high scattering properties. This explains the presence of a high-intensity homogeneous but rapidly decaying OCT signal in both co- and cross-polarization.

Gliomas

In gliomas the tissue elements are discohesive and disordered (**Figures 4C2–C4**); although there are a few elements with high-scattering properties (**Figure 4C5**). Therefore, the CP OCT images of tumorous tissue are characterized by low signal intensities in co- (**Figures 4A2–A5**) and cross-polarizations (**Figures 4B2–B5**). Grades I-III astrocytomas on the CP OCT images are represented by low intensity and slowly attenuating signals (**Figures 4A2–A4,B2–B4**), however the signal may be homogeneous (**Figures 4A2,A4,B2,B4**) or heterogeneous in the presence of cysts, calcification, and hemorrhaging (**Figures 4A3,B3**). The CP OCT signal of a glioblastoma is of low intensity, and heterogeneous with tessellated areas of high intensity (**Figures 4A5,B5**) corresponding to areas of high cell density, necrosis or hemorrhaging (**Figure 4C5**). The attenuation rate of the CP OCT signal may be high or low with the attenuation along the inferior border of the image being uniform or non-uniform.

The initial comparative analysis of CP OCT images of brain specimens with typical histological structures has demonstrated the capability of OCT to differentiate between white matter and tumorous tissue. However, there are no clear criteria for distinguishing between white matter and tumorous tissue due to the variability of the signal characteristics of the gliomas. Therefore, it is also evident that OCT cannot be used for the intraoperative grading of gliomas.

Visual Assessment Criteria for CP OCT Images for Distinguishing Between White Matter and Gliomal Tissue

Between all investigators the values of the coefficients Q and φ were high for the parameter "signal intensity" in co- and cross-polarization ($Qco = 0.91–0.92$; $\varphi co = 0.64–0.65$; $Qcross = 0.92–0.94$; $\varphi cross = 0.64–0.70$) and also statistically significant for the parameters "the homogeneity of intensity" ($Qco = 0.86–0.94$; $\varphi co = 0.47–0.50$) and "the uniformity of attenuation" ($Qco = 0.58–0.82$; $\varphi co = 0.30–0.44$) in co-polarization. The inter-rater reliability between investigators was perfect for the parameter "signal intensity" in both polarizations ($\kappa = 0.90$; $\alpha = 0.90$) and substantial for "the homogeneity of intensity" ($\kappa = 0.79$; $\alpha = 0.79$) and "the uniformity of attenuation" ($\kappa = 0.75$; $\alpha = 0.75$) in co-polarization (**Table 1**).

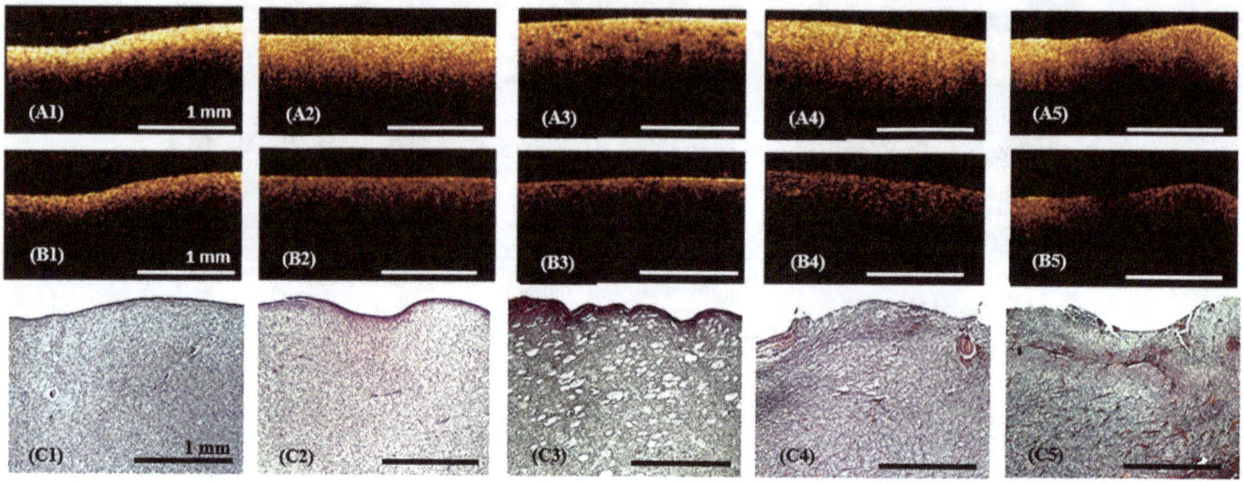

FIGURE 4 | *Ex vivo* CP OCT images **(A1–A5)**, **(B1–B5)** and corresponding histology **(C1–C5)** of white matter **(A1–C1)**, diffuse astrocytoma Grade II **(A2–C2)**, **(A3–C3)**, diffuse astrocytoma Grade III **(A4–C4)** and glioblastoma **(A5–C5)**; on the CP OCT image of diffuse astrocytoma Grade II can be seen microcysts typical for this type of tumor **(A3,C3)**; **(A1–A5)**—CP OCT images in co-polarization and **(B1–B5)**—in cross-polarization. Histological images **(C1–C5)**-hematoxylin and eosin staining.

TABLE 1 | Visual assessment criteria of CP OCT images for distinguishing between white matter and glioma tissue.

CP OCT image parameter	White matter	Tumor
MAIN CRITERIA		
The signal intensity in co-polarization	*Intense*	*Non-intense*
The signal intensity in cross-polarization	*Intense*	*Non-intense*
ADDITIONAL CRITERIA		
The homogeneity of intensity in co-polarization	Homogeneous	Heterogeneous
The uniformity of attenuation in co-polarization	Uniform	Un-uniform

TABLE 2 | The results of diagnostic test by visual assessment of the CP OCT images.

Polarization	Inter-rater reliability rate	Sensitivity, %	Specificity, %	Diagnostic accuracy, %
Co-	0.83/0.83	89–93	67–73	83–84
Cross-	0.86/0.86	80–87	75–89	82–83
Co- and cross-simultaneously	0.92/0.91	82–85	92–94	87–88

Based on the results of the first test the most powerful criteria for the visual assessment of microstructural CP OCT images to enable differentiation between glial tumor tissue and white matter are the CP OCT signal intensities in co- and cross-polarization. Also for this aim, the homogeneity of intensity and the uniformity of attenuation can be used as additional criteria.

Diagnostic Accuracy of CP OCT Based on Visual Assessment of Images

The results of the second set of tests, using the identified main and additional criteria, separately in co- and cross-polarization and simultaneously in co- and cross-polarization (**Table 2**) demonstrate their great inter-rater reliability. The test based on simultaneously assessing CP OCT images in co- and cross-polarization showed a higher diagnostic accuracy (87–88%).

Using co-polarization showed higher sensitivity (89–93%); therefore using this regimen allows minimization of the risk of failure of tumor detection. The high specificity of 92–94% that can be achieved by using simultaneous visual assessment of the images in co- and cross-polarization is associated with the low risk of misguided white matter resection.

Intraoperative Visual Assessment of the CP OCT Images

The intraoperative *in vivo* CP OCT images of white matter and tumors obtained by the certified OCT system with the handled probe show full structural similarity to the *ex vivo* CP OCT images of brain specimens obtained using the laboratory OCT setup, however, owing to differences in image processing between the OCT systems the intensity of the intraoperative images in co- and cross-polarization are lower (~4 times).

The cortex is characterized by specific vertical striations arising as the "shadows" of the blood vessels located just under the tissue surface (**Figures 5A1, 6A1**), and these striations can be considered as a specific cortex-indicator. The white matter tissue is characterized by its high attenuation, although the intensity is lower in cross-polarization than for the signal in co-polarization (**Figures 5B1,B2, 6B1**). Regardless of the glioma grade, the tumorous tissue is characterized by low-intensity, homogeneous or heterogeneous signals with low attenuation rate in co-polarization (**Figures 5C1, 6A2,A3**, images in co-polarization). Since the OCT device approved for clinical use only provides imaging at low intensity the signal in cross-polarization is therefore almost absent from the tumor (**Figures 5C2, 6A2,A3,**

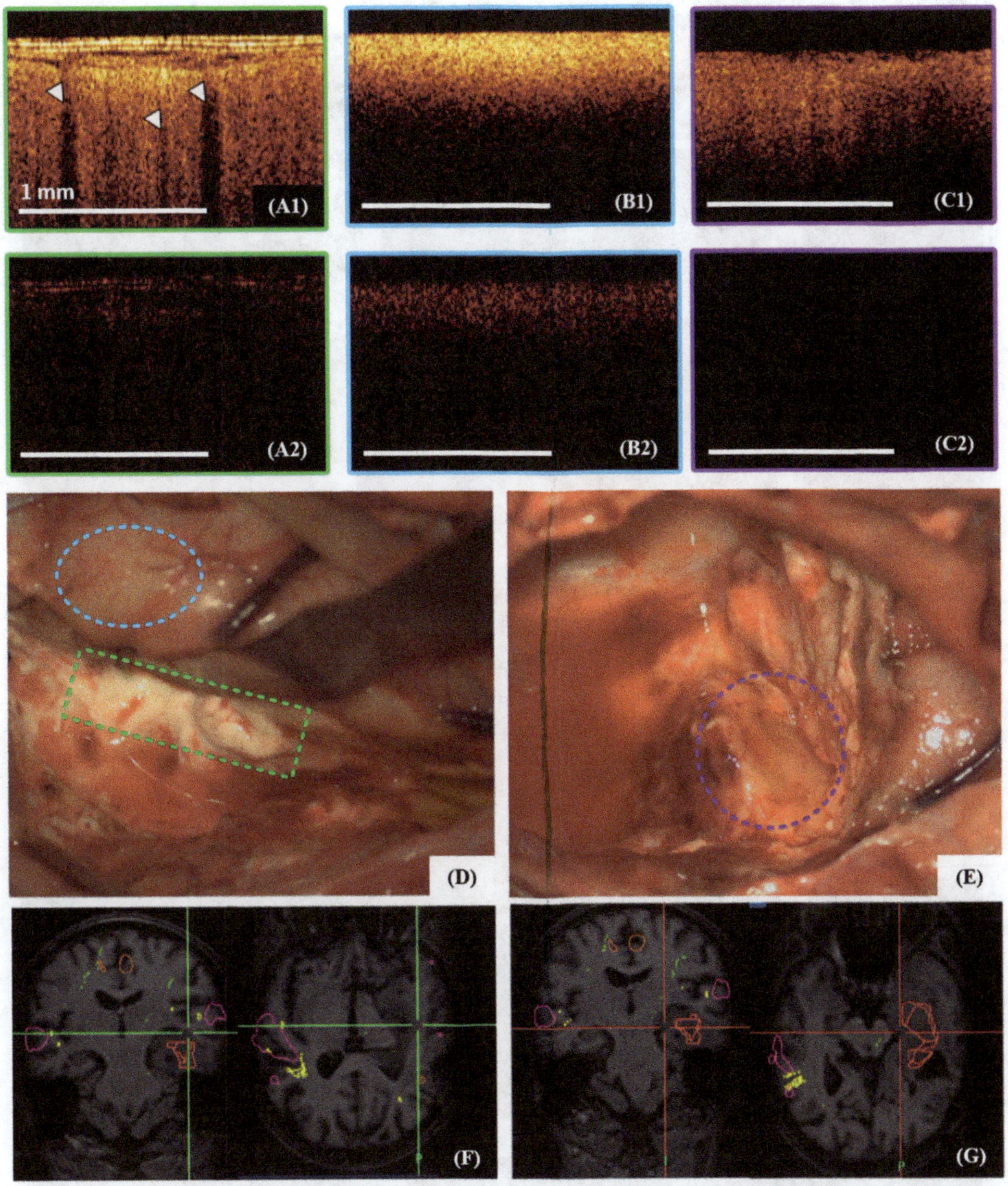

FIGURE 5 | Intraoperative CP OCT images of cortex **(A1,A2)**, white matter **(B1,B2)** and diffuse astrocytoma Grade II **(C1,C2)**; the scanning areas of the corresponding tissue types in the surgical field are marked with green **(A1,A2)**, blue **(B1,B2)** and violet **(C1,C2)** dotted lines **(D,E)**, and interrelated with the neuronavigation data **(F,G)**; **(A1–C1)**—CP OCT images in co-polarization and **(A2–C2)**—in cross-polarization. The white arrows show characteristic vertical striations arising from "shadows" of the blood vessels located just under the tissue surface.

images in cross-polarization) and very low from the cortex (**Figures 5A2**, **6A1**, images in cross-polarization). The scanning areas of the corresponding tissue types in the surgical field are marked with green (cortex, **Figures 5A1,A2**), blue (white matter, **Figures 5B1,B2**) and violet (diffuse astrocytoma Grade II, **Figures 5C1,C2**) dotted lines (**Figures 5D,E**) and interrelated with the neuronavigation data (**Figures 5F,G**).

OCT scanning of the cortex was performed in 9 cases (53%). In all the comparisons, the OCT and neuronavigation data showed that the tumor had widened through the tumor margin that can be detected under the white light of the operating microscope. In the case of visible cortical invasion by the tumor the OCT scanning was performed from this area to visually healthy brain tissue. In the case of visually intact cortex, the scanning was started from the central part of the tumor as detected by the neuronavigation system.

Taking into account the variability of the CP OCT images for a variety of different reasons (e.g., brain swelling), when distinguishing white matter and tumor it is better to commence the OCT scanning of white matter from a control area (where

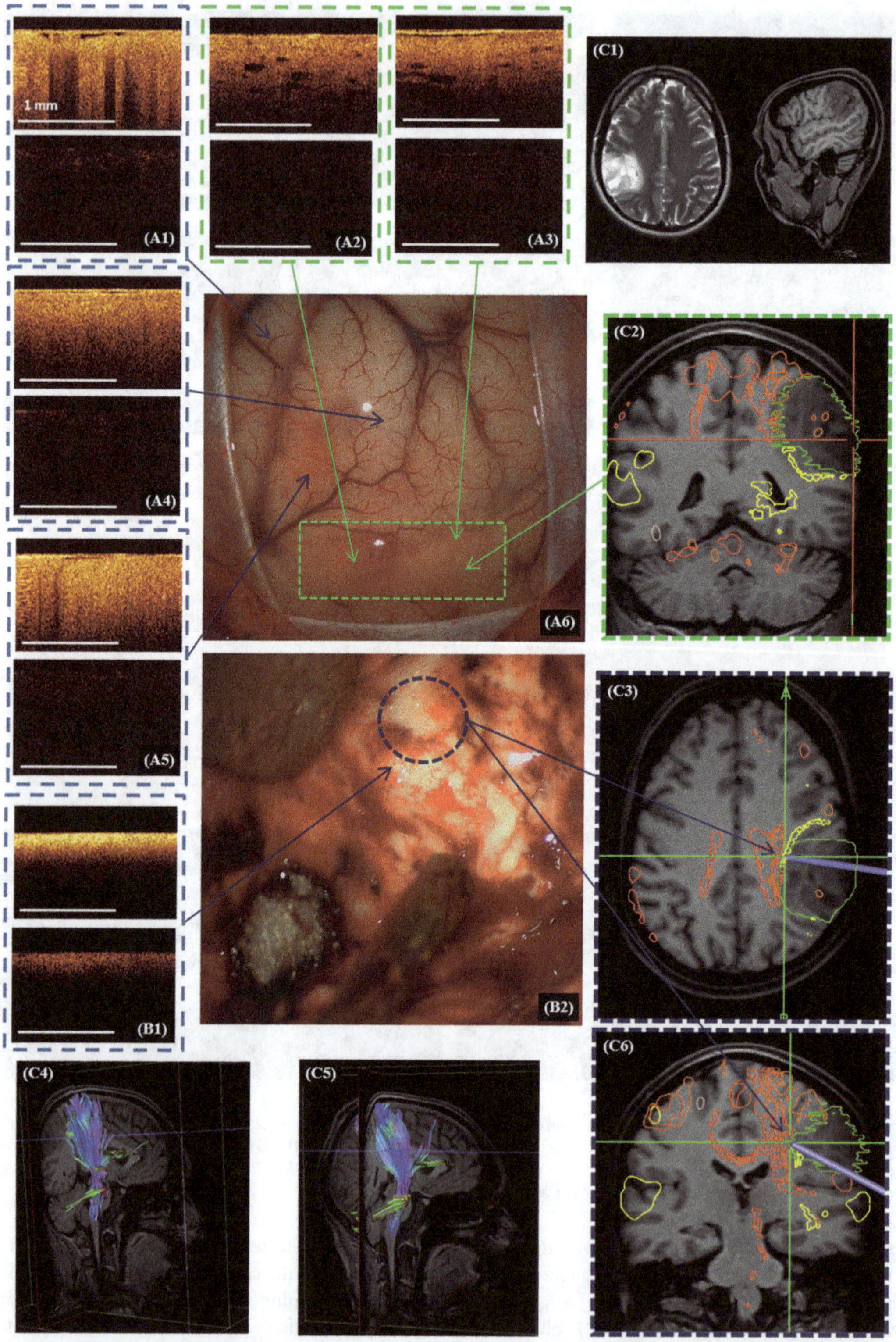

FIGURE 6 | Intraoperative CP OCT images in a patient with diffuse astrocytoma (Grade II): of the cortex **(A1)** with well-defined **(A2,A3; A6**—green dotted line) and invisible **(A4,A5)** tumor invasion, white matter **(B1)** close to the right corticospinal tract (**B2**—blue color dotted line; **C3,C4**—marked by red color); the scanning areas of corresponding tissue types in the surgical field **(A6,B2)** are marked with green **(A6)** and, blue **(B2)** dotted lines and interrelated with the neuronavigation data, where the tumor is marked with a green line and the corticospinal tract with a red line **(C2,C3,C6)**. Preoperative MRI in T1 and T2 **(C1)** and the corticospinal tract reconstruction based on the DTI before **(C4)** and after **(C5)** operation. **(A1–A5,B1)**—CP OCT images in co-polarization (upper image) and cross-polarization (lower image).

there is no doubt about the histology) to enable comparison of this scan with following images. In our study scanning of control area before tumor resection was performed only in 9 patients (53%), while in the other cases the identified criteria (**Table 1**) and standard CP OCT images of white matter (**Figures 4A1,B1, 5B1,B2**) were used.

Perfect detection of white matter by OCT can be useful when tumor resection is performed close to white matter tracts. **Figure 6** shows the process of removal of a diffuse astrocytoma (Grade II) in the right parietal lobe. The preoperative diffusion tensor imaging (DTI) data uploaded in the neuronavigation system demonstrated that the tumor was closely adjacent to right cortico-spinal tract (**Figures 6C2–C4**). Electrical stimulation in this region had shown a response at a current of 5 mA (pulse frequency of 60 Hz, with a single phase duration of 1 ms in trains lasting 4 s), that meant the approximate distance to the tract was about 5 mm. Based on the identified criteria, OCT scanning demonstrated the presence of white matter in this region. It was taken decision to stop further resection. On post-operative DTI, no change in the corticospinal tract was detected. Therefore, the simultaneous use of subcortical electrostimulation and OCT was able to define more exactly the required extent of resection close to eloquent white matter tracts.

DISCUSSION

During surgery of infiltrative brain tumors the benefits of novel intraoperative imaging technologies are self-evident, due to the lack of resolving capacity of the operating microscope for distinguishing tumorous and non-tumorous tissues and the detection of any residual tumor (24–27). In order to overcome this problem, at present, the most commonly used technologies are fluorescent visualization with 5-ALA (28–30) and intraoperative MRI (31, 32). However, these methods have some limitations; therefore, the development of novel intraoperative technologies has become particularly relevant. OCT appears to provide a very promising method for routine neurosurgical practice due to the clear benefits of this method such as: safety (using a near infrared light source does not risk tissue damage); accuracy (high resolution ∼10 micron) the absence of a requirement for contrast agents; imaging depths of more than 1 mm; the ability to obtain images at a distance and therefore the opportunity for integration into a surgical microscope or endoscope (2, 3).

Obviously, the increased interest in OCT has been the result of the continuing improvements in several aspects of OCT, such as imaging speed, sensitivity, the development of functional OCT extensions and signal data processing. The quantitative assessment of OCT with the determination of various optical coefficients such as backscattering (33) and attenuation (4, 10, 34) coefficients provides higher diagnostic accuracy compared with the qualitative assessment of OCT images. Kut et al. have demonstrated the high diagnostic accuracy of OCT for distinguishing tumors from white matter on the basis of the optical attenuation coefficient: for patients with higher-grade tumors the sensitivity/specificity reached 92%/100%; for low-grade tumors sensitivity/specificity values were 100%/80% (4). Unfortunately, at present, clinically approved OCT systems can provide only visual assessment, although that has been sufficient to improve readability for neurosurgeons. Additionally, such visual assessment for distinguishing white matter from tumor tissue also provides high sensitivity of (82–85%), specificity (92–94%), and diagnostic accuracy (87–88%). Therefore, it can be proposed for routine clinical use, although with some restrictions.

This paper deliberately references previously published data (20) with regard to intraoperative approval of the visual CP OCT criteria identified for distinguishing white matter from tumor tissue. These criteria have been specified in place of the previously suggested "loss of normal attenuation" from the tumorous tissue (9, 10). However, this criterion remains relevant for the detection of tumor invasion into the cortex, which is characterized by a "typical view" of vertical striations, disappearing in cases where there are any changes of cortical microarchitecture. The result of this study questions the significance of the "homogeneous" criterion for distinguishing tumor and white matter because of the variability of the characteristics of the OCT signal from gliomas. For example, tumorous tissue may have a quite homogeneous OCT signal, while, on the other hand, white matter in the vicinity of necrotic areas or hematomas can lose its homogeneity.

The study has shown that CP OCT, as an extension of OCT, broadens the functionality of the method. The assessment of CP OCT images simultaneously in co- and cross-polarization has shown a higher specificity (92–94% against 67–73%) and diagnostic accuracy (87–88% against 83–84%) compared with conventional OCT. Therefore, this mode is effective to use during tumor resection closely adjacent to eloquent white matter tracts. Using CP OCT, based on visual assessment along with co-polarization, shows high sensitivity (89–93% against 82–85% when using co- and cross-polarization simultaneously) and therefore it is effective in improving identification of the necessary extent of resection in non-eloquent brain areas.

In this study, discrete histological tissue types such as cortex, white matter and tumor have been described. The formation of the OCT signal and its differences between tumor and white matter can be explained using a simple model of the structural organization of the tissue: tumorous tissue can be represented as an assembly of tumor cells that are characterized by low attenuation, compared to the high attenuation of myelin. However, differentiation using visual assessment can be difficult when comparing white matter with structureless (or intact) myelin and tumorous tissue with necrosis (or necrosis alone), due to their similarity in optical properties. Tumorous tissue without necrosis forms the typical structure of all Grade I-III astrocytomas and the peripherial area of glioblastomas (Grade IV). Necrotic areas characterized by high attenuation (forward cross-scattering) always present in (1) the glioblastoma core, (2) tissues after radiotherapy (e.g., in the case of recurrent astrocytoma after combination treatment) and (3) tissues following bipolar coagulation (total necrosis). The high attenuation (forward cross-scattering) of white matter is the result of the high-density packaging of its myelin fibers. Some events such as structural damage of the myelin, or cerebral edema related to tumor growth, can lead to a significant decrease of attenuation and of forward cross-scattering (35). These myelin changes are typical of the peritumoral area of high-grade astrocytomas. Probably, improvements in the quantitative assessment of OCT data will allow these tissue types to be clearly distinguished.

At the moment, in all doubtful cases, consideration must be given to the patient‘s preoperative data, localization of the OCT scanning area, and the distance from eloquent brain areas. For example, if the preoperative clinical data is indicative of a low-grade glioma, during tumor resection no necrotic areas or myelin damage would be expected, so the surgeon would not expect to find necrotic areas or dramatic changes in the myelin structure, meaning that distinguishing between white matter and tumor is not an issue In the case of a glioblastoma, the white matter in the peritumoral area might be characterized by low attenuation and forward cross-scattering, so the intensity of the CP OCT signal could decrease in co- and cross-polarization. On the other hand in the case where there has been previous radiation therapy (e.g., recurrent glioblastoma) the tumor mass could include a vast amount of necrotic tissue and be characterized by high intensity in the CP OCT images. Therefore, in both cases the differentiation between white matter and tumorous tissue can be difficult. Consequently, in these doubtful cases, decisions about the extent of resection should primarily be based on the distance from eloquent brain areas. Hemorrhages can also compromise the interpretability of the OCT signals (10), therefore, before scanning, they should be removed together with any necrotic areas associated with bipolar coagulation.

In contrast to white matter, the cortex does not contain densely packed myelin fibers that might lead to difficulties in distinguishing between cortex and tumor, although tumor is characterized by higher cellularity and nuclear density comparing to cortex. Visual assessment of OCT signals based on the criterion "loss of normal attenuation" allows tumors to be distinguished from the cortex during *in vivo* scanning (10, 23). Probably, additional *in vivo* studies would enable clearer determination of the optical differences between cortex and tumor and offer better definitions for the quantitative OCT criteria (23).

This study was based on *ex vivo* brain specimens for a number of reasons: (1) the possibility of carrying out maximally targeted histological examinations to appropriately validate the OCT; (2) the absence of strict time limitations, which made it possible to perform multiple scans to monitor the image quality. The previously performed comparative analysis of the optical properties of white matter and tumorous tissues of the brain allow us to conclude that the CP OCT images obtained *ex vivo* show a full qualitative similarity to the *in vivo* CP OCT images (23). However, *ex vivo* study is not representative for the cortex by reason of the disappearance of the unique characteristics of the CP OCT signal in *ex vivo* CP OCT images.

The study has several limitations. One of them is the use of different CP OCT devices in the preclinical part and during the intraoperative scanning. Although the experimental device has some advantages due to a better signal characteristics and a more detailed computer processing of the OCT data, using it during surgical procedures was not possible due to its novel character and the absence of permission for its clinical use. Therefore, the study demonstrates the advantages of CP OCT on fresh pathological specimens, but not for intraoperative CP OCT data. In the *ex vivo* CP OCT study based on fresh specimens it is easier to "target" the region of interest and therefore provide advanced histological validation of CP OCT image in comparison with *in vivo* CP OCT study, where image interpretation can be complicated by the impact of several factors such as tissue deformation during its removal, difficulties in access to the region of interest where the white matter is infiltrated by tumor, active bleeding and use of hemostatic materials affecting the quality of the CP OCT images. However, the promising results of this study allow us to recommend implementing a clinical CP OCT prototype based on the experimental one used in this study.

Further, only three raters were tested, therefore the results may be considered as preliminary. Increasing the number of raters may improve the results in terms of visual assessment, diagnostic accuracy, sensitivity and specificity for CP OCT for distinguishing white matter from tumor tissue.

The limitation of the intraoperative phase of the study was lack of morphological verification of scanning areas. Using image guiding under neuronavigation system and high magnification of surgical microscope doesn‘t provide exact information about tissue morphology.

Nevertheless, while OCT does not provide molecular information and cannot detect individual tumor cells, it looks promising in assisting navigation during neurosurgical procedures such as glioma resection, stereotactic biopsy and the placement of electrodes for deep brain stimulation. For clinical translation, OCT can be integrated into standard operating equipment such as surgical microscopes (6, 7), and probes for stereotactic procedures (36). For the purposes of glioma surgery, the cross-polarization mode provides a good illustration of a functional extension to OCT, which can offer opportunities to improve the visual assessment of OCT data.

CONCLUSION

CP OCT based on the visual assessment of obtained images is a promising imaging tool for distinguishing tumorous and non-tumorous tissues during glioma resection. The most powerful criteria are the signal intensities in co- and cross-polarization. Further to this purpose, additional criteria such as the homogeneity of intensity and the uniformity of attenuation can also be used. The simultaneous assessment of CP OCT images in co- and cross-polarization has demonstrated better diagnostic accuracy for distinguishing white matter from tumor tissue than OCT alone. Differentiation between cortex and white matter can be performed based on the criterion "loss of normal attenuation" (loss of the "typical view" of vertical striations on CP OCT images). In distinguishing white matter and tumors the diagnostic accuracy using the visual CP OCT criteria was 87–88%. The CP OCT data is easily associated with intraoperative neurophysiological and neuronavigation findings and can provide supplementary information for neurosurgeons during tumor resection.

AUTHOR CONTRIBUTIONS

KY, EK, AM, and NG: study concept and design. KY, EG, PS, IM, and LK: data acquisition and quality control of data. KY, AM, SK, GG, and EK: data analysis and interpretation. KY, EK, AM, and NG: manuscript preparation. AP, EZ, and NG: manuscript review.

ACKNOWLEDGMENTS

We thank Dr. Nikolay N. Karyakin (rector of PRMU, Nizhny Novgorod, Russia) for active supporting translation of CP OCT into clinical usage.

REFERENCES

1. Jenkinson MD, Barone DG, Bryant A, Vale L, Bulbeck H, Lawrie TA, et al. Intraoperative imaging technology to maximise extent of resection for glioma. *Cochrane Database Syst Rev.* (2018) 22:Cd012788. doi: 10.1002/14651858.CD012788.pub2
2. Yashin KS, Kravets LY, Gladkova ND, Gelikonov GV, Medyanik IA, Karabut MM, et al. [Optical coherence tomography in neurosurgery]. *Zhu Vopr Neirokhir Im N N Burdenko.* (2017) 81:107–15. doi: 10.17116/neiro2017813107-115
3. Valdes PA, Roberts DW, Lu FK, Golby A. Optical technologies for intraoperative neurosurgical guidance. *Neurosurg Focus.* (2016) 40:E8. doi: 10.3171/2015.12.FOCUS15550
4. Kut C, Chaichana KL, Xi J, Raza SM, Ye X, McVeigh ER, et al. Detection of human brain cancer infiltration *ex vivo* and *in vivo* using quantitative optical coherence tomography. *Sci Transl Med.* (2015) 7:292ra100. doi: 10.1126/scitranslmed.3010611
5. Sun C, Lee KKC, Vuong B, Cusimano M, Brukson A, Mariampillai A, et al., editors. Neurosurgical hand-held optical coherence tomography (OCT) forward-viewing probe. In: *Proceedings Volume 8207, Photonic Therapeutics and Diagnostics VIII.* San Francisco: *SPIE BiOS* (2012).
6. Lankenau E, Klinger D, Winter C, Malik A, Müller H, Oelckers S, et al. Combining optical coherence tomography (OCT) with an operating microscope. In: Buzug T, Holz D, Bongartz J, Kohl-Bareis M, Hartmann U, Weber S, editors. *Advances in Medical Engineering. Springer Proceedings in Physics.* Vol. 114. Berlin; Heidelberg: Springer (2007). p. 343–8. doi: 10.1007/978-3-540-68764-1_57
7. Lankenau EM, Krug M, Oelckers S, Schrage N, Just T, Hüttmann G. iOCT with surgical microscopes: a new imaging during microsurgery. *Adv Opti Technol.* (2013) 2:233–39. doi: 10.1515/aot-2013-0011
8. Kiseleva EB, Yashin KS, Moiseev AA, Snopova LB, Gelikonov GV, Medyanik IA, et al. Quantitative cross-polarization optical coherence tomography detection of infiltrative tumor margin in a rat glioma model: a pilot study. *Sovremennye Tehnol Med.* (2018) 10:6–14. doi: 10.17691/stm2018.10.1.01
9. Bohringer HJ, Boller D, Leppert J, Knopp U, Lankenau E, Reusche E, et al. Time-domain and spectral-domain optical coherence tomography in the analysis of brain tumor tissue. *Lasers Surg Med.* (2006) 38:588–97. doi: 10.1002/lsm.20353
10. Bohringer HJ, Lankenau E, Stellmacher F, Reusche E, Huttmann G, Giese A. Imaging of human brain tumor tissue by near-infrared laser coherence tomography. *Acta Neurochim.* (2009) 151:507–17; discussion 17. doi: 10.1007/s00701-009-0248-y
11. Baumann B. Polarization sensitive optical coherence tomography: a review of technology and applications. *Appl Sci.* (2017) 7:474. doi: 10.3390/app70 50474
12. de Boer JF, Hitzenberger CK, Yasuno Y. Polarization sensitive optical coherence tomography – a review [Invited]. *Biomed Opt Express.* (2017) 8:1838–73. doi: 10.1364/BOE.8.001838
13. Wang H, Akkin T, Magnain C, Wang R, Dubb J, Kostis WJ, et al. Polarization sensitive optical coherence microscopy for brain imaging. *Opt Lett.* (2016) 41:2213–6. doi: 10.1364/OL.41.002213
14. Boas DA, Wang H, Magnain C, Fischl B. Polarization-sensitive optical coherence tomography of the human brain connectome. *SPIE Newsroom.* (2017). doi: 10.1117/2.1201701.006834
15. Wang H, Zhu J, Akkin T. Serial optical coherence scanner for large-scale brain imaging at microscopic resolution. *NeuroImage.* (2014) 84:1007–17. doi: 10.1016/j.neuroimage.2013.09.063
16. Wang H, Zhu J, Reuter M, Vinke LN, Yendiki A, Boas DA, et al. Cross-validation of serial optical coherence scanning and diffusion tensor imaging: a study on neural fiber maps in human medulla oblongata. *NeuroImage.* (2014) 100:395–404. doi: 10.1016/j.neuroimage.2014.06.032
17. Gubarkova EV, Dudenkova VV, Feldchtein FI, Timofeeva LB, Kiseleva EB, Kuznetsov SS, et al. Multi-modal optical imaging characterization of atherosclerotic plaques. *J Biophoton.* (2016) 9:1009–20. doi: 10.1002/jbio.201500223
18. Gladkova N, Kiseleva E, Robakidze N, Balalaeva I, Karabut M, Gubarkova E, et al. Evaluation of oral mucosa collagen condition with cross-polarization optical coherence tomography. *J Biophoton.* (2013) 6:321–9. doi: 10.1002/jbio.201200059
19. Schmitt JM, Xiang SH. Cross-polarized backscatter in optical coherence tomography of biological tissue. *Optics Lett.* (1998) 23:1060–62. doi: 10.1364/OL.23.001060
20. Yashin K, Kiseleva EB, Gubarkova EV, Moiseev AA, Kuznetsov SS, Medyanik IA, et al. Visual assessment criteria of microstructural *ex vivo* co-and cross-polarized optical coherence tomography images in gliomas. In: *Proceedings of SPIE*, Vol 10685. Bellingham, WA (2018). p. 106853F.
21. Gelikonov VM, Gelikonov GV, Shilyagin PA. Linear-wavenumber spectrometer for high-speed spectral-domain optical coherence tomography. *Optics Spectroscopy.* (2009) 106:459–65. doi: 10.1134/S0030400X09030242
22. Moiseev AA, Gelikonov GV, Terpelov DA, Shilyagin PA, Gelikonov VM. Noniterative method of reconstruction optical coherence tomography images with improved lateral resolution in semitransparent media. *Laser Phys Lett.* (2013) 10:125601. doi: 10.1088/1612-2011/10/12/125601
23. Kiseleva EB, Yashin KS, Moiseev AA, Sirotkina MA, Timofeeva LB, Fedoseeva VV, et al. Cross-polarization optical coherence tomography in comparative *in vivo* and *ex vivo* studies of the optical properties of normal and tumorous brain tissues. *Sovremennye Tehnol Med.* (2017) 9:177. doi: 10.17691/stm2017.9.4.22
24. Berger MS. Malignant astrocytomas: surgical aspects. *Sem Oncol.* (1994) 21:172–85.
25. Ducray F, Dutertre G, Ricard D, Gontier E, Idbaih A, Massard C. [Advances in adults' gliomas biology, imaging and treatment]. *Bull du Cancer.* (2010) 97:17–36. doi: 10.1684/bdc.2009.1019
26. Robins HI, Lassman AB, Khuntia D. Therapeutic advances in malignant glioma: current status and future prospects. *Neuroimaging Clin North Am.* (2009) 19:647–56. doi: 10.1016/j.nic.2009.08.015
27. Sanai N, Berger MS. Glioma extent of resection and its impact on patient outcome. *Neurosurgery.* (2008) 62:753–64; discussion 264–6. doi: 10.1227/01.neu.0000318159.21731.cf
28. Hadjipanayis CG, Widhalm G, Stummer W. What is the surgical benefit of utilizing 5-aminolevulinic acid for fluorescence-guided surgery of malignant gliomas? *Neurosurgery.* (2015) 77:663–73. doi: 10.1227/NEU.0000000000000929
29. Potapov AA, Gavrilov AG, Goriainov SA, Gol'bin DA, Zelenkov PV, Kobiakov GL, et al. [Intraoperative fluorescent visualization and laser spectroscopy in intrinsic brain tumor surgery]. *Zh Vopr Neirokhi Im N N Burdenko.* (2012) 76:3–11; discussion 12.
30. Potapov AA, Goryaynov SA, Okhlopkov VA, Pitskhelauri DI, Kobyakov GL, Zhukov VY, et al. [Clinical guidelines for the use of intraoperative fluorescence diagnosis in brain tumor surgery]. *Zh Vopr Neirokhi Im N N Burdenko.* (2015) 79:91–101 doi: 10.17116/neiro201579591-101
31. Fahlbusch R, Samii A. Intraoperative MRI. *Neurosurgical Focus.* (2016) 40:E3. doi: 10.3171/2015.12.FOCUS15631

32. Eljamel MS, Mahboob SO. The effectiveness and cost-effectiveness of intraoperative imaging in high-grade glioma resection; a comparative review of intraoperative ALA, fluorescein, ultrasound and MRI. *Photodiagno Photodyn Ther.* (2016) 16:35–43. doi: 10.1016/j.pdpdt.2016.07.012
33. Boppart SA, Brezinski ME, Pitris C, Fujimoto JG. Optical coherence tomography for neurosurgical imaging of human intracortical melanoma. *Neurosurgery.* (1998) 43:834–41. doi: 10.1097/00006123-199810000-00068
34. Yuan W, Kut C, Liang W, Li X. Robust and fast characterization of OCT-based optical attenuation using a novel frequency-domain algorithm for brain cancer detection. *Sci Rep.* (2017) 7:44909. doi: 10.1038/srep44909
35. Rodriguez CL, Szu JI, Eberle MM, Wang Y, Hsu MS, Binder DK, et al. Decreased light attenuation in cerebral cortex during cerebral edema detected using optical coherence tomography. *Neurophotonics.* (2014) 1:025004. doi: 10.1117/1.NPh.1.2.025004
36. Liang CP, Wierwille J, Moreira T, Schwartzbauer G, Jafri MS, Tang CM, et al. A forward-imaging needle-type OCT probe for image guided stereotactic procedures. *Optics Express.* (2011) 19:26283–94. doi: 10.1364/OE.19.026283

14

Enhancing Safety in Reconstructive Microsurgery Using Intraoperative Indocyanine Green Angiography

Ingo Ludolph*, Raymund E. Horch, Andreas Arkudas and Marweh Schmitz

Department of Plastic and Hand Surgery and Laboratory for Tissue Engineering and Regenerative Medicine, University Hospital of Erlangen, Friedrich-Alexander-University of Erlangen-Nuernberg FAU, Erlangen, Germany

****Correspondence:***
Ingo Ludolph
ingo.ludolph@uk-erlangen.de

Intraoperative assessing and postoperative monitoring of the viability of free flaps is of high relevance in reconstructive microsurgery. Today different methods for the evaluation of tissue perfusion are known. Indocyanine Green angiography is an emerging technique among plastic surgeons with a broad scope of applications especially in microsurgical free flap transfer. We demonstrate the value and clinical application of this technique based on representative selected cases where Indocyanine Green angiography was used in microsurgical free flap transfers from different anatomic donor sites during the operation. Hereby perforator selection, flap tailoring, changes of blood flow and patency of anastomoses was judged and decision making was based on the angiographic findings. This method has proven to be valid, reproducible and easy to use. The application is not limited to the evaluation of skin perfusion, but is also applicable to muscle tissue or chimeric or composite flaps. Reliable judgement is especially given for the extent of arterially perfused tissue following complete flap dissection. Moreover, this real-time angiography revealed a high sensitivity for the detection of poorly perfused flap areas, thus supporting the conventional clinical judgement and reducing complications. In summary Indocyanine Green angiography has the potential to reduce flap related complications and to contribute to enhancing and extending the possibilities of free flap surgery.

Keywords: ICG, Indocyanine Green angiography, microsurgery, free flap, imaging

INTRODUCTION

In plastic reconstructive surgery, the number of free tissue transfers has increased significantly in recent decades. Given the appropriate indication recent advancements in operative techniques and imaging modalities have facilitated microvascular reconstructions to become safer, more reliable procedures almost independent from the patient's age (1–4).

Preoperative assessment of the microvasculature anatomy at the tissue harvesting site with advanced imaging modalities has assisted surgeons in the appropriate selection of the donor site, perforator, and flap and has led to an overall improvement in the flap outcomes (1, 5). Furthermore, the question of the intraoperative decision making especially in critically large free flaps, the individual intraoperative perforator constellation and the patency of anastomoses is as relevant as the question of the postoperative flap monitoring. Since the early days of microsurgical reconstructive procedures postoperative flap monitoring in particular is of high relevance for a successful outcome. Hence many clinical and experimental studies deal with this issue. Therefore, modern imaging devices ideally should address the entire scope of a reconstructive procedure, from the planning to the postoperative perfusion monitoring. Today several different techniques are available, all of them with the aim of decreasing flap associated complications.

Laser assisted Indocyanine Green angiography (ICG angiography) in its advanced technical version provides real-time angiography, which enables decision making on tissue perfusion in free and pedicled flaps to be made with high reliability both intraoperatively and postoperatively. ICG was introduced into clinical routine in the 1950's. It was initially used in hepatology as a function test, in cardiologic diagnostics and later by ophthalmologists as it shows less leakage from blood vessels as compared to fluorescein (6, 7). In ophthalmology it is valuable because it remains for a long time in more blood-perfused tissues such as the choroid and the blood vessels.

In this study we give insight into the spectrum of the application of ICG angiography in plastic reconstructive surgery based on representative and selected clinical cases and demonstrate the advantages and disadvantages of this procedure in the context of the current literature.

MATERIALS AND METHODS

Among the variety of more than 150 free flaps and pedicled flaps performed in our institution per year four representative clinical cases with different indications for a reconstructive procedure at varying anatomical locations were selected to highlight the status of ICG angiography.

Written informed consent was obtained from all patients in accordance with the Declaration of Helsinki and ICG measurements were performed within a study protocol which was approved by the institutional Review Board (registration number 85_13 B).

As a method for skin perfusion analysis we used ICG-angiography (SPY Elite System, Novadaq Technologies Inc., Toronto, Canada) which has been utilized by our group in more than 300 cases since 2014. Exclusion criteria were solely based on contraindications for the application of Indocyanine Green, e.g., iodine allergy, autonomous adenoma of thyroid gland, hyperthyroidism or due to refusal by the patient. In all free flaps, independent of the anatomic region or the tissue included, it was routinely performed in a standard mode using a 12.5 mg bolus of ICG dye through a venous line.

After intravenous injection of ICG dye, it binds to plasma proteins. The short plasma half-life period of ICG of 3 to 4 min allows repeated injections. It is not metabolized and is excreted by the liver into bile. At the area of interest the ICG is excited by a near-infrared laser. The laser device has no potential for causing damage to the tissue or the observer. The fluorescent substance displays an absorption maximum at 805 nm and an emission maximum at 835 nm. Light at a wavelength of 800 nm in the near-infrared range is minimally absorbed by water or hemoglobin and is not scattered by tissues, which allows visualization of blood vessels (7). The dye highlights vessels up to a minimum of 3 to 5 mm in the tissue. The perfusion pattern, the intensity of the fluorescence as an indicator for dye uptake and the clearance within the tissue is displayed on a video monitor. Well-perfused areas appear bright due to dye uptake, whereas mal-perfused areas are relatively dark. In a standard mode the device displays the video in a gray scale. An additional analysis tool provides color modes and calculation of ingress and egress rates in absolute or relative values. Furthermore, contour levels can be defined for determination of perfusion areas in relation to an automatically or individually set references point in the field of interest. The analysis tool allows the user to work on the videos and pictures at a later time.

RESULTS

Case 1

A 71 year old male patient suffered from an extensive tissue defect at the dorsum of the left hand as a result of a bicycle incident. After multiple debridement and wound conditioning using negative pressure wound therapy the defect had to be reconstructed by a large free anterior lateral thigh flap from the left thigh. During flap harvesting two distant main perforators were detected, located very lateral within the flap. Following complete flap dissection the first ICG measurement was performed with the flap left in place at the thigh. Thus, the special perforator constellation and the borders of the adjacent perforasomes could be determined. **Figure 1** clearly displays the perforasome border nourished by the proximal perforator in the flap which was not to judge sufficiently by clinical signs. After a few seconds the distal perforasome was also perfused shown by an uptake of the ICG dye. Due to this analysis both perforators were then included in the flap.

The flap was anastomosed to the left radial artery in an end-to-side fashion as well as to concomitant recipient veins. Hereupon another ICG measurement revealed a well-perfused flap without changes of blood flow pattern compared to the point after flap harvesting. The perforasome constellation was confirmed and the flap exactly trimmed to the defect size dependent on the ICG perfusion pattern (**Figure 1**).

Case 2

A 49 year old female patient presented a progressive lymphedema at the right leg refractory to conservative measures. In the medical history 4 years ago a laparoscopic hysterectomy and adnexectomy as well as a radical pelvic lymphadenectomy on the right side were performed because of a uterine cervical carcinoma. Despite conservative treatment the lymphedema exacerbated resulting in functional impairment and loss of quality of life. After inconspicuous follow up care and lymphoscintigraphy scan a microsurgically transplanted omentum majus flap containing lymph nodes and lymph vessles was planned. Using a laparoscopic approach the omentum majus flap was raised including the right gastroepiploic artery and vein. The flap was then anastomosed to the right femoral artery and vein. **Figure 2** shows the ICG measurement after anastomosis. The well-perfused vessel arcades via the right gastroepiploic artery could be defined, whereas ICG angiography revealed the mal-perfused parts of the omentum majus which

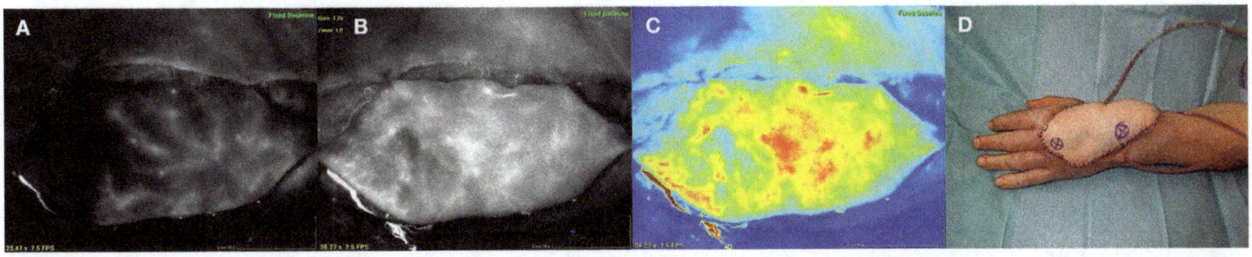

FIGURE 1 | Free anterior lateral thigh flap (ALT) for reconstruction of the dorsum of the left hand. **(A)** (left) ALT flap after harvesting at the left thigh. ICG angiography marking the perforasome perfused by the proximal perforator revealing a distinct perfusion border. **(B)** (middle left) Flap perfused via a proximal and distal perforator showing perfusion of adjacent perforasomes. **(C)** (middle right) ICG angiography color mode. **(D)** (right) ALT flap after inset at the left hand. Asterix within the flap marking the distal (right) and proximal (left) perforator.

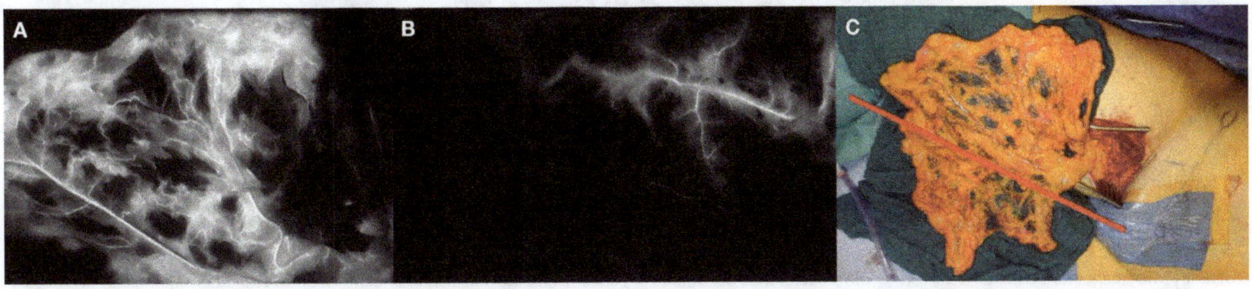

FIGURE 2 | Free omentum majus flap at the right inguinal region. **(A)** (left) ICG angiography of the omentum majus after anastomosis to the femoral vessels showing exact perfusion of the vessel arcades and the adjacent tissue. **(B)** (middle) Mal-perfused part of the omentum majus flap. **(C)** (right) Flap at the inguinal region after anastomosis. Red bar indicates the border between well-perfused (top) and mal-perfused (bottom) parts of the omentum majus defined by ICG angiography.

could not be determined by clinical signs. Especially in free flaps where no skin is included and peripheral bleeding on the wound edges is not common as well as residual perfusion is not sufficient for tissue survival, conventional clinical judgement by means of capillary refill or color change is not a reliable option. Discarding of too much or too less tissue is the possible consequence in these cases. Finally after discarding mal-perfused tissue parts the omentum majus was placed and spread out in the subcutaneous tissue to enable lymph vessels to grow in and establish a new lymph collector for the right lower extremity.

Case 3

In a 55 year old female patient invasive breast cancer was diagnosed in her right breast. Neoadjuvant chemotherapy was recommended followed by modified radical mastectomy and radiotherapy. After an uneventful follow up period without tumor relapse during 1 year after mastectomy the patient presented for autologous breast reconstruction with abdominal tissue. A preoperative computed tomography angiography showed a strong lateral perforator from the inferior epigastric artery. Finally a so called DIEP flap (deep inferior epigastric artery perforator flap) was harvested based on the aforementioned lateral perforator on the left side of the abdomen. Because it was hypothesized that lateral located perforators do not constantly perfuse the flap tissue across the midline and often a possibly large flap volume is necessary especially in thin patients, ICG measurement is used to define the perfusion pattern.

In this case ICG angiography showed a well perfused flap area across the midline and flap shaping was performed due to the ICG dye uptake to gain the maximum flap tissue. After anastomosis of the flap to the internal mammary artery and vein in an end-to-end fashion the repeated ICG measurement presented patent anastomoses and a well perfused DIEP flap also in the peripheral zones with no relevant change of the blood flow pattern (**Figure 3**).

Case 4

An 83 year old female patient presented with a skin necrosis at the right knee and an infection of her knee joint prosthesis after multiple operations necessitating replacement of the joint prosthesis due to relapsing implant infections in the past. Because a total knee arthrodesis was not possible due to relevant shortening of the lower extremity and a high risk of osteomyelitis, wound conditioning using negative pressure wound therapy and defect reconstruction was planned to salvage the knee prosthesis and to prevent limb amputation as an ultima ratio procedure. In an interdisciplinary approach with the department of orthopedic surgery the mobile parts of the prosthesis were changed and the defect was closed with a free myocutaneous latissimus dorsi flap. The whole latissimus dorsi muscle was harvested with a large cutaneous flap island as this was necessary due to the defect size. Also in this case ICG measurement was done after harvesting and after anastomosis to the superficial femoral artery and vein.

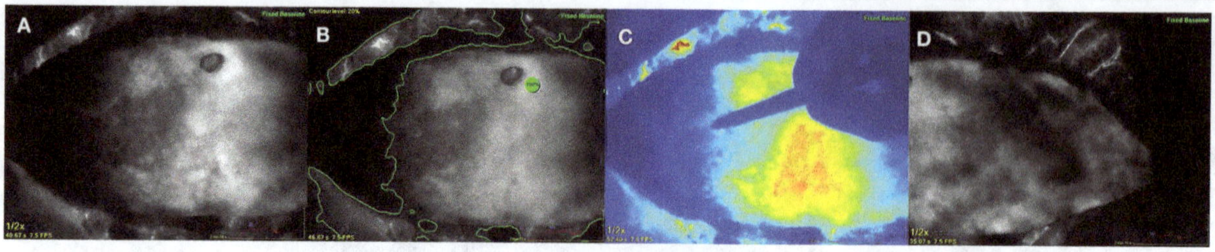

FIGURE 3 | Deep inferior epigastric perforator flap after complete harvesting at the abdomen based on a single lateral located perforator. **(A)** (left) ICG angiography showing the perfusion pattern on the contralateral side of the perforator across the midline. **(B)** (middle left) Analysis by using a contour level of 20% in relation to a reference point of maximum fluorescence within the flap. **(C)** (middle right) Color mode showing the surgeons hand marking the flap borders due to the ICG perfusion pattern. **(D)** (right) ICG angiography of the ipsilateral part of the flap indicating excellent perfusion.

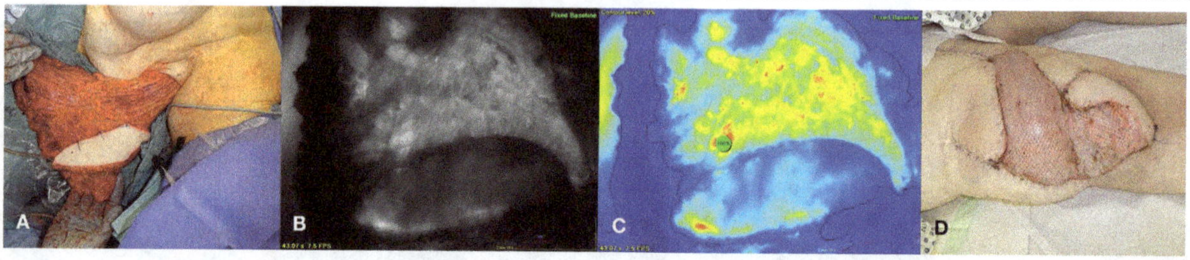

FIGURE 4 | Myocutaneous latissimus dorsi flap for coverage of a defect at the right knee. **(A)** Latissimus flap after complete harvesting at the left axilla. **(B)** (middle left) ICG angiography revealing mal-perfused flap areas at the periphery. **(C)** (middle right) Color mode and contour level at 20% in relation to a reference point of maximum fluorescence within the flap. **(D)** (right) Flap after inset and anastomosis at the right knee.

Based on the perfusion analysis the very peripheral parts of the muscle had to be discarded, whereas the cutaneous island showed normal dispersion of the dye indicating normal perfused tissue (**Figure 4**).

DISCUSSION

Due to technical advancements and the increased knowledge in the field of plastic reconstructive surgery within the last 2–3 decades, the possibilities of microsurgically free tissue transfers have increased massively. As a result, free tissue transfers on the one hand and pedicled flaps on the other hand are now so called standard procedures in a high volume center almost independent of the patient's age (2, 3). In particular, plastic reconstructive surgeons have dealt with the question of flap monitoring since the beginning of microsurgery. In the early 1980s plastic surgeons were already aware of the importance of flap monitoring, which then relied on clinical observation (8). It is generally accepted that nowadays the intraoperative analysis of flap perfusion becomes more and more important in addition to the preoperative perfusion assessment, e.g., the so-called perforator mapping (1, 9–12). Besides the perfusion assessment after flap harvesting and anastomosis, the intraoperative use of imaging techniques is of particular interest in complex constellations of the donor vessels, especially when large flaps are required that challenge the classical perforasomes. It has added a highly valuable tool for intraoperative flap shaping and designing the flaps according to their optimal perfusion zones. Only few imaging methods are actually evaluated and established in clinical routine (9–11, 13, 14). The most common methods today are the laser assisted Indocyanine Green angiography, thermography, combined laser Doppler spectrophotometry, the laser speckle contrast imaging, hyperspectral imaging or near infrared spectroscopy, respectively (15–22). Most techniques are predominantly used in the context of experimental or clinical studies and have their own advantages and disadvantages in the context of the abovementioned fields of application. The ideal monitoring instrument should primarily meet the following requirements: non-invasive and contactless, spatial resolution about the flap, accurate, and easy to use even for inexperienced personnel and providing timely information (17).

ICG angiography has been used for more than 50 years in the clinical assessment of cardiovascular function, hepatic clearance, and retinal angiography. Up to now, it is well-standardized and the laser technologies as well as the analysis options have evolved significantly. The ICG dye itself has proofed to be safe and it features for assessing tissue perfusion have enabled to develop other applications in various surgical procedures, especially in plastic surgery (10).

Denneny et al. performed an experimental study in 1983 (8) using neurovascular island flaps in rats which were transected and re-anastomosed after flap harvesting. Hereafter Fluorescein dye was injected and uptake and elimination of the dye was visualized by a fiberoptic perfusion fluorometer. They stated that this method provides reliable data about flap perfusion and predicts viability. In recent years more studies concerning tissue perfusion analysis were published (23–25). Especially in the field of immediate alloplastic breast reconstruction the perfusion of the mastectomy skin flap was evaluated using ICG angiography, because judgement of inadequate microcirculatory perfusion can be difficult and may result in skin flap or fat necrosis and reoperation. Nevertheless, for the application in free flap surgery there is still a lack of literature.

As presented in our study the advantages of this method, however, are obvious. ICG angiography offers a real-time determination of tissue vascularity and perfusion, showing a high sensitivity especially in the arterial phase of dye distribution (13). The selected representative cases prove the reproducible practicability for intraoperative perforasome definition in perforator flaps and individualized flap tailoring as well as for the judgement of muscle flaps or even the omentum majus flap.

In autologous breast reconstruction after mastectomy due to breast cancer, microsurgically transplanted tissue from the abdomen, the so-called DIEP- or muscle sparing TRAM flap, represents the gold standard today. Particularly in obese patients or in DIEP flaps where the perforator distribution and the vascular pattern within the fat layer is not predictable, clinical flap tailoring according to the zonal classification by Hartrampf or Holm might be misleading (26, 27). As shown in case 3, individual flap planning is possible by ICG angiography with a high sensitivity for mal-perfused tissue parts. Therefore, partial flap necrosis or fat necrosis can be reduced.

As we could observe in our patients, the initial phase of dye uptake within the flap tissue can be defined as safely perfused tissue. The method is independent of the investigator, reproducible as well as contactless and with a high spatial and temporal resolution. It is an external device and therefore the use is not limited to the operating room. Due to the short half-life, multiple measurements are possible at short intervals. Additionally it can be applied for postoperative flap monitoring in critical cases or if flap perfusion is not distinct by using other methods.

The application possibilities in plastic reconstructive surgery are manifold. Thus, ICG angiography can be applied not only to assess skin or muscle flaps, but also to chimeric flaps, e.g., osteomyocutaneous as well as free vascularized bone grafts such as the free medial femoral condyle bone graft or even after finger replantation (28, 29). If the technique can also contribute to judge flap autonomisation and further clarify the long term vascular changes in transplanted flaps in the long term run seems evident, but is not completely clear yet (30, 31). Further studies are required to address this topic.

However, some inherent limitations regarding ICG angiography need to be discussed also. It represents an invasive procedure in which the intravenous application of a dye is required. Throughout the years of experience with ICG the incidence of adverse effects of the dye has been infrequent and they have generally been of low severity (32, 33). Relative contraindications such as iodide allergy or severe renal failure have to be considered. In addition, the venous phase after dye uptake in the tissue is not comparable in its precision to the very sensitive arterial uptake phase. Thus, the judgement of a venous congestion is more difficult and requires more general experiences with the technique. In addition increasing background fluorescence develops in the tissue when measurements are taken repeatedly in short intervals. The latter can lead to an indistinct perfusion assessment. By using ICG angiography intraoperatively different factors could potentially influence skin perfusion. These included variables such as the use of epinephrine containing tumescent solution, administration of vasopressors, blood pressure, oxygen saturation, fraction of inspired oxygen, temperature and hematocrit as well as individual anatomical differences (34).

Despite the broad application, still no absolute or relative perfusion levels correlating with fluorescence intensity of the dye—which would allow defining parts of the tissue as well-perfused or mal-perfused, respectively—have been standardized. In our experience, a "relative perfusion level" between 20 and 30% in relation to the most fluorescent area within the relevant tissue turned out to be safely perfused tissue. Concerning the postoperative monitoring the non-continuous nature of capturing data and the large size of the device we used the application for a routine bedside monitoring postoperatively is limited (35). Nevertheless, frequent measurements are possible in principle also on the ward or in an outpatient setting.

CONCLUSION

ICG angiography enables a standardized and reproducible real-time angiography of different tissues and provides a high sensitivity in detecting well-perfused and non-perfused tissue in the field of plastic reconstructive surgery. It has the potential to reduce flap related complications and to optimize and extend the possibilities of free flap surgery. Further studies in different applications fields are required to standardize application and enhance the possibilities of this method in plastic surgery.

ETHICS STATEMENT

Written informed consent was obtained from all patients in accordance with the Declaration of Helsinki and ICG measurements were performed within a study protocol which was approved by the institutional Review Board (registration number 85_13 B).

AUTHOR CONTRIBUTIONS

IL: study conception. IL, RH, AA, and MS: acquisition of data. IL, RH, and MS: analysis and interpretation. IL and RH: drafting of manuscript. IL, RH, AA, and MS: critical revision.

REFERENCES

1. Chae MP, Hunter-Smith DJ, Rozen WM. Comparative analysis of fluorescent angiography, computed tomographic angiography and magnetic resonance angiography for planning autologous breast reconstruction. *Gland Surg.* (2015) 4:164–78. doi: 10.3978/j.issn.2227-684X.2015.03.06
2. Ludolph I, Lehnhardt M, Arkudas A, Kneser U, Pierer G, Harder Y, et al. [Plastic reconstructive microsurgery in the elderly patient - consensus

statement of the German Speaking Working Group for Microsurgery of the Peripheral Nerves and Vessels]. *Handchir Mikrochir Plast Chir.* (2018) 50:118–25. doi: 10.1055/s-0043-115730

3. Fried FW, Beier JP, Bohr C, Iro H, Horch RE, Arkudas A. Free latissimus dorsi myocutaneous flap in a 6-month-old child for reconstruction of a temporal fossa defect after teratoma resection. *Ann Plast Surg.* (2019) 82:62–3. doi: 10.1097/SAP.0000000000001629
4. Steiner D, Horch RE, Eyupoglu I, Buchfelder M, Arkudas A, Schmitz M, et al. Reconstruction of composite defects of the scalp and neurocranium-a treatment algorithm from local flaps to combined AV loop free flap reconstruction. *World J Surg Oncol.* (2018) 16:217. doi: 10.1186/s12957-018-1517-0
5. Mathes DW, Neligan PC. Current techniques in preoperative imaging for abdomen-based perforator flap microsurgical breast reconstruction. *J Reconstruct Microsurg.* (2010) 26:3–10. doi: 10.1055/s-0029-1244806
6. Lohman RF, Ozturk CN, Ozturk C, Jayaprakash V, Djohan R. An analysis of current techniques used for intraoperative flap evaluation. *Ann Plast Surg.* (2015) 75:679–85. doi: 10.1097/SAP.0000000000000235
7. Liu DZ, Mathes DW, Zenn MR, Neligan PC. The application of indocyanine green fluorescence angiography in plastic surgery. *J Reconstruct Microsurg.* (2011) 27:355–64. doi: 10.1055/s-0031-1281515
8. Denneny JC III, Weisman RA, Silverman DG. Monitoring free flap perfusion by serial fluorometry. *Otolaryngol Head Neck Surg.* (1983) 91:372–6. doi: 10.1177/019459988309100405
9. Bellamy JL, Mundinger GS, Flores JM, Wimmers EG, Yalanis GC, Rodriguez ED, et al. Do adjunctive flap-monitoring technologies impact clinical decision making? an analysis of microsurgeon preferences and behavior by body region. *Plast Reconstruct Surg.* (2015) 135:883–92. doi: 10.1097/PRS.0000000000001064
10. Burnier P, Niddam J, Bosc R, Hersant B, Meningaud JP. Indocyanine green applications in plastic surgery: a review of the literature. *J Plast Reconstruct Aesthet Surg.* (2017) 70:814–27. doi: 10.1016/j.bjps.2017.01.020
11. Smit JM, Negenborn VL, Jansen SM, Jaspers MEH, de Vries R, Heymans MW, et al. Intraoperative evaluation of perfusion in free flap surgery: a systematic review and meta-analysis. *Microsurgery.* (2018) 38:804–18. doi: 10.1002/micr.30320
12. Saint-Cyr M, Wong C, Schaverien M, Mojallal A, Rohrich RJ. The perforasome theory: vascular anatomy and clinical implications. *Plast Reconstruct Surg.* (2009 124:1529–44. doi: 10.1097/PRS.0b013e3181b98a6c
13. Ludolph I, Arkudas A, Schmitz M, Boos AM, Taeger CD, Rother U, et al. Cracking the perfusion code?: Laser-assisted Indocyanine Green angiography and combined laser Doppler spectrophotometry for intraoperative evaluation of tissue perfusion in autologous breast reconstruction with DIEP or ms-TRAM flaps. *J Plast Reconstruct Aesthet Surg.* (2016) 69:1382–8. doi: 10.1016/j.bjps.2016.07.014
14. Hauck T, Horch RE, Schmitz M, Arkudas A. Secondary breast reconstruction after mastectomy using the DIEP flap. *Surg Oncol.* (2018) 27:513. doi: 10.1016/j.suronc.2018.06.006
15. Beier JP, Horch RE, Arkudas A, Dragu A, Schmitz M, Kneser U. Decision-making in DIEP and ms-TRAM flaps: the potential role for a combined laser Doppler spectrophotometry system. *J Plast Reconstruct Aesthet Surg.* (2013) 66:73–9. doi: 10.1016/j.bjps.2012.08.040
16. Rothenberger J, Amr A, Schaller HE, Rahmanian-Schwarz A. Evaluation of a non-invasive monitoring method for free flap breast reconstruction using laser doppler flowmetrie and tissue spectrophotometry. *Microsurgery.* (2013) 33:350–7. doi: 10.1002/micr.22096
17. Holmer A, Marotz J, Wahl P, Dau M, Kammerer PW. Hyperspectral imaging in perfusion and wound diagnostics - methods and algorithms for the determination of tissue parameters. *Biomed Tech Biomed Eng.* (2018) 63:547–56. doi: 10.1515/bmt-2017-0155
18. Holm C, Mayr M, Hofter E, Dornseifer U, Ninkovic M. Assessment of the patency of microvascular anastomoses using microscope-integrated near-infrared angiography: a preliminary study. *Microsurgery.* (2009) 29:509–14. doi: 10.1002/micr.20645
19. Hardwicke JT, Osmani O, Skillman JM. Detection of perforators using smartphone thermal imaging. *Plast Reconstruct Surg.* (2016) 137:39–41. doi: 10.1097/PRS.0000000000001849
20. Draijer M, Hondebrink E, van Leeuwen T, Steenbergen W. Review of laser speckle contrast techniques for visualizing tissue perfusion. *Lasers Med Sci.* (2009) 24:639–51. doi: 10.1007/s10103-008-0626-3
21. Briers D, Duncan DD, Hirst E, Kirkpatrick SJ, Larsson M, Steenbergen W, et al. Laser speckle contrast imaging: theoretical and practical limitations. *J Biomed Opt.* (2013) 18:066018. doi: 10.1117/1.JBO.18.6.066018
22. Rother U, Gerken ALH, Karampinis I, Klumpp M, Regus S, Meyer A, et al. Dosing of indocyanine green for intraoperative laser fluorescence angiography in kidney transplantation. *Microcirculation.* (2017) 24:1–7. doi: 10.1111/micc.12392
23. Casey WJ III, Connolly KA, Nanda A, Rebecca AM, Perdikis G, Smith AA. Indocyanine green laser angiography improves deep inferior epigastric perforator flap outcomes following abdominal suction lipectomy. *Plast Reconstruct Surg.* (2015) 135:491e-7e. doi: 10.1097/PRS.0000000000000964
24. Swanson E. Comparison of limited and full dissection abdominoplasty using laser fluorescence imaging to evaluate perfusion of the abdominal skin. *Plast Reconstruct Surg.* (2015) 136:31e-43e. doi: 10.1097/PRS.0000000000001376
25. Preidl RH, Schlittenbauer T, Weber M, Neukam FW, Wehrhan F. Assessment of free microvascular flap perfusion by intraoperative fluorescence angiography in craniomaxillofacial surgery. *J Cranio-Max-Facial Surg.* (2015) 43:643–8. doi: 10.1016/j.jcms.2015.03.013
26. Holm C, Mayr M, Hofter E, Ninkovic M. Perfusion zones of the DIEP flap revisited: a clinical study. *Plast Reconstruct Surg.* (2006) 117:37–43. doi: 10.1097/01.prs.0000185867.84172.c0
27. Hartrampf CR, Scheflan M, Black PW. Breast reconstruction with a transverse abdominal island flap. *Plast Reconstruct Surg.* (1982) 69:216–25. doi: 10.1097/00006534-198202000-00007
28. Gould DJ, Mehrara BJ, Neligan P, Cheng MH, Patel KM. Lymph node transplantation for the treatment of lymphedema. *J Surg Oncol.* (2018) 118:736–42. doi: 10.1002/jso.25180
29. Valente SA, Al-Hilli Z, Radford DM, Yanda C, Tu C, Grobmyer SR. Near infrared fluorescent lymph node mapping with indocyanine green in breast cancer patients: a prospective trial. *J Am Coll Surg.* (2018) 228:672-678. doi: 10.1016/j.jamcollsurg.2018.12.001
30. Granzow J, Li AI, Caton A, Boyd JB. Free flap survival following failure of the vascular pedicle. *Ann Plast Surg.* (2015) 75:44–8. doi: 10.1097/SAP.0000000000000136
31. Yoon AP, Jones NF. Critical time for neovascularization/angiogenesis to allow free flap survival after delayed postoperative anastomotic compromise without surgical intervention: a review of the literature. *Microsurgery.* (2016) 36:604–12. doi: 10.1002/micr.30082
32. Newman MI, Samson MC. The application of laser-assisted indocyanine green fluorescent dye angiography in microsurgical breast reconstruction. *J Reconstruct Microsurg.* (2009) 25:21–6. doi: 10.1055/s-0028-1090617
33. Hope-Ross M, Yannuzzi LA, Gragoudas ES, Guyer DR, Slakter JS, Sorenson JA, et al. Adverse reactions due to indocyanine green. *Ophthalmology.* (1994) 101:529–33. doi: 10.1016/S0161-6420(94)31303-0
34. Munabi NC, Olorunnipa OB, Goltsman D, Rohde CH, Ascherman JA. The ability of intra-operative perfusion mapping with laser-assisted indocyanine green angiography to predict mastectomy flap necrosis in breast reconstruction: a prospective trial. *J Plast Reconstruct Aesthet Surg.* (2014) 67:449–55. doi: 10.1016/j.bjps.2013.12.040
35. Karinja SJ, Lee BT. Advances in flap monitoring and impact of enhanced recovery protocols. *J Surg Onco.* (2018) 118:758–67. doi: 10.1002/jso.25179

15

Development of a Simulation Model for Fluorescence-Guided Brain Tumor Surgery

Daniel Valli [1†], Evgenii Belykh [1†], Xiaochun Zhao [1], Sirin Gandhi [1], Claudio Cavallo [1], Nikolay L. Martirosyan [2], Peter Nakaji [1], Michael T. Lawton [1] and Mark C. Preul [1]*

Department of Neurosurgery, Barrow Neurological Institute, St. Joseph's Hospital and Medical Center, Phoenix, AZ, United States, [2] Department of Neurosurgery, University of Arizona, Tucson, AZ, United States

***Correspondence:** Mark C. Preul neuropub@barrowneuro.org*

†Co-first authors

Objective: Fluorescence dyes are increasingly used in brain tumor surgeries, and thus the development of simulation models is important for teaching neurosurgery trainees how to perform fluorescence-guided operations. We aimed to create a tumor model for fluorescence-guided surgery in high-grade glioma (HGG).

Methods: The tumor model was generated by the following steps: creating a tumor gel with a similar consistency to HGG, selecting fluorophores at optimal concentrations with realistic color, mixing the fluorophores with tumor gel, injecting the gel into fresh pig/sheep brain, and testing resection of the tumor model under a fluorescence microscope. The optimal tumor gel was selected among different combinations of agar and gelatin. The fluorophores included fluorescein, indocyanine green (ICG), europium, chlorin e6 (Ce6), and protoporphyrin IX (PpIX). The tumor model was tested by neurosurgeons and neurosurgery trainees, and a survey was used to assess the validity of the model. In addition, the photobleaching phenomenon was studied to evaluate its influence on fluorescence detection.

Results: The best tumor gel formula in terms of consistency and tactile response was created using 100 mL water at 100°C, 0.5 g of agar, and 3 g of gelatin mixed thoroughly for 3 min. An additional 1 g of agar was added when the tumor gel cooled to 50°C. The optimal fluorophore concentration ranges were fluorescein 1.9×10^{-4} to 3.8×10^{-4} mg/mL, ICG 4.9×10^{-3} to 9.8×10^{-3} mg/mL, europium 7.0×10^{-2} to 1.4×10^{-1} mg/mL, Ce6 2.2×10^{-3} to 4.4×10^{-3} mg/mL, and PpIX 1.8×10^{-2} to 3.5×10^{-2} mg/mL. No statistical differences among fluorophores were found for face validity, content validity, and fluorophore preference. Europium, ICG, and fluorescein were shown to be relatively stable during photobleaching experiments, while chlorin e6 and PpIX had lower stability.

Conclusions: The model can efficiently highlight the "tumor" with 3 different colors—green, yellow, or infrared green with color overlay. These models showed high face and content validity, although there was no significant difference among the models regarding the degree of simulation and training effectiveness.

They are useful educational tools for teaching the key concepts of intra-axial tumor resection techniques, such as subpial dissection and nuances of fluorescence-guided surgery.

Keywords: europium, fluorescein, fluorescence-guided tumor surgery, fluorophores, high-grade glioma, indocyanine green, protoporphyrin IX, tumor model

INTRODUCTION

Neurosurgery has entered a new era with the application of fluorescence guidance technologies, which are widely applicable in multiple surgical disciplines. To achieve maximal resection, several fluorophores have been introduced into tumor surgery.

1. Fluorescein is a fluorescent dye with an excitation wavelength range of 460–500 nm and emission range of 540–690 nm. It can be visualized under the Yellow 560 filter of the operating microscope. Fluorescein has been used to improve the resection of malignant gliomas by targeting the tumor and margins with doses ranging from 2 to 20 mg/kg administered intravenously (1–3).
2. Indocyanine green (ICG) is widely used in vascular neurosurgery to identify and evaluate the vascular pattern, but it has also been also used for malignant glioma surgeries. It has a peak excitation at a wavelength of 750–800 nm and is visualized by near-infrared cameras at an emission maximum of 850 nm. The usual administration of ICG for vascular application is an intravenous bolus of 5–25 mg, with some tumors remaining fluorescent for about 10 min (4–6). Higher doses of ICG (5 mg/kg) imaged with more sensitive cameras have been used in fluorescence-guided brain tumor resection (6, 7).
3. Protoporphyrin IX (PpIX) is produced from the bioconversion of 5-aminolevulinic acid (5-ALA), which is administered orally at doses of 10–50 mg 4 h before surgery (8). PpIX accumulates in high-grade glioma (HGG) cells and demonstrates red fluorescence with peak emission around 630 nm under blue light (405 nm) excitation, which allows for tumor cells targeted by fluorescence (9–14).
4. Chlorin e6 (Ce6) is a red fluorescent dye, a second-generation photosensitizer, which can be excited with blue light and has an absorption peak of 400 nm. It can be used to target malignant brains tumors or for photodynamic therapy with a dose of 40 mg/m^2 body surface (15–18). Ce6 can be used for fluorescence guidance, but, unlike 5-ALA, its mechanism is not related to bioconversion; rather, similar to fluorescein and ICG, it is related to passive accumulation in the tumor (16, 19, 20).
5. Europium is a photoluminescent lanthanide that emits red light under blue light excitation. It is highly stable and may be used to target tumors in nanoparticles, which can be used in experimental models (21–24). We have demonstrated that europium-based materials have high photostability and can be used for calibration and normalization of quantitative PpIX fluorescence (9).

It is increasingly important to develop simulative models to educate neurosurgical residents and trainees and to help them develop surgical skills in a safe environment. However, for tumor models, it is challenging to construct a model that can mimic the intra-axial tumor resection process under fluorescence guidance in a laboratory environment. Such teaching models help the trainee to understand the key steps and nuances in fluorescence-assisted tumor resection to achieve maximal resection, especially in the case of invasive tumors, such as malignant gliomas.

In this study, we developed a "tumor gel" based on different combinations of gelatin and agar to mimic the consistency of HGG. Different fluorescent dyes were also tested to simulate the visible fluorescence under microscope magnification. We also built a training model by injecting the tumor gel into fresh sheep/pig brains to simulate a realistic tumor resection (25, 26).

MATERIALS AND METHODS

The development of this model involved two major components: the tumor gel for the consistency of the tumor and the dye for the fluorescent effect. Additionally, we tested the photobleaching effect in the models. Finally, we injected the combination of tumor gel and fluorescent agents into fresh sheep and pig brains and tested the model among neurosurgeons and neurosurgical trainees using a scoring system.

Tumor Gel

A tumor gel was developed based on different combinations of agar (Landor Trading Co. Agar Powder) and gelatin (Knox Original Gelatin, Unflavored) to simulate the consistency and firmness of HGG.

A preliminary experiment was performed to find the optimal proportions of agar and gelatin by mixing different amounts with 100 mL of boiling water. Agar and gelatin were tested separately with amounts of 0.2, 0.3, 0.4, 0.5, and 1–5 g in 0.5 g increments and together in various proportions (**Figure 1**). The powder was dissolved thoroughly in boiling water for 3 min to generate a homogeneous polymer.

After elimination of clearly unworkable combinations (too soft or too hard), 12 different combinations of agar or gelatin or both were included in subsequent tests. Six neurosurgeons with broad experience in brain tumor surgery tested and scored all 12 combinations, using a scoring system from 0 to 10 (10 meant the best simulation of an HGG). Equipment and instruments used to assess the gels included those that would normally be used for resecting an invasive brain tumor, such as operating microscope,

Abbreviations: 5-ALA, 5-aminolevulinic acid; Ce6, chlorin e6; FNa, fluorescein; FTG, fluorescent tumor gel; HGG, high-grade glioma; ICG, indocyanine green; PpIX, protoporphyrin IX.

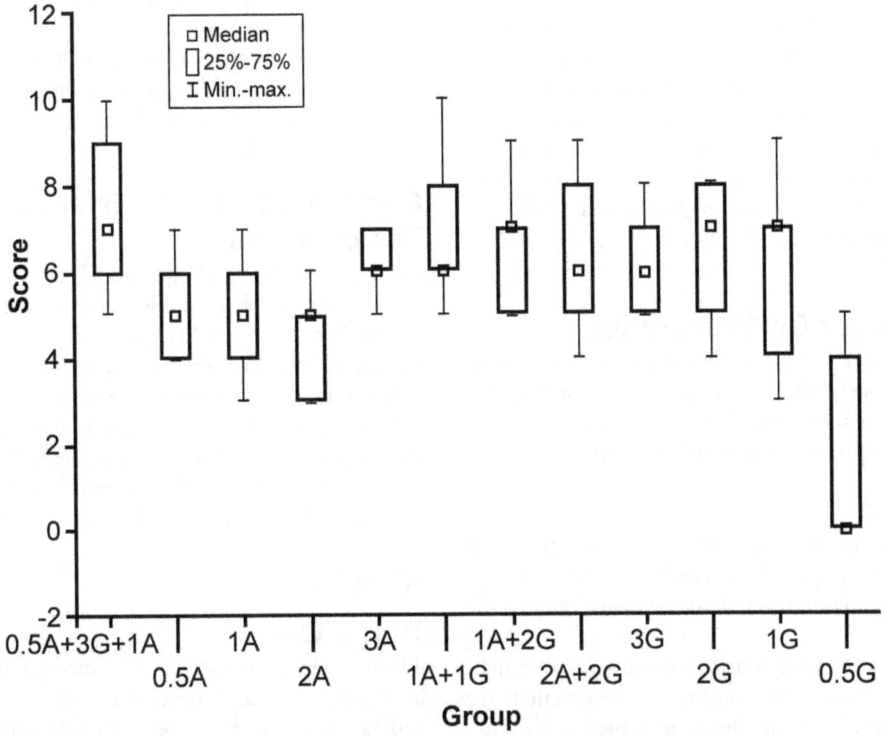

FIGURE 1 | Box plot comparison of 12 solutions with different formulas (horizontal axis) and their scores (0–10, vertical axis). The formula with the highest score was 0.5 g agar and 3 g gelatin with 100 mL boiling water, with additional 1 g of Agar added at 50°C. A, agar; G, gelatin; min-max, minimum to maximum values. *Used with permission from Barrow Neurological Institute, Phoenix, Arizona.*

bipolar forceps, microdissectors, microsuction, microscissors, and microforceps.

To increase the granulation to mimic a real tumor, an additional 1 g of agar was added to the tumor gel (100 mL solution) during cooling (at 50°C).

Optimal Concentrations of Fluorescent Agents

We acquired images of the following dyes at different concentrations: fluorescein (AK-FLUOR Fluorescein Injection, USP), ICG (Cardiogreen Sigma-Aldrich I2633), europium (Sigma-Aldrich), Ce6 (Frontier Scientific), and PpIX (free acid, Enzo Life Sciences). Serial dilutions of the fluorescent dyes were performed to obtain solutions at different concentrations. Normal saline was used as a control for fluorescein and ICG, and dimethyl sulfoxide was used as a control for the remaining three fluorophores. Fluorescein was diluted into 24 shares with concentrations ranging from 1.5×10^{-6} to 12.5 mg/mL. ICG was diluted into 17 shares with concentrations ranging from 3.1×10^{-4} to 10 mg/mL. Europium was diluted into 18 shares with concentrations ranging from 5.5×10^{-4} to 36 mg/mL. Ce6 was diluted into 23 shares with concentrations ranging from 8.6 $\times 10^{-6}$ to 36 mg/mL. PpIX was diluted into 22 shares with concentrations ranging from 1.7×10^{-5} to 36 mg/mL.

Images were captured with an operating microscope (Kinevo 900 OPMI, Carl Zeiss, Oberkochen, Germany) and a camera attached to the observing ocular lens of the microscope (Cannon EOS Rebel T2i, Tokyo, Japan). Different filters of the operating microscope were used with the filters: Blue 400 was used in the analysis of europium, Ce6, and PpIX; Yellow 560 for fluorescein; and Infrared 800 with and without overlay for ICG. A long-wave pass (LWP) filter (B+W F-Pro 58 090 5×E, Schneider Kreuznach, Bad Kreuznach, Germany) was attached to the external camera to accurately measure and analyze PpIX, Ce6, and europium fluorescence.

Settings of the microscope were focus 5× and distance 200 mm, with additional light used when applicable (Blue 400 and Yellow 560), and 1/15 s shutter speed (for the microscope's internal camera) for all images. Procedures using ICG were performed at 25% light intensity (68 mW/cm^2), and the procedures using fluorescein were performed using a Yellow 560 filter at 20% light intensity (9.7 mW/cm^2). The external camera was set at 1/4 s exposure and light sensitivity of the imaging sensor of ISO (International Organization for Standartization) 100 for ICG and fluorescein. Procedures using europium, Ce6, and PpIX were performed under a Blue 400 filter at 100% light intensity (13.4 mW/cm^2), with the red filter attached on the external camera set to 4/5 s exposure and ISO 400. Irradiance was measured using an S120VC photodiode power sensor and a PM400 power meter calibrated to 405 nm for Blue 400, 532 nm for Yellow 560, and 785 nm for Infrared 800 mode (Thorlabs, Dachau, Germany) (9).

Optimal dye concentrations used in the preparation of the fluorescent tumor gels (FTG) were selected by comparing the colors directly under the ocular lens of the microscope. Images were then analyzed in Fiji (27) using the mean pixel signal intensity of the region of interest to confirm the relationship between the relative fluorescence intensity and concentration to select the optimal concentration. Multichannel analysis was used for ICG and single-channel analysis in the others—the green channel for fluorescein and the red channel for europium, Ce6, and PpIX.

Fluorescent Tumor Gel Preparation

The FTG was created by mixing the selected fluorescent dye with the tumor gel immediately after the addition of booster agar at 50°C (see above). To generate the FTG, 5 mL of tumor gel was mixed with each dye at previously selected concentrations.

Photobleaching

A known phenomenon that may affect the interpretation of fluorescence during a period of continuous observation, photobleaching was taken into account and compared among the different FTGs.

Different types of FTG were tested under microscope light with corresponding filters with continuous observation for 5 min, which corresponds to the clinically expected duration of the imaging before altering the microscope position. The photobleaching effect in ICG was recorded using ICG angiography mode as videos, whereas for the remainder of the dyes, a series of images was acquired every 6 s using the external camera. Frames of the ICG video were extracted as images every 6 s using GOM Lab (Gom & Company, South Korea). The settings of the microscope, filter, and camera were the same as above.

The light intensity of each image was extracted during the 5-min continuous observation using Fiji in the region of interest with the same methods as described above.

Tumor Model Preparation

Cooled sheep and pig brains, purchased from a local meat source, were used for the final tumor model preparation to simulate brain tumor resection. A total of 5 mL FTG solution (5 mL FTG and dye at its corresponding concentration) was aspirated in a 5 mL syringe attached to a 21-gauge needle. The FTG was subsequently injected into a fresh sheep and pig brain subcortically; only 1.5–2 mL of the FTG was injected because the size of sheep and pig brain is less than the size of a human brain. The injection was performed meticulously to avoid leakage using a previously described technique (28).

Tumor Model Resection

Three fully trained neurosurgeons and 2 neurosurgical residents (PGY1 and PGY6) assessed the tumor model. Their general information and experience of neurosurgery were collected. They performed simulative tumor resection under microscopic magnification (Kinevo 900 OPMI, Carl Zeiss, Oberkochen, Germany) with and without the assistance of fluorescence guidance. The participants were instructed to perform subpial dissections and to preserve the normal brain tissue. All FTGs were tested by all participants under the corresponding microscopic filters. The simulative operative procedure included operating microscope, and instruments including bipolar forceps, microdissectors, microsuction, microscissors, and microforceps.

Questionnaire of Satisfaction About the Tumor Model

Participants evaluated the model using a questionnaire with items about the face validity, content validity, and white light comparison. Face validity questions evaluate the realism of the model, whereas content validity is a qualitative measure of the appropriateness of the model as a teaching modality (29). The answering system was structured with scores 1–5, in which 1 means "strongly disagree" and 5 means "strongly agree" for all but one question, in which 1 means "easier" and 5 means "more difficult." The questionnaire is shown in **Supplemental Figure 1**.

RESULTS

Tumor Gel

Results of the comparison of all tumor gel formulas are illustrated in **Figure 1**. The best tumor gel formula in terms of consistency and tactile response similar to HGG was the first formula in **Figure 1**: 100 mL 100°C water, 0.5 g of agar, and 3 g of gelatin mixed thoroughly for 3 min ($P_{Kruskal-Wallis} = 0.048$). One gram of agar was added when the tumor gel was at 50°C during the cooling down period.

Optimal Concentrations of Fluorescent Agents

The optimal concentration range of fluorescein was 1.9×10^{-4} to 3.8×10^{-4} mg/mL (**Figure 2**), of ICG was 4.9×10^{-3} to 9.8×10^{-3} mg/mL (**Figure 3**), of europium was 7.0×10^{-2} to 1.4×10^{-1} mg/mL (**Figure 4A**), of Ce6 was 2.2×10^{-3} to 4.4×10^{-3} mg/mL (**Figure 4B**), and of PpIX was 1.8×10^{-2} to 3.5×10^{-2} mg/mL (**Figure 4C**).

During observation of ICG, as the concentration of ICG increased, the fluorescent intensity increased to oversaturation at first, and then decreased as the concentration increased. Two different concentrations produced similar optimal intensity (**Figure 3**), but the solution with a lower concentration was selected for convenience (ICG 4.9×10^{-3} to 9.8×10^{-3} mg/mL).

Because fluorescence intensity was lower in the agar solution than in the normal saline or dimethyl sulfoxide, the following concentrations were selected to create the FTGs: FNa-TG at the concentration of 2.44×10^{-4} mg/mL, ICG-TG 2.5×10^{-2} mg/mL, Eu-TG 1.44×10^{-1} mg/mL, and Ce6-TG 1.125×10^{-2} mg/mL. These FTGs were used to test the effect of photobleaching.

PpIX demonstrated unexpected behavior when mixed with the tumor gel—the red fluorescence disappeared very quickly, with the gel appearing somewhat brown-black. Hydrochloric acid (12M) was added to the FTG in a 1:10 ratio before the dye was mixed (PpIX, 1.1×10^{-3} mg/mL)

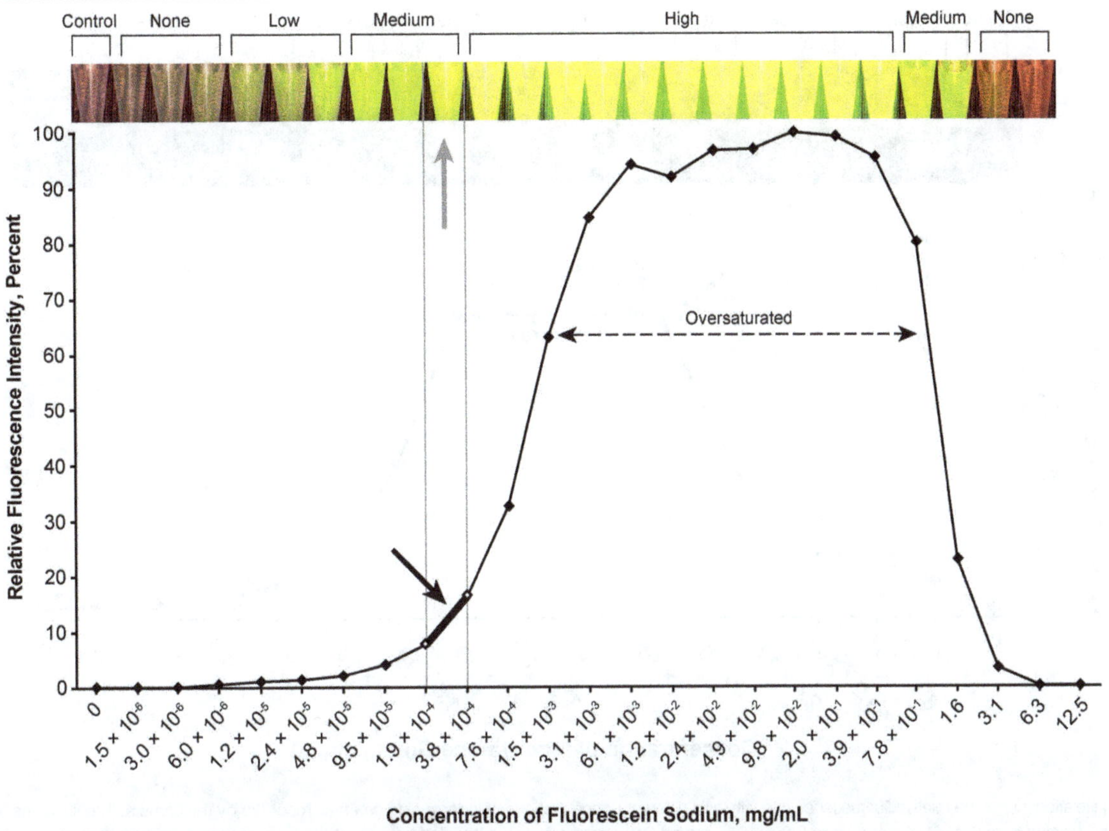

FIGURE 2 | Relationship of relative fluorescence intensity and different concentrations of fluorescein as recorded by the camera. The fluorescence with the concentration ranging from 6.1×10^{-3} mg/mL to ~4.0 mg/mL is oversaturated. The heading bar shows the fluorescence color and intensity at different concentrations (*gray arrow* indicates optimal intensity). A concentration of 1.9×10^{-4} to 3.8×10^{-4} mg/mL was subjectively selected as the optimal concentration for the tumor model (*black arrow*) by observing the color. *Used with permission from Barrow Neurological Institute, Phoenix, Arizona.*

to circumvent this behavior based on the pH-sensitive property of 5-ALA (30), which eventually prevented the color change.

Photobleaching

During the 5-min photobleaching test, we observed decreases of 22.3% in fluorescein (**Figure 5A**), 10% in ICG (**Figure 5B**), 17.57% in europium (**Figure 5C**, red), 37.56% in Ce6 (**Figure 5C**, orange), and 44.84% in PpIX (**Figure 5C**, light purple). The rate of bleaching effect was higher for PpIX than the rates for europium and Ce6.

Tumor Model Resection Test

Five neurosurgeons and neurosurgical trainees aged 28–37 years tested the tumor model. Every participant performed 5 resections (1 operation per fluorophore). Three out of 5 had at least 2 years of experience in microneurosurgery including glioma resection experience. None had previous experience with any tumor model for resection training. The tumor models under different stages of resection and under different fluorescent modes are shown in **Figure 6**.

Face Validity

Mean scores of the questions for face validity are shown in **Figure 7**. On average, participants answered with a high degree of agreement on the first four questions, which indicates high face validity of the developed model. There were no significant differences among the different dyes for each individual face validity question or for the sum of the four scores ($P_{Kruskal-Wallis} > 0.05$ for all, see **Supplemental Figures 2, 3**).

Content Validity

Mean scores for the questions for content validity are shown in **Figure 8**. On average, participants answered with a high degree of agreement on the six questions regarding the content validity of the model, which indicates high content validity of the developed model for the purpose of simulating fluorescence-guided surgical tumor resection. There were no significant differences among the different dyes for each individual content validity question or for the sum of the four scores ($P_{Kruskal-Wallis} > 0.05$ for all, see **Supplemental Figure 4**).

Fluorophores Preferences

Results of the subjective comparative evaluation between the fluorophores are shown in **Figure 9**. On average, participants

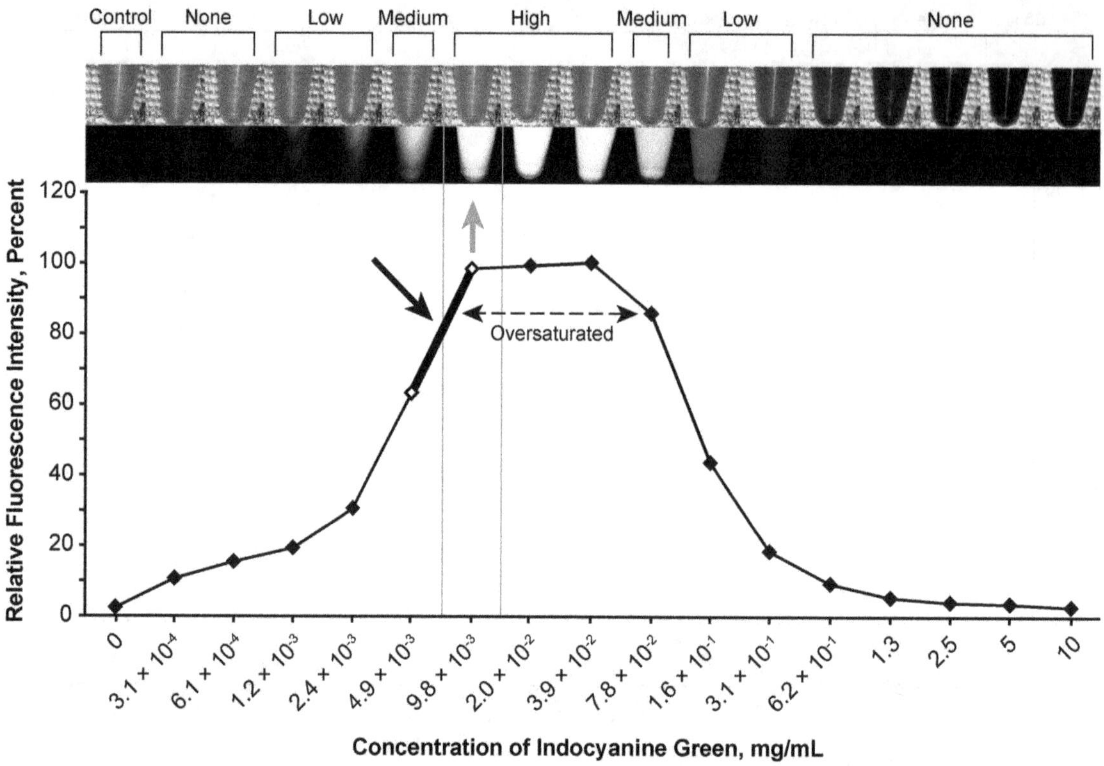

FIGURE 3 | Relationship of the relative fluorescence intensity and different concentrations of indocyanine green as recorded by the camera. The fluorescence with the concentration ranging from 2.0×10^{-2} mg/mL to 3.9×10^{-2} mg/mL is oversaturated. The heading bar shows the fluorescence color and intensity at different concentrations (*gray arrow* indicates optimal intensity). A concentration of 4.9×10^{-3} to 9.8×10^{-3} mg/mL was subjectively selected as the optimal concentration for the tumor model (*black arrow*) by observing the color. *Used with permission from Barrow Neurological Institute, Phoenix, Arizona.*

answered with a high degree of agreement on the questions regarding the convenience, effectiveness, and visual appeal of the fluorescence-guidance of the model. Moreover, when ranking the fluorophores, no fluorophore was significantly better or worse than the others. There were no significant differences among the different dyes for each of the final five questions ($P_{Kruskal-Wallis} > 0.05$ for all, see **Supplemental Figure 5**), indicating that there was no fluorophore that was subjectively superior or inferior to others among the participants.

DISCUSSION

For educational purposes, it is of paramount importance to learn and practice tumor resection prior to a real surgery. Length of survival has been correlated to extent and volume of tumor resection for HGG. Fluorescence techniques add a layer of complexity interpreting tumor boundary in brain tumor surgery, especially for HGG. Previous studies have shown that realistic tumor models can be used in training neurosurgery residents to help them learn the concepts of glioma surgery and the application of fluorescence in neurosurgery (25, 26).

However, those reported models did not include all of the features, such as in real brain tissue simulation and realistic colors of fluorescence-guided tumor surgery (fluorescein, ICG, and europium) along with different filters used in real surgeries. It would arguably be more valuable to have all characteristics in one model to mimic a real neurosurgical scenario. To the best of our knowledge, this is the first report of an in-brain tumor model resembling HGG combined with the use of fluorescence. The tumor model contains 3 parts: the tumor gel, which can offer a tactile response similar to a real tumor during the resection; fluorescent dyes, which can mimic the realistic application of fluorescence; and the actual sheep or pig brains. The FTG was injected in the pig and sheep brains to create a simulation model that replicates the properties of HGG and surrounding brain tissue in a human brain.

Consistency of the Tumor Gel

A tumor model should offer realistic tactile feedback when appropriate instruments are used to help the trainees acquire a simulative experience. We developed a tumor model to simulate HGG. The consistency of HGG may vary from firm to gelatinous and, in general, demonstrates a degree of firmness between normal parenchyma and a firmer, harder metastatic lesion. During the preparation of our tumor gel formula, we created different types of tumor gels of different firmness and consistencies, including those that resemble the metastatic lesions (the solutions of 3 g agar in 100 mL water or 2 g agar plus 2 g gelatin in 100 mL water). The latter recipe results

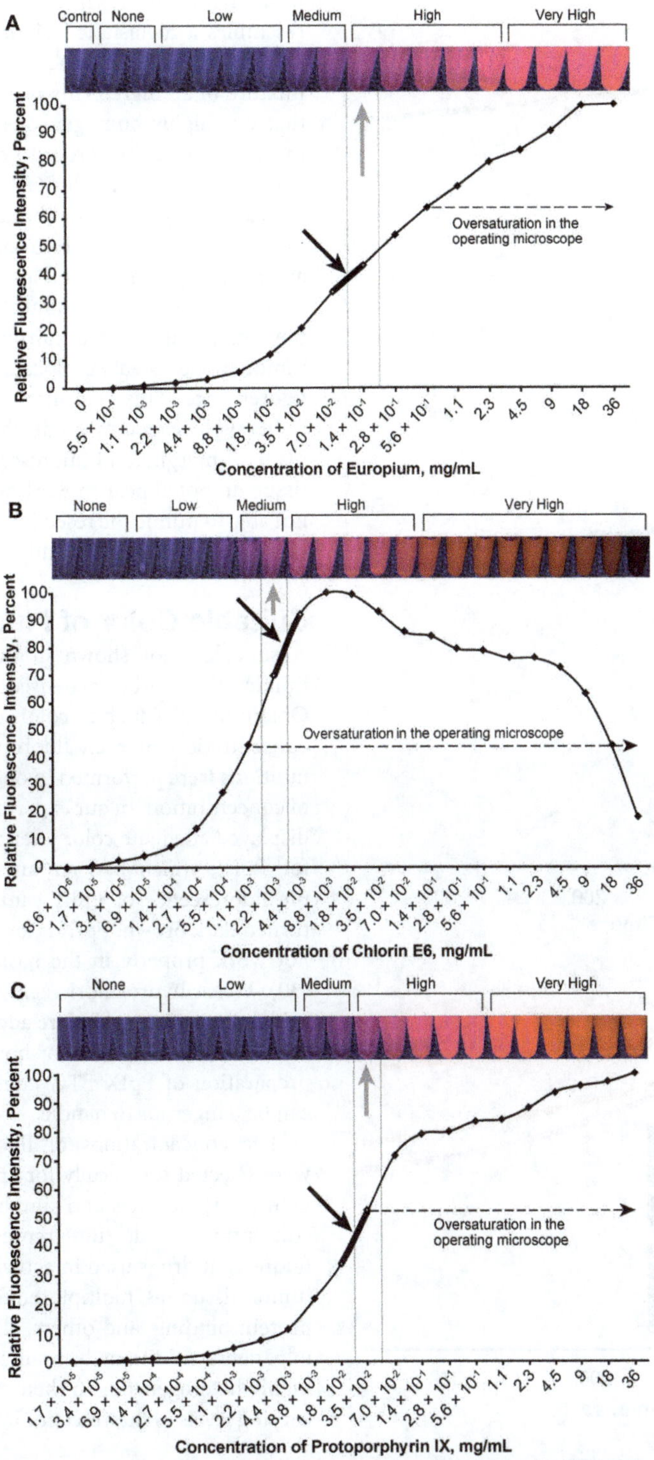

FIGURE 4 | Relationship of the relative fluorescence intensity and different concentrations of europium **(A)**, chlorin e6 **(B)**, and protoporphyrin IX **(C)**. The heading bars show the fluorescence color and intensity at different concentrations (*gray arrows* indicate optimal intensity). For europium **(A)**, the fluorescence was oversaturated when the concentration was higher than 5.6×10^{-1} mg/mL, and the concentration range of 7.0×10^{-2} to 1.4×10^{-1} mg/mL was subjectively selected as the optimal concentration for the tumor model (*black arrow*) by observing the color. For chlorin e6 **(B)**, the fluorescence was oversaturated as recorded through the operating microscope camera when the concentration was above 1.1×10^{-3} mg/mL, and the concentration range of 2.2×10^{-3} to 4.4×10^{-3} mg/mL was subjectively selected as the optimal concentration for the tumor model (*black arrow*) by observing the color. For protoporphyrin IX **(C)**, the fluorescence was oversaturated as recorded by the microscope camera when the concentration was higher than 3.5×10^{-2} mg/mL, and the concentration range of 1.8×10^{-2} to 3.5×10^{-2} mg/mL was subjectively selected as the optimal concentration for the tumor model (*black arrow*) by observing the color. *Used with permission from Barrow Neurological Institute, Phoenix, Arizona.*

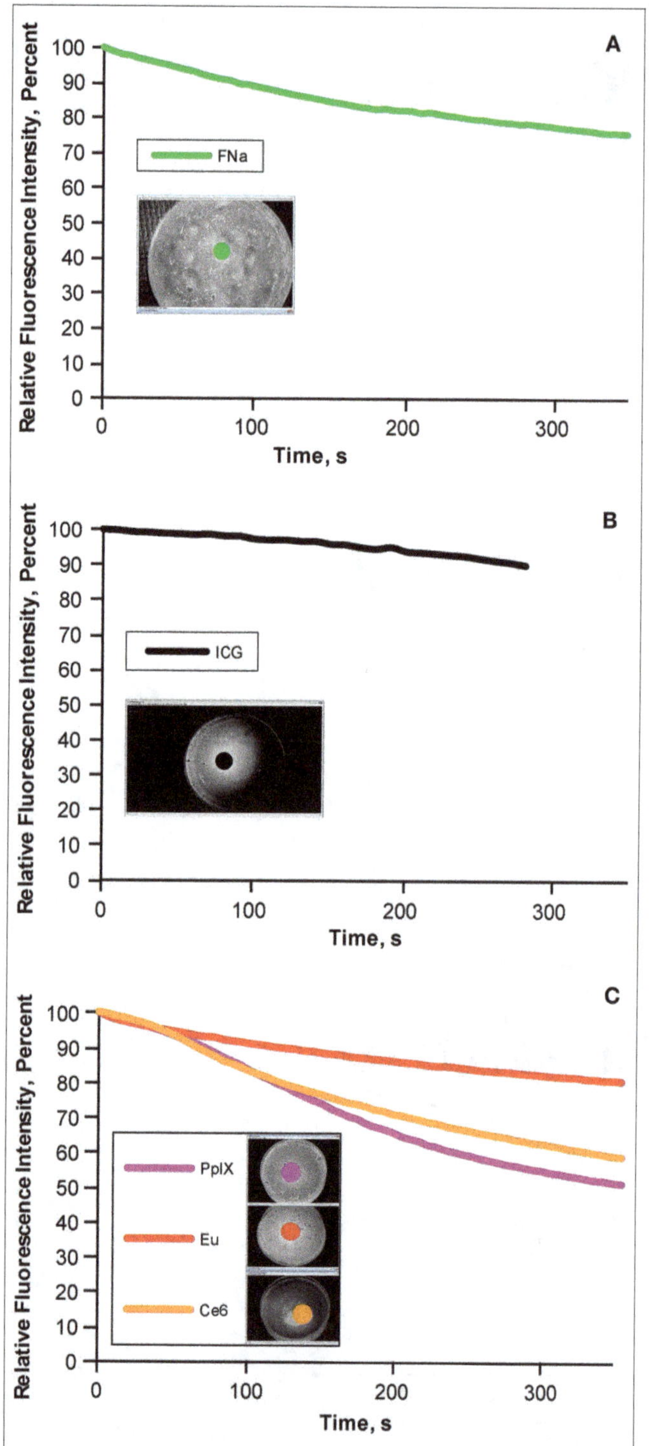

FIGURE 5 | Bleaching phenomena: brightness decrease in different fluorescent tumor gels. **(A)** Fluorescein (FNa); **(B)** indocyanine green (ICG); and **(C)** protoporphyrin IX (PpIX), europium (Eu), and chlorin e6 (Ce6), which are demonstrated together because the same filter was used for all three. During the 5-min (300-s) observation, the decrease in relative fluorescence intensity was approximately 20% for fluorescein, 10% for ICG, 45% for PpIX, 10% for europium, and 35% for Ce6. Inset photographs in each graph show the regions of interests (indicated by colored dots) used to quantify the fluorescence intensity over time. *Used with permission from Barrow Neurological Institute, Phoenix, Arizona.*

in a slightly firmer, more solid consistency that more closely resembles a metastatic lesion, rather than an invading glioma. During preparation of the gel, we also noticed that the thorough mixture of all ingredients in 100°C water produced a tumor gel that was highly homogeneous, whereas a real glioma would be more granulated. In order to create the granularity, we added a booster dose of agar at 50°C during the cooling-down period.

During any intra-axial brain tumor resection, identifying the margin of the tumor and working in the plane between the tumor and normal parenchyma is almost always the principle goal. This technique requires the tumor model to have a similar, but not the same, consistency as normal parenchyma. The margin of the tumor model is easy to locate, especially with the assistance of fluorescence. This goal may be realistic in HGG or metastatic tumors; however, low-grade glioma usually does not have a clear plane of margin, and fluorescence techniques to identify tumor tissue do not appear to work well in such tumors. Our model is not able to mimic the resection of low-grade glioma, which is one of the limitations of the study.

Suitable Color of Fluorescence

A suitable color shown in the tumor model can realistically mimic the fluorescence used in fluorescence-guided surgery. Obtaining a suitable color requires choosing the optimal concentration of each fluorophore. In our study, a series of dilutions were performed to obtain solutions with different levels of concentration. In our experiment, all fluorophores successfully displayed adequate color after mixing with the tumor gel except for PpIX, which had an unexpected behavior. After mixing, the fluorescence of PpIX vanished quickly and the tumor gel turned dark brown. PpIX is an acidophilic substance, which may not work properly in the basic environment of the tumor gel (30). When hydrochloric acid was added into the tumor gel to acidify the tumor gel before adding PpIX, the gel was fluorescent and used in the resection; however, this extra step makes the preparation of PpIX FTG cumbersome, and hydrochloric acid can be dangerous to handle.

The concentrations of fluorophores chosen in our study were selected specifically for application and their functionality with the tumor gels and simulation model development. These concentrations do not represent the concentration of the fluorescent drugs used in actual surgery and accumulated in the tumor tissue, as multiple environmental factors, such as pH, protein binding, and others, affect actual fluorescence intensity in patients. Additionally, brain tumors, especially HGG, are often highly heterogeneous in their cytoarchitecture and present with varying levels of fluorescence intensity within the tumor (31–33).

Advantages and Disadvantages of Fluorophores

Fluorescence techniques are widely used in neurosurgical subdisciplines, and learning to operate under fluorescence is increasingly important for neurosurgeons. The different fluorophores have advantages and disadvantages, and the features of each fluorophore should be well-understood by any neurosurgeon using fluorescent techniques. Recent excellent

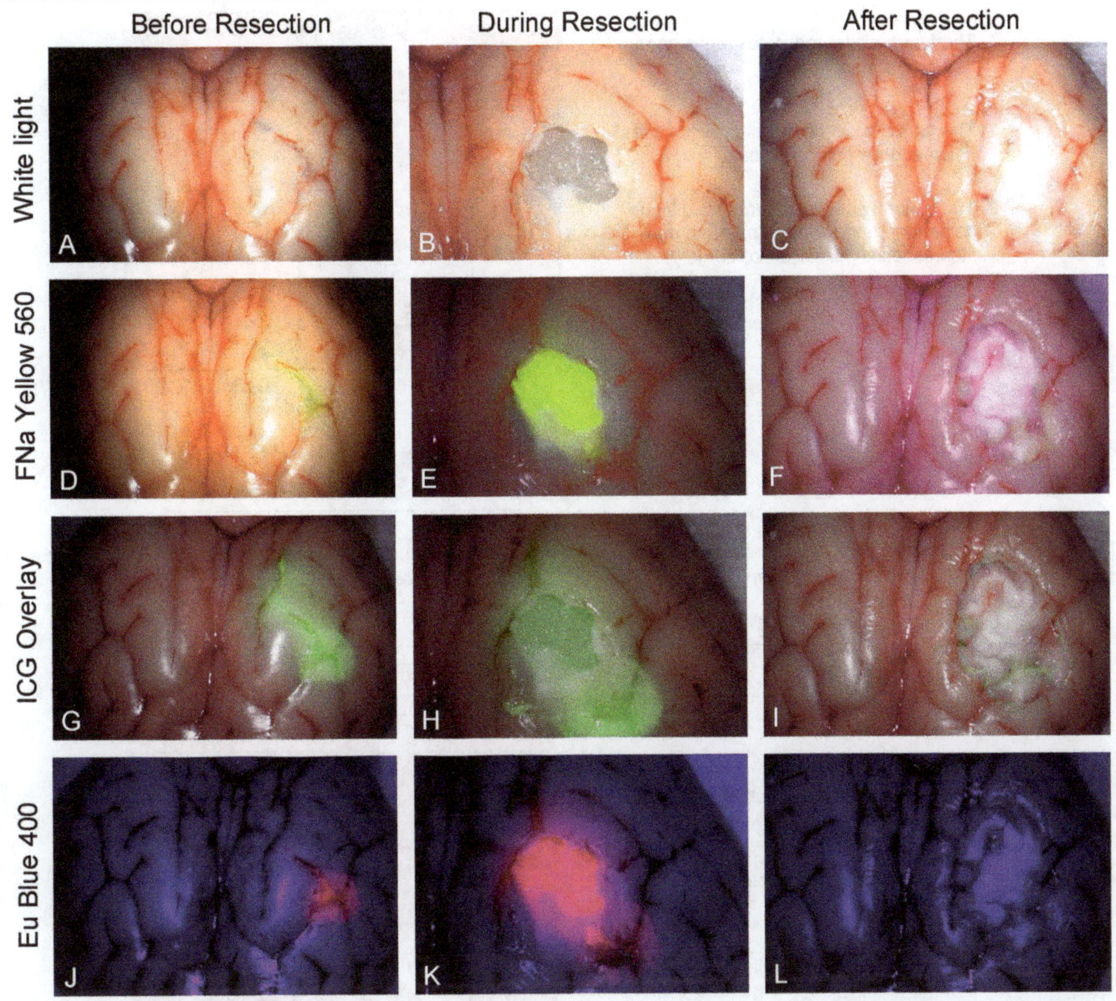

FIGURE 6 | Tumor model in a pig brain at different stages of resection viewed under white light and with the various fluorophores (fluorescein [FNa], indocyanine green [ICG], and europium [Eu]) viewed under their corresponding filters. Tumor model viewed under white light **(A)** before, **(B)** during, and **(C)** after resection. Tumor model after application of fluorescein **(D)** before, **(E)** during, and **(F)** after resection under Yellow 560 filter. Tumor model after application of ICG **(G)** before, **(H)** during, and **(I)** after resection in the ICG overlay mode. Tumor model after application of europium **(J)** before, **(K)** during, and **(L)** after resection under Blue 400 filter. *Used with permission from Barrow Neurological Institute, Phoenix, Arizona.*

reviews discuss fundamental aspects of fluorescence-guided surgery in greater detail (34–36).

Fluorescein is a bright yellow fluorophore used off-label for tumor labeling in neurosurgery, with a growing body of evidence suggesting that its use improves achievement of gross total resection (37–39). Advanced illumination capabilities of the latest operating microscopes allow neurosurgeons to work directly under the Yellow 560 filter throughout the tumor resection (40).

ICG is used in vascular neurosurgery to evaluate the patterns of the vasculature (41), and recent studies suggest its feasibility for brain tumor fluorescence-guided surgery (42). New operating microscopes provide the function of real-time ICG overlay (**Figures 6G–I**), in which the ICG signal is injected into the original white light optical pathway as a semitransparent green overlay (43–45). This enables undistracted continuous manipulations and observation of both normal anatomy and ICG signal, which would be ideal for fluorescence-guided surgery of brain tumors. ICG allows for subsurface imaging as demonstrated by **Figure 6H**. Additionally, there was a tiny rim of residual ICG signal (**Figure 6I**), which represents staining of the pia. Whether this finding represents better sensitivity in detecting ICG signal compared with other fluorophores requires further investigation.

Europium, Ce6, and PpIX are all red fluorophores that can be used for simulation models. We used europium because of its fluorescence spectral similarity to PpIX and the additional benefit that, unlike PpIX, europium is not fast bleaching and can be observed for a relatively longer period than PpIX fluorescence. Ce6 is a photosensitizer that has also been explored which has the same fluorescent color and works under the Blue 400 filter, the illumination of which is blue. Therefore, even though the tumor can be illuminated by fluorescence, it might be challenging

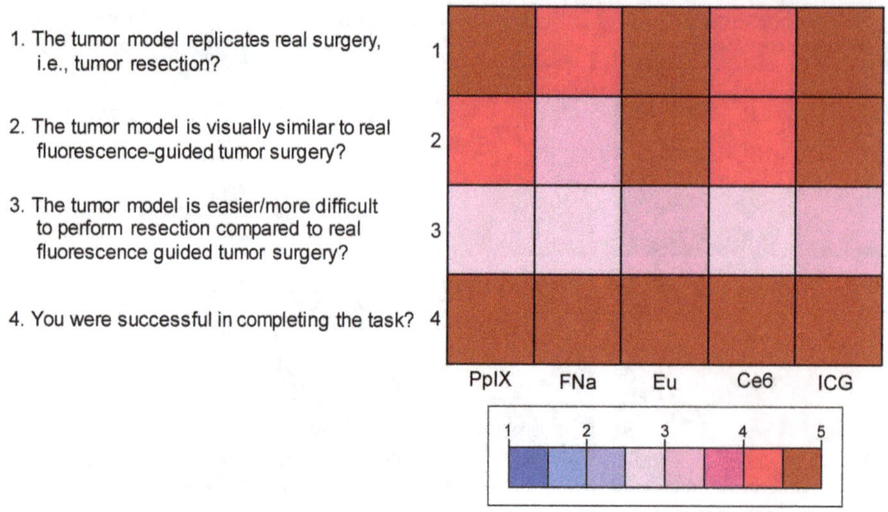

FIGURE 7 | Color-coded plot for questions about face validity. The colored bar shows the scores and their corresponding colors; the score for each question was the average score based on the questionnaire. *Used with permission from Barrow Neurological Institute, Phoenix, Arizona.*

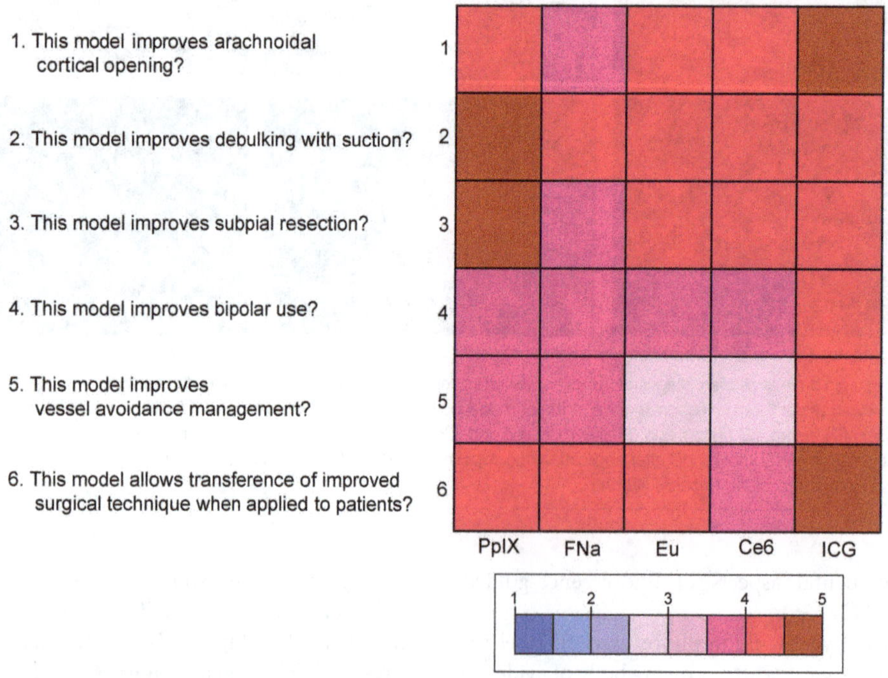

FIGURE 8 | Color-coded plot for questions about content validity. The colored bar shows the scores and their corresponding colors; the score for each question was the average score based on the questionnaire. *Used with permission from Barrow Neurological Institute, Phoenix, Arizona.*

to continuously operate under fluorescence because blood is difficult to visualize. As well, switching between the Blue 400 filter and white light illumination is imperative in real surgery. In our tumor model, there is no bleeding, thus the participants were able to perform the tumor resection under Blue 400 filter without switching, which is not realistic and is one of the major limitations of this model.

Fluorescein and 5-ALA are observed through two separate optical pathways, and therefore can be visualized in stereoscopic three-dimensional mode, which can offer the perception of depth to the observers of the operation. However, ICG, with or without the overlay, is detected through a single optical pathway, and therefore can only be visualized as a two-dimensional image or a semi-transparent pseudo-colored overlay, which lacks

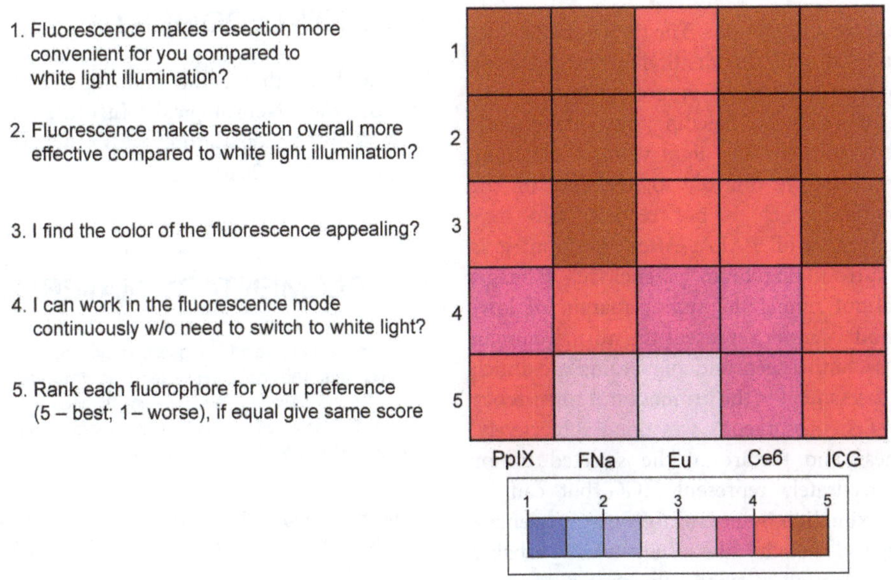

FIGURE 9 | Color-coded plot for questions about fluorophore preferences. The colored bar shows the scores and their corresponding colors; the score for each question was the average score based on the questionnaire. *Used with permission from Barrow Neurological Institute, Phoenix, Arizona.*

depth, making it disadvantageous in terms of practical and educational purposes.

Fluorescence intensity does not necessarily have a linear correlation with the concentration of the fluorophore, which necessitates careful dose selection. With increased concentration, after reaching a peak of fluorescence intensity, all fluorophores are amenable to concentration-dependent quenching, the effect of decreased fluorescence when the concentration of the fluorophore is too high (35). **Figures 2–6** demonstrate this concentration-dependent quenching phenomenon.

Satisfaction scores were relatively high for all the fluorophores. This could mean that, if the tumor cells are labeled with different colors, this sole difference in labeling color would not be likely to affect the efficacy of the resection.

Significance of Photobleaching in Fluorescence Application

Photobleaching is a well-known phenomenon in which the intensity of fluorescence may decrease as the fluorophore is exposed under the excitation light during a prolonged period. This phenomenon may interfere with the interpretation of the fluorescence as the intensity is altered.

Our results demonstrated that fluorescein, ICG, and europium were relatively stable regarding the fluorescence intensity. Among the 3 fluorophores that can mimic the color of 5-ALA, europium is the most stable, which makes it a superior choice for the red fluorescence model.

Realistic Brain Tumor Model: Significance in Practical Education

This project has a potential educational impact for less experienced neurosurgical trainees. They can practice the simulative tumor resection to understand the key concepts of intra-axial brain tumor resection. Subpial resection is a method that can maximize the resection of the lesion while minimizing the risk of damage to the nearby gyrus. It can be deleterious to practice such techniques in real situations, because beginners may not understand the difference between the consistencies of lesions and normal parenchyma. It is certainly valuable for the trainee or less experienced neurosurgeon to practice such concepts prior to the real operation (28).

Because they are hazardous materials, fluorescent dyes are not always available in a laboratory situation for practice. In the tumor model, we created a FTG, that can be shaped and injected easily. Neurosurgical beginners can learn the variations in appearance of fluorescence of different dyes at various positions and light intensities of the microscope while handling a model with a similar consistency to human tissue. The FTG can be widely used in courses because it is an affordable option, is quick and easy to prepare, and has a formula that is replicable. Based on the formula, future models of different types of brain tumors with different consistencies (i.e., metastatic tumor) can be reproduced following the same steps.

Although we did not assess the long-term stability of the FTGs, if necessary, they can be kept in air-tight bags to prevent drying. After being stored for 1 month in a light-protected place, the gels were still fluorescent; however, we believe that freshly prepared gels are better because the tumor gel may dry up, and the concentration of the fluorophore may alter during long-term preservation. Also, sodium azide can be added to the tumor gel to make a 0.01% (weight/volume) solution in order to prevent the growth of mold over time. Caution should be exercised because sodium azide is toxic.

Limitations

The tumor model has several limitations. The tumor model does not permit the practice of skills in identifying and handling vessels; therefore, control of bleeding cannot be taught with this model. Because there is no bleeding, the participants can perform the resection under blue light without switching back to white light (blood is difficult to visualize in the dark fluorescence mode), which is not realistic and may have biased the effectiveness of 5-ALA. After resection, it is difficult to evaluate surrounding brain parenchyma damage. The tumor model cannot mimic the tumor margin of low-grade gliomas. This model cannot represent the normal human brain anatomy because both sheep and pig brains are much smaller. Additionally, assessment of the firmness and consistency of the tumor gels by 6 neurosurgeons was done subjectively. Therefore, the firmness and texture of the selected tumor gel recipe may not accurately represent HGG but can be viewed as a close approximation by neurosurgeons experienced in brain tumor surgery. Finally, the study was probably underpowered for the detection of small subjective differences among the fluorophores. The absence of significant differences among the tested fluorophores reflects the heterogeneity in the questionnaire responses regarding these fluorophores (5-ALA, fluorescein, and to a lesser extent ICG) in the neurosurgical literature (46, 47).

CONCLUSION

In this paper, we present and compare 5 simulation models for fluorescence-guided brain tumor surgery, specifically of HGG. The models efficiently highlighted the "tumor" with 3 different colors—green, yellow, or infrared pseudocolored in green—and multicolor labeling is possible. These models exhibited high face and content validity, and there was no significant difference in the fluorescence-guided surgery performance or fluorescence appearance scores between the models. These models may be effective educational tools for learning the key concepts and technical nuances of fluorescence-guided brain tumor surgery associated with intra-axial tumor resection.

AUTHOR CONTRIBUTIONS

EB and MP: conception and design of the study. DV, EB, and XZ: developed the tumor gels and assessed fluorescence measures. SG, CC, NM, PN, EB, and DV: assessed the tumor model. DV and XZ: wrote the first draft of the manuscripts. EB and DV: performed the statistical analysis. PN, ML, and MP: contributed funding, resources acquisition, and supervision. All authors contributed to manuscript revision and read and approved the submitted version.

ACKNOWLEDGMENTS

The authors thank the staff of Neuroscience Publications at Barrow Neurological Institute for assistance with manuscript preparation. EB acknowledges scholarship support SP-2240.2018.4.

SUPPLEMENTARY MATERIAL

Supplemental Figure 1 | The questionnaire about the tumor model administered to participants. The answering system was structured with scores 1–5, in which 1 means "strongly disagree" and 5 means "strongly agree" for all but one question, in which 1 means "easier" and 5 means "more difficult." *Used with permission from Barrow Neurological Institute, Phoenix, Arizona.*

Supplemental Figure 2 | Mean scores of answers to questionnaire. *Used with permission from Barrow Neurological Institute, Phoenix, Arizona.*

Supplemental Figure 3 | Scores for the 4 questions for face validity of the tumor model. Scores for the question "The tumor model replicates real surgery?" ranged from 4.4 to 4.8 (highest score was for ICG); from 4 to 5 for the question "The tumor model is visually similar to real fluorescence-guided tumor surgery?" (highest for europium [Eu]); from 2.6 to 3 (3 meaning the most adequate) for the question "The tumor model is easier/more difficult to perform resection compared to real fluorescence-guided tumor surgery?" (most adequate was ICG); and from 4.6 to 5 for the question "You were successful in completing the task?" (highest for ICG). No comparison reached statistical significance. *Used with permission from Barrow Neurological Institute, Phoenix, Arizona.*

Supplemental Figure 4 | Scores for the 6 questions for content validity of the tumor model. Scores for the question "This model improves arachnoidal cortical opening?" ranged from 3.8 to 4.8 (highest score was ICG); from 4 to 4.8 for the question "This model improves debulking with suction?" (highest for ICG); from 3.8 to 4.6 for the question "This model improves subpial resection?" (highest for PpIX); from 3.6 to 4 for the question "This model improves bipolar use?" (highest for ICG); from 3.2 to 4 for the question "This model improves vessel avoidance/management?" (highest for ICG); and from 3.8 to 4.8 for the question "This model allows transference of improved surgical technique when applied to patients?" (highest for ICG). No comparison reached statistical significance. *Used with permission from Barrow Neurological Institute, Phoenix, Arizona.*

Supplemental Figure 5 | Scores for the 5 questions for comparing the fluorophores. The highest and lowest scores for the question "The fluorescence makes resection more convenient for you compared to white light illumination?" were 4.8 (ICG) and 4.2 (europium [Eu]); 5 (ICG) and 4.4 (europium) for the question "The fluorescence makes resection overall more effective compared to white light illumination?"; 4.8 (fluorescein sodium [FNa] and ICG) and 4.2 (chlorin e6 and PpIX) for the question "You find the color of the fluorescence appealing?"; and 4.4 (ICG) and 3.6 (europium and chlorin e6) for the question "You can work in the fluorescence mode continuously without need to switch to white light?" For the question asking participants to rank the fluorophores in order of preference (5 being the best and 1 the worst), ICG had the highest score, followed by PpIX, Ce6, fluorescein sodium, and europium. No comparison reached statistical significance. *Used with permission from Barrow Neurological Institute, Phoenix, Arizona.*

REFERENCES

1. Neira JA, Ung TH, Sims JS, Malone HR, Chow DS, Samanamud JL, et al. Aggressive resection at the infiltrative margins of glioblastoma facilitated by intraoperative fluorescein guidance. *J Neurosurg.* (2017) 127:111–22. doi: 10.3171/2016.7.JNS16232
2. Francaviglia N, Iacopino DG, Costantino G, Villa A, Impallaria P, Meli F, et al. Fluorescein for resection of high-grade gliomas: a safety study control in a single center and review of the literature. *Surg Neurol Int.* (2017) 8:145. doi: 10.4103/sni.sni_89_17
3. Schwake M, Stummer W, Suero Molina EJ, Wölfer J. Simultaneous fluorescein sodium and 5-ALA in fluorescence-guided glioma surgery. *Acta Neurochir.*

(2015) 157:877–9. doi: 10.1007/s00701-015-2401-0

4. Senders JT, Muskens IS, Schnoor R, Karhade AV, Cote DJ, Smith TR, et al. Agents for fluorescence-guided glioma surgery: a systematic review of preclinical and clinical results. *Acta Neurochir.* (2017) 159:151–67. doi: 10.1007/s00701-016-3028-5
5. Belykh E, Martirosyan NL, Yagmurlu K, Miller EJ, Eschbacher JM, Izadyyazdanabadi M, et al. Intraoperative fluorescence imaging for personalized brain tumor resection: current state and future directions. *Front Surg.* (2016) 3:55. doi: 10.3389/fsurg.2016.00055
6. Zeh R, Sheikh S, Xia L, Pierce J, Newton A, Predina J, et al. The second window ICG technique demonstrates a broad plateau period for near infrared fluorescence tumor contrast in glioblastoma. *PLoS ONE.* (2017) 12:e0182034. doi: 10.1371/journal.pone.0182034
7. Li C, Sullivan PZ, Cho S, Nasrallah MP, Buch L, Isaac Chen HC, et al. Intraoperative molecular imaging with second window ICG facilitates confirmation of contrast-enhancing tissue during intracranial stereotactic needle biopsy: a case series. *World Neurosurg.* (2019). doi: 10.1016/j.wneu.2019.02.231. [Epub ahead of print].
8. Michael AP, Watson VL, Ryan D, Delfino KR, Bekker SV, Cozzens JW. Effects of 5-ALA dose on resection of glioblastoma. *J Neurooncol.* (2019) 141:523–31. doi: 10.1007/s11060-019-03100-7
9. Belykh E, Miller EJ, Patel AA, Bozkurt B, Yagmurlu K, Robinson TR, et al. Optical characterization of neurosurgical operating microscopes: quantitative fluorescence and assessment of PpIX photobleaching. *Sci Rep.* (2018) 8:12543. doi: 10.1038/s41598-018-30247-6
10. Colditz MJ, Leyen K, Jeffree RL. Aminolevulinic acid (ALA)-protoporphyrin IX fluorescence guided tumour resection. Part 2: theoretical, biochemical and practical aspects. *J Clin Neurosci.* (2012) 19:1611–6. doi: 10.1016/j.jocn.2012.03.013
11. Díez Valle R, Hadjipanayis CG, Stummer W. Established and emerging uses of 5-ALA in the brain: an overview. *J Neurooncol.* (2019) 141:487–94. doi: 10.1007/s11060-018-03087-7
12. Lakomkin N, Hadjipanayis CG. Fluorescence-guided surgery for high-grade gliomas. *J Surg Oncol.* (2018) 118:356–61. doi: 10.1002/jso.25154
13. Pustogarov N, Panteleev D, Goryaynov SA, Ryabova AV, Rybalkina EY, Revishchin A, et al. Hiding in the shadows: CPOX expression and 5-ALA induced fluorescence in human glioma cells. *Mol Neurobiol.* (2017) 54:5699–708. doi: 10.1007/s12035-016-0109-7
14. Hadjipanayis CG, Stummer W. 5-ALA and FDA approval for glioma surgery. *J Neurooncol.* (2019) 141:479–86. doi: 10.1007/s11060-019-03098-y
15. Akimoto J. Photodynamic therapy for malignant brain tumors. *Neurol Med Chir.* (2016) 56:151–7. doi: 10.2176/nmc.ra.2015-0296
16. Shimizu K, Nitta M, Komori T, Maruyama T, Yasuda T, Fujii Y, et al. Intraoperative photodynamic diagnosis using talaporfin sodium simultaneously applied for photodynamic therapy against malignant glioma: a prospective clinical study. *Front Neurol.* (2018) 9:24. doi: 10.3389/fneur.2018.00024
17. Namatame H, Akimoto J, Matsumura H, Haraoka J, Aizawa K. Photodynamic therapy of C6-implanted glioma cells in the rat brain employing second-generation photosensitizer talaporfin sodium. *Photodiagnosis Photodyn Ther.* (2008) 5:198–209. doi: 10.1016/j.pdpdt.2008.08.001
18. Tsutsumi M, Miki Y, Akimoto J, Haraoka J, Aizawa K, Hirano K, et al. Photodynamic therapy with talaporfin sodium induces dose-dependent apoptotic cell death in human glioma cell lines. *Photodiagnosis Photodyn Ther.* (2013) 10:103–10. doi: 10.1016/j.pdpdt.2012.08.002
19. Tzerkovsky DA, Osharin VV, Istomin YP, Alexandrova EN, Vozmitel MA. Fluorescent diagnosis and photodynamic therapy for C6 glioma in combination with antiangiogenic therapy in subcutaneous and intracranial tumor models. *Exp Oncol.* (2014) 36:85–9.
20. Akimoto J, Fukami S, Ichikawa M, Mohamed A, Kohno M. Intraoperative photodiagnosis for malignant glioma using photosensitizer talaporfin sodium. *Front Surg.* (2019) 6:12. doi: 10.3389/fsurg.2019.00012
21. Hu Z, Chi C, Liu M, Guo H, Zhang Z, Zeng C, et al. Nanoparticle-mediated radiopharmaceutical-excited fluorescence molecular imaging allows precise image-guided tumor-removal surgery. *Nanomedicine.* (2017) 13:1323–31. doi: 10.1016/j.nano.2017.01.005
22. Binnemans K. Interpretation of europium(III) spectra. *Coord Chem Rev.* (2015) 295:1–45. doi: 10.1016/j.ccr.2015.02.015
23. Zeng H, Li X, Sun M, Wu S, Chen H. Synthesis of europium-doped fluorapatite nanorods and their biomedical applications in drug delivery. *Molecules.* (2017) 22:753. doi: 10.3390/molecules22050753
24. Galimov DI, Bulgakov RG. The first example of fluorescence of the solid individual compounds of Eu2+ ion: EuCl2, EuI2, EuBr2. *J Luminescence.* (2019) 34:127–9. doi: 10.1002/bio.3580
25. Kamp MA, Knipps J, Steiger HJ, Rapp M, Cornelius JF, Folke-Sabel S, et al. Training for brain tumour resection: a realistic model with easy accessibility. *Acta Neurochir.* (2015) 157:1975–81; discussion 1981. doi: 10.1007/s00701-015-2590-6
26. Mashiko T, Oguma H, Konno T, Gomi A, Yamaguchi T, Nagayama R, et al. Training of intra-axial brain tumor resection using a self-made simple device with agar and gelatin. *World Neurosurg.* (2018) 109:e298–e304. doi: 10.1016/j.wneu.2017.09.162
27. Schindelin J, Arganda-Carreras I, Frise E, Kaynig V, Longair M, Pietzsch T, et al. Fiji: an open-source platform for biological-image analysis. *Nat Methods.* (2012) 9:676–82. doi: 10.1038/nmeth.2019
28. Sabel M. *Getting Ready for Brain Tumor Surgery.* New York, NY: Thieme (2017). doi: 10.1055/b-006-149701
29. Kirkman MA, Ahmed M, Albert AF, Wilson MH, Nandi D, Sevdalis N. The use of simulation in neurosurgical education and training. A systematic review. *J Neurosurg.* (2014) 121:228–46. doi: 10.3171/2014.5.JNS131766
30. Sharma M, Graham JY, Walczak PA, Nguyen R, Lee LK, Carson MD, et al. Optical pH measurement system using a single fluorescent dye for assessing susceptibility to dental caries. *J Biomed Optics.* (2019) 24:017001. doi: 10.1117/1.JBO.24.1.017001
31. Martinez-Moreno M, Kiesel B, Woehrer A, Mischkulnig M, Furtner J, Timelthaler G, et al. *Ex-vivo* analysis of quantitative 5-ALA fluorescence intensity in diffusely infiltrating gliomas with a handheld spectroscopic probe: correlation with histopathology, proliferation and microvascular density. *Photodiagnosis Photodyn Ther.* (2019) 27:354–61. doi: 10.1016/j.pdpdt.2019.05.013
32. Widhalm G, Wolfsberger S, Minchev G, Woehrer A, Krssak M, Czech T, et al. 5-Aminolevulinic acid is a promising marker for detection of anaplastic foci in diffusely infiltrating gliomas with nonsignificant contrast enhancement. *Cancer.* (2010) 116:1545–52. doi: 10.1002/cncr.24903
33. Ross JL, Cooper LAD, Kong J, Gutman D, Williams M, Tucker-Burden C, et al. 5-Aminolevulinic acid guided sampling of glioblastoma microenvironments identifies pro-survival signaling at infiltrative margins. *Sci Rep.* (2017) 7:15593. doi: 10.1038/s41598-017-15849-w
34. Zhang DY, Singhal S, Lee JYK. Optical principles of fluorescence-guided brain tumor surgery: a practical primer for the neurosurgeon. *Neurosurgery.* (2018). doi: 10.1093/neuros/nyy315. [Epub ahead of print].
35. Gioux S, Choi HS, Frangioni JV. Image-guided surgery using invisible near-infrared light: fundamentals of clinical translation. *Mol Imaging.* (2010) 9:237–55. doi: 10.2310/7290.2010.00034
36. Wei L, Roberts DW, Sanai N, Liu JTC. Visualization technologies for 5-ALA-based fluorescence-guided surgeries. *J Neurooncol.* (2019) 141:495–505. doi: 10.1007/s11060-018-03077-9
37. Kaneko S, Eljamel MS. Fluorescence image-guided neurosurgery. *Future Oncol.* (2017) 13:2341–8. doi: 10.2217/fon-2017-0194
38. Acerbi F, Broggi M, Schebesch KM, Hohne J, Cavallo C, De Laurentis C, et al. Fluorescein-guided surgery for resection of high-grade gliomas: a multicentric prospective phase II study (FLUOGLIO). *Clin Cancer Res.* (2018) 24:52–61. doi: 10.1158/1078-0432.CCR-17-1184
39. Xiang Y, Zhu XP, Zhao JN, Huang GH, Tang JH, Chen HR, et al. Blood-brain barrier disruption, sodium fluorescein, and fluorescence-guided surgery of gliomas. *Br J Neurosurg.* (2018) 32:141–8. doi: 10.1080/02688697.2018.1428731
40. Belykh EG, Zhao X, Cavallo C, Bohl MA, Yagmurlu K, Aklinski JL, et al. Laboratory evaluation of a robotic operative microscope-visualization platform for neurosurgery. *Cureus.* (2018) 10:e3072. doi: 10.7759/cureus.3072
41. Ewelt C, Nemes A, Senner V, Wölfer J, Brokinkel B, Stummer W, et al. Fluorescence in neurosurgery: its diagnostic and therapeutic use. Review of the literature. *J Photochem Photobiol B.* (2015) 148:302–9. doi: 10.1016/j.jphotobiol.2015.05.002
42. Acerbi F, Vetrano IG, Sattin T, de Laurentis C, Bosio L, Rossini Z, et al. The role of indocyanine green videoangiography with FLOW 800 analysis for the

surgical management of central nervous system tumors: an update. *Neurosurg Focus.* (2018) 44:E6. doi: 10.3171/2018.3.FOCUS1862

43. Martirosyan NL, Skoch J, Watson JR, Lemole GM Jr, Romanowski M, Anton R. Integration of indocyanine green videoangiography with operative microscope: augmented reality for interactive assessment of vascular structures and blood flow. *Neurosurgery.* (2015) 11(Suppl. 2):252–7; discussion 257–8. doi: 10.1227/NEU.0000000000000681
44. Watson JR, Gainer CF, Martirosyan N, Skoch J, Lemole GM Jr, Anton R, et al. Augmented microscopy: real-time overlay of bright-field and near-infrared fluorescence images. *J Biomed Opt.* (2015) 20:106002. doi: 10.1117/1.JBO.20.10.106002
45. Nickele C, Nguyen V, Fisher W, Couldwell W, Aboud E, David C, et al. A pilot comparison of multispectral fluorescence to indocyanine green videoangiography and other modalities for intraoperative assessment in vascular neurosurgery. *Operat Neurosurg.* (2018) 17:103–9. doi: 10.1093/ons/opy237
46. Liu JT, Meza D, Sanai N. Trends in fluorescence image-guided surgery for gliomas. *Neurosurgery.* (2014) 75:61–71. doi: 10.1227/NEU.0000000000000344
47. Brawanski A, Acerbi F, Nakaji P, Cohen-Gadol A, Schebesch KM. Poor man-rich man fluorescence. Is this really the problem? *Acta Neurochir.* (2015) 157:1959–61. doi: 10.1007/s00701-015-2553-y

16

Surgery for Malignant Brain Gliomas: Fluorescence-Guided Resection or Functional-Based Resection?

Hugues Duffau [1,2*]

[1] *Department of Neurosurgery, Montpellier University Medical Center, Gui de Chauliac Hospital, Montpellier, France,* [2] *Team "Plasticity of Central Nervous System, Stem Cells and Glial Tumors," U1051 Laboratory, National Institute for Health and Medical Research (INSERM), Institute for Neurosciences of Montpellier, Montpellier University Medical Center, Montpellier, France*

Correspondence:
Hugues Duffau
h-duffau@chu-montpellier.fr

Keywords: fluorescence imaging, glioblastoma, functional-based resection, fluorescence-guided resection, brain glioma

The goal of surgery for malignant brain glioma is to optimize the extent of resection (EOR) while preserving the quality of life. A meta-analysis evidenced that gross total resection improves progression free survival and overall survival (OS) in glioblastomas (1). In a consecutive cohort with 500 newly diagnosed glioblastomas, a significant survival benefit was noted with as little as 78% EOR, and stepwise improvement in OS was observed even in the 95–100% EOR range (2). Interestingly, in 243 glioblastomas, survival advantages from total resection remained significant in multivariate analysis after adjustment for bias (3). Concerning anaplastic gliomas, the volume of residual neoplasm on postoperative MRI predicts the time to tumor progression and OS (4).

However, maximal resection can be challenging because it may be difficult to identify the boundaries of glioma due to its infiltrative feature, especially with a white-light microscope. Therefore, to improve the intraoperative real-time visualization of malignant gliomas, the use of fluorescence-guided surgery (FGS) has been advocated, with 5-aminolevulinic acid (5-ALA) as the first option (5, 6). Intrasurgical fluorescence imaging allowed an increase of EOR in high-grade gliomas compared to conventional microsurgery with white-light, as demonstrated by a seminal randomized controlled trial (7). The great merit of this study was also to emphasize the need to objectively assess the EOR on postoperative MRI following glioblastoma surgery. In this Frontiers issue, applications of fluorescence and other optical imaging technology in oncological surgery have been highlighted, especially for malignant brain tumor. Nonetheless, despite a prolific literature on this topic in the past decade, the actual benefit of FGS for glioma patients may be discussed, due to substantial limitations.

From an oncological perspective, beyond the fact that 5-ALA is not adapted to show diffused low-grade gliomas, FGS may paradoxically restrict EOR in high-grade gliomas. Indeed, it has recently been suggested that supracomplete resection, which consists on the removal of a margin around the enhancement, may improve OS in glioblastomas (8). This original concept is based upon the fact that relapses mostly occur at the periphery of the operating cavity, where specific tumor and stromal cells that promote glioblastoma growth and invasion exist (9). In a cohort with 1229 glioblastomas, Li et al. reported a significantly longer OS of 20.7 months when a resection of $\geq$ 53.21% of the surrounding FLAIR-weighted MRI abnormalities was performed in addition to the total contrast-enhancing removal, versus 15.5 months in the case of excision of the enhancement alone (10). Consequently, even though 5-ALA goes beyond the borders of contrast enhancement, because its diffusion is nonetheless reduced, the tumorological risk intrinsically related to this method is to prematurely stop the resection around the tumor mass identified by fluorescence—while optionally, a lobectomy with a (sub)total resection of the FLAIR abnormalities would have been possible in non-eloquent areas, thus with a better impact on OS. From a functional

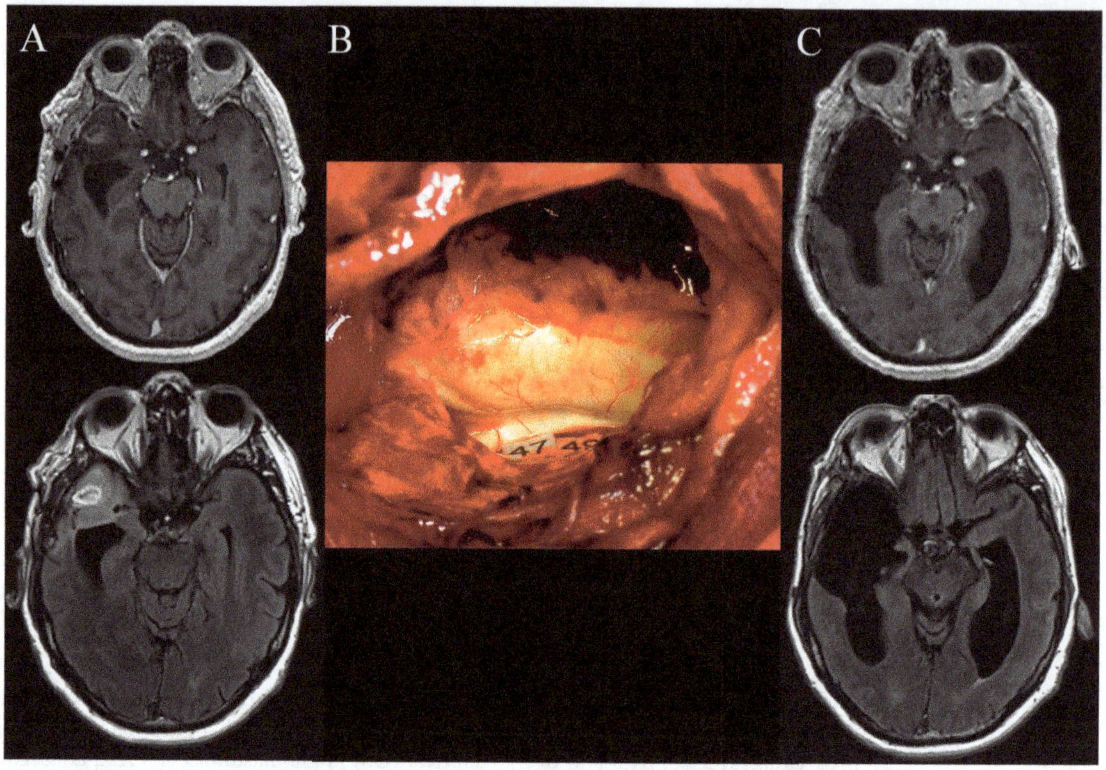

FIGURE 1 | (A) Preoperative axial enhanced T1-weighted MRI (upper) and FLAIR-weighted MRI (lower) achieved in a 50-year-old right-handed man who experienced seizures that allowed the discovery of a right anterior temporal high-grade glioma. The patient underwent a previous "minimal-invasive image-guided surgery" performed under general anesthesia in another hospital with a partial resection of the enhancement and the FLAIR hypersignal. An anaplastic astrocytoma was diagnosed. At that time, the patient was referred to our department and a reoperation was proposed with awake mapping in order to achieve a supratotal resection according to functional boundaries. The neurological examination was normal. Nonetheless, the preoperative neuropsychological evaluation revealed a slight deficit of higher-cognitive functions, that is, theory of mind and semantic processing. **(B)** Intraoperative view after resection, achieved up to eloquent structures, especially at the subcortical level. Indeed, direct electrostimulation of white matter tracts enabled the identification of the subcortical neural networks involved in theory of mind (mentalizing) (tag 47) and non-verbal semantics (tag 49) - which have been mapped according to the results of the presurgical neurocognitive assessment. **(C)** Postoperative axial enhanced T1-weighted MRI (upper) and FLAIR-weighted MRI (lower) (performed 3 months after resection) demonstrating a supracomplete resection of both the enhancement and the FLAIR hypersignal. The patient recovered, with an improvement of the neuropsychological examination thanks to a post-surgical cognitive rehabilitation. A diffuse WHO grade III astrocytoma (IDH1 mutated, non-codeleted) was diagnosed, and postoperative chemotherapy was administrated, with no radiotherapy. The imaging is stable with 4 years of follow-up, and the patient continues to enjoy a normal life, with no symptoms.

point of the view, the same property of 5-ALA going beyond the enhanced part of the glioma can result in permanent neurological deterioration for tumors involving structures essential for brain functions. For example, Díez Valle et al. reported a rate of new or increased neurological worsening of 8.2% in a series with glioblastomas operated on using 5-ALA (11), that is, a higher rate in comparison with series using intraoperative electrical mapping −3.4% in a recent meta-analysis (12).

Therefore, an alternative to overcome these limitations is to switch from a FGS to a functional-guided resection by means of direct electrical stimulation (DES) (13). Indeed, the meta-analysis by De Witt et al. in which the benefit of intraoperative electrical mapping on glioma surgery outcome was investigated on the basis of over 8,000 patients, evidenced that the surgical excision of both high-grade gliomas and low-grade gliomas using DES was correlated with more radical resections and with a significantly lower rate of severe permanent impairment—even for tumors located in eloquent regions (12). It is necessary to stress that such a demonstration of an improved EOR associated with a simultaneous decrease of neurological morbidity thanks to the use of fluorescence *per se*, compared with results reported in series using intraoperative functional mapping [currently considered as the standard of care of glioma surgery (12)], is still lacking.

Of note, it has been proposed to combine 5-ALA and electrophysiological mapping, especially for gliomas invading critical areas (14–17). However, even if technically there is not antagonism to use both methods, FGS is conceptually incompatible with functional mapping-based resection. Indeed, although the aim of 5ALA-guided surgery is to remove the enhanced part of the glioma, with the double risk not to achieve a supramarginal resection when functionally feasible or to induce a persistent deficit in eloquent structures (since it is in essence unable to provide functional information), the purpose of mapping-guided surgery is not to achieve a ≪tumorectomy≫ but to perform the most extensive resection of the parenchyma invaded by a diffuse tumoral disease—on the condition that this part of the brain is not critical for neural functions (8, 18). In other words, the aim is to push the resection until eloquent structures have been encountered, both at cortical and subcortical levels, with no margin left around these functional boundaries (13). In practice, if there are discrepancies in information given by 5-ALA and DES, neurosurgeons should rely on functional mapping. For instance, if fluorescence reveals residual glioma but electrical mapping shows that it invades functional tissue, resection must be stopped to preserve the neural networks (19). On the other hand, if 5-ALA demonstrates a ≪complete≫ tumoral removal, but the eloquent structures have not yet been reached according to DES, resection should be pursued up to functional limits in order to achieve a supratotal excision (20) (**Figure 1**).

In summary, with the ultimate goal of optimizing the onco-functional balance, namely, to improve both OS and quality of life in patients with malignant brain gliomas, FGS can be questioned by (re)opening the door to functional mapping-guided resection, to be able to maximize the benefit/risk ratio of surgery in high-grade gliomas (12, 18, 21)—as already extensively demonstrated in diffuse low-grade gliomas (22).

AUTHOR CONTRIBUTIONS

The author confirms being the sole contributor of this work and has approved it for publication.

REFERENCES

1. Brown TJ, Brennan MC, Li M, Church EW, Brandmeir NJ, Rakszawski KL, et al. Association of the extent of resection with survival in glioblastoma: a systematic review and meta-analysis. *JAMA Oncol.* (2016) 2:1460–9. doi: 10.1001/jamaoncol.2016.1373
2. Sanai N, Polley MY, McDermott MW, Parsa AT, Berger MS. An extent of resection threshold for newly diagnosed glioblastomas. *J Neurosurg.* (2011) 115:3–8. doi: 10.3171/2011.2.JNS10998
3. Stummer WW, Reulen HJ, Meinel T, Pichlmeier U, Schumacher W, Tonn JC, et al. Extent of resection and survival in glioblastoma multiforme: identification of and adjustment for bias. *Neurosurgery.* (2008) 62:564–76. doi: 10.1227/01.neu.0000317304.31579.17
4. Keles GE, Chang EF, Lamborn KR, Tihan T, Chang CJ, Chang SM, et al. Volumetric extent of resection and residual contrast enhancement on initial surgery as predictors of outcome in adult patients with hemispheric anaplastic astrocytoma. *J Neurosurg.* (2006) 105:34–40. doi: 10.3171/jns.2006.105.1.34
5. Halani SH, Adamson DC. Clinical utility of 5-aminolevulinic acid HCl to better visualize and more completely remove gliomas. *Onco Targets Ther.* (2016) 9:5629–42. doi: 10.2147/OTT.S97030
6. Stummer W, Suero Molina E. Fluorescence imaging/agents in tumor resection. *Neurosurg Clin N Am.* (2017) 28:569–83. doi: 10.1016/j.nec.2017.05.009
7. Stummer W, Pichlmeier U, Meinel T, Wiestler OD, Zanella F, Reulen HJ. Fluorescence-guided surgery with 5-aminolevulinic acid for resection of malignant glioma: a randomised controlled multicentre phase III trial. *Lancet Oncol.* (2006) 7:392–401. doi: 10.1016/S1470-2045(06)70665-9
8. Duffau H. Is supratotal resection of glioblastoma in noneloquent areas possible? *World Neurosurg.* (2014) 82:e101–3 doi: 10.1016/j.wneu.2014.02.015
9. Petrecca K, Guiot MC, Panet-Raymond V, Souhami L. Failure pattern following complete resection plus radiotherapy and temozolomide is at the resection margin in patients with glioblastoma. *J Neurooncol.* (2013) 111:19–23. doi: 10.1007/s11060-012-0983-4
10. Li YM, Suki D, Hess K, Sawaya R. The influence of maximum safe resection of glioblastoma on survival in 1229 patients: can we do better than gross-total resection? *J Neurosurg.* (2016) 124:977–88. doi: 10.3171/2015.5.JNS 142087
11. Díez Valle R, Tejada Solis S, Idoate Gastearena MA, García de Eulate R, Domínguez Echávarri P, Aristu Mendiroz J. Surgery guided by 5-aminolevulinicfluorescence in glioblastoma: volumetric analysis of extent of resection insingle-center experience. *J Neurooncol.* (2011) 102:105–13. doi: 10.1007/s11060-010-0296-4
12. De Witt Hamer PC, Gil Robles S, Zwinderman A, Duffau H, Berger MS. Impact of intraoperative stimulation brain mapping on glioma surgery outcome: a meta-analysis. *J Clin Oncol.* (2012) 30:2559–65. doi: 10.1200/JCO.2011.38.4818
13. Duffau H. Mapping the connectome in awake surgery for gliomas: an update. *J Neurosurg Sci.* (2017) 61:612–30. doi: 10.23736/S0390-5616.17.04017-6
14. Della Puppa A, Pellegrin S, d'Avella E, Gioffrè G, Rossetto M, Gerardi A, et al. 5-aminolevulinic acid (5-ALA) fluorescence guided surgery of high-grade gliomas in eloquent areas assisted by functional mapping. Our experience and review of the literature. *Acta Neurochir.* (2013) 155:965–72. doi: 10.1007/s00701-013-1660-x
15. Schucht P, Seidel K, Beck J, Murek M, Jilch A, Wiest R, et al. Intraoperative monopolar mapping during 5-ALA-guided resections of glioblastomas adjacent to motor eloquent areas: evaluation of resection rates and neurological outcome. *Neurosurg Focus.* (2014) 37:E16. doi: 10.3171/2014.10.FOCUS14524
16. Picart T, Armoiry X, Berthiller J, Dumot C, Pelissou-Guyotat I, Signorelli F, et al. Is fluorescence-guided surgery with 5-ala in eloquent areas for malignant gliomas a reasonable and useful technique? *Neurochirurgie.* (2017) 63:189–96. doi: 10.1016/j.neuchi.2016.12.005
17. Corns R, Mukherjee S, Johansen A, Sivakumar G. 5-aminolevulinic acid guidance during awake craniotomy to maximise extent of safe resection of glioblastoma multiforme. *BMJ Case Rep.* (2015) 2015:bcr2014208575. doi: 10.1136/bcr-2014-208575
18. Ferracci FX, Duffau H. Improving surgical outcome for gliomas with intraoperative mapping. *Exp Rev Neurother.* (2018) 18:333–41. doi: 10.1080/14737175.2018.1451329
19. Feigl GC, Ritz R, Moraes M, Klein J, Ramina K, Gharabaghi A, et al. Resection ofmalignant brain tumors in eloquent cortical areas: a new multimodal approachcombining 5-aminolevulinic acid and intraoperative monitoring. *J Neurosurg.* (2010) 113:352–7. doi: 10.3171/2009.10.JNS09447
20. Yordanova YN, Duffau H. Supratotal resection of diffuse gliomas - an overview of its multifaceted implications. *Neurochirurgie.* (2017) 63:243–9. doi: 10.1016/j.neuchi.2016.09.006
21. Sanai N, Berger MS. Surgical oncology for gliomas: the state of the art. *Nat Rev Clin Oncol.* (2018) 15:112–25. doi: 10.1038/nrclinonc.2017.171
22. Duffau H. Diffuse low-grade glioma, oncological outcome and quality of life: a surgical perspective. *Curr Opin Oncol.* (2018) 30:383–9. doi: 10.1097/CCO.0000000000000483

17

Fluorescence Image Histology Pattern Transformation Using Image Style Transfer

Mohammadhassan Izadyyazdanabadi[1,2], *Evgenii Belykh*[2], *Xiaochun Zhao*[2], *Leandro Borba Moreira*[2], *Sirin Gandhi*[2], *Claudio Cavallo*[2], *Jennifer Eschbacher*[3], *Peter Nakaji*[3], *Mark C. Preul*[2] *and Yezhou Yang*[1*]

[1] *School of Computing, Informatics, and Decision System Engineering, Arizona State University, Tempe, AZ, United States,* [2] *The Loyal and Edith Davis Neurosurgery Research Laboratory, Department of Neurosurgery, St. Joseph's Hospital and Medical Center, Barrow Neurological Institute, Phoenix, AZ, United States,* [3] *Department of Neuropathology, St. Joseph's Hospital and Medical Center, Barrow Neurological Institute, Phoenix, AZ, United States*

***Correspondence:**
Yezhou Yang
yz.yang@asu.edu

Confocal laser endomicroscopy (CLE) allow on-the-fly *in vivo* intraoperative imaging in a discreet field of view, especially for brain tumors, rather than extracting tissue for examination *ex vivo* with conventional light microscopy. Fluorescein sodium-driven CLE imaging is more interactive, rapid, and portable than conventional hematoxylin and eosin (H&E)-staining. However, it has several limitations: CLE images may be contaminated with artifacts (motion, red blood cells, noise), and neuropathologists are mainly trained on colorful stained histology slides like H&E while the CLE images are gray. To improve the diagnostic quality of CLE, we used a micrograph of an H&E slide from a glioma tumor biopsy and image style transfer, a neural network method for integrating the content and style of two images. This was done through minimizing the deviation of the target image from both the content (CLE) and style (H&E) images. The style transferred images were assessed and compared to conventional H&E histology by neurosurgeons and a neuropathologist who then validated the quality enhancement in 100 pairs of original and transformed images. Average reviewers' score on test images showed 84 out of 100 transformed images had fewer artifacts and more noticeable critical structures compared to their original CLE form. By providing images that are more interpretable than the original CLE images and more rapidly acquired than H&E slides, the style transfer method allows a real-time, cellular-level tissue examination using CLE technology that closely resembles the conventional appearance of H&E staining and may yield better diagnostic recognition than original CLE grayscale images.

Keywords: confocal laser endomicroscopy, fluorescence, digital pathology, brain tumor imaging, deep learning, image style transfer

INTRODUCTION

Confocal laser endomicroscopy (CLE) is undergoing rigorous assessment for its potential to assist neurosurgeons to examine tissue *in situ* during brain surgery (1–5). The ability to scan tissue or surgical resection bed on-the-fly essentially producing optical biopsies, compatibility with different fluorophores, miniature size of the probe and the portability of the system are essential features of this promising technology. Currently, the most frequent technique used for neurosurgical intraoperative diagnosis is examination of frozen section hematoxylin and eosin (H&E)-stained histology slides.

Figure 1A shows an example image from a glioma acquired by CLE (left) and a micrograph of an H&E slide (right), acquired by conventional light microscopy. Although generating CLE images is much faster than H&E slides (1 s per image compared to about 20 min per slide), many CLE images may be non-optimal and can be obscured with artifacts including background noise, blur, and red blood cells (6). The histopathological features of gliomas are often more identifiable in the H&E slide images compared to the CLE images generated using non-specific fluorescent dyes such as fluorescein sodium (FNa). Neuropathologists as well are used to evaluating detailed histoarchitecture colorfully stained with H&E for diagnoses, especially for frozen section biopsies. Fluorescent images from intraoperative neurosurgical application present a new digital gray scale (monochrome) imaging environment to the neuropathologist for diagnosis that may include hundreds of images from one case. Recently, the U.S. FDA has approved a blue laser range CLE system primarily utilizing FNa for use in neurosurgery.

Countervailing these diagnostic and visual deficiencies in CLE images requires a rapid, automated transformation that can: (1) remove the occluding artifacts, and (2) add (amplify) the histological patterns that are difficult to recognize in the CLE images. Finally, this transformation should avoid removing the critical details (e.g., cell structures, shape) or adding unreal patterns to the image, to maintain the integrity of the image content. Such a method may present "transformed" CLE images to the neuropathologist and neurosurgeon that may resemble images based on familiar and standard, even colored, appearances from histology stains, such as H&E.

One method for implementing this transformation could be supervised learning, however, supervised learning requires paired images (from the same object and location) to learn the mapping between the two domains (CLE and H&E). Creating a dataset of colocalized H&E and CLE images is infeasible because of problems in exact co-localization and intrinsic tissue movements, although small, and artifacts introduced during H&E slide preparation. "Image style transfer," first introduced by Gatys et al. (7), is an image transformation technique that blends the content and style of two separate images to produce the target image. This process minimizes the distance between feature maps of the source and target images using a pretrained convolutional neural network (CNN).

In this study, we aimed to remove the inherent occlusions and enhance the structures that were problematical to recognize in CLE images. Essentially, we attempted to make CLE images generated from non-specific FNa application during glioma surgery appear like standard H&E-stained histology and evaluate the accuracy and usefulness. We used the image style transfer method since it extracts abstract features from the CLE and H&E image that are independent of their location in the image and thus can operate on the images that are not from the same location. More details about the image style transfer algorithm and the quality assessment protocol follow in section Methods. Our results from a test dataset showed that on average, the diagnostic quality of stylized images was higher than the original CLE images, although there were some cases where the transformed image showed new artifacts.

METHODS

Image Style Transfer

Image style transfer takes a content and style image as input and produces a target image that shows the structures of the content image and the general appearance of the style image. This is achieved through four main components: (1) a pretrained CNN that extracts feature maps from source and target images, (2) quantitative calculation of the content and style representations for source and target images, (3) a loss function to capture the difference between the content and style representation of source and target images, and (4) an optimization algorithm to minimize the loss function. In contrast to CNN supervised learning, where the model parameters are updated to minimize the prediction error, image style transfer modifies the pixel values of the target image to minimize the loss function while the model parameters are fixed.

A 19-layer visual geometry group network (VGG-19), that is pretrained on ImageNet dataset, extracts feature maps from CLE, H&E, and target images. Feature maps in layer "Conv4_2" of VGG-19 are used to calculate the image content representation, and a list of gram matrices from feature maps of five layers ("ReLU1_1", "ReLU2_1", ..., "ReLU5_1") are used to calculate the image style representation. To examine the difference between the target and source images, the following loss function was used:

$$Loss_{Total} = \underbrace{\frac{1}{2}\sum\left(C_{CLE} - C_{Target}\right)^2}_{\text{Content Loss: difference between content representation of the CLE and target image}} + \underbrace{\alpha \times \sum_{i=1}^{5} w^i \times \sum\left(S^i_{H\&E} - S^i_{Target}\right)^2}_{\text{Style Loss: difference between style representation of the H\&E and target image}}$$

C_{CLE} and C_{Target} are the content representations of the CLE and target image, $S^i_{H\&E}$ and S^i_{Target} are the style representations of the H&E and target image based on the feature maps of the ith layer, and w^i (weight of ith layer in the style representation) equals 0.2. The parameter α determines relative weight of style loss in the total loss and is set to 100. A limited memory optimization algorithm [L-BFGS (8)] minimizes this loss.

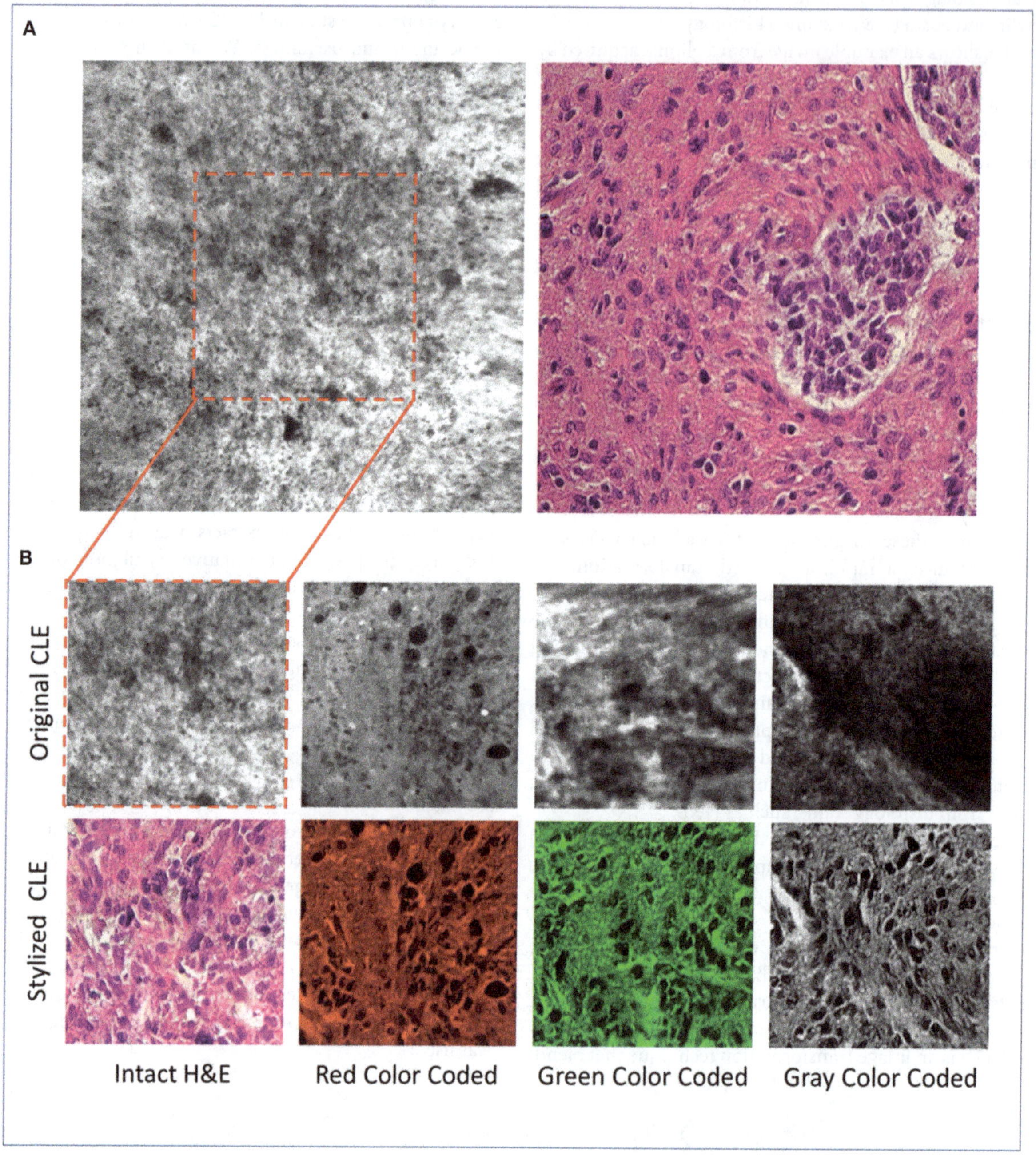

FIGURE 1 | (A) Representative CLE (Optiscan 5.1, Optiscan Pty., Ltd.) and H&E images from glioma tumors. **(B)** Original and stylized CLE images from glioma tumors, in 4 color coding: gray, green, red, intact H&E.

For the experiment, 100 CLE images [from a recent study by Martirosyan et al. (5)] were randomly selected from 15 subjects with glioma tumors as content images. A single micrograph of an H&E slide from a glioma tumor biopsy of a different patient (not one of the 15 subjects) was used as the style image (**Figure 1A**, right). For each CLE image, the optimization process was run for 1,600 iterations and the target image was saved for evaluation and referred to as the "stylized image" in the following sections.

Evaluation

Although the stylized images presented the same histological patterns as H&E images and seemed to contain similar structures to those present in the corresponding original CLE images, a quantitative image quality assessment was performed to rigorously evaluate the stylized images. Five neurosurgeons independently assessed the diagnostic quality of the 100 pairs of original and stylized CLE images. For each pair, the reviewers sought to examine two properties in each stylized image and provided a score for each property based on their evaluation: (1) whether the stylization process removed any critical structures (negative impact) or artifacts (positive impact) that were present in the original CLE image, and (2) whether the stylization process added new structures that were not present (negative impact) or were difficult to notice (positive impact) in the original CLE image. The scores are between 0 and 6 with the following annotations: 0, extreme negative impact; 1, moderate negative impact; 2, slight negative impact; 3, no significant impact; 4, slight positive impact; 5, moderate positive impact; and 6, extreme positive impact (Further information and instructions about the quality assessment survey is available in the **Supplementary Materials**).

Since the physicians were more familiar with the H&E than the CLE images, it was possible that the reviewers would overestimate the quality of stylized images merely due to their color resemblance to H&E images (during style transfer the color of CLE image is also changed to pink and purple). To explore how the reviewers' scores would change if the stylized images were presented in a different color other than the pink and purple (the common color for H&E images), the stylized images were processed in four different ways: (I) 25 stylized images were converted into gray-scale images (averaging the three red, green, and blue channels), (II) 25 stylized images were color-coded in green (first converted the image to gray-scale and then set red and blue channels to zero), (III) 25 stylized images were color-coded as red (similar approach), and (IV) 25 stylized images were used without any further changes (intact H&E). Since there are too many structures in each CLE image, and to examine the images more precisely, we used the center-crop of each original CLE and its stylized version for evaluation. **Figure 1B** shows some example stylized images used for evaluation.

RESULTS AND ANALYSIS

Figure 2A shows a histogram of all reviewers' scores for the removed artifacts (blue bars) and added structures (orange bars) in the stylized images with different colors. Overall, the number of stylized CLE images that have higher diagnostic quality than the original images (score >3) was significantly larger than those with equal or lower diagnostic quality for both removed artifacts and added structures scores (one-way chi square test $p < 0.001$). Results from stylized images that were color-coded (gray, green, red) showed the same trend for the added structures scores, indicating that the improvement was not just because of color resemblance.

There was significant difference between how much the model added structures and removed artifacts. For all the color-coded and intact stylized images, the average of added structures scores was larger than the removed artifacts scores (t-test $p < 0.001$). This suggests that the model was better at enhancing the structures that were challenging to recognize than removing the artifacts.

Figure 2B shows the frequency of different combinations of scores for removed artifacts and added structures in an intensity map. Each block represents how many times a rater scored an image with the corresponding values on the x (improvement by added structures) and y (improvement by removed artifacts) axes for that block. The most frequent incident across all the stylized images is the coordinates (5,4), which means moderately adding structures and slightly removing artifacts, followed by (5,5) meaning moderately adding structures and removing artifacts. Although the intensity maps derived from different color-coded images were not exactly similar, the most frequent combination in each group still indicated positive impact in both properties. The most frequent combination of scores, for each of the color-coded images, was as follows: gray = (5,4), green = (5,5), red = (5,4), and intact = (5,4).

As a further analysis, we counted the number of images that had an average score of below three to see how often the algorithm removed critical structures or added artifacts that were misleading to the neurosurgeons. From the 100 tested images, 3 images had only critical structures removed, 4 images had only artifacts or unreal added structures, and 2 images had both artifacts added and critical structures removed. On the contrary, 84 images showed improved diagnostic quality through both removed artifacts and added structures that were hard to recognize, 6 images had only artifacts removed, and 5 images had only critical structures added. **Figure 1B** shows some example stylized images with improved quality compared to the original CLE, and **Figure 2C** shows two stylized images with decreased diagnostic quality through removed critical structures (top) and added artifacts (bottom).

DISCUSSION

In this study, image style transfer method was used to improve the diagnostic quality of CLE images from glioma tumors by transforming the histology patterns in CLE images of fluorescein sodium-stained tissue into the ones in conventional H&E-stained tissue slides. From the 100 test images, 90 images showed reduced artifacts and 89 images showed improvement in difficult structures (more identifiable) after the transformation, confirmed by five neurosurgeon reviewers. Similar results in color coded images (gray, green, red) suggested that the improvement was not solely because of the color resemblance of stylized images to the H&E slide images. The same method could be used to transform CLE videos as shown in the **Supplementary Materials**.

In a related study by Gu et al. (9), cycle-consistent generative adversarial network (CycleGAN) was used as a data synthesis method to overcome the limited size of dataset in probe-based CLE (pCLE). A real dataset of pCLE images and histology slide images were used to train a generative model that transformed the histology slide images into pCLE. The pCLE dataset was then augmented with the synthesized images to train a computer aided diagnostic system for classification of breast lesions that are stained with acriflavine hydrochloride. However, for use in the *in vivo* brain, fluorophores are currently extremely limited—only three are approved: 5-ALA, indocyanine green, and fluorescein sodium. Currently CLE in the brain only uses fluorescein sodium. Each of these fluorophores yields completely unique unrelated appearances. However, our aim was to evaluate the diagnostic

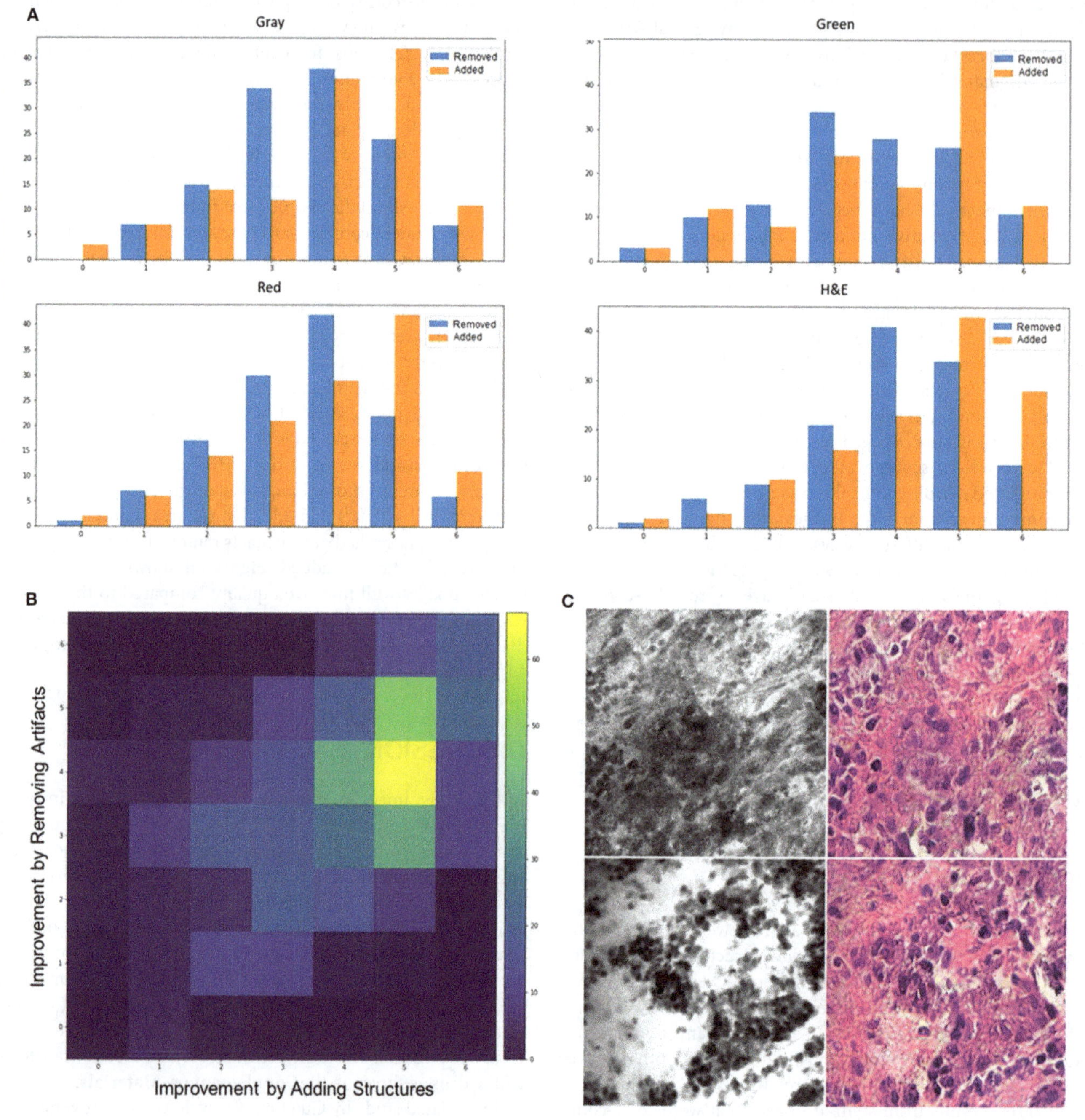

FIGURE 2 | (A) Histogram of scores for added structures and removed artifacts from different color—coded images. **(B)** An intensity map showing the frequency of different combinations of scores for adding structures (x axis) and removing artifacts (y axis). **(C)** Two example images that the stylization process removed some critical details (top) or added unreal structures (bottom).

quality of images that are obtained using fluorescein sodium stained biopsy tissue of brain lesions acquired during intracranial surgery. Fluorescein sodium is a non-specific stain which collects in the tissue background or extracellular space, thus does not produce images such as are stained with acriflavine, which is more specific and stains intracellular structures. Such a situation using fluorescein is thus even more of a diagnostic challenge and for transforming patterns from the CLE image domain to one of the familiar H&E histopathology images.

Although other studies have used CycleGAN for medical domain adaptation (9–11), none has applied "image style transfer" method for transforming CLE to H&E. Despite CycleGAN requirement of many images from both modalities (CLE and H&E) to train the model, image style transfer can produce transformed images with a single image of each modality. This aspect of efficiency may have an important impact in surgery or pathology interpretation where there is a limited number of images available. Such an aspect of efficiency may lend itself better for inclusion into the CLE operating system for automated decision-making.

The purpose of our study was to evaluate the impact of image style transfer on the diagnostic quality of CLE brain and brain tumor (glioma) images from the neurosurgeons' perspectives. While studies like (9) explore the impact of synthesized data on computer-aided diagnostic methods, our study focused on improving the quality of CLE images from the physician point of view. Due to the intrinsic differences and mechanical limitations between the intraoperative CLE with a field of view of only 400 microns, neurosurgical biopsy instruments that acquire about 1 mL of tissue at minimum, normal physiologic brain movements, and light microscopy imaging of histology sections and slides, it is nearly impossible to image and correlate the same exact location with the two modalities. This limited us to compare the transformed CLE images with the potential real H&E stained sections of the same area, using measures such as structural similarity as performed by Shaban et al. (11) in their study. Indeed, the only available ground truth is the original CLE image (before transformation) which could be used to examine if any critical structures are removed or if unreal cellular architecture is added.

CONCLUSIONS

In this study, image style transfer was applied to CLE images from gliomas to enhance their diagnostic quality. Style transfer with an H&E-stained slide image had an overall positive impact on the diagnostic quality of CLE images. The improvement was not solely because of the colorization of CLE images; even the stylized images that were converted to gray, red, and green, reported improved diagnostic quality compared to the original CLE images. Employment of more specific clinical tasks to explore the advantage of stylization in diagnosing gliomas and other tumor types is underway based on this preliminary success. The fact that the style transfer is based on permanent histology H&E, provides an intraoperative advantage. Initial pathology diagnosis for brain tumor surgery is usually based on frozen section histology, with formal diagnosis awaiting the inspection of permanent histology slides requiring one to several days. The style transfer is based on rapidly acquired, on-the-fly (i.e., real time) *in vivo* intraoperative CLE images that most resemble the permanent histology; therefore, it is a significant advantage for interpretation. Frozen section histology often involves freezing artifact, cutting problems, and may have inconsistent staining for histological characteristics that are important for diagnosis. Style transferred CLE images are then most comparable to the permanent histology, and may be even better because CLE is imaging live tissue without such architectural disturbance.

In the future, application of more advanced methods for transferring patterns in the histology slides to the CLE images will be used to improve their interpretability. Because of the high number of CLE images acquired during a single case, style transfer could add value to such fluorescence images, and allows for computer-aided techniques to play a meaningful, convenient, and efficient role to aid the neurosurgeon and neuropathologist in analysis of CLE images and to more rapidly determine diagnosis.

AUTHOR'S NOTE

This research article was part of a Ph.D. dissertation (12).

AUTHOR CONTRIBUTIONS

MI, EB, YY, and MP conceived and wrote the article. MI and YY formulated computer learning systems. LM, XZ, SG, CC, and EB assessed the quality of images. PN acquired images from neurosurgical cases. JE examined the CLE and histology images.

REFERENCES

1. Martirosyan NL, Georges J, Eschbacher JM, Cavalcanti DD, Elhadi AM, Abdelwahab MG, et al. Potential application of a handheld confocal endomicroscope imaging system using a variety of fluorophores in experimental gliomas and normal brain. *Neurosurg Focus.* (2014) 36:E16. doi: 10.3171/2013.11.FOCUS13486
2. Foersch S, Heimann A, Ayyad A, Spoden GA, Florin L, Mpoukouvalas K, et al. Confocal laser endomicroscopy for diagnosis and histomorphologic imaging of brain tumors *in vivo*. *PLoS ONE.* (2012) 7:e41760. doi: 10.1371/journal.pone.0041760
3. Belykh E, Miller EJ, Patel AA, IzadyYazdanabadi M, Martirosyan NL, Yagmurlu K, et al. Diagnostic accuracy of the confocal laser endomicroscope for *in vivo* differentiation between normal and tumor tissue during fluorescein-guided glioma resection: laboratory investigation. *World Neurosurg.* (2018) 115:e337–48. doi: 10.1016/j.wneu.2018.04.048
4. Izadyyazdanabadi M, Belykh E, Mooney M, Martirosyan N, Eschbacher J, Nakaji P, et al. Convolutional neural networks: ensemble modeling, fine-tuning and unsupervised semantic localization for neurosurgical CLE images. *J Vis Commun Image Represent.* (2018) 54:10–20. doi: 10.1016/j.jvcir.2018.04.004
5. Martirosyan NL, Eschbacher JM, Kalani MYS, Turner JD, Belykh E, Spetzler RF, et al. Prospective evaluation of the utility of intraoperative confocal laser endomicroscopy in patients with brain neoplasms using fluorescein sodium: experience with 74 cases. *Neurosurg Focus.* (2016) 40:E11. doi: 10.3171/2016.1.FOCUS15559
6. Izadyyazdanabadi M, Belykh E, Martirosyan N, Eschbacher J, Nakaji P, Yang Y, et al. Improving utility of brain tumor confocal laser endomicroscopy: objective value assessment and diagnostic frame detection with convolutional neural networks. In: *Progress in Biomedical Optics and Imaging - Proceedings of SPIE* (Orlando, FL), (2017).

7. Gatys LA, Ecker AS, Bethge M. Image Style Transfer using convolutional neural networks. In: *2016 IEEE Conference on Computer Vision and Pattern Recognition (CVPR)* (Las Vegas, NV), (2016).
8. Zhu C, Byrd RH, Lu P, Nocedal J. Algorithm 778: L-BFGS-B: fortran subroutines for large-scale bound-constrained optimization. *ACM Trans Math Softw.* (1997) 23:550–60. doi: 10.1145/279232.279236
9. Gu Y, Vyas K, Yang J, Yang G. Transfer recurrent feature learning for endomicroscopy image recognition. *IEEE Trans Med Imaging.* (2019) 38:791–801. doi: 10.1109/TMI.2018.2872473
10. Rivenson Y, Wang H, Wei Z, de Haan K, Zhang Y, Wu Y, et al. Virtual histological staining of unlabelled tissue-autofluorescence images via deep learning. *Nat Biomed Eng.* (2019) 3:466–77. doi: 10.1038/s41551-019-0362-y
11. Shaban MT, Baur C, Navab N, Albarqouni S. Staingan: stain style transfer for digital histological images. *arXiv [Preprint]. arXiv:180401601.* (2018). Available online at: https://arxiv.org/abs/1804.01601
12. Yazdanabadi MI. *Confocal laser endomicroscopy image analysis with deep convolutional neural networks* (Doctoral dissertation). Arizona State University, Tempe, AZ, United States (2019).

18

Indocyanine-Green for Fluorescence-Guided Surgery of Brain Tumors: Evidence, Techniques and Practical Experience

Steve S. Cho [1,2]***, Ryan Salinas*** [2] ***and John Y. K. Lee*** [2*]

[1] Perelman School of Medicine at the University of Pennsylvania, Philadelphia, PA, United States, [2] Department of Neurosurgery at the Hospital of the University of Pennsylvania, Philadelphia, PA, United States

***Correspondence:**
John Y. K. Lee
leejohn@uphs.upenn.edu

The primary treatment for brain tumors often involves surgical resection for diagnosis, relief of mass effect, and prolonged survival. In neurosurgery, it is of utmost importance to achieve maximal safe resection while minimizing iatrogenic neurologic deficit. Thus, neurosurgeons often rely on extra tools in the operating room, such as neuronavigation, intraoperative magnetic resonance imaging, and/or intraoperative rapid pathology. However, these tools can be expensive, not readily available, time-consuming, and/or inaccurate. Recently, fluorescence-guided surgery has emerged as a cost-effective method to accurately visualize neoplastic areas in real-time to guide resection. Currently, 5-aminolevulinic-acid (5-ALA) remains the only fluorophore that has been approved specifically for fluorescence-guided tumor resection. Its use has demonstrated improved resection rates and prolonged progression-free survival. However, protoporphyrin-IX, the metabolic product of 5-ALA that accumulates in neoplastic cells, fluoresces in the visible-light range, which suffers from limited tissue penetration and significant auto-fluorescence. Near-infrared fluorescence, on the other hand, overcomes these problems with ease. Since 2012, researchers at our institution have developed a novel technique using indocyanine-green, which is a well-known near-infrared fluorophore used traditionally for angiography. This Second-Window-ICG (SWIG) technique takes advantage of the increased endothelial permeability in peritumoral tissue, which allows indocyanine-green to accumulate in these areas for intraoperative visualization of the tumor. SWIG has demonstrated utility in gliomas, meningiomas, metastases, pituitary adenomas, chordomas, and craniopharyngiomas. The main benefits of SWIG stem from its highly sensitive detection of neoplastic tissue in a wide variety of intracranial pathologies in real-time, which can help neurosurgeons both during surgical resections and in stereotactic biopsies. In this review of this novel technique, we summarize the development and mechanism of action of SWIG, provide evidence for its benefits, and discuss its limitations. Finally, for those interested in near-infrared fluorescence-guided surgery, we provide suggestions for maximizing the benefits while minimizing the limitations of SWIG based on our own experience thus far.

Keywords: indocyanine-green, near-infrared, tumor resection, enhanced-permeability and retention effect, fluorescence-guided surgery

INTRODUCTION

Surgical resection of brain tumors remains an important part of cancer care for pathologic diagnosis, relief of mass effect, and survival benefit (1–9). However, radical resections, such as those practiced in other surgical fields, in the brain could result in neurologic morbidity that may outweigh the benefits of surgery (10). Neurosurgeons must thus balance the goals of maximal resection with minimizing neurologic deficits, which is a difficult task. Indeed, gross-total-resection (GTR) rates for intracranial tumors range from <30% for glioblastoma-multiforme (GBM) and other high-grade gliomas (HGG) to ~70% for benign meningiomas or pituitary adenomas, and tumors recur even after perceived GTR (11–16). Therefore, it is of paramount importance that neurosurgeons intraoperatively distinguish neoplasm from benign brain parenchyma and surrounding tissue. In addition to enhanced illumination, magnification, and experienced interpretation of tissue color and texture, neurosurgeons often rely on extra tools in the operating room, such as neuronavigation, intraoperative magnetic resonance imaging (MRI), intraoperative rapid pathology, and/or intraoperative ultrasound (17, 18). However, these modalities can have significant drawbacks, such as brain-shifts for neuronavigation and low availability, high cost, and high false-positive rate for intraoperative MRI (17–21). Recently, fluorescence-guided surgery (FGS) has emerged as a rapid and cost-effective alternative to these techniques.

In June 2017, the US Food and Drug Administration (FDA) approved 5-aminolevulinic-acid (5-ALA) as an agent for fluorescence-guided neurosurgery. First tried in neurosurgery in 1998, 5-ALA is a prodrug that leads to selective accumulation of a fluorophore, protoporphyrin IX (PpIX), in malignant cells, which can then be visualized intraoperatively using blue-light excitation (22–28). In a pivotal randomized-control study, Stummer et al. demonstrated that 5-ALA fluorescence-guided surgery led to a 65% GTR rate, compared to 36% in the control group in patients with high-grade gliomas (29). Other studies have replicated the benefits of 5-ALA in high-grade gliomas, as well as potential benefit in other intracranial tumors, such as meningiomas and pituitary adenomas (30–32). Despite the rigorous evidence that 5-ALA use is advantageous, it has visible-light emission that is significantly absorbed by endogenous fluorophores (i.e., heme), limiting its tissue penetration. Furthermore, the brain has numerous endogenous fluorophores, such as lipofuscin or flavin, with excitation/emission spectra that can overlap significantly with PpIX, reducing contrast between the tumor and the background brain (**Figure 1A**).

Fluorescein is another FDA-approved fluorophore that has traditionally been used for angiography in ophthalmology but with recent applications in tumor surgery. Studies have demonstrated that a bolus injection of fluorescein during the operation leads to fluorescein accumulating in areas of blood-brain-barrier breakdown in the peritumoral tissue. Fluorescein has demonstrated a range of sensitivity and specificity for intracranial tumors in prior studies, with generally high sensitivity but lower specificity compared to 5-ALA (33–39). Like 5-ALA, fluorescein is a visible-light fluorophore and suffers from limited visualization through tissue and weak contrast from surrounding normal brain (**Figure 1B**). Some have attempted dual-injections of 5-ALA and fluorescein to enhance detection of neoplastic tissue by increasing the contrast between the neoplastic tissue that uptake 5-ALA and the peritumoral area that uptake fluorescein (40).

More recently, indocyanine-green (ICG), a near-infrared (NIR) fluorophore (peak excitation = 805 nm, peak emission = 835 nm), has demonstrated utility in labeling tumor tissue. Unlike the conventional use of ICG as an angiographic agent, a novel technique using ICG, termed the Second Window ICG (SWIG), has been demonstrated in recent years. Due to the limitations of 5-ALA and fluorescein mentioned earlier, we have focused on NIR fluorophores. Thus, we investigated SWIG in various intracranial tumors, including high-grade gliomas, meningiomas, brain metastases, and pituitary adenomas. In this article, we review the brief history and hypothesized mechanism of action behind SWIG, examine the evidences supporting its use neurosurgery, detail specific operative techniques to minimize errors, and describe our group's practical experience with this novel technique.

HISTORY AND MECHANISM OF ACTION OF SWIG IN INTRACRANIAL TUMORS

Neurosurgeons are familiar with ICG and its role as an angiographic agent since the 1960s. ICG is a small, amphiphilic molecule (<800 daltons) that, when injected intravenously, normally remains within the blood vessel mostly bound to albumin and other plasma proteins. It is removed by biliary excretion and has a very short half-life of <180 s. Due to this short half-life, ICG is usually given as a bolus dose of <0.5 mg/kg and NIR imaging is performed immediately afterwards to delineate the vasculature.

In 1993, Hansen et al. described a technique using ICG boluses to create contrast between neoplastic tissue and brain parenchyma in rat models, rather than just visualizing vasculature (41); this was soon followed by another study by Haglund et al. in rats (42) and in human patients (43). In this last study, patients received a bolus of ICG at 1 mg/kg and then were imaged for up to 10 min after the bolus dosing, allowing ICG to accumulate in the tumor while washing out of the surrounding parenchyma. In patients with HGG, significant contrast between tumor and background was detected, while in patients with low-grade gliomas (LGG), this contrast decreased significantly between 4 and 10 min after ICG injection.

Finally, in a 2012 study, Madajewski et al. proposed that a high-dose infusion of ICG (7.5 mg/kg) given 24 h prior to surgery allows ICG to accumulate in areas of neoplasm, facilitating detection of residual neoplasm after standard resection in murine flank tumor models (44). This effect was confirmed in a follow-up dose-confirmation study in a murine flank tumor model (45) and was further demonstrated in a murine intracranial tumor model by our lab (46). It has been hypothesized that the accumulation of ICG occurs through the well-described enhanced permeability and retention (EPR) effect, which stipulates that solid tumors

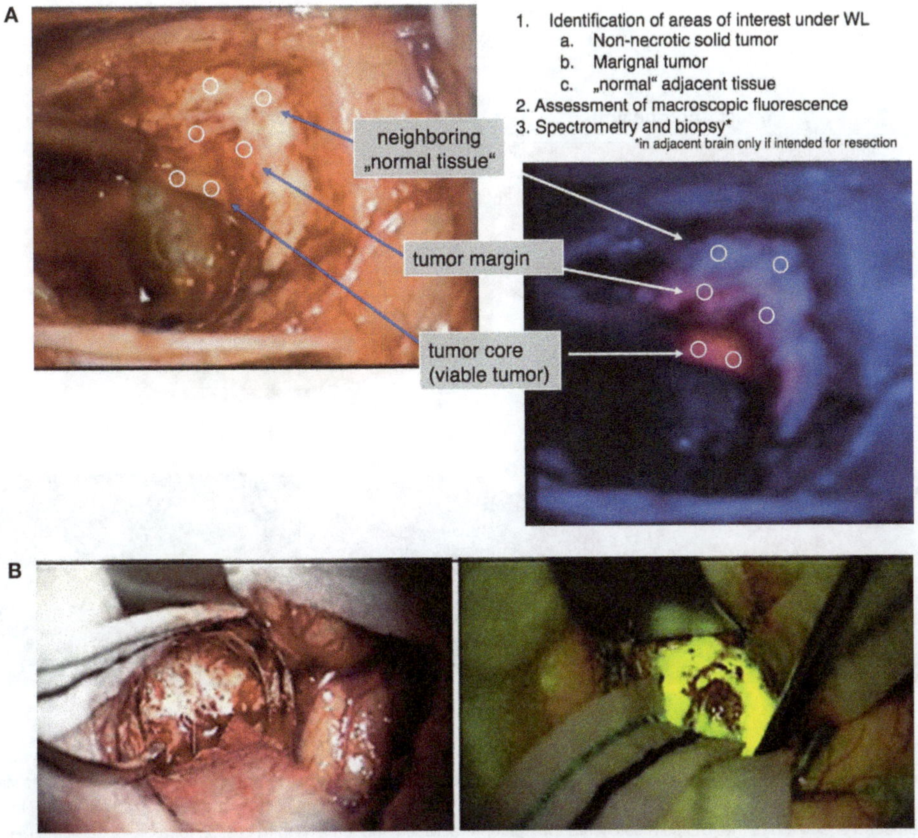

FIGURE 1 | Examples of visible light fluorophores used in brain tumor resection. **(A)** 5-ALA is an oral prodrug that is converted to proptoporphyrin-IX, a visible light fluorophore with red emission, in high-grade neoplastic cells. Under blue-light excitation (400–410 nm), pink areas correspond to areas of neoplasm against the dark-blue background (28). **(B)** Fluorescein is a visible-light fluorophore with yellow emission that highlights areas of blood-brain-barrier damage. When injected intravenously 1–3 h prior to tumor exposure, areas of tumor can be visualized in yellow using yellow-green (460–500 nm) excitation (38).

possess enhanced vascular permeability due to defective vascular structures, impaired lymphatic drainage systems, and increased permeability mediators (47). ICG then accumulates in these areas of enhanced vascular permeability and can be visualized 24-h later (**Figure 2**) (48).

EVIDENCE AND POTENTIAL BENEFITS OF SWIG

SWIG has been investigated in various intracranial applications (**Table 1**). We summarize the results below and discuss potential implications.

Intra-Axial Brain Tumors: Gliomas and Metastases

In 2016, we published the results of the first SWIG study in 15 patients with gliomas (49). An important discovery was that the strongest predictor of positive intraoperative NIR fluorescence was contrast-enhancement on preoperative MRI (p-value = 0.03) (**Figure 3A**). NIR fluorescence could be detected from tumors >1 cm deep and in 8 patients, the tumor could be detected prior to durotomy. In contrast-enhancing gliomas (12/15 in this study), SWIG demonstrated 98% sensitivity, 45% specificity, 82% positive-predictive-value (PPV) and 90% negative-predictive-value (NPV) for detecting areas of neoplasm in biopsy specimens, with an area under the receiver operating characteristic curve (AUROC) of 0.715. In comparison, white-light alone was 84% sensitive and 80% specific for neoplasm, with a PPV of 92%, NPV of 67%, and AUROC of 0.822. Updated data from our group that is yet unpublished shows that SWIG has a PPV of 88% and NPV of 63% for margin specimens in contrast-enhancing gliomas, compared to white-light alone with a PPV of 100% and NPV of 38%. Furthermore, data currently under review for publication suggests that NIR imaging of the surgical bed after resection can increase the surgeon's confidence that GTR has been achieved if there are no residual areas of NIR fluorescence (**Figures 3B–E**).

The utility of SWIG was also investigated in 13 patients with various intracranial metastases in a 2017 study (50). SWIG demonstrated higher sensitivity (96 vs. 82%) and NPV (75 vs. 67%) but lower specificity (27 vs. 91%) and PPV (77 vs. 96%). AUROC with SWIG was 0.619, whereas AUROC with white-light alone was 0.865. NIR signal was visualized through the dura in 11 patients and in patients with sub-surface tumors, NIR signal could be visualized at least to a depth of 6.8 mm below the cortex (**Figure 4**).

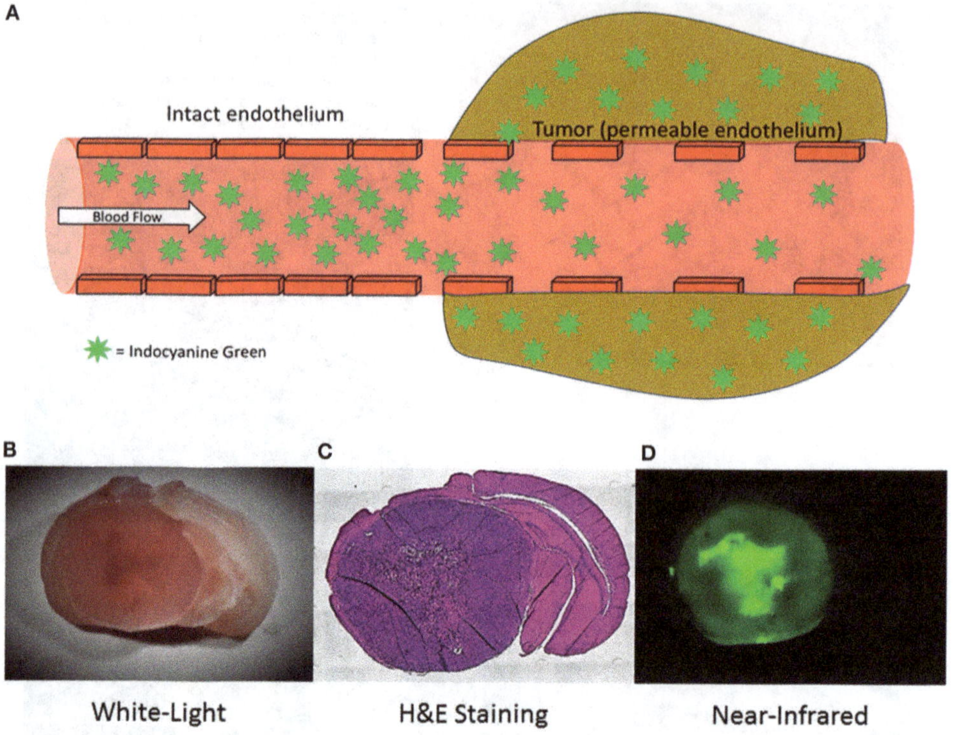

FIGURE 2 | Mechanism of action for Second Window Indocyanine Green (SWIG) **(A)** ICG is hypothesized to accumulate in neoplastic areas via the enhanced permeability and retention effect. In areas of normal brain, with intact endothelium, the ICG remains intravascular and washes away quickly. In areas of tumor, which often have permeable/damaged endothelium, the ICG permeates into the peritumoral tissue and remains in the tissue for a prolonged time (54). **(B–D)** SWIG in murine model of GBM (U87 cells). Under white-light alone **(B)**, it is difficult to visualize the full extent of the tumor, which is demonstrated by hematoxylin and eosin (H&E) staining **(C)**. With SWIG **(D)**, however, both the core of the tumor and the margin are delineated under near-infrared fluorescence.

TABLE 1 | Summary of studies investigating near-infrared fluorescence guided neurosurgery with second-window ICG.

References	Tumor type (n)	Sensitivity (WL, NIR)	Specificity (WL, NIR)	PPV (WL, NIR)	NPV (WL, NIR)
Lee et al. (49)	Gliomas (15)	84% 98%	80% 45%	92% 82%	67% 90%
Lee et al. (50)	Metastases (13)	82% 96%	91% 27%	96% 77%	67% 75%
Lee et al. (51)	Meningiomas (18)	82% 96%	100% 39%	100% 71%	78% 88%
Cho et al. (52)	Varied (6)	NA	NA	NA	NA
Jeon et al. (53)	Skull-base Tumors (15)	NA	NA	NA	NA
Cho et al. (54)	Pituitary Adenomas (16)	88% 100%	90% 29%	96% 82%	73% 100%

NA, Not applicable; NIR, Near-infrared; NPV, Negative-predictive value; PPV, Positive-predictive value; WL, White-light.

The latest application for SWIG under investigation is in stereotactic biopsies of intracranial tumors. Currently, stereotactic brain biopsies may have prolonged operative time due to the need for confirmation of abnormal tissue from frozen pathology. If the result is inconclusive, this may require further biopsy specimens in the operating room. However, using SWIG, the neurosurgeon can examine biopsied specimens *ex-vivo* for NIR fluorescence in the operating room. If the tissue is non-fluorescent, chances are very high that the specimen is not neoplastic or otherwise abnormal due to the highly sensitive nature of SWIG for neoplasm, and thus, another biopsy should be taken; conversely, with fluorescent tissue, the surgeon can be confident that abnormal tissue was biopsied (data under review) (**Figure 5**). Thus, SWIG offers an affordable, rapid, and accurate adjunct to stereotactic biopsies to increase the neurosurgeons' confidence and reduce operating length.

Extra-Axial Brain Tumors: Meningiomas, Pituitary Adenomas, and Others

SWIG has demonstrated sensitive detection of neoplasm in extra-axial tumors as well. In a 2017 study of SWIG in 18 meningioma patients (15 grade I, 3 grade II), NIR imaging detected strong fluorescence in 14 tumors (51). It was noted that 4 tumors demonstrated "inverse" NIR fluorescence, in which the background signal was higher than the signal within the tumor, and linear regression suggested that time from ICG injection was negatively correlated with NIR fluorescence contrast (p-value $= 0.022$, $R^2 = 0.2876$); we have hypothesized that this inverse fluorescence may be due to either quenching of ICG that can occur at concentrations >125 ug/L (52) or the slow permeation of ICG out of the neoplastic tissue into the surrounding area

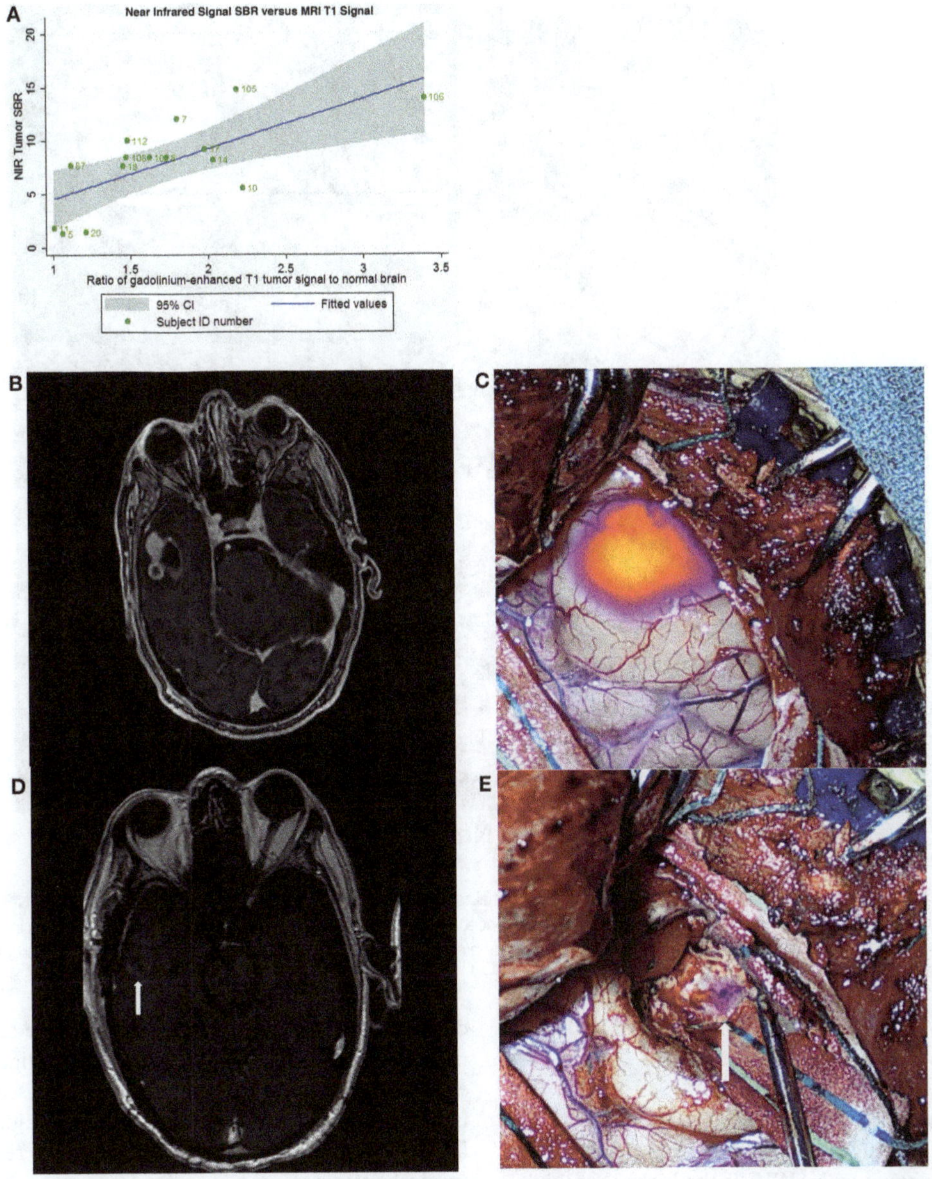

FIGURE 3 | Utility of SWIG in patients with GBM. **(A)** The amount of near-infrared fluorescence detected in tumors after SWIG administration positively correlates with contrast-enhancement on preoperative MRI (p-value 0.03), suggesting that SWIG can label contrast-enhancing tissue in real-time (49). **(B,C)** A contrast-enhancing GBM demonstrates strong NIR fluorescence in the operating room after durotomy. This technique does not suffer from brain-shifts, unlike neuronavigation. **(D,E)** After standard resection, NIR imaging of the surgical bed demonstrates no residual areas of strong NIR fluorescence. Postoperative day-1 MRI demonstrates postoperative changes with gross-total resection. Arrows indicate the orientation of the surgical bed. In patients whom post-resection NIR imaging does not demonstrate residual NIR fluorescence, the neurosurgeon can be more confident that gross-total resection has been achieved.

after 24 h, although neither has been definitively demonstrated. Overall, SWIG demonstrated 96% sensitivity, 39% specificity, 71% PPV, and 88% NPV for detecting neoplasm in these meningioma patients with an AUROC of 0.677, compared to white-light alone, which showed 82% sensitivity, 100% specificity, 100% PPV, and 78% NPV with an AUROC of 0.911.

Finally, SWIG is applicable to skull base tumors, such as pituitary adenomas, chordomas, and craniopharyngiomas, which were accessed via the transnasal/transsphenoidal approach. A 2018 study of 8 pituitary adenomas, 3 craniopharyngiomas, and 4 chordomas demonstrated that all the tumors demonstrated NIR fluorescence (**Figure 6**) (53). Again, contrast-enhancement on preoperative MRI was the best predictor of NIR fluorescence contrast to normal background (p-value = 0.0003). In pituitary adenomas, SWIG demonstrated 100% sensitivity, 20% specificity, 71% PPV, and 100% NPV for neoplasm in biopsy specimens, compared to white-light alone with 90% sensitivity, 100% specificity, 100% PPV, and 83% NPV (n = 15). A more recent study shows that SWIG had 100% sensitivity, 29% specificity, 82% PPV, and 100% NPV (n = 30), whereas white-light

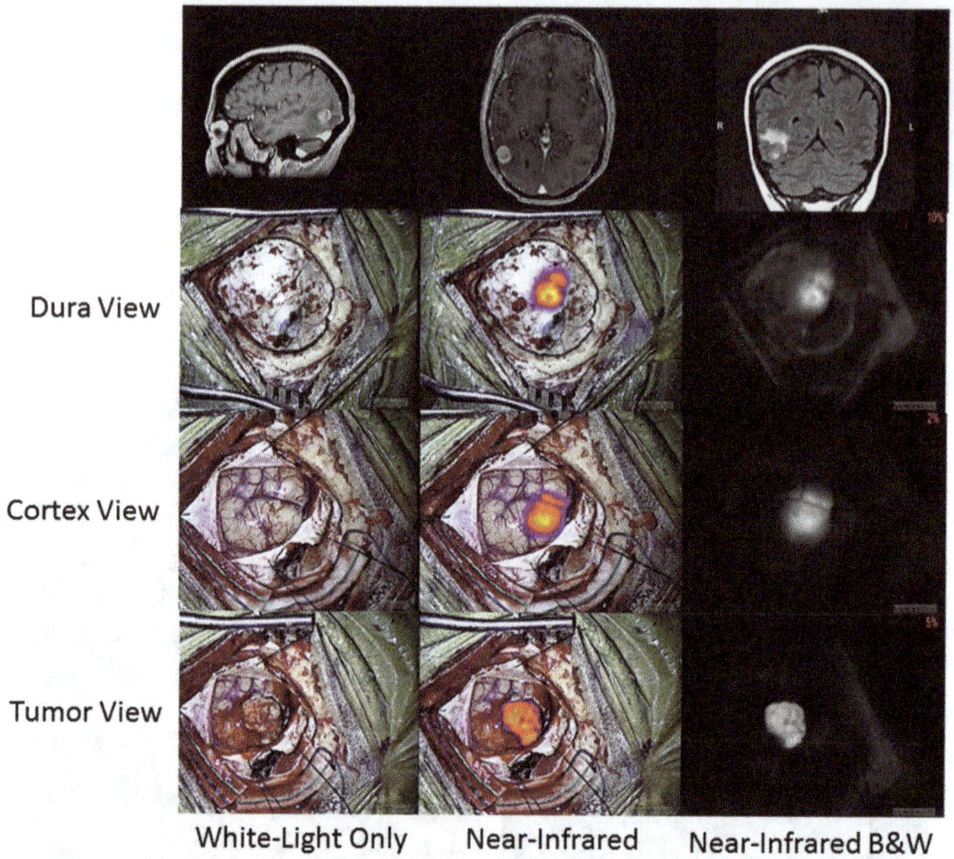

FIGURE 4 | Further clinical applications of SWIG in neurosurgery—trans-dural visualization. In this patient with a subcortical brain metastasis, NIR imaging localized the tumor through intact dura as well as intact cortex. Unlike visible-light fluorescence, NIR fluorescence can travel through tissue up to >1 cm in the brain. Since NIR imaging provides real-time localization of tumor, this can help neurosurgeons better plan the access through the dura and minimize cortical disruption (50).

had 88% sensitivity, 90% specificity, 96% PPV, and 73% NPV ($n = 78$) (54).

Benefits of SWIG in Neurosurgery

Overall, these studies suggest that the main benefit of intraoperative NIR imaging with SWIG is the higher sensitivity and NPV for detecting neoplastic tissue, which may allow surgeons to detect more residual neoplasm at the margins after resection than with white-light alone, increasing the chances of achieving GTR. SWIG studies thus far are all limited by the fact that the scope of surgery was not changed depending on NIR imaging, as SWIG was a technique under investigation at the time. In other words, even if the senior surgeon observed residual areas of fluorescent tissue after standard resection, further resection was not performed. Therefore, it is currently difficult to quantify the effects NIR imaging with SWIG on surgical outcomes. However, given that 5-ALA, with lower sensitivity (~70–90%), similar PPV (>95%), and much lower NPV (19–24%) has demonstrated benefit in increasing GTR rates and progression-free survival (29), it is not unreasonable to expect that fluorescence-guided surgery with SWIG would lead to equally improved, if not better, surgical outcomes compared to surgery with 5-ALA. Furthermore, the results demonstrating correlation between absence of fluorescence and GTR in HGG is encouraging as well. A study to investigate changing the extent of surgery according to NIR fluorescence with SWIG is currently under way and will better elucidate the effects of fluorescence-guided surgery with SWIG on resection rates and surgical outcomes.

In contrast to PpIX or fluorescein, SWIG imaging utilizes NIR fluorescence, leading to great tissue penetration. The longer NIR wavelength allows the photons to travel further in the body, especially in less dense tissue, because there is less absorption by hemoglobin and other proteins (55, 56). Thus, as demonstrated in the above studies, NIR fluorescence from subcortical tumors can be imaged through intact dura and cortex, which is not possible with white-light visualization or with 5-ALA, except under very limited circumstances with specialized equipment (57). Furthermore, since NIR imaging is performed in real-time, SWIG does not suffer from brain shifts and other inaccuracies in directing the surgeon toward the tumor bulk as can be seen in neuronavigation. Both the deeper tissue signal and the real-time feedback can benefit the surgeon in accurately planning access through the dura and minimizing cortical disruption.

Finally, a defining feature of SWIG is its widespread applicability. Unlike receptor-targeted dyes or metabolic dyes,

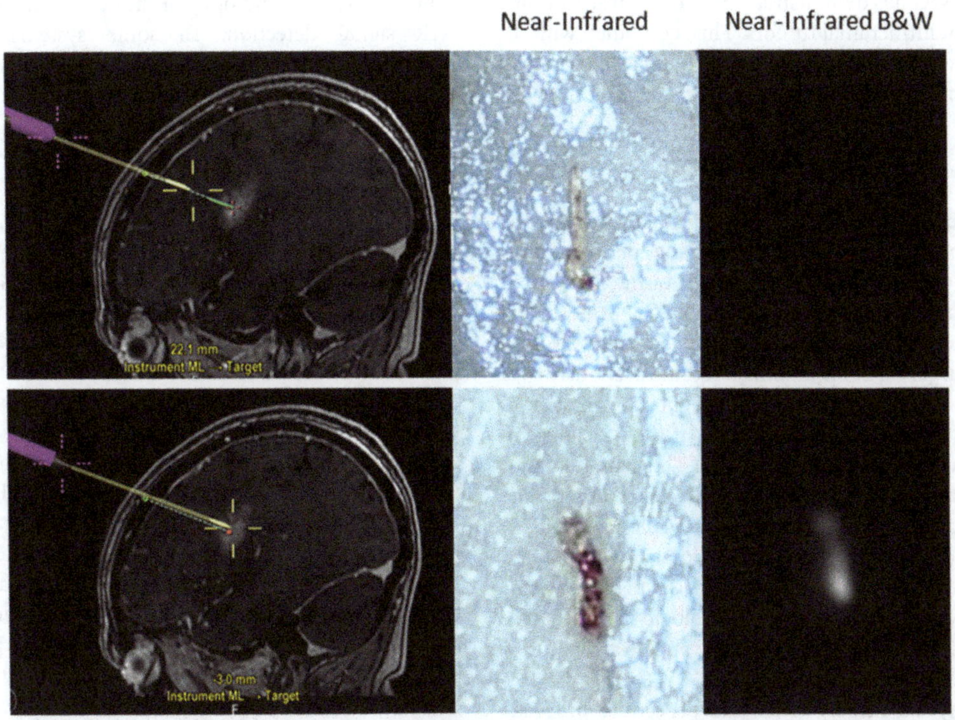

FIGURE 5 | Application of SWIG for stereotactic biopsies. Stereotactic biopsies with SWIG offer rapid confirmation that abnormal tissue was biopsied. When a sample was biopsied outside the contrast-enhancing legion using neuronavigation (top row), it did not demonstrate NIR fluorescence and was normal tissue on the frozen pathology. On the contrary, when a sample was biopsied within the contrast-enhancement (bottom row), it demonstrated NIR fluorescence and pathology diagnosis was GBM. Thus, SWIG offers an affordable, rapid, and accurate adjunct to stereotactic biopsies to reduce operating length.

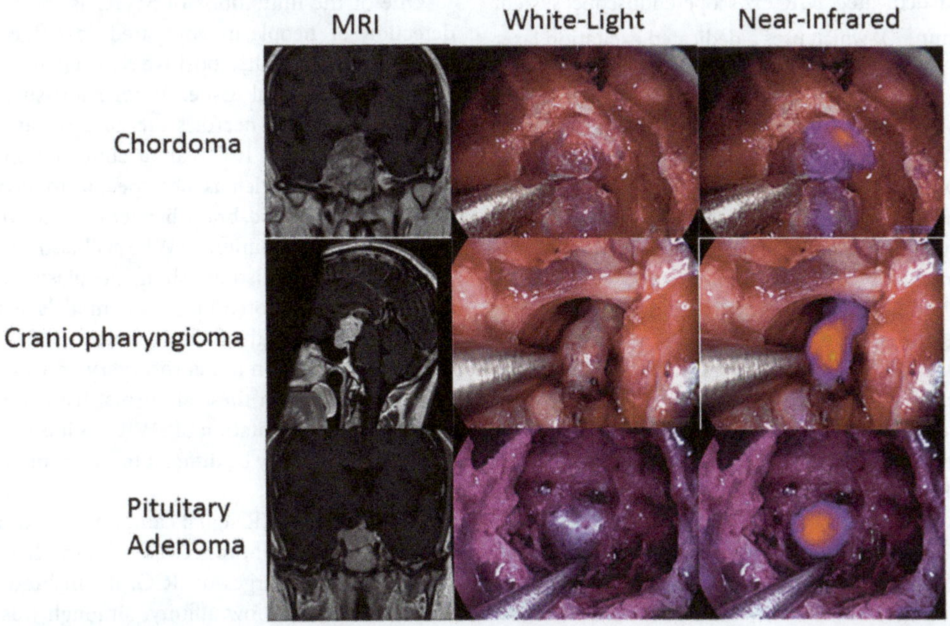

FIGURE 6 | SWIG in extra-axial brain tumors. Patients with chordomas (top row), craniopharyngiomas (middle row), and pituitary adenomas (bottom row) all demonstrate NIR fluorescence with SWIG. Visualization was performed with a NIR-sensitive endoscope system (53).

such as 5-ALA, SWIG has demonstrated nearly equivalent utility in a wide variety of intracranial tumors. This, combined with the high availability of ICG, makes SWIG an easily accessible adjunct to the armamentarium of neurosurgeons world-wide.

TECHNICAL CONSIDERATIONS

SWIG is fundamentally different from traditional angiography with ICG or the minimally delayed imaging performed by Haglund et al. In order to take full advantage of the EPR effect, ICG must be administered between 16 and 30 h prior to the surgery (46). Generally, patients receive an outpatient infusion the day prior to surgery. ICG is administered intravenously over 1 h, at a dose of 5 mg per kg of body weight. The patient is closely monitored throughout the duration of the infusion and for 30 min afterwards for any adverse events. Thus, far, no major complications from ICG administration has been reported. The patient then returns the next day for the surgery. Of note, in a few recent cases, including a spinal cord meningioma and peripheral nerve schwannoma, ICG was administered 6–8 h prior to tumor exposure. While NIR imaging detected pathologic tissue in these cases, there is still insufficient evidence to validate this shorter time window in humans.

Intraoperatively, the surgery setup and procedure proceeds as per standard of care, with the one exception of having a dedicated NIR imaging device present in the operating room. While conventional surgical microscopes have add-on modules that allow NIR imaging of ICG, these were designed for ICG angiography with a much higher concentration of ICG. These modules are not sensitive enough to low concentrations of ICG and do not have a wide dynamic range. Our group uses a dedicated NIR exoscope/endoscope system (VisionSense Iridium™), which uses a dedicated excitation laser and an integrated post-acquisition image processing. This allows simultaneous visualization of visual light, NIR signal alone, and an overlaid augmented-reality type display of both signals simultaneously. This system was identified as having superior sensitivity and dynamic range compared to other commercial NIR imaging platforms in a comparison study by DSouza et al. (58). Our group further compared the dedicated NIR exoscope system to a commercial neurosurgical microscope module and demonstrated that for SWIG fluorescence-guided surgery, the dedicated NIR system is more suitable, as it can more reliably detect NIR fluorescence through the dura and detect NIR signal from neoplastic tissue with a higher tumor-to-brain contrast over a larger dynamic range of NIR fluorescent signal (**Figure 7**) (52). Other dedicated NIR imaging platforms with strong excitation and high-quality image-processing may also be viable options. More sophisticated add-on modules for surgical microscopes are emerging as well.

In order to minimize background and maximize signal detection, ambient light should be minimized. During the SWIG visualization of the procedure, both room and overhead operating lights are turned off as even these lights can lead to some degree of NIR signal detection. Furthermore, careful consideration should be made if simultaneous neuronavigation is utilized. It has been noted that neuronavigation systems utilizing NIR technology for fiducial detection interfere with NIR signal detection. In some systems, a pulsing NIR light is generated from the neuronavigation "camera" and is visualized by the NIR imaging system as a pulsing, high background signal. Therefore, the neuronavigation camera should be directed away from the field while using any SWIG detection system.

After craniotomy but before durotomy, the NIR imaging modules is introduced into the field to assess whether the tumor can be visualized through the dura. In many cases of superficial tumors, the tumor boundary can be easily delineated through the dura. Durotomy is then performed and repeat NIR imaging is performed to confirm tumor location. In cases of deep tumors, neuronavigation is used to locate and expose the tumor. Once the tumor is exposed, NIR fluorescence of the gross tumor specimen is measured. Then, resection of the tumor proceeds in the standard of care manner, without NIR imaging. After the senior neurosurgeon is satisfied with the resection, NIR imaging is again performed to assess for residual fluorescence. Depending on the protocol, any areas of residual fluorescence can be simply recorded, biopsied, or completely removed. Closure is then performed in a standard manner and the patient undergoes postoperative MRI to assess the extent of resection.

PRACTICAL EXPERIENCE

During our experience with SWIG over the past 4 years, we have come to better understand the various factors that can help or hinder surgeons utilizing SWIG fluorescence-guided surgery, which we detail below.

One of the limitations of SWIG is the higher false-positive detection of neoplasm compared to surgeon judgment with white-light alone. False-positive NIR signal can come from either abnormal or normal tissue. Abnormal tissue, such as neoplasm, inflammation, and necrosis are all associated with endothelial damage and thus, ICG can accumulate in these tissues via the EPR effect, which is not specific to neoplasm, but rather targets areas of blood-brain-barrier breakdown. Since these areas enhance with gadolinium, SWIG will also highlight these areas. The difficulty in distinguishing neoplasm from inflammation and necrosis was noted in murine models as well as canine and human patients with thoracic cancers (59). We have noted a similar phenomenon in neurosurgery, in which SWIG could not distinguish between these abnormal tissues (unpublished data). This is the main limitation of SWIG, as it is not a tumor-targeting dye, and it will likely be difficult to overcome without developing targeting moieties.

False-positive NIR signal can occur in normal tissues as well, especially in the skin, mucosa, and dura. It is believed that due to the negative charges on ICG, it can bind nonspecifically to these tissue with a low affinity, although this has not yet been definitively demonstrated as the cause. Thus, in many cases, we have observed NIR signal from skin, mucosa, and/or dura that are certainly not neoplastic. There are two steps that the surgeon can take in the operating room to minimize these false-positive signals.

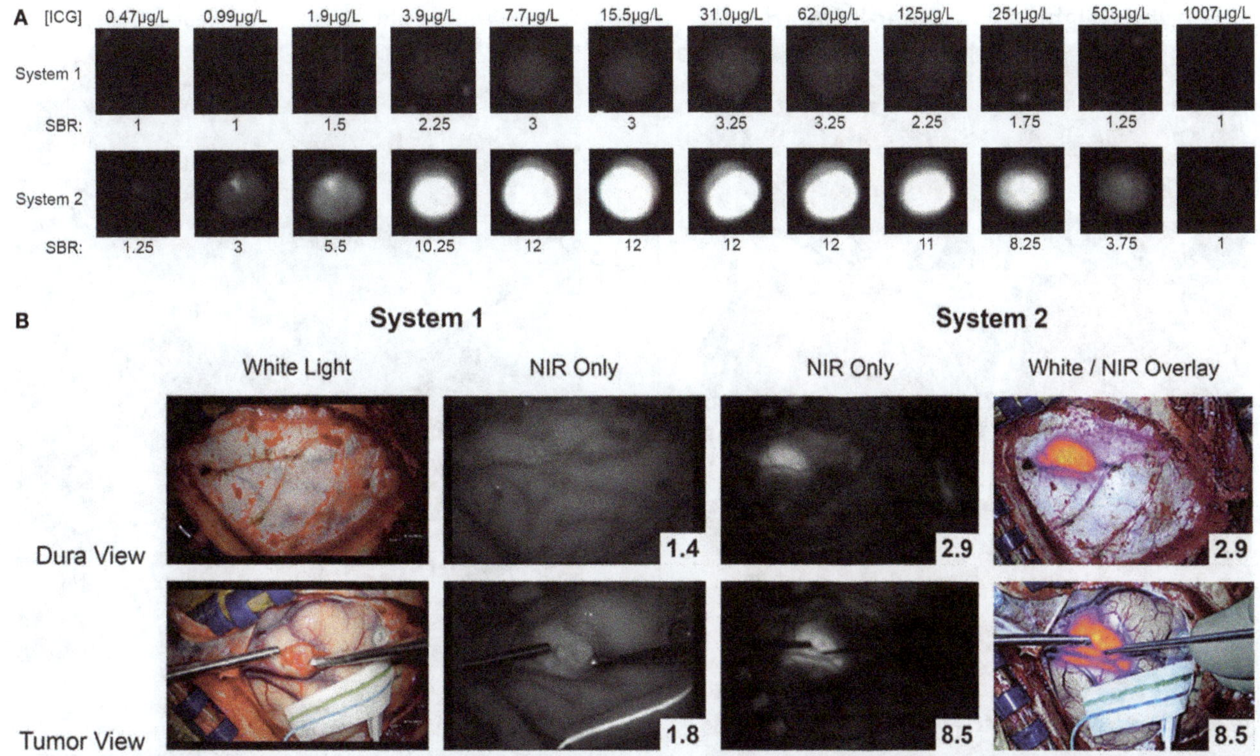

FIGURE 7 | A prior study compared a conventional state-of-the-art microscope (System 1) with a NIR-detecting module to a dedicated NIR-imaging system (System 2). In both *ex-vivo* **(A)** and *in-vivo* visualizations of ICG (**B**; NIR signal-to-background ratio in bottom right corner), System 2 was much more sensitive to NIR fluorescence, with a greater dynamic range. Furthermore, only System 2 was capable of imaging NIR fluorescence through the dura. Thus, for successful surgeries with SWIG, a sensitive, dedicated NIR imaging system is necessary (52).

Many NIR imaging systems have variable gains, which reflect the sensitivity of the camera sensor to the emission photons, that can be adjusted and fixed by the operator. The higher the gain, the more sensitive the camera, and the weaker the signals that can be detected. Thus, a gain that is set too high can result in detection of NIR fluorescence that isn't true neoplasm (**Figures 8A–D**) (51). One way to avoid this problem is to note the gain setting when the tumor is first exposed and then to fix the gain at that level throughout the rest of the surgery. The surgeon can then be confident that any NIR fluorescence that is detected is at the same level of fluorescence as the tumor, increasing the likelihood that the area of fluorescence is neoplastic.

Another factor that can contribute to false-positive NIR signals is the distance between the sensor and the tissue. This is more of a factor with endoscopic surgeries, as the scope is often brought to very close proximity to the tissue of interest for optimal visualization. Since optical signal decays as a factor of distance-squared, simply halving the distance between the endoscope and the tissue of interest can elevate the detected NIR signal 16-fold (4-fold increase in excitation strength, 4-fold increase in emission detection). Thus, similar to the gain above, having the endoscope too proximal to the tissue can cause falsely elevated NIR signal to be detected. In order to avoid this, the surgeon should attempt to visualize areas of suspected NIR fluorescence from a set distance. With the VisionSense Iridium endoscope in transsphenoidal surgeries for pituitary adenomas using a related NIR dye, we demonstrated that having the endoscope at a distance that maintains the distance between the two medial opticocarotid recesses to be <50% of the field of view is ideal for minimizing false-positive NIR signals (**Figures 8E–H**) (60, 61). Endoscopes that offer more precise distance measurements could further help the neurosurgeon to acquire more accurate NIR signals.

Furthermore, there are two factors that can hinder the surgeon's ability to detect true-positive NIR fluorescence: strong signal in the surrounding normal tissue and pooled blood. If the gain is properly set as described above, the surgeon should be able to detect residual areas of NIR fluorescence that is at the same level of fluorescence as the tumor, and thus, likely to be residual neoplasm. However, if there is a significant amount of fluorescence in the skin, mucosa, or dura surrounding the surgical bed, the NIR camera may not properly detect smaller areas of fluorescence. If the surrounding area is covered with surgical towels or gauze to isolate the surgical bed, small areas of residual fluorescence can be detected more easily (**Figures 9A–D**). Pooled blood can also often obscure areas of NIR fluorescence by physically blocking the excitation and emission lights (**Figures 9E,F**). Thus, when imaging for NIR

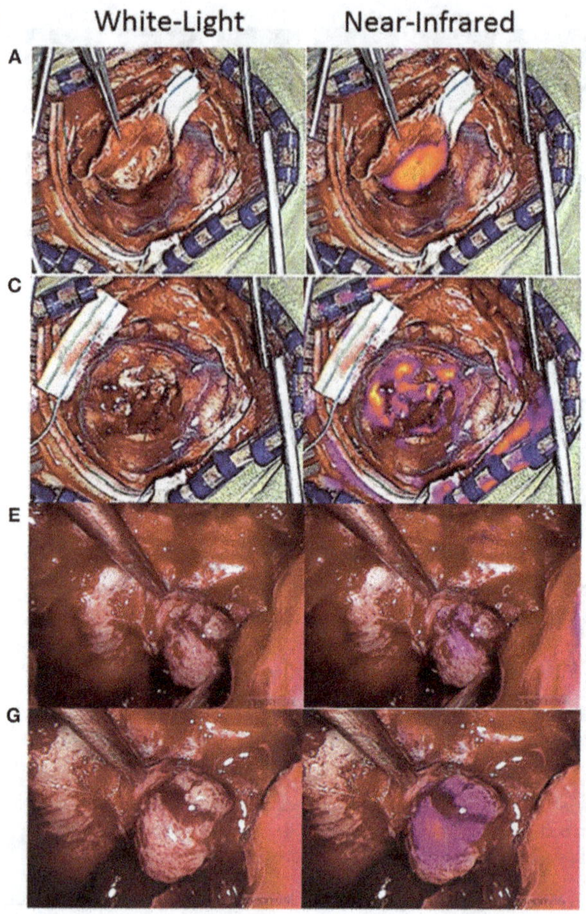

FIGURE 8 | False-positive NIR signal using SWIG. There are two main sources of false-positive signals that may arise during NIR imaging: high gain settings and small distance between the NIR sensor and the tissue. **(A–D)** Some NIR imaging systems have adjustable gain (NIR sensitivity) that need to be fixed in order to avoid detecting false-positive signals. When the tumor was first exposed in this patient with a meningioma **(A)**, the gain was at 15% and strong NIR fluorescence was detected from the tumor **(B)**. After resection **(C)**, NIR fluorescence was again detected, but the gain was at 71% **(D)**. Once the gain was adjusted down to 15%, those areas of NIR fluorescence disappeared, suggesting that the NIR signal had been false-positives (51). **(E–H)** In endoscopic fluorescence-guided surgery, the distance between the scope and the tissue of interest is important as well. Since optical signal decays as a factor of distance-squared, bringing the scope in close proximity to any tissue can result in fluorescence detection. This patient with a pituitary adenoma received a folate-receptor targeted near-infrared dye, but postoperative immunohistochemistry demonstrated no folate-receptor expression; thus, the tumor should not have demonstrated fluorescence. When the tumor was visualized from a distance **(E,F)**, there was minimal NIR signal; however, when the scope was brought closer to the tissue **(G,H)**, the tumor seemed to fluoresce. Thus, maintaining the proper distance between the endoscope and the tissue is of paramount importance in avoiding false-positive NIR signals (61).

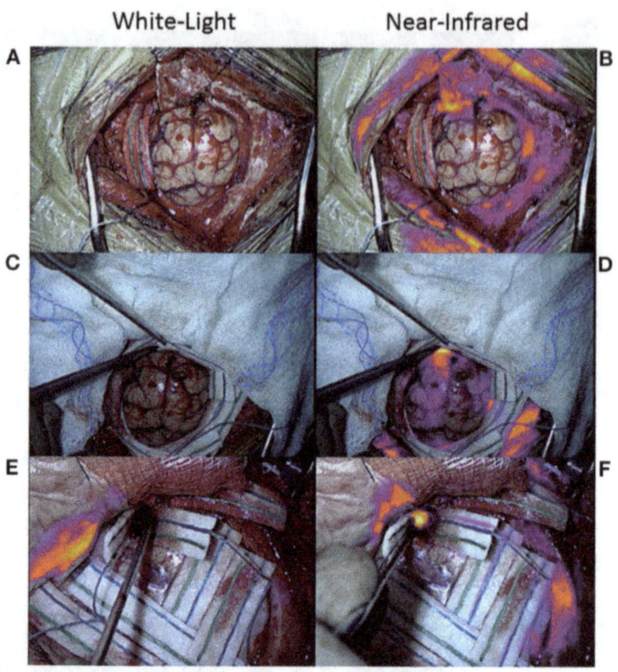

FIGURE 9 | False-negative NIR signal using SWIG. There are two main sources of false-negative signals that may arise during NIR imaging: surrounding, nonspecific NIR signal and blood/fluid. **(A–D)** Upon durotomy in this patient with a GBM, strong but nonspecific NIR signal was observed in the skin and dura, which masked any NIR signal coming from the actual tumor. Once the nonspecific signals were obscured by the surgeon, the NIR fluorescence from the tumor could be detected properly. **(E,F)** Blood and other fluids can obscure NIR fluorescence. In this patient, after standard resection, no NIR fluorescence was detected in the surgical bed initially. However, after removing blood and fluid, the underlying NIR fluorescence was detected.

fluorescence, it is important to achieve hemostasis to clear the field of blood and place the tissue of interest in direct line of the excitation light.

Overall, fluorescence-guided surgery using SWIG has technical intricacies that may require a learning curve. We have detailed the steps that neurosurgeons can take in the operating room to both minimize false-positive signals and to elucidate true-positive signals.

Finally, a consideration for neurosurgeons interested in the technique is the cost of SWIG. As mentioned previously, SWIG requires sensitive NIR imaging capabilities, which is best achieved with a dedicated imaging system, such as the VisionSense Iridium; this system currently costs approximately \$100–150 K depending on whether the endoscope function is available. The cost of ICG may vary by institution; a typical patient may need 350–400 mg of ICG (5 mg/kg bodyweight).

FUTURE RESEARCH

There are two main directions in which future research can improve NIR fluorescence-guided neurosurgery. One is improving the specificity of NIR imaging. Despite its potential benefits in the operating room, SWIG is limited mainly by its low specificity as it works through the EPR effect, which is not tumor-specific. One way to overcome this limitation may be to conjugate novel NIR dyes that target specific receptors on neoplastic cell surfaces. In fact, multiple such conjugates are currently being investigated in preclinical and clinical trials for different intracranial tumors. For instance, folate-receptor overexpression on nonfunctional pituitary adenomas and meningiomas may provide targets for sensitive and specific detection of these tumors in real-time (54, 60–62). An alternative is to use imaging apparatus with higher resolution for fluorescence, which may better distinguish true areas of fluorescence from areas of false-positive fluorescence. This has been demonstrated in murine models with fluorescein and ICG using confocal microscopy and may become applicable clinically (63, 64).

Another limitation of NIR imaging in the operating room is the low sensitivity of the imaging equipment. It is well-acknowledged, and our group has demonstrated, that conventional surgical microscopes with add-on NIR modules are significantly less sensitive for NIR fluorescence, especially at lower concentrations, than dedicated NIR imaging modules. Integrating the high NIR sensitivity into conventional microscopes will hugely increase the applicability of NIR fluorescence-guided neurosurgery, further increasing the potential benefits of this novel technique to improve patient outcomes.

CONCLUSION

Fluorescence-guided surgery with SWIG is a widely applicable technique that allows neurosurgeons to visualize tumors and residual neoplasm at the margins with greater sensitivity than with white-light and microscopy alone. In this review, we have explained the mechanism of SWIG and its potential benefits, as well as steps that neurosurgeons can take to maximize the utility of this novel technique. Results with SWIG thus far are encouraging and suggest potential benefit in improving patient outcomes in neurosurgery.

AUTHOR CONTRIBUTIONS

SC drafted the manuscript and prepared the figures and tables. RS and JL provided critical revisions for the manuscript. All authors agree to be accountable for the contents of this work.

ACKNOWLEDGMENTS

We would like to thank Jun Jeon, BS, and Carrie Li, BS who provided some of the figures for this review.

REFERENCES

1. Hammouche S, Clark S, Wong AH, Eldridge P, Farah JO. Long-term survival analysis of atypical meningiomas: survival rates, prognostic factors, operative and radiotherapy treatment. *Acta Neurochir.* (2014) 156:1475–81. doi: 10.1007/s00701-014-2156-z
2. Lacroix M, Abi-Said D, Fourney DR, Gokaslan ZL, Shi W, DeMonte F., et al. A multivariate analysis of 416 patients with glioblastoma multiforme: prognosis, extent of resection, and survival. *J Neurosurg.* (2001) 95:190–8. doi: 10.3171/jns.2001.95.2.0190
3. Patchell RA. The management of brain metastases. *Cancer Treat Rev.* (2003) 29:533–40.
4. Sanai N, Polley, M.-Y., McDermott MW, Parsa AT, Berger MS. An extent of resection threshold for newly diagnosed glioblastomas. *J Neurosurg.* (2011) 115:3–8. doi: 10.3171/2011.2.JNS10998
5. SIMPSON D. The recurrence of intracranial meningiomas after surgical treatment. *J Neurol Neurosurg Psychiatry.* (1957) 20:22–39.
6. Ezzat S, Asa SL, Couldwell WT, Barr CE, Dodge WE, Vance ML, et al. The prevalence of pituitary adenomas. *Cancer.* (2004) 101:613–9. doi: 10.1002/cncr.20412
7. Greenman Y, Cooper O, Yaish I, Robenshtok E, Sagiv N, Jonas-Kimchi T., et al. Treatment of clinically nonfunctioning pituitary adenomas with dopamine agonists. *Eur J Endocrinol.* (2016) 175:63–72. doi: 10.1530/EJE-16-0206
8. Lee JYK, Bohman, L-E, Bergsneider M. Contemporary neurosurgical techniques for pituitary tumor resection. *J Neurooncol.* (2014) 117:437–44. doi: 10.1007/s11060-013-1315-z
9. Stummer W, Kamp MA. The importance of surgical resection in malignant glioma. *Curr Opin Neurol.* (2009) 22:645–9. doi: 10.1097/WCO.0b013e3283320165
10. Zhang C, Zhao Y, Zhang H, Chen X, Zhao N, Tan D., et al. The application of heptamethine cyanine dye DZ-1 and indocyanine green for imaging and targeting in xenograft models of hepatocellular carcinoma. *Int J Mol Sci.* (2017) 18:1332. doi: 10.3390/ijms18061332
11. Schucht P, Beck J, Abu-Isa J, Andereggen L, Murek M, Seidel K., et al. Gross total resection rates in contemporary glioblastoma surgery. *Neurosurgery.* (2012) 71:927–36. discussion 935–6. doi: 10.1227/NEU.0b013e31826d1e6b
12. Pereira BJA, de Almeida AN, Paiva WS, de Aguiar PHP, Teixeira MJ, et al. Natural history of intraventricular meningiomas: systematic review. *Neurosurg Rev.* (2018). doi:10.1007/s10143-018-1019-0. [Epub ahead of print].
13. Aizer AA, Bi WL, Kandola MS, Lee EQ, Nayak L, Rinne ML, et al. Extent of resection and overall survival for patients with atypical and malignant meningioma. *Cancer.* (2015) 121:4376–81. doi: 10.1002/cncr.29639
14. Berkmann S, Schlaffer S, Nimsky C, Fahlbusch R, Buchfelder M. Follow-up and long-term outcome of nonfunctioning pituitary adenoma operated by transsphenoidal surgery with intraoperative high-field magnetic resonance imaging. *Acta Neurochir.* (2014) 156:2233–43; discussion 2243.doi: 10.1007/s00701-014-2210-x
15. Almutairi RD, Muskens IS, Cote DJ, Dijkman MD, Kavouridis VK, Crocker E., et al. Gross total resection of pituitary adenomas after endoscopic vs. microscopic transsphenoidal surgery: a meta-analysis. *Acta Neurochir.* (2018) 160:1005–21. doi: 10.1007/s00701-017-3438-z
16. Seltzer J, Wedemeyer MA, Bonney PA, Carmichael JD, Weiss M, Zada G. Outcomes following transsphenoidal surgical management of incidental pituitary adenomas: a series of 52 patients over a 17-year period. *J Neurosurg.* (2018) 1:1–9.doi: 10.3171/2017.11.JNS171485
17. Wirtz CR, Albert FK, Schwaderer M, Heuer C, Staubert A, Tronnier VM., et al. The benefit of neuronavigation for neurosurgery analyzed by its impact on glioblastoma surgery. *Neurol Res.* (2000) 22:354–60.
18. Sherman JH, Hoes K, Marcus J, Komotar RJ, Brennan CW, Gutin PH. Neurosurgery for brain tumors: update on recent technical advances. *Curr Neurol Neurosci Rep.* (2011) 11:313–9. doi: 10.1007/s11910-01 1-0188-9
19. Berkmann S, Schlaffer S, Nimsky C, Fahlbusch R, Buchfelder M. Intraoperative high-field MRI for transsphenoidal reoperations of nonfunctioning pituitary adenoma. *J Neurosurg.* (2014) 121:1–10. doi: 10.3171/2014.6.JNS131994
20. Kuo JS, Barkhoudarian G, Farrell CJ, Bodach ME, Tumialan LM, Oyesiku NM., et al. Congress of neurological surgeons systematic review and evidence-based guideline on surgical techniques and technologies for the management of patients with nonfunctioning pituitary adenomas. *Neurosurgery.* (2016) 79:E536–8. doi: 10.1227/NEU.0000000000001390.
21. Sheehan J, et al. Congress of neurological surgeons systematic review and evidence-based guideline for the management of patients with residual or recurrent nonfunctioning pituitary adenomas. *Neurosugery.* (2016) 79:539–40. doi: 10.1227/NEU.0000000000001385
22. Layer G, Reichelt J, Jahn D, Heinz DW. Structure and function of enzymes in heme biosynthesis. *Protein Sci.* (2010) 19:1137–61. doi: 10.1002/pro.405
23. Tran TT, Mu A, Adachi Y, Adachi Y, Taketani S. Neurotransmitter transporter

family including SLC6A6 and SLC6A13 contributes to the 5-aminolevulinic acid (ALA)-induced accumulation of protoporphyrin IX and photodamage, through uptake of ALA by cancerous cells. *Photochem Photobiol.* (2014) 90:1136–43. doi: 10.1111/php.12290
24. Nakai Y, Tatsumi Y, Miyake M, Anai S, Kuwada M, Onishi S., et al. Expression of ferrochelatase has a strong correlation in protoporphyrin IX accumulation with photodynamic detection of bladder cancer. *Photodiagnosis Photodyn Ther.* (2016) 13:225–32. doi: 10.1016/j.pdpdt.2015.07.174
25. Collaud S, Juzeniene A, Moan J, Lange N. On the selectivity of 5-aminolevulinic acid-induced protoporphyrin IX formation. *Curr Med Chem Anticancer Agents.* (2004) 4:301–16.
26. Schwake M, Günes D, Köchling M, Brentrup A, Schroeteler J, Hotfilder M., et al. Kinetics of porphyrin fluorescence accumulation in pediatric brain tumor cells incubated in 5-aminolevulinic acid. *Acta Neurochir (Wien).* 156:1077–84.doi: 10.1007/s00701-014-2096-7
27. Stummer W, Stocker S, Wagner S, Stepp H, Fritsch C, Goetz C., et al. Intraoperative detection of malignant gliomas by 5-aminolevulinic acid-induced porphyrin fluorescence. *Neurosurgery.* (1998) 42:518–25; discussion 525–6. doi: 10.1097/00006123-199803000-00017
28. Stummer W, Stepp H, Wiestler OD, Pichlmeier U. Randomized, prospective double-blinded study comparing 3 different doses of 5-aminolevulinic acid for fluorescence-guided resections of malignant gliomas. *Neurosurgery.* (2017) 81:230–9. doi: 10.1093/neuros/nyx074
29. Stummer W, Pichlmeier U, Meinel T, Wiestler OD, Zanella F, Reulen HJ, et al. Fluorescence-guided surgery with 5-aminolevulinic acid for resection of malignant glioma: a randomised controlled multicentre phase III trial. *Lancet Oncol.* (2006) 7:392–401. doi: 10.1016/S1470-2045(06)70665-9
30. Eljamel MS, Leese G, Moseley H. Intraoperative optical identification of pituitary adenomas. *J Neurooncol.* (2009) 92:417–21. doi: 10.1007/s11060-009-9820-9
31. Coluccia D, Fandino J, Fujioka M, Cordovi S, Muroi C, Landolt H. Intraoperative 5-aminolevulinic-acid-induced fluorescence in meningiomas. *Acta Neurochir.* (2010) 152:1711–9. doi: 10.1007/s00701-010-0708-4
32. Valdes PA, Bekelis K, Harris BT, Wilson BC, Leblond F, Kim A., et al. 5-Aminolevulinic acid-induced protoporphyrin IX fluorescence in meningioma: qualitative and quantitative measurements *in vivo.* *Neurosurgery.* (2014) 10(Suppl. 1):74–82; discussion 82–3. doi: 10.1227/NEU.0000000000000117
33. Okuda T, Yoshioka H, Kato A. Fluorescence-guided surgery for glioblastoma multiforme using high-dose fluorescein sodium with excitation and barrier filters. *J Clin Neurosci.* (2012) 19:1719–22. doi: 10.1016/j.jocn.2011.12.034
34. Acerbi F, Broggi M, Eoli M, Anghileri E, Cavallo C, Boffano C, et al. Is fluorescein-guided technique able to help in resection of high-grade gliomas? *Neurosurg. Focus.* (2014) 36:E5. doi: 10.3171/2013.11.FOCUS 13487
35. Okuda T, Kataoka K, Yabuuchi T, Yugami H, Kato A. Fluorescence-guided surgery of metastatic brain tumors using fluorescein sodium. *J Clin Neurosci.* (2010) 17:118–121. doi: 10.1016/j.jocn.2009.06.033
36. Chen B, Wang H, Ge P, Zhao J, Li W, Gu H., et al. Gross total resection of glioma with the intraoperative fluorescence-guidance of fluorescein sodium. *Int J Med Sci.* (2012) 9:708–714. doi: 10.7150/ijms.4843
37. Akçakaya MO, Göker B, Kasimcan MÖ, Hamamcioglu MK, Kiriş T. Use of sodium fluorescein in meningioma surgery performed under the YELLOW-560 nm surgical microscope filter: feasibility and preliminary results. *World Neurosurg.* (2017) 107:966–73. doi: 10.1016/j.wneu.2017.07.103
38. Francaviglia N, Iacopino DG, Costantino G, Villa A, Impallaria P, Meli F., et al. Fluorescein for resection of high-grade gliomas: a safety study control in a single center and review of the literature. *Surg Neurol Int.* (2017) 8:145. doi: 10.4103/sni.sni_89_17
39. Bowden SG, Neira JA, Gill BJA, Ung TH, Englander ZK, Zanazzi G., et al. Sodium fluorescein facilitates guided sampling of diagnostic tumor tissue in nonenhancing gliomas. *Neurosurgery.* (2018) 82:719–27. doi: 10.1093/neuros/nyx271
40. Suero Molina E, Wölfer J, Ewelt C, Ehrhardt A, Brokinkel B, Stummer W. Dual-labeling with 5-aminolevulinic acid and fluorescein for fluorescence-guided resection of high-grade gliomas: technical note. *J Neurosurg.* (2018) 128:399–405. doi: 10.3171/2016.11.JNS161072
41. Hansen DA, Spence AM, Carski T, Berger MS. Indocyanine green (ICG) staining and demarcation of tumor margins in a rat glioma model. *Surg Neurol.* (1993) 40:451–6.
42. Haglund MM, Hochman DW, Spence AM, Berger MS. Enhanced optical imaging of rat gliomas and tumor margins. *Neurosurgery.* (1994) 35:930-40; discussion 940–1.
43. Haglund MM, Berger MS, Hochman DW. Enhanced optical imaging of human gliomas and tumor margins. *Neurosurgery.* (1996) 38:308–17.
44. Madajewski B, Judy BF, Mouchli A, Kapoor V, Holt D, Wang MD., et al. Intraoperative near-infrared imaging of surgical wounds after tumor resections can detect residual disease. *Clin Cancer Res.* (2012) 18:5741–51. doi: 10.1158/1078-0432.CCR-12-1188
45. Jiang JX, Keating JJ, Jesus EM, Judy RP, Madajewski B, Venegas O., et al. Optimization of the enhanced permeability and retention effect for near-infrared imaging of solid tumors with indocyanine green. *Am J Nucl Med Mol Imaging.* (2015) 5:390–400.
46. Zeh R, Sheikh S, Xia L, Pierce J, Newton A, Predina J., et al. The second window ICG technique demonstrates a broad plateau period for near infrared fluorescence tumor contrast in glioblastoma. *PLoS ONE.* (2017) 12:e0182034. doi: 10.1371/journal.pone.0182034
47. Maeda H, Wu J, Sawa T, Matsumura Y, Hori K. Tumor vascular permeability and the EPR effect in macromolecular therapeutics: a review. *J Control Release.* (2000) 65:271–84.
48. Ergin A, Wang M, Zhang JY, Bruce JN, Fine RL, Bigio IJ., et al. The feasibility of real-time *in vivo* optical detection of blood-brain barrier disruption with indocyanine green. *J Neurooncol.* (2012) 106:551–60. doi: 10.1007/s11060-011-0711-5
49. Lee JYK, Thawani JP, Pierce J, Zeh R, Martinez-Lage M, Chanin M, et al. Intraoperative near-infrared optical imaging can localize gadolinium-enhancing gliomas during surgery. *Neurosurgery.* (2016) 79:856–71. doi: 10.1227/NEU.0000000000001450
50. Lee JYK, Pierce JT, Zeh R, Cho SS, Salinas R, Nie S, et al. Intraoperative near-infrared optical contrast can localize brain metastases. *World Neurosurg.* (2017) 106:120–30. doi: 10.1016/j.wneu.2017.06.128
51. Lee JYK, Pierce JT, Thawani JP, Zeh R, Nie S, Martinez-Lage M, et al. Near-infrared fluorescent image-guided surgery for intracranial meningioma. *J Neurosurg.* (2018) 128:380–90. doi: 10.3171/2016.10.JNS 161636
52. Cho SS, Zeh R, Pierce JT, Salinas R, Singhal S, Lee JYK. Comparison of near-infrared imaging camera systems for intracranial tumor detection. *Mol Imaging Biol.* (2018) 20:213–20. doi: 10.1007/s11307-017-1107-5
53. Jeon JW, Cho SS, Nag S, Buch L, Pierce J, Su YS, et al. Near-infrared optical contrast of skull base tumors during endoscopic endonasal surgery. *Oper. Neurosurg.* (2018) 1–11. doi: 10.1093/ons/opy213. [Epub ahead of print].
54. Cho SS, Jeon J, Buch L, Nag S, Nasrallah M, Low PS, et al. Intraoperative near-infrared imaging with receptor-specific versus passive delivery of fluorescent agents in pituitary adenomas. *J Neurosurg.* (2018) 1:1–11. doi: 10.3171/2018.7.JNS181642.
55. Frangioni JV. *In vivo* near-infrared fluorescence imaging. *Curr Opin Chem Biol.* (2003) 7:626–34.
56. Padalkar M V,Pleshko N. Wavelength-dependent penetration depth of near infrared radiation into cartilage. *Analyst.* (2015) 140:2093–100. doi: 10.1039/c4an01987c
57. Roberts DW, Olson JD, Evans LT, Kolste KK, Kanick SC, Fan X., et al. Red-light excitation of protoporphyrin IX fluorescence for subsurface tumor detection. *J Neurosurg.* (2018) 128:1690–7. doi: 10.3171/2017.1.JNS1 62061
58. Dsouza AV, Lin H, Henderson ER, Samkoe KS, Pogue BW. Review of fluorescence guided surgery systems: identification of key performance capabilities beyond indocyanine green imaging. *J Biomed Opt.* 21:80901.doi: 10.1117/1.JBO.21.8.080901
59. Hekman MCH, Rijpkema M, Bos DL, Oosterwijk E, Goldenberg DM, Mulders PFA., et al. Intraoperative near-infrared imaging can distinguish cancer from normal tissue but not inflammation. *PLoS ONE.* (2014) 9:e103342. doi: 10.1371/journal.pone.0103342
60. Cho SS, Zeh R, Pierce JT, Jeon J, Nasrallah M, Adappa ND., et al. Folate receptor near-infrared optical imaging provides sensitive and specific intraoperative visualization of nonfunctional pituitary adenomas. *Oper Neurosurg.* (2018) 16:59–70.doi: 10.1093/ons/opy034

61. Lee JY. K. et al. Folate receptor overexpression can be visualized in real time during pituitary adenoma endoscopic transsphenoidal surgery with near-infrared imaging. *J Neurosurg.* (2017) 129:390–403. doi: 10.3171/2017.2.JNS163191
62. Pierce JT, Cho SS, Nag S, Zeh R, Jeon J, Holt D, et al. Folate receptor overexpression in human and canine meningiomas—immunohistochemistry and case report of intraoperative molecular imaging. *Neurosurgery.* (2018) 1–10. doi: 10.1093/neuros/nyy356. [Epub ahead of print].
63. Belykh E, Miller EJ, Patel AA, Yazdanabadi MI, Martirosyan NL, Yagmurlu K., et al. Diagnostic accuracy of a confocal laser endomicroscope for *in vivo* differentiation between normal injured and tumor tissue during fluorescein-guided glioma resection: laboratory investigation. *World Neurosurg.* (2018) 115:e337–48. doi: 10.1016/j.wneu.2018.04.048
64. Martirosyan NL, Cavalcanti DD, Eschbacher JM, Delaney PM, Scheck AC, Abdelwahab MG., et al. Use of *in vivo* near-infrared laser confocal endomicroscopy with indocyanine green to detect the boundary of infiltrative tumor. *J Neurosurg.* (2011) 115:1131–8. doi: 10.3171/2011.8.JNS11559

19

Delta-Aminolevulinic Acid-Mediated Photodiagnoses in Surgical Oncology

Joseph F. Georges[1,2*], *Amber Valeri*[1,2], *Huan Wang*[3], *Aaron Brooking*[1,2], *Michael Kakareka*[1,2], *Steve S. Cho*[4,5], *Zein Al-Atrache*[6], *Michael Bamimore*[6], *Hany Osman*[7], *Joseph Ifrach*[6], *Si Yu*[3], *Carrie Li*[4], *Denah Appelt*[1], *John Y. K. Lee*[5], *Peter Nakaji*[8], *Kristin Brill*[9] and *Steven Yocom*[2]

[1] Department of Neurosurgery, Philadelphia College of Osteopathic Medicine, Philadelphia, PA, United States, [2] Department of Neurosurgery, Cooper University Healthcare, Philadelphia, PA, United States, [3] School of Medicine, Cooper Medical School of Rowan University, Camden, NJ, United States, [4] Perelman School of Medicine, University of Pennsylvania, Philadelphia, PA, United States, [5] Department of Neurosurgery, Hospital of the University of Pennsylvania, Philadelphia, PA, United States, [6] School of Medicine, Philadelphia College of Osteopathic Medicine, Philadelphia, PA, United States, [7] Wellman Center for Photomedicine, Massachusetts General Hospital, Boston, MA, United States, [8] Department of Neurosurgery, St. Joseph's Hospital and Medical Center, Barrow Neurological Institute, Phoenix, AZ, United States, [9] Department of Surgery, MD Anderson Cancer Center at Cooper Health Systems, Camden, NJ, United States

***Correspondence:**
Joseph F. Georges
joseph.georges@asu.edu

Fluorescence imaging is an emerging clinical technique for real-time intraoperative visualization of tumors and their boundaries. Though multiple fluorescent contrast agents are available in the basic sciences, few fluorescence agents are available for clinical use. Of the clinical fluorophores, delta aminolevulinic acid (5ALA) is unique for generating visible wavelength tumor-specific fluorescence. In 2017, 5ALA was FDA-approved for glioma surgery in the United States. Additionally, clinical studies suggest this agent may have utility in surgical subspecialties outside of neurosurgery. Data from dermatology, OB/GYN, urology, cardiothoracic surgery, and gastrointestinal surgery show 5ALA is helpful for intraoperative visualization of malignant tissues in multiple organ systems. This review summarizes data from English-language 5ALA clinical trials across surgical subspecialties. Imaging systems, routes of administration, dosing, efficacy, and related side effects are reviewed. We found that modified surgical microscopes and endoscopes are the preferred imaging devices. Systemic dosing across surgical specialties range between 5 and 30 mg/kg bodyweight. Multiple studies discussed potential for skin irritation with sun exposure, however this side effect is infrequently reported. Overall, 5ALA has shown high sensitivity for labeling malignant tissues and providing a means to visualize malignant tissue not apparent with standard operative light sources.

Keywords: fluorescence, 5ALA, protoporphyrin IX, surgery, neurosurgery, glioma

INTRODUCTION

Surgeons have utilized light to better visualize their surgical fields since antiquity. Fluorescence, a relatively new discovery, has been studied since the early-to-mid twentieth century as a means for providing better contrast of structures during surgery. Reports from the late twentieth century showing fluorescence contrast could improve intraoperative visualization of tumors during surgery has fueled a renewed interest in further developing clinical fluorescence imaging techniques.

In the United States, few agents are clinically approved for generating intraoperative fluorescence contrast (1). Though novel agents are in various stages of clinical trials, the three agents currently approved for clinical use are fluorescein, indocyanine green, and delta-aminolevulinic acid (5ALA), and of these, only 5ALA has a specific FDA clinical indication for CNS use (2). Of these, 5ALA is also the only agent that produces intracellular tumor-specific fluorescence. Delta-aminolevulinic acid generates this fluorescence by causing tumor-specific accumulation of the fluorescent molecule protoporphyrin IX (PpIX).

Delta-aminolevulinic acid is produced by the condensation of succinate and glycine, and was first reported in a Nature article in 1953 (3, 4). Studies with radiolabeled carbon showed this molecule was involved in porphyrin synthesis (3). Studies during the 1950s and 1960s focused on the role of 5ALA in the heme synthesis pathway (5, 6). The first human studies with 5ALA were conducted in 1956, and were devised to study 5ALA metabolism. In these studies, 5ALA was given orally (7). Skin sensitivity, a well-known complication of 5ALA, was first reported in 1956 (7). This phenomenon occurred 2–11 h after 5ALA administration.

Porphyrin-mediated fluorescence was first reported in the late nineteenth century. However, the potential role porphyrins would have in tumor visualization would not be reported until half a century later in lab-based studies. The earliest clinical studies of 5ALA-mediated tumor visualization were reported for dermatology and urology in 1990 and 1994, respectively (8–10). Throughout the remaining twentieth century and early twenty first century, clinicians and scientists continued to evaluate the role of 5ALA-mediated fluorescence for intraoperative photodiagnosis of neoplasms in neurosurgery, head and neck surgery, cardiothoracic surgery, gastrointestinal surgery and OB/GYN.

This review provides a history of notable findings for 5ALA-mediated photodiagnosis across surgical subspecialties. The information is derived from a PubMed search of all English language clinical trials published between 1950 and 2018. Basic science and animal studies are excluded from this review.

NEUROSURGERY

First Application of 5ALA in Neurosurgery

The first study investigating 5ALA in neurosurgery was published by Stummer et al. (11). In this seminal study, Stummer administered 10 mg/kg of 5ALA orally to 9 patients with high-grade gliomas (HGG) 3 h prior to induction of anesthesia. Using a 375–440 nm bandpass filter, Stummer was able to provide blue-light excitation. A long-pass filter >455 nm blocked the reflected excitation light and allowed the emitted protoporphyrin IX fluorescence to be visualized. From the 9 patients, Stummer took a total of 89 biopsies; in these specimens, 5ALA fluorescence demonstrated 85% sensitivity, 100% specificity, and 90% accuracy. The major contributors to the false-negatives were areas of low-density infiltrates of malignant cells and necrotic areas of the tumors. At the 10 mg/kg dose, no adverse effects were recorded. This study, while small, established the utility of 5ALA as an intraoperative imaging agent and began a new era for fluorescence-guided neurosurgery studies.

Landmark 5ALA Studies in Neurosurgery

Since the first paper in 1998, Stummer et al. and other groups have continued to investigate various aspects of 5ALA in neurosurgery. In 2000, Stummer et al. published a study in a larger cohort of 52 patients with HGGs, this time stratifying fluorescence subjectively into strong, vague, and none (12). The study demonstrated again that 5ALA was highly sensitive and specific for neoplasm and that residual fluorescence after standard resection predicted subtotal resection, seen on postoperative MRI as residual enhancement. The most impactful clinical neurosurgery 5ALA study was the 2006 randomized, controlled, multi-center trial by Stummer et al. (13). In the study, 270 HGG patients were randomized to either fluorescence-guided surgery with 5ALA or conventional surgery with white-light alone. Importantly, the study demonstrated that those in the 5ALA arm achieved gross total resection (GTR) at a much higher rate (65% vs. 36%, $p < 0.0001$) and had significantly higher progression-free survival (PFS) at 6 months (41% vs. 21.1%, $p = 0.0003$) without significant changes in postoperative neurologic deficits. Although the study was underpowered to demonstrate effects on overall survival, the results were nonetheless encouraging. In 2014, Coburger further demonstrated that 5ALA was more accurate than intraoperative MRI for detecting neoplasm at the infiltration zone, establishing 5ALA as both a more cost-effective and superior alternative (14).

Appropriate 5ALA Dose and Route of Administration

The current accepted dose for 5ALA administration in neurosurgery is an oral dose of 20 mg/kg bodyweight ~3 h before induction of anesthesia, translating to roughly 4–5 h before tumor exposure. In Stummer et al.'s first study in 1998, the dose used was 10 mg/kg. Two later studies investigated different doses of 5ALA in neurosurgery: a 2017 study by Stummer et al. (15) and another 2017 study by Eljamel et al. (16). Stummer et al. studied the efficacy of 0.2, 2, and 20 mg/kg in a total of 21 patients with HGGs and demonstrated that a 10-fold increase in dosage from 2 to 20 mg/kg yielded only a 4-fold increase in signal. They concluded that a dose higher than 20 mg/kg was unlikely to yield significant benefits. Eljamel et al. on the other hand, investigated doses from 10 to 50 mg/kg in 10 mg/kg increments in 19 patients with HGGs. They concluded that a dose of up to 50 mg/kg was safe in patients and suggested that higher doses of 5ALA may increase tumor fluorescence, although their results were not statistically significant in their small sample population. Considering these results, most groups, including Stummer et al.

have transitioned to 20 mg/kg, which seems to be both safe and effective.

In terms of route of administration, 5ALA has always been administered orally for neurosurgical patients. Preclinical studies, and studies in healthy patients, have established that oral 5ALA is rapid and effective (17). Thus, changes to the route of administration have not been considered for 5ALA in neurosurgery.

Imaging 5ALA Fluorescence in Neurosurgery

Neurosurgeons have relied heavily on surgical microscopes for intracranial surgeries since the 1950s (18). Hence, the majority of 5ALA visualization in neurosurgery has been performed with surgical microscopes (**Figure 1A**). In general, add-on modules are attached to existing microscopes to achieve blue-light excitation. Initially, when Stummer et al. first described their experience with 5ALA, a 375–440 nm bandpass filter was placed in front of the Xenon light, which provided UV and blue-light excitation. A long-pass >455 nm filter was used to block the reflected excitation light, in order to better detect the red PpIX fluorescence. This setup was used by Stummer's group and other groups until the mid-2000's, when Zeiss introduced its Blue400 module, which uses a 400–410 nm filter for excitation and 620–710 nm filter for emission and can rapidly toggle between white-light and blue-light illumination. Band pass emission filters at 620–710 nm were initially utilized to specifically visualize the peak red emission of PpIX; however, most surgeons found it difficult to operate with red light only. Hence, emission filters in the next generation of microscopes were changed from the narrow band pass filter to a 444 nm long pass filter. Although the field is illuminated only with blue light, autofluorescence in green and mild yellow provide the surgeon with illumination of surrounding background structures while resecting pink/red fluorescent tissue (**Figure 1B**). Leica has recently offered its FL400 module (380–430 nm excitation filter with a 444 nm long pass emission filter), which, similar to the Zeiss module, provides intraoperative visualization of PpIX.

Although exoscopes are a relatively new addition to the neurosurgeons' armamentarium, at least one group has attempted 5ALA visualization using an exoscope. Piquer et al. demonstrated that a commercial exoscope fitted with a 380–430nm excitation filter and >444 nm emission filter could be used to visualize 5ALA fluorescence reliably in the operating room (19, 20). Their study remains one of few studies to visualize 5ALA fluorescence without standard microscope equipment.

Current Status of 5ALA

In June 2017, 5ALA was FDA-approved as an intraoperative visualizing agent for patients with HGGs. Although 5ALA has been difficult for U.S. neurosurgeons to access outside of research studies, that is slowly changing as of April 2019 (2).

Future Applications of 5ALA Fluorescence in Neurosurgery

Though most clinical 5ALA studies have focused on patients with HGGs, some groups have investigated its application in other intracranial tumors. For instance, Widhalm et al. (21, 22) demonstrated that non-enhancing gliomas are poor targets for 5ALA and Valdes et al. (23) concluded that conventional 5ALA imaging was of limited use in patients with low-grade gliomas. On the other hand, Valdes et al. (24) and Coluccia et al. (25) investigated the utility of 5ALA in meningiomas and concluded that most meningiomas (80 and 94%, respectively) demonstrated PpIX fluorescence. Similarly, Eljamel et al. concluded that 5ALA fluorescence was useful in pituitary adenomas of various subtypes (26). These studies offer encouraging evidence that 5ALA fluorescence may be applicable to other intracranial tumors and may further help neurosurgeons visualize tumors in the operating room.

Technological advances are improving clinical 5ALA fluorescence detection. Thus far, most neurosurgeons have relied on qualitative grading of PpIX fluorescence (i.e., strong, vague, none), which is limited in objectivity and sensitivity. Multiple groups have demonstrated that quantitative grading of fluorescence, achieved with an intraoperative spectrometry probe, increases the sensitivity and accuracy of 5ALA fluorescence (23, 24, 27). Furthermore, an important limitation in 5ALA fluorescence is the micron-scale tissue penetration by ultraviolent excitation light, which can hinder sensitive tumor detection. Therefore, to increase depth penetration of excitation light, Roberts et al. recently demonstrated that using red-light excitation (620–640 nm) and a sensitive spectrally-resolved camera to take advantage of 5ALA's second, smaller excitation/emission peak, neoplastic areas could be visualized up to 5 mm below the tissue surface (28).

Conclusion

Overall, 5ALA has demonstrated utility in increasing GTR rates and PFS in patients with HGGs and may be applicable to other intracranial tumors as well. Along with potential advances in intraoperative visualization techniques, 5ALA may ultimately improve patient outcomes in neurosurgery.

UROLOGY

First Application of 5ALA in Urology

The first study to evaluate 5ALA in Urology was published by Kriegmair et al. (9). In this study, an intravesicular application of 1.5 g of 5ALA dissolved in 50 ml of sodium bicarbonate was instilled. Time of exposure of 5ALA ranged from 15 to 360 min. The mean time between instillation and fluorescence cystoscopy was 204 min. Urologic surgery was performed under violet light from a krypton ion laser with 406.7 nm excitation. This provided visualization of red fluorescence from protoporphyrin IX in the urothelium of the bladder to perform biopsies of the bladder wall in 68 patients who were suspected to have bladder cancer. In this study, photodynamic diagnosis utilizing 5ALA fluorescence-directed urothelium biopsy diagnosed bladder cancer with a high sensitivity of 100% and specificity of 68.5%. No serious side effects were observed with intravesicular instillation of 5ALA. This study generated confidence that 5ALA could provide highly

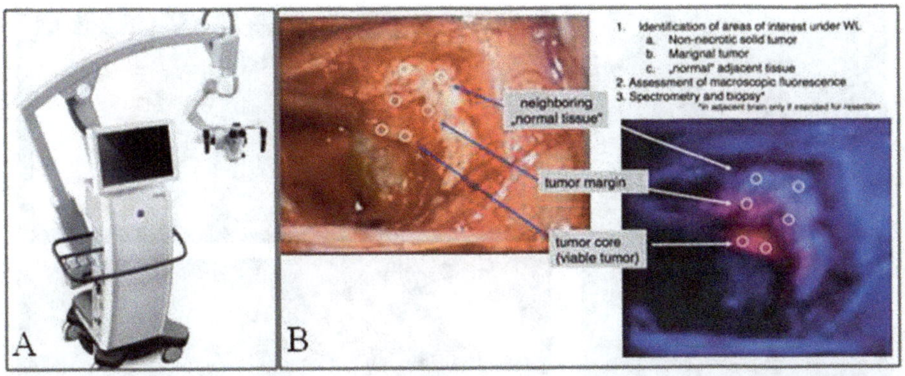

FIGURE 1 | Fluorescence imaging in neurosurgery. **(A)** Zeiss Pentero fluorescence surgical microscope used for intraoperative imaging. **(B)** Brightfield illumination compared to PpIX fluorescence from a malignant glioma, note fluorescence signal of the tumor compared to tumor margin and normal adjacent brain [Intraoperative images courtesy of Stummer et al. (15)].

sensitive visualization and improved resection of difficult-to-detect lesions, such as carcinoma *in situ* and urothelial dysplasia, resulting in diminished recurrence rates.

Appropriate 5ALA Dose and Route of Administration

5ALA can be administered via two routes for the diagnosis of urologic malignancies. In early studies, a 1.5 g, 3% solution of 5ALA was given almost exclusively by direct intravesicular instillation 2–3 h before biopsy was performed. In more recent studies, researchers have transitioned to administering a 20 mg/kg body weight oral solution of 5ALA 3–4 h before biopsy is performed. Inoue et al. evaluated the safety and efficacy of 10 mg/kg vs. 20 mg/kg of oral 5ALA in white light vs. fluorescence cystoscopy in a total of 62 patients (29). The rates of carcinoma *in situ* and high grade non-invasive papillary urothelial carcinoma detected only by white light cystoscopy was 4.0 and 0.0%, respectively in the 10 and 20 mg/kg groups vs. 16.0 an 36.1%, respectively in the 10 and 20 mg/kg fluorescence cystoscopy groups. Inoue et al. performed a follow-up study in 2016 which demonstrated that sensitivity increased in a dose-dependent manner with fluorescence cystoscopy, reporting 83.7% at $\geqq$ 10 mg/kg and <15 mg/kg, 86.4% at $\geqq$ 15 mg/kg and <20 mg/kg, and 96.3% at $\geqq$ 20 mg/kg (30).

Imaging 5ALA Fluorescence in Urology

In the first study to document the results of 5ALA photodynamic diagnostics in urologic malignancy, Kriegmair et al. utilized a krypton ion laser 406.7 nm excitation. The majority of studies published in this field utilize a xenon arc lamp with a 370–440 nm bandpass filter, with or without long-pass filter to detect the red PpIX fluorescence. A fluorescence cystoscope, sometimes the help of a 0 or 30 telescope is typically employed (**Figure 2**) (32, 33). Fukuhara et al. published a study in 2015 reporting the utility of a flexible fluorescence-cystoscope with a twin-mode monitor in 5ALA photodynamic diagnosis of bladder cancer (31). In this particular study, a new PDD system consisting of a fluorescence endoscope with a SAFE-3000 processor and flexible cystoscope with a xenon lamp and semiconductor laser. Fluorescence images were observed with a charge coupled device image processor. A twin-mode monitor allowed a white light image and fluorescent image to be visualized simultaneously.

Adverse Effects of 5ALA

Intravesicular application of 5ALA is overall, well-tolerated with minimal side effects. Multiple studies reported transient urinary urgency, pollakisuria, and alginuresis (34, 35). With the oral administration of 5ALA, patients are often described as having transient hypotension, transaminitis and skin photosensitivity (29, 31, 36).

Limitations of 5ALA in Diagnosis of Bladder Cancer

Speiss et al. reported in 2006 that fluorescence cystoscopy with 5ALA can have a false-positive rate as high as 40% (37). Possible causes of a false-positive result include: inflammation, urothelial hyperplasia, recent urethral stents, bacteriuria, previous intravesicular therapy within the previous 3 months, and inexperience of the performing Urologist (38, 39).

Current Status of 5ALA in Urology

The United Stated Food and Drug Administration approved 5ALA for intra-operative photodynamic diagnosis of bladder cancers in 1999. Currently, studies are being conducted regarding the use of a 5ALA ester, hexyl aminolevulinate, to compare efficacy and diagnostic accuracy.

Conclusion

Overall, 5ALA has demonstrated increased sensitivity in diagnosis of bladder cancers compared to white-light cystoscopy, especially in the case of carcinoma *in situ* and dysplasia. It has shown to improve visualization of surgical margins at resection and to decrease recurrence rates.

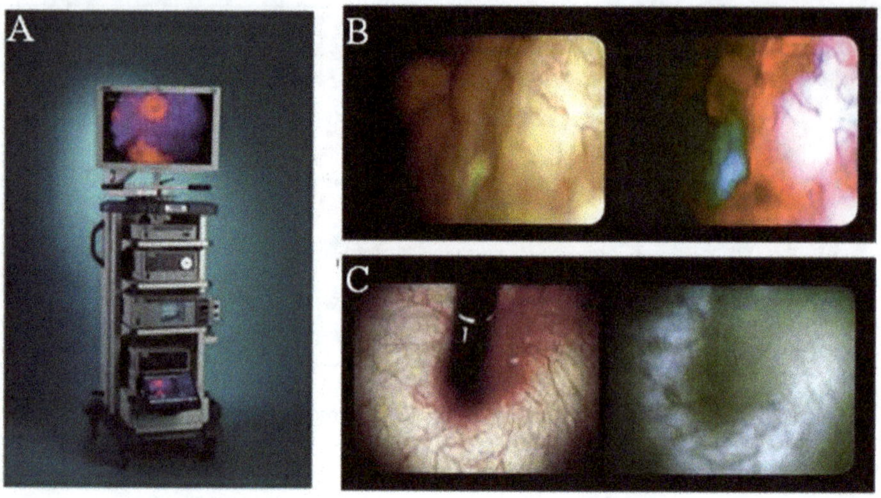

FIGURE 2 | Fluorescence imaging in urology. **(A)** Karl Stortz D-light C used for blue-light cystoscopy as an adjunct to white-light cystoscopy for detection of non-muscle invasive bladder cancer in patients with suspected or known lesion(s). **(B)** White light mode (left side) and blue light mode (right side) images of bladder cancer simultaneously observed using twin mode monitor. Flat lesions show red florescence. **(C)** White light mode (left side) and blue light mode (right side) images of bladder neck using turned back flexible cystoscopy in a vertical direction. No red fluorescence observed [Intraoperative images courtesy of Fukuhara et al. (31)].

DERMATOLOGY

First Application in Clinical Dermatology

The first study investigating 5ALA in dermatology was published by Kennedy et al. (40). Though this study was designed to evaluate the role of 5ALA in photodynamic therapy, fluorescence was reported from tumor areas. In this study, 5ALA was applied topically in a 20% solution to basal cell carcinoma (BCC) lesions. After waiting 3 h, the lesions underwent light exposure. Their initial results were promising. In the first 80 lesions that were treated using this technique, 90% of the lesions had a complete response rate and 7.5% had a partial response rate following a single treatment (40). Significant interest in the dermatologic utility of 5ALA has steadily grown since the work of Kennedy et al.

Landmark 5ALA Studies in Dermatology

Szeimies et al. evaluated tissue localization of protoporphyrin (Pp IX) after topical application of ALA by measuring the fluorescence in different histological types of BCC lesions in 1994. These investigators used a 10% 5ALA and 10% CAB-OSIL M-5 (highly dispersed SiO2, CAB-OSIL Division, Cabot GmbH, Hanau, Germany) in propylene glycol ointment on fifteen patients with BCC lesions undergoing Mohs microsurgical resection (MMS). The area was bandaged after applying 5ALA ointment. Patients then underwent MMS 4–12 h after applying the 5ALA ointment. The control patients did not receive 5ALA prior to MMS. A microscope equipped with a 515–560 nm excitation filter was used during the MMS. The site of red fluorescence was compared to the histopathology. The results showed that tumors undergoing resection after waiting only 4 h had no significant fluorescence, whereas, tumors that underwent resection after 12 h showed a strong tumor-specific red fluorescence (10). These results differed from Kennedy et al. group who appreciated fluorescence of BCC tissue only after 3 h from the application of topical 5ALA. The optimal time required from the application of 5ALA to treatment was still unclear and further clinical studies were needed. The addition of solvents, such as Dimethyl sulfoxide (DMSO) and Ethylenediaminetetraacetic acid (EDTA) to the topical ointment was investigated by Peng et al. to determine if the use of these solvents can enhance the absorbability and specificity of 5ALA in tumor cells. They compared the topical application of 5ALA containing 20% 5ALA alone to 20% 5ALA plus 20% DMSO and 4% EDTA in patients with BCC lesions. They found that 5ALA alone was only located in the superficial layers in the lesion at 3 h post-application and both the penetration into the deeper parts of the lesion along with the degree of fluorescence was improved in the patients who received 20% 5ALA plus 20% DMSO and 4% EDTA after similarly evaluating lesions 3 h post-application. A 99% DMSO wash for 15 min prior to the application of 20% DMSO and 4% EDTA further enhanced the degree of penetration and fluorescence.

Despite apparent accumulation in tumors and improvement in surgical outcomes, 5ALA often showed poor delineation of tumors from normal tissue (41). Poor correlation often results from extension of the PpIX fluorescence beyond the true margins of the tumor and non-specific accumulation in benign lesions such as scars, sebaceous hyperplasia and others (42, 43). A few studies have shown that the accumulation of 5ALA in tumors with an intact epidermis which is usually seen in nodular BCC lesions is less compared to other types of BCC lesions that typical have epidermal ulcerations. This suggests that at the cellular level, the accumulation of 5ALA is not tumor specific but may be related to increased epidermal permeability and cellularity of tumors (44, 45). The use of esters of ALA, such as Methyl-ALA (MAL) improved delineation and specificity of the BCC lesions most likely secondary to the increased permeability of the molecule (43, 46, 47). Liposome encapsulation of 5ALA further enhances the lipophilicity of 5ALA and requires less time for maximal fluorescence (~2 h). Although better demarcation of non-melanotic skin lesions was found using liposome encapsulated 5ALA, the increased lipophilicity increases false positives due to the accumulation of Pp IX in sebaceous lesions, such as sebaceous hyperplasia along with viral warts, lichenoid inflammation and melanocytic nevi. Dense hairy areas also showed increased background fluorescence suggesting that this method is not suitable in regions with excess hair (42).

In addition to utility in BCC, topical 5ALA has also been found useful for the demarcation of squamous cell carcinomas (SCC) (48, 49). Delineation and complete excision of SCC lesions can be more challenging compared to BCC lesions due to its frequent irregular margins. Jeon et al. evaluated the use of 5ALA in delineating tumor margins in 64 patients undergoing MMS. Before the application of 5ALA, excessive crusts or scales were scraped off the lesion without causing bleeding and then the lesion cleaned with saline gauze. Nineteen patients received 20% 5ALA, 19 patients received 16% MAL and the remaining control patients did not receive a photosensitizer. The incubation period for the patients that received topical 5ALA was 6 h compared to 3 h for the patients received topical MAL. After the incubation period, a Wood lamp (ultraviolet examination light, model 31602, 356 nm; Burton Medical Products Corp., Chatsworth, CA) was used to determine the margins of the SCC lesion for MMS. The results showed that after MMS, the number of stages required for complete tumor removal was lower in the patients that received either 5ALA or MAL. There was no significant difference between 5ALA and MAL in terms of surgical benefits. A surgical benefit was not seen in all patients that had high-risk histologically SCC features, which may be due to irregular infiltrative patterns for these, PpIX may not penetrate the deeper layers and/or these cells do not produce as much PpIX compared to the cells with histologically low-risk SCC features (48).

Appropriate 5ALA Dose and Route of Administration in Dermatology

As discussed above, topical use is the most common application of 5ALA in dermatology. Prior studies have used 5ALA or methyl ALA, mixed with DMSO/EDTA and or liposomal ALA. Further clinical studies, however, are warranted to determine the optimal clinical dermatology agent that should be used.

Imaging 5ALA Fluorescence in Dermatology

Future development of imaging hardware and techniques to improve PpIX visualization and differentiation of abnormal tissue from normal tissue would be useful. Studies suggest auto-fluorescence is reduced within tumor cells with an excitation wavelength ~370 nm and an emission wavelength around 455 nm which is different compared to normal tissue (50–52). A few studies have shown improved 5ALA demarcation of BCC lesions when measured in concert with reduced background auto-fluorescence (50–52).

Conclusions and Future Applications of 5ALA Fluorescence in Dermatology

Studies have shown improved surgical outcomes with the use of 5ALA in both photodynamic therapy and delineating tumor margins in MMS, especially in BCC lesions. Fewer studies to date have evaluated the use of 5ALA for SCC, though these studies have shown that 5ALA has potential for improve visualization of SCC. With a better understanding of the kinetics of 5ALA, along with advancements in imaging techniques, 5ALA-mediated visualization has potential for becoming standard practice in the treatment of BCC and SCC lesions, along with expanding use to other skin lesions such as melanoma (**Figure 3**).

OBSTETRICS AND GYNECOLOGY

First Application of 5ALA Imaging in OB/GYN

Use of 5ALA in gynecologic cases now covers a broad spectrum of procedures (54–56) since PpIX was shown to accumulate in endometrial cancer cells by Wyss-Desserich and colleagues at non-toxic doses in 1996 (57). In this study, fluorescence was observed *in vitro* with best results found at 1 mg/ml incubated for 24 h and excited at 488 nm.

There is variation with the amount of 5ALA induced PpIX fluorescence in endometrium throughout the menstrual cycle. Highest fluorescence values are seen in secretory endometrium, followed by hyperplastic endometrium. In atrophic and proliferative phase endometrium fluorescence intensity and rate are the lowest (58).

Landmark Studies and Appropriate 5ALA Dose/Route of Administration

Topical absorption of 5ALA is effective in patients with cervical neoplasia (CIN) II and III, as well as with lichen planus (55, 56). A cervical cap with 2–4 mL of 200 mg/ml 5ALA placed for 1.5 h demonstrates that dysplastic cervical tissue consistently has greater fluorescence than normal tissue. This persists at 1.5, 3, and 6 h after exposure (55). In Women with verified genital erosive lichen planus, 2 ml vaginal suppository of 6.25 mg/ml Hexyl 5-aminolevulinate applied for 3 h shows successful conversion and accumulation PpIX. Superficial fluorescence increases significantly in affected areas, and while this is not statistically significant at 30 min, it becomes so at 3 h. On microscopy, affected mucosa has strong fluorescence originating in submucosal inflammatory cells below the basal membrane (56).

Ovarian carcinoma is a good candidate for early detection with PpIX fluoroscopy as it commonly presents late in course and metastasizes. After initial tumor removal, second look operations can prevent recurrence. Intraperitoneal 5ALA solution given at a concentration of 30 mg/kg 5 h before laparoscopy has been evaluated as a route for administration and has shown systemic distribution comparable to oral/topical preparations. In a third

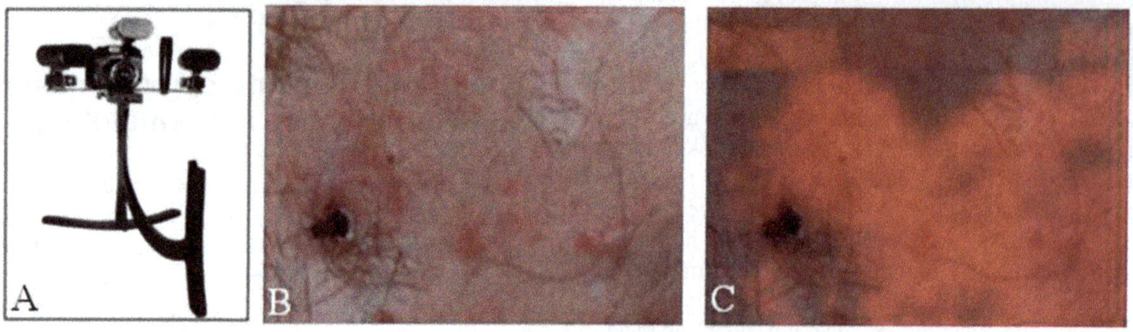

FIGURE 3 | Fluorescence imaging in dermatology. **(A)** Clearstone UV-DA, DigiMed Systems-Medical digital imaging system with ability to take ultraviolet photos. Courtesy of DigiMed Systems. **(B)** Brightfield illumination vs. **(C)** fluorescence-overlay imaging of a facial basal cell carcinoma. [Intraoperative images courtesy of Wan et al. (53)].

of patients with metastases seen at second look operations, PpIX fluorescence was able to detect tumor in a majority of cases that would otherwise have been missed with brightfield illumination alone (59).

5ALA has also been used to delineate peritoneal endometriosis, occasionally as an incidental finding. At doses as low as 10 mg/kg administered orally 4–5 h before laparoscopy there is increased concentration of PpIX fluorescence in peritoneal lesions. These lesions are typically difficult to visualize. 5ALA utility in OB/GYN is limited by increased PpIX concentration in fimbriae and tubal tissue with unknown effects on fertility (54).

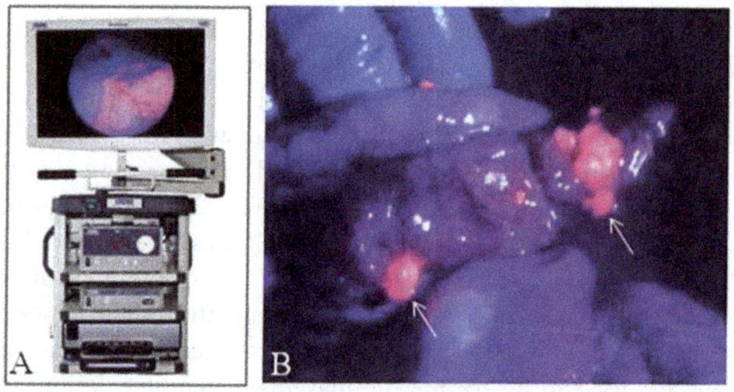

FIGURE 4 | Fluorescence imaging in obstetrics and gynecology. **(A)** Karl Storz D-Light fluorescence endoscopy system. **(B)** Laparoscopic image of peritoneum with ovarian cancer metastases with fluorescence-overlay imaging, Sote small fluorescent metastases (arrows) were histologically consistent with tumor. [Intraoperative images courtesy of Yonemura et al. (60)].

Conclusion and Future Applications of 5ALA Fluorescence in OB/GYN

Overall these early studies have shown 5ALA-mediated fluorescence in abnormal ovarian, endometrial, peritoneum and vulva tissue (**Figure 4**). There is potential for widespread and standardized use of 5ALA in OB/GYN especially as it pertains to second look operations in ovarian carcinoma. Further clinical studies are warranted to determine the safety and efficacy of 5ALA-mediated tumor visualization in OB/GYN.

HEAD AND NECK SURGERY

First Application of 5ALA in Head and Neck Surgery

Identifying innovative approaches to labeling and visualizing the borders of oropharynx and laryngeal neoplasms is a significant area of interest in head and neck surgery. The incidence of these neoplasms has increased during the last 2–3 decades secondary to alcohol and tobacco abuse (61). Studies show that survival rates increase with early stage carcinomas; however, the diagnosis of a tumor at the primary stage can be challenging. Earlier researchers used toluidine blue staining and auto-fluorescence imaging to visualize these lesions. However, Sabes et al. found a high false positive and false negative rate with the use of toluidine blue for detecting oral lesions which limited its widespread use. Similarly, Leunig et al. found that autofluorescence between normal and malignant tissue varied significantly between patients. Therefore, toluidine blue staining and autofluorescence never became popular in clinical use. Leunig et al. investigated the local use of 5ALA in patients with head and neck tumors. In this study, 16 patients with histologically confirmed oral SCC were given an oral rinse of 200 mg 5ALA dissolved in 50 ml of mineral oil. A zero- degree endoscope (Art, Nr. 7200 A; Storz, Tuttlingen, Germany) with ultraviolet light filtered xenon-arc lamp system along with an optimal multichannel analyzer (O-SMA 3; SI Instruments, Gilching, Germany) was used to measure the fluorescence contrast between tumor and normal tissue. In all patients, protoporphyin IX fluorescence was detected and significantly higher in the tumor compared to the surrounding healthy tissue. Therefore, the use of oral 5ALA potentially represented a new method for the early detection of oral dysplastic and malignant lesions (61). This study's promising results initiated further research in the use of 5ALA in head and neck surgery.

Landmark 5ALA Studies in Head and Neck Surgery

Since the first paper evaluating the use of 5ALA in head and neck surgery in 1996, Leunig and other groups have continued to investigate the use of 5ALA in head and neck surgery. In 2000, Leunig et al. assessed the use of 5ALA for the detection of oral SCC in 58 patients. These patients rinsed with a 0.4% solution of 5ALA dissolved in mineral oil for 15 min while closely being supervised. After waiting for a 1 to 2.5 h period for incubation, biopsies were taken from red fluorescence areas presumed to represent tumor tissue along with tumor boundaries and normal tissue using a modified 0°degree endoscope equipped with a filter (OG515, Schott, Mainz, Germany). In this study, the topical use of 5 ALA had a sensitivity of 99% and a specificity of 60% in detecting oral squamous cell cancer and dysplasia with no direct side effects of 5 ALA. This study suggests 5ALA can be a useful tool in the early detection of oral malignancy, but further clinical studies were warranted (62). Zheng et al. later further evaluated the use of 5ALA in detecting oral cancer lesions. Their study included 49 patients with either clinically suspicious lesions or pathologically proven malignancies of the oral cavity. The patients rinsed with a 0.4% rinsing solution of 5 ALA dissolved in mineral oil for 15 min. After waiting for an incubation period of 1.5 to 2 h, all patients underwent fluorescence endoscopic-guided biopsies. The malignant and dysplastic histological findings closely correlated with PpIX fluorescence The sensitivity and specificity with the use of 5ALA for separating benign tissue from dysplasia was 92 and 96%, respectively. A sensitivity of 98% and a specificity of 96% was achieved in distinguishing carcinoma *in situ* from SCC with the use of 5ALA, and a sensitivity of 98% and specificity of 92% for distinguishing carcinoma *in situ* and squamous cell carcinoma from dysplasia was achieved with the use of 5ALA (63).

The use of 5ALA for distinguishing laryngeal CA from benign tissue has also been closely evaluated. Mehlmann et al. used a 5 ml 0.9% NaCl solution of 5ALA topically applied in 16 patients with suspected or histologically proven malignancies of the larynx via a nebulized inhaler 1–2 h prior to a microlarnyngoscopy. Microlaryngoscopy was performed through an optimized endoscope (Hopkins 0, Art. No. KSTEXB001-3 or 27005AI, Storz, Tuttlingen German) equipped with a special filter system (D-light, Art No. 20133201, Storz) that was attached to a footswitch that allowed switching between brightfield illumination and fluorescence imaging. Forty-five biopsies were taken. Areas of normal tissue appeared green in color whereas malignant sites showed a strong red fluorescence. The sensitivity and specificity of 5- ALA in separating normal tissue for malignant tissue was 95 and 80%, respectively (64). This was the first clinical study that showed 5ALA utility for the detection of laryngeal cancer. Csanady et al. later further investigated the use of 5ALA in detecting pharyngeal cancer. This study included 31 patients with either precancerous, malignant or benign lesions of the laryngeal or hypopharyngeal cavities. Patients received topical application of 1% 5ALA solution diluted with 0.9% saline solution via nebulizer. After a 1.5–2 h incubation period, fluorescence-guided endoscopic biopsies were performed. With the use of 5ALA, the sensitivity and specificity of detecting laryngeal and pharyngeal cancer from normal tissue was 96 and 76%, respectively. Hence, the laryngeal and hypopharyngeal tumors and their margins were found to be accurately outlined under fluorescence imaging showing the usefulness of 5ALA for intraoperative visualization of neoplastic tissue (65).

Visualizing the parathyroid gland while operating in a small space can be challenging, even for the most experienced surgeons (66). Methylene blue was initially used for identifying the parathyroid gland intraoperatively. However, its clinical use is limited as it is associated with serious side effects including: vascular pain, staining of the skin and urine, and neurological toxicity (66). This intrigued Prosst et al. to investigate the use of 5ALA in a 52 y.o female with refractory secondary hyperparathyroidism for identifying the parathyroid glands. The patient received 30 mg/kg of body weight of 5ALA dissolved in water given orally 4 h prior to surgery. After anterior cervical neck surgical exposure by an otolaryngologists, a 4 mm scope (30; Hopkins II; Karl Stortz CO) connected to D-light fluorescence system was brought into the operative field. Though the parathyroid glands were unable to be identified under white-light mode, they became clearly visible by their typical red fluorescence under 635 nm illumination. The patient did not experience any side effects from 5ALA (67). Suzuki et al. also investigated 5ALA's fluorescence in normal parathyroid glands in 13 patients with thyroid disease undergoing hemithyroidectomy. Patients were orally administered 20 mg/kg body weight of 5ALA dissolved in 10% glucose 5 h prior to surgery. After anterior neck exposure, the room was darkened and the incision was illuminated with a violet-blue light of 405 nm. In all 13 patients, parathyroid glands were easily identified by their red fluorescence, even when they could not be detected under normal light conditions (66). Takeuchi et al. further evaluated the use of 5ALA for identifying parathyroid gland tissue in 20 patients with primary hyperparathyroidism, 6 patients with secondary hyperparathyroidism, and 3 patients with thyroid tumors and normal parathyroid glands. All patients were administered oral 20 mg/kg 45 min to 5 h prior to surgery. In the majority of the cases, 5ALA accurately identified both normal and abnormal parathyroid glands (68).

Appropriate 5ALA Dose and Route of Administration

The preferred application of 5ALA fluorescence during head and neck surgeries depends on the area of surgical interest. For oral lesions, a 0.4% oral solution of 5ALA dissolved in mineral oil rinsed for 15 min followed by 1 to 2.5 h incubation prior to illumination is the most common regime used (61–63). A 0.4–1.0% 5ALA solution diluted with 0.9% saline topically applied via a nebulized inhaler with an incubation period of 1–2 h prior to a microlarnyngoscopy has been reported for oral and pharyngeal lesions (64, 65). Whereas, for parathyroid and thyroid surgery, 20–30 mg/kg of 5ALA given orally with an incubation period between 45 min to 5 h has been reported (66–68). The safety of 5ALA, regardless of the administration route, has been questioned. Some studies suspected an increase in serum creatinine levels after 5ALA administration; however, this was refuted by Quon et al. when they concluded that the increased creatinine levels represented a false elevation due to substrate competition (69). Evidence in head and neck surgery shows that 5ALA is safe with little to no side effects, with the precaution to avoid sun exposure 24 to 48 h after ingesting 5ALA to avoid the risk of skin bleaching and other phototoxic effects on the skin and eyes (63, 70).

Imaging 5ALA Fluorescence in Head and Neck Surgery

At the molecular level, 5ALA is metabolized by neoplastic or highly metabolic tissues into protoporphyrin IX, a photosensitive metabolite that is excited between wavelengths 375–440 nm and subsequently emits fluorescence between 635 and 700n m (71). The use of an endoscope equipped with a special filter system attached to a footswitch that allows changing between brightfield illumination and fluorescence excitation is the preferred method for detecting the red fluorescence when 5ALA is applied in head and neck surgery.

Conclusions and Future Applications of 5ALA in Head and Neck Surgery

The above studies suggest that 5ALA has potential for improving the early detection of suspected oral and pharyngeal cancerous lesions and may reduce operative time and rate of reoperation in patients with parathyroid and thyroid disease. The disadvantage of 5ALA is the need for patients to avoid sun exposure 24 to 48 h after exposure to 5ALA. More clinical studies are needed to further validate the surgical benefits of 5ALA compared to routine surgery before the use of 5ALA can become FDA-approved for clinical practice in head and neck surgery.

GASTROINTESTINAL SURGERY

First Application of 5ALA in Gastrointestinal (GI) Surgery

The use of 5ALA for photodiagnosis in gastroenterology and gastrointestinal surgery, while broad and encompassing esophageal, gastric, hepatic, and colorectal pathologies, has not yet replaced established standard practice in this field. Interestingly, its first use was aimed at a predominantly preventive strategy during screening colonoscopies to identify mucosal adenomas with malignant potential. Although adenomas are benign, there is no method to distinguish between benign and malignant lesions by conventional colonoscopy. Therefore, Eker et al. (72) described the use of 5ALA to aid in the differentiation of mucosal tissue, potentially as a means to decrease cost and labor involved in removing benign lesions. Of 57 selected patients undergoing laser-induced fluorescence colonoscopy, 41 were ultimately included. Patients were given oral ALA at 5 mg/kg and underwent the study after 2–3 h. A nitrogen laser was tested at excitation wavelengths of 337, 504, and 436 nm. The excitation of tissues at 337 nm was used, as that wavelength yielded the maximum difference in emission between normal and adenomatous tissue. All patient groups were combined at the 337 nm wavelength, including patients who were treated with 5ALA and those who were not. When excited at 337 nm, the sensitivity for adenoma detection was 100% and the specificity was 96%. At the other wavelengths of 405 and 463 nm, the sensitivity and specificity were also higher for 5ALA-treated patients than those without.

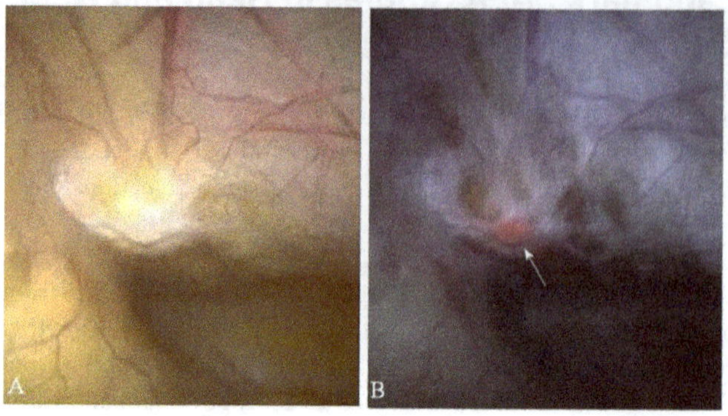

FIGURE 5 | Fluorescence imaging in Gastrointestinal Surgery. **(A)** Non-specific peritoneal area under white light illumination. **(B)** Corresponding fluorescence overlay image shows fluorescence foci histologically consistent with metastatic gastric cancer (arrow). Images obtained with Karl Storz D-light endoscope system. [Intraoperative images courtesy of Namikawa et al. (74)].

The application of 5ALA in predicting the malignant potential of dysplastic epithelial cells associated with ulcerative colitis also demonstrated an efficacious use of the fluorescent molecule. One group evaluated the use of 5ALA to enhance the detection of dysplastic tissue that may otherwise be missed from the conventional standard of care, which is four-quadrant random colon biopsies. In this study, 37 patients underwent 54 colonoscopies and received systemic oral ingestion, a local enema, or a local catheter-directed spray form of 5ALA. The local spray had the highest sensitivity of 100% for detecting malignant tissue. Overall, this serves as a promising modality to increase detection of dysplasia with a reduction of sampling error and unnecessary random biopsies (73).

Landmark 5ALA Studies in GI Surgery

Similar to its use for colorectal cancer, endoscopic 5ALA fluorescence has been explored as a surveillance method for detecting dysplastic, pre-malignant tissue of the esophagus (Barret's), and more recently, assisting in laparoscopy-guided resection of gastric and hepatic malignancies (**Figure 5**). These studies have highlighted the growing number of 5ALA applications in GI surgery while also demonstrating the mild, transient adverse reaction profile with oral administration.

Much of the data pertaining to the use of 5ALA is for the diagnosis and detection of dysplastic tissue in Barrett's esophagus during upper endoscopy. Barrett's esophagus is the replacement of normal esophageal epithelium (stratified squamous) to colonic epithelium (simple columnar), typically due to chronic exposure to acid reflux from the stomach. It is considered a premalignant lesion and requires endoscopic surveillance with biopsy. The biopsy for Barrett's esophagus is extensive: it involves obtaining 4 random quadrant biopsies for every 2 cm length of the Barrett's esophagus. The tissue within Barrett's esophagus can be classified as a range: nondysplastic, low grade dysplasia, high grade dysplasia, to adenocarcinoma, but these cannot be distinguished by gross examination with standard endoscopy. Given the time and cost required to biopsy Barrett's esophagus via the conventional method, alternative methods are investigated to better pinpoint dysplastic lesions, such as the use of ALA.

Brand et al. (75) evaluated the use of 5ALA to identify dysplasia within Barrett's esophagus, high grade dysplasia in particular. Twenty patients with known Barrett's esophagus were given 5ALA at 10 mg/kg dissolved in orange juice 3 h prior to endoscopy. A nitrogen laser at excitation of 400 nm was used at a total of 97 mucosal sites. The use of 5ALA provided detection of high grade dysplasia from normal tissue at 77% sensitivity and 71% specificity. In nodular high grade dysplasia the sensitivity and specificity of 5ALA-mediated photodiagnosis approaches 100%. Although the use of fluorescence endoscopy may assist in identification of these high grade lesions, there is no definitive data that suggest its use is superior to random biopsies.

Stepinac et al. (76) performed a similar study investigating the fluorescence detection of dysplasia and early cancer in Barrett's esophagus using 20 mg/kg of 5ALA vs. conventional random four-quadrant biopsy. Twenty-eight patients with known Barrett's esophagus were selected for the study. All patients first underwent conventional endoscopy with random four quadrant biopsies at 1 cm intervals approximately 4–6 weeks prior to fluorescence endoscopy. A total of 532 biopsies were taken. During fluorescence endoscopy, a total of 178 biopsies were taken, 81 in fluorescent regions and 97 in non-fluorescent regions. The sensitivity and specificity of fluorescence-guided biopsies were 100 and 63%, respectively. Fluorescence endoscopy identified 5 low grade dysplasia lesions that were not identified by conventional biopsy. Conventional biopsy identified 3 low grade dysplasia lesions that were not detected during fluorescence endoscopy. Both the conventional and 5ALA methods were able to identify high grade dysplasia and adenocarcinoma, but neither is ideal for identification of low grade dysplasia. However, the use of ALA and fluorescence endoscopy may result in fewer biopsies needed to achieve the same diagnosis (81 biopsies vs. 531).

Although the incidence of gastric cancer has decreased overall, it remains one of the most common cancers worldwide. It commonly spreads by peritoneal seeding. The presence of peritoneal dissemination can alter the treatment decision-making between surgery and chemotherapy. In patients with locally advanced disease, performing a staging laparoscopy can help guide treatment. Staging laparoscopy has a sensitivity of ~30–40% for peritoneal seeding. Kishi et al. (77) has evaluated the use of 5ALA to enhance the tumor detection rate in advanced gastric cancer. Thirteen patients with known gastric cancer were selected to undergo staging laparoscopy. They are given 1 g 5ALA 4 h prior to laparoscopy. The detection rate for metastatic lesions using 5ALA had a sensitivity of 93% and a specificity of 100%. However, there were inconsistencies in the detection of the primary tumors. Although all primary tumors with serosal invasion were detected, 5ALA failed to help identify two primary tumors without serosal invasion and two primary tumors with adjacent organ invasion. This emphasizes the limitation of the use of visible wavelength fluorescence imaging, for while it is useful in detecting surface tumors, it may not visualize tumors that are deeply embedded in tissue.

In 2017, Ushimaru et al. (78) performed 5ALA-assisted staging laparoscopy on 113 patients with advanced gastric cancer and based their treatment strategies on the results of the laparoscopy. They retrospectively evaluated the outcomes, and identified predictive factors for peritoneal metastasis. All patients were given 1 g 5ALA 3–5 h prior to laparoscopy. Observation of abdominal cavity using white light and blue light was done using the Storz D-light System laparoscope. Patients noted to have peritoneal metastasis and/or positive cytology, as diagnosed by 5ALA staging laparoscopy, underwent chemotherapy and an interval gastrectomy if a later laparoscopy revealed negative peritoneal disease. Those without metastasis or cytology underwent definitive gastrectomy during the same procedure. Patients with no peritoneal metastasis had a similar estimated survival than patients with peritoneal metastasis only seen with 5ALA. Factors that were predictive for metastasis were advanced T stage, diffuse-type histology, ascites, and female sex. This study suggests that the use of staging laparoscopy with 5ALA may enhance the diagnostic accuracy for advanced gastric cancer patients and thereby improve their overall treatment outcome.

5ALA-mediated photodiagnosis of hepatic tumors is currently being explored. Kaibori et al. (79) evaluated a total of 134 patients undergoing hepatic resections. They compared the utility of both 5ALA and Indocyanine Green for the intraoperative detection of tumors. Although Indocyanine Green had higher sensitivity of tumor detection (96% vs. 57%), the specificity of detection by 5ALA was 100%. One limitation of photodiagnosis for solid organ tumors is short distance of penetration. 5ALA mediated fluorescence only penetrates 2–5 mm of tissue, limiting its use to superficial tumors. The adverse effects, while transient and self-limited, may also deter patient participation.

A serious complication of hepatic resection is postoperative bile leak. Inoue et al. (80) evaluated 737 patients who underwent hepatic resections. Of these, 109 patients were given oral 1 g 5ALA dissolved in 20 ml of 50% glucose approximately 3 h prior to hepatic resection, which is excreted in the bile. Intraoperatively, patients were evaluated for leaks after resection, first by gross evaluation then by blue light (405 nm) illumination. Fluorescence imaging using 5ALA increased the intraoperative detection rate of bile leaks from 8.3 to 13.7%. Given the mildly increased detection rate, more studies will be needed to justify routine use of 5ALA.

Appropriate Dose of 5ALA and Route of Administration

The optimal dosing of 5ALA in the upper and lower GI tract did not vary significantly from that which was historically used in non-GI related malignancies. Since its earlier application for the photodiagnosis of colorectal (72, 73) and esophageal carcinoma (75, 76), oral administration of 5 and 10 mg/kg, respectively, demonstrated superior sensitivity and specificity in identifying neoplastic tissue on par with that of tradition biopsy-based surveillance methods. Oral administration of even greater amounts of 5ALA up to 1 g for its more recent gastric and hepatic applications (77–80), including the fluorescence of post-resection bile leaks, has shown equal efficacy.

Conclusions and Future Applications of 5ALA in GI Surgery

Although there is promising data regarding the use of photodiagnosis in gastroenterology and general surgery, there lacks conclusive data to push its use into standard practice. More randomized control trials with larger patient samples are still needed at this time.

CARDIOTHORACIC SURGERY SECTION

First Application of 5ALA in Cardiothoracic Surgery

The first study examining 5ALA's ability to detect early stage lung cancer was published in 1996 by Baumgartner et al. (81). In this study, Baumgartner administered 5–10 wt% (250–500 mg 5ALA in 0.5 ml isotonic saline) through a medical nebulizer to 7 patients with positive or suspicious sputum cytology, but negative white light bronchoscopy, for inhalation for 30–40 min followed by fluorescence bronchoscopy after 3 h. An ultraviolet light with 406.7–413.5 nm was used for excitation. A target integrating color CCD video camera was adapted to the bronchoscope and captured emission wavelength of 635 nm and 705 nm. Baumgartner calculated that the amount of 5ALA inhaled within lung tissue was independent of patients' breathing patterns. Thus, patients can have a wide range of pulmonary function without concern for variability in 5ALA concentration. A peak plasma blood PpIX concentration was found at 3.5 h after inhalation. No side-effects were observed in the 7 patients. A total of 30 tissue samples were taken which showed nine tumors, including seven carcinoma *in situ*, by PpIX fluorescence. Sensitivity was 100% and specificity ranged from 30 to 50% due to five tissue samples exhibiting weak fluorescence with indeterminate diagnoses. This study showed that 5ALA inhalation was safe, could mediate detection of carcinoma *in situ* within lung tissue, and may be used to assist diagnosing early bronchial malignancies.

Follow-Up Study Using Inhaled 5ALA for Bronchial Tumors

Following Baumgartner's study of 7 patients, Piotrowski et al. performed a perspective feasibility study on safety and efficacy of 5ALA for diagnosing bronchial neoplasms (82). Forty-nine patients, divided into four groups, inhaled either 5 or 10 ml of 5ALA solution 3 h before bronchoscopy examination. Xenon short arc lamp with a special filter system was used for fluorescence excitation ($\lambda ex = 375–440$ nm) along with an integrated filter that blocked remitted excitation (long pass = 440 nm). Groups consisted of laryngo-tracheo-bronchial tumors that were previously diagnosed by conventional diagnostic modes ($n = 17$); patients with prior surgery due to bronchial tumors ($n = 6$), patients with prior surgery for laryngeal cancer ($n = 4$); and present or ex-heavy smokers without signs of tumor in conventional examinations ($n = 22$). There was no significant difference between pre and post FEV1 values. The overall sensitivity of 5ALA was 82% and specificity was 62% for all groups, PPV of 45% and NPV of 90%. When brightfield illumination (WLB) plus 5ALA was compared with brightfield alone, there was an increase in sensitivity by 2.1% and NPV by 6%, but decreased specificity by 35.4% and PPV by 53.1%. When the heavy smoker group was excluded (due to increased number of false positives), the WLB+5ALA sensitivity increased by 22% and NPV by 34%, whereas specificity decreased by 26% and PPV by 35%. Due to its higher sensitivity, 5ALA was able to identify recurrent SCC in one patient and a synchronous lesion in another patient that were WLB-negative. Because of the high number of false positive samples, authors concluded that 5ALA should not be used for screening. Rather in combination with WLB, it could be used to guide the physician in choosing proper sites for biopsy due to its higher sensitivity and NPV. Additionally, in this study 5ALA induced transient bronchial obstruction in 2 patients from the heavy smokers group that was reversed with short acting beta agonists.

5ALA Fluorescence for Staging Pleural Malignancies in Patients With Inconclusive Pleural Effusions

Thoracoscopy is often used in patients with negative pleural fluid examinations for staging of malignancies. However, some cases still remain undiagnosed or understaged (83). In 2006, Baas et al. in a feasibility study, incorporated fluorescence and white light inspection on 26 patients with non-diagnostic pleural effusions to test 5ALA's efficacy in diagnosing and staging of pleural malignancies. Three patients were excluded either due to multiple adhesions within thoracic cavity or inability to perform endoscopic inspection. Patients ingested a 2,000 to 2,500 mg capsule of 5ALA depending on body weight followed by thoracoscopy 3–4 h later. Fluorescence images were recorded using the D-LIGHT System with <500 nm for excitation and long-pass filter (470 nm long-pass). In 23 patients, a total of 111 biopsies were taken. Fifteen patients were diagnosed with malignant mesothelioma, 5 with metastases. Three patients had benign plaques and one with empyema. One patient who did not receive initial diagnosis developed mesothelioma 6 months later. A discrepancy between white light and 5ALA occurred in 37 biopsies and further analysis showed there was no improvement using 5ALA to obtain diagnosis. However, with 5ALA, 4 patients upstaged their diagnosis through detection of small lesions (<3 mm) throughout the parietal and visceral pleura as well as the collapsed lung. Complications occurred in 3 patients from thoracoscopy. No side-effects were reported using 5ALA besides grade 1 skin burn in 3 patients 28 to 36 h after 5ALA intake. Authors showed that 5ALA can help improve staging in patients with pleural malignancy and could help guide in choosing proper biopsy sites during thoracoscopy.

In another study of undiagnosed pleural effusions by Pikin et al. 23 patients with non-conclusive pleural effusions received 25 mg/kg of 5ALA 3 h before video-assisted bronchoscopy (84). A total of 118 biopsies were taken. Both white light and fluorescence thoracoscopy detected pleural deposits in 20 patients but fluorescence was able to detect additional lesions in 12 of the 20 patients. In three other patients with macroscopically normal pleura by white-light mode, 5ALA detected micrometastases in one patient that was metastatic lung adenocarcinoma by histological examination. Results from combined conventional and florescence thoracoscopy showed specificity of 88.4%, sensitivity of 89.1% and diagnostic accuracy of 88.9%—results much higher than other studies. Authors pointed out that detecting additional lesions in patients with macroscopic pleural spread does not influence outcome in the majority of cases. However, detection of pleural micometastases in patients with peripheral lung cancer and visceral pleural invasion could improve pre-operative approaches and possible outcomes.

Pharmacokinetics of Inhaled 5ALA for Optimum 5ALA-Induced Protoporphyrin IX Fluorescence in Bronchial Tissue

In Baumgartner et al.'s 1996 study, he first showed that 5ALA was safe for inhalation. In a follow-up study, Hautmann et al. examined *in vivo* kinetics of inhaled 5ALA that generate the greatest difference in fluorescence between tumor and adjacent bronchial tissue. Nineteen patients with known or suspected bronchial carcinoma are given 200 mg of 5ALA dissolved in 5 ml of isotonic NaCl via inhalation. Patients are then randomized to 1,2,3,4, or 6 h before bronchoscopy under local anesthesia.

Excitation wavelength of 380–440 nm was used and emission greater 630 nm, with a peak emission at 635, were measured using Optical Multichannel Analyzer (OMA). Spectroscopy was then analyzed on all macroscopically suspicious areas and areas showing porphyrin fluorescence. A total of 38 biopsies were taken that showed sensitivity that is almost twice that of white light, but with a significant decrease in specificity. This decrease in specificity was explained by the uptake of 5ALA by inflammatory lesions. Spectroscopy showed that normal tissue showed a maximum fluorescence 200 min after 5ALA application and lesions with moderate dysplasia at 160 min after 5ALA application. The spectral data showed significant difference between lesions with moderate dysplasia and normal, as well as lesions with moderate dysplasia and lesions with mild dysplasia 80 to 270 min after 5ALA inhalation. During this time interval, 5ALA fluorescence in lesions with moderate dysplasia can exhibit fluorescence values 5 times higher compared to the normal tissue. No difference was seen in lesions with mild dysplasia and normal tissue (85).

5ALA Facilitates Differentiation of Primary Lung Cancer With Pleural Invasion

Kitada et al. recruited a total of 40 patients diagnosed pre-operatively with lung cancer to undergo white light and 5ALA-mediated photodiagnosis. Patients consisted of 28 cases with primary lung cancer, 8 with metastatic lung tumors, 2 with malignant pleural tumors, and 2 with benign tumors. All lung metastases on the pleural surface, pleural malignant mesotheliomas and benign tumors were visualized under red fluorescence. For primary lung tumors, red fluorescence was confirmed in 15 of 28 patients (53.5%). All P11–P13 (ranging from tumor invading beyond elastic layer to tumors invading parietal pleura) tumors were visualized (10/10). However, visualization decreased to 5/18 (27.7%) for p10 cases (tumor within subpleural parenchyma or superficial invasion of pleural connective tissue). These 5 cases had been previously diagnosed as p11. Authors showed that 5ALA enhances accurate diagnosis of malignant lesions on the pleural surface as well as detection and localization of small disseminated lesions and small metastatic tumors to the lung (86).

Current Status and Future Directions of 5ALA in Cardiothoracic Surgery

Currently, 5ALA is still used as a research tool for photodynamic diagnosis in cardiothoracic surgery. Future direction of 5ALA includes a possible of direct comparison of brightfield vs. 5ALA-mediated fluorescence bronchoscopy in a randomized control trial to determine which yields higher sensitivity and/or specificity.

Conclusion

Clinical studies show 5ALA photodynamic diagnosis yields higher sensitivity but lower specificity in identifying lung and pleural malignancies. When added with conventional brightfield illumination, 5ALA can help visualize small primary tumors (<3 mm), small lung metastases and primary lung cancer with pleural invasions. 5ALA may prove useful for guiding surgeons to specific biopsy sites and in the upstaging of tumors.

DISCUSSION

The clinical use of fluorescent molecules dates back to the start of the twentieth century. Coined "Photodynamic Wirkung," or photodynamic phenomenon, European scientists first described how to utilize these molecules to macroscopically label abnormal tissue (87). While initially a conceptual application, this methodology has driven numerous oncologic investigations of naturally derived fluorescent molecules. Hematoporphyrin derivatives were introduced in the mid-twentieth century as potentially valuable diagnostic tools and treatment modalities. Early studies conducted by Lipson and colleagues (88) using rudimentary, yet novel, endoscopic devices to differentiate neoplastic cells from normal tissue further developed our understanding of hematoporphyrin derivatives in the surgical setting. Currently FDA-approved for its use is glioma surgery, 5ALA has undergone significant advances in its applications to include neurosurgical, head and neck, urological, cardiothoracic, gastrointestinal, and OB/GYN surgery. This historical review of clinical studies highlights the rapidly expanding role of 5ALA in the diagnosis and treatment of neoplastic disease.

Within each surgical field, studies have outlined the advantages and disadvantages 5ALA-mediated photodiagnosis. Due to its ubiquity in the heme synthesis pathway of all cells, and preferential accumulation of PpIX within neoplastic cells, the route and dosage of 5ALA has minimally varied. Intra-venous, oral, intra-peritoneal, intra-vaginal, inhaled, and topically administered 5ALA all demonstrate a similar optimal dosing (5–30 mg/kg), and often, dose-dependent responses. For many 5ALA applications, maximum dose are determined not by increased adverse reactions, but rather plateauing of sensitivity and specificity in neoplastic cell labeling. This phenomenon seems intuitive given 5ALA's role as a naturally occurring PpIX precursor. Studies have noted relatively benign and avoidable adverse reactions including bronchospasm with inhaled variants, and photosensitivity most prevalent with topical and oral administration of 5ALA. Regardless of route of administration, the sensitivity of 5ALA photodiagnosis has varied from 83% with low doses in urologic dysplasia to 100% for most other applications. Albeit rare, a notable disadvantage of using 5ALA is represented in its poor specificity in differentiating moderate dysplasia or cells exhibiting inflammatory changes from normal tissue or higher-grade dysplastic lesions. This limitation is most apparent in labeling urothelial carcinoma and BCC/SCC, resulting in high false positive rates due to epithelial hypercellularity or inadequate depth of topical penetration, respectively. In order to ameliorate non-specific labeling observed with these applications, the composition of 5ALA delivery systems (liposomal) and solvents (EDTA or DMSO) are continuing to be evaluated.

Imaging devices used to visualize 5ALA uptake and PpIX fluorescence are also advancing in their design and implementation. In early clinical applications of hematoporphyrin derivatives, such as PpIX, for malignancies of the upper GI and cardiopulmonary systems, a 400-watt mercury lamp transmitted white light via glass fiber cables through which excitatory (~400 nm) wavelengths were separated by a quartz rod placed in a rigid bronchoscope (88). Using optical filters in the form of glasses or eye-shields, the surgeon would then visualize only red-fluorescence wavelengths corresponding to PpIX. Current-day fluorescence-guided surgery using commercially available wide-field microscopes is significantly less cumbersome and utilizes more sensitive short pass and long pass filters integrated within the system. Additional imaging hardware designs have aimed to improve on the historical limitations of using 5ALA in its various surgical contexts. While still investigational, newer imaging hardware optimizes the resolution of PpIX in either islands of neoplastic cells or areas of lower-grade lesions where PpIX fluorescence may not be as robust as that of higher-grade lesions. The largest obstacles toward this goal have been to mitigate signal-to-noise ratio of autofluorescent tissue and to achieve a greater sensitivity in localizing deep, labeled tissue (89).

Administration of 5ALA has granted surgeons within multiple subspecialties the ability to more accurately visualize malignant tissue during surgery. The vast data from studies collected during the past 6–7 decades is representative of 5ALA's small side effect profile and reliable efficacy. The growth of 5ALA's intraoperative applications during this timeframe has been paralleled by advancements in imaging technology focused on improving PpIX visualization. These clinical trials suggest 5ALA is a relatively safe molecule for generating intraoperative photodiagnosis of malignant tissues across multiple surgical-oncology subspecialties.

AUTHOR CONTRIBUTIONS

JG, AV, HW, AB, MK, SC, ZA-A, MB, HO, JI, SYu, and CL wrote key portions of the manuscript and created the figures. DA, JL, PN, KB, and SYo oversaw the writing process, provided mentorship, edited, and contributed to manuscript.

REFERENCES

1. Mooney MA, Zehri AH, Georges JF, Nakaji P. Laser scanning confocal endomicroscopy in the neurosurgical operating room: a review and discussion of future applications. *Neurosurg Focus.* (2014) 36:E9. doi: 10.3171/2013.11.FOCUS13484
2. Hadjipanayis CG, Stummer W. 5-ALA and FDA approval for glioma surgery. *J Neurooncol.* (2019) 141:479–86. doi: 10.1007/s11060-019-03098-y
3. Neuberger A, Scott JJ. Aminolaevulinic acid and porphyrin biosynthesis. *Nature.* (1953) 172:1093–4. doi: 10.1038/1721093a0
4. Schiffmann E, Shemin D. Further studies on the utilization of delta-aminolevulinic acid for porphyrin synthesis. *J Biol Chem.* (1957) 225:623–8.
5. Granick S. Porphyrin biosynthesis in erythrocytes. I. Formation of gamma-aminolevulinic acid in erythrocytes. *J Biol Chem.* (1958) 232:1101–17.
6. Granick S, Mauzerall D. Pbrphyrin biosynthesis in erythrocytes. II. Enzymes converting gamma-aminolevulinic acid to coproporphyrinogen. *J Biol Chem.* (1958) 232:1119–40.
7. Berlin NI, Neuberger A, Scott JJ. The metabolism of delta -aminolaevulic acid. 1. Normal pathways, studied with the aid of 15N. *Biochem J.* (1956) 64:80–90. doi: 10.1042/bj0640080
8. Kriegmair M, Baumgartner R, Knuchel R, Ehsan A, Steinbach P, Lumper W, et al. [Photodynamic diagnosis of urothelial neoplasms after intravesicular instillation of 5-aminolevulinic acid]. *Urologe A.* (1994) 33:270–5.
9. Kriegmair M, Baumgartner R, Knuechel R, Steinbach P, Ehsan A, Lumper W, et al. Fluorescence photodetection of neoplastic urothelial lesions following intravesical instillation of 5-aminolevulinic acid. *Urology.* (1994) 44:836–41. doi: 10.1016/S0090-4295(94)80167-3
10. Szeimies RM, Sassy T, Landthaler M. Penetration potency of topical applied delta-aminolevulinic acid for photodynamic therapy of basal cell carcinoma. *Photochem Photobiol.* (1994) 59:73–6. doi: 10.1111/j.1751-1097.1994.tb05003.x
11. Stummer W, Stocker S, Wagner S, Stepp H, Fritsch C, Goetz C, et al. Intraoperative detection of malignant gliomas by 5-aminolevulinic acid-induced porphyrin fluorescence. *Neurosurgery.* (1998) 42:518–25.
12. Stummer W, Novotny A, Stepp H, Goetz C, Bise K, Reulen HJ. Fluorescence-guided resection of glioblastoma multiforme by using 5-aminolevulinic acid-induced porphyrins: a prospective study in 52 consecutive patients. *J Neurosurg.* (2000) 93:1003–13. doi: 10.3171/jns.2000.93.6.1003
13. Stummer W, Pichlmeier U, Meinel T, Wiestler OD, Zanella F, Reulen HJ, et al. Fluorescence-guided surgery with 5-aminolevulinic acid for resection of malignant glioma: a randomised controlled multicentre phase III trial. *Lancet Oncol.* (2006) 7:392–401. doi: 10.1016/S1470-2045(06)70665-9
14. Coburger J, Engelke J, Scheuerle A, Thal DR, Hlavac M, Wirtz CR, et al. Tumor

detection with 5-aminolevulinic acid fluorescence and Gd-DTPA-enhanced intraoperative MRI at the border of contrast-enhancing lesions: a prospective study based on histopathological assessment. *Neurosurg Focus.* (2014) 36:E3. doi: 10.3171/2013.11.FOCUS13463

15. Stummer W, Stepp H, Wiestler OD, Pichlmeier U. Randomized, prospective double-blinded study comparing 3 different doses of 5-aminolevulinic acid for fluorescence-guided resections of malignant gliomas. *Neurosurgery.* (2017) 81:230–9. doi: 10.1093/neuros/nyx074
16. Eljamel S, Petersen M, Valentine R, Buist R, Goodman C, Moseley H, et al. Comparison of intraoperative fluorescence and MRI image guided neuronavigation in malignant brain tumours, a prospective controlled study. *Photodiagn Photodyn Ther.* (2013) 10:356–61. doi: 10.1016/j.pdpdt.2013.03.006
17. Loh CS, MacRobert AJ, Bedwell J, Regula J, Krasner N, Bown SG. Oral versus intravenous administration of 5-aminolaevulinic acid for photodynamic therapy. *Br J Cancer.* (1993) 68:41–51. doi: 10.1038/bjc.1993.284
18. Kriss TC, Kriss VM. History of the operating microscope: from magnifying glass to microneurosurgery. *Neurosurgery.* (1998) 42:899–907. doi: 10.1097/00006123-199804000-00116
19. Belloch JP, Rovira V, Llacer JL, Riesgo PA, Cremades A. Fluorescence-guided surgery in high grade gliomas using an exoscope system. *Acta Neurochir* (2014) 156:653–60. doi: 10.1007/s00701-013-1976-6
20. Piquer J, Llacer JL, Rovira V, Riesgo P, Rodriguez R, Cremades A. Fluorescence-guided surgery and biopsy in gliomas with an exoscope system. *BioMed Res Int.* (2014) 2014:207974. doi: 10.1155/2014/207974
21. Widhalm G, Wolfsberger S, Minchev G, Woehrer A, Krssak M, Czech T, et al. 5-Aminolevulinic acid is a promising marker for detection of anaplastic foci in diffusely infiltrating gliomas with nonsignificant contrast enhancement. *Cancer.* (2010) 116:1545–52. doi: 10.1002/cncr.24903
22. Widhalm G, Kiesel B, Woehrer A, Traub-Weidinger T, Preusser M, Marosi C, et al. 5-Aminolevulinic acid induced fluorescence is a powerful intraoperative marker for precise histopathological grading of gliomas with non-significant contrast-enhancement. *PloS ONE.* (2013) 8:e76988. doi: 10.1371/journal.pone.0076988
23. Valdes PA, Jacobs V, Harris BT, Wilson BC, Leblond F, Paulsen KD, et al. Quantitative fluorescence using 5-aminolevulinic acid-induced protoporphyrin IX biomarker as a surgical adjunct in low-grade glioma surgery. *J Neurosurg.* (2015) 123:771–80. doi: 10.3171/2014.12.JNS14391
24. Valdes PA, Bekelis K, Harris BT, Wilson BC, Leblond F, Kim A, et al. 5-Aminolevulinic acid-induced protoporphyrin IX fluorescence in meningioma: qualitative and quantitative measurements *in vivo. Neurosurgery.* (2014) 10(Suppl. 1):74–82. doi: 10.1227/NEU.0000000000000117
25. Coluccia D, Fandino J, Fujioka M, Cordovi S, Muroi C, Landolt H. Intraoperative 5-aminolevulinic-acid-induced fluorescence in meningiomas. *Acta Neurochir (Wien).* (2010) 152:1711–9. doi: 10.1007/s00701-010-0708-4
26. Eljamel MS, Leese G, Moseley H. Intraoperative optical identification of pituitary adenomas. *J Neurooncol.* (2009) 92:417–21. doi: 10.1007/s11060-009-9820-9
27. Stummer W, Tonn JC, Goetz C, Ullrich W, Stepp H, Bink A, et al. 5-Aminolevulinic acid-derived tumor fluorescence: the diagnostic accuracy of visible fluorescence qualities as corroborated by spectrometry and histology and postoperative imaging. *Neurosurgery.* (2014) 74:310–9. doi: 10.1227/NEU.0000000000000267
28. Roberts DW, Olson JD, Evans LT, Kolste KK, Kanick SC, Fan X, et al. Red-light excitation of protoporphyrin IX fluorescence for subsurface tumor detection. *J Neurosurg.* (2018) 128:1690–7. doi: 10.3171/2017.1.JNS162061
29. Inoue K, Anai S, Fujimoto K, Hirao Y, Furuse H, Kai F, et al. Oral 5-aminolevulinic acid mediated photodynamic diagnosis using fluorescence cystoscopy for non-muscle-invasive bladder cancer: a randomized, double-blind, multicentre phase II/III study. *Photodiagn Photodyn Ther.* (2015) 12:193–200. doi: 10.1016/j.pdpdt.2015.03.008
30. Inoue K, Matsuyama H, Fujimoto K, Hirao Y, Watanabe H, Ozono S, et al. The clinical trial on the safety and effectiveness of the photodynamic diagnosis of non-muscle-invasive bladder cancer using fluorescent light-guided cystoscopy after oral administration of 5-aminolevulinic acid (5-ALA). *Photodiagn Photodyn Ther.* (2016) 13:91–6. doi: 10.1016/j.pdpdt.2015.12.011
31. Fukuhara H, Kureishi M, Khoda T, Inoue K, Tanaka T, Iketani K, et al. The utility of a flexible fluorescence-cystoscope with a twin mode monitor for the 5-Aminolevulinic acid-mediated photodynamic diagnosis of bladder cancer. *PloS ONE.* (2015) 10:e0136416. doi: 10.1371/journal.pone.0136416
32. Colombo R, Naspro R, Bellinzoni P, Fabbri F, Guazzoni G, Scattoni V, et al. Photodynamic diagnosis for follow-up of carcinoma *in situ* of the bladder. *Ther Clin Risk Manage.* (2007) 3:1003–7.
33. D'Hallewin MA, Vanherzeele H, Baert L. Fluorescence detection of flat transitional cell carcinoma after intravesical instillation of aminolevulinic acid. *Am J Clin Oncol.* (1998) 21:223–5. doi: 10.1097/00000421-199806000-00002
34. Frimberger D, Zaak D, Hofstetter A. Endoscopic fluorescence diagnosis and laser treatment of transitional cell carcinoma of the bladder. *Semin Urol Oncol.* (2000) 18:264–72.
35. Kriegmair M, Baumgartner R, Knuchel R, Stepp H, Hofstadter F, Hofstetter A. Detection of early bladder cancer by 5-aminolevulinic acid induced porphyrin fluorescence. *J Urol.* (1996) 155:105–9. doi: 10.1097/00005392-199601000-00038
36. Osman E, Alnaib Z, Kumar N. Photodynamic diagnosis in upper urinary tract urothelial carcinoma: a systematic review. *Arab J Urol.* (2017) 15:100–9. doi: 10.1016/j.aju.2017.01.003
37. Spiess PE, Grossman HB. Fluorescence cystoscopy: is it ready for use in routine clinical practice? *Curr Opin Urol.* (2006) 16:372–6. doi: 10.1097/01.mou.0000240312.16324.9a
38. Draga RO, Grimbergen MC, Kok ET, Jonges TN, Bosch JL. Predictors of false positives in 5-aminolevulinic acid-induced photodynamic diagnosis of bladder carcinoma: identification of patient groups that may benefit most from highly specific optical diagnostics. *Urology.* (2009) 74:851–6. doi: 10.1016/j.urology.2009.04.095
39. Kata SG, Aboumarzouk OM, Zreik A, Somani B, Ahmad S, Nabi G, et al. Photodynamic diagnostic ureterorenoscopy: a valuable tool in the detection of upper urinary tract tumour. *Photodiagn Photodyn Ther.* (2016) 13:255–60. doi: 10.1016/j.pdpdt.2015.08.002
40. Kennedy JC, Pottier RH, Pross DC. Photodynamic therapy with endogenous protoporphyrin IX: basic principles and present clinical experience. *J Photochem Photobiol B Biol.* (1990) 6:143–8. doi: 10.1016/1011-1344(90)85083-9
41. Fritsch C, Becker-Wegerich PM, Menke H, Ruzicka T, Goerz G, Olbrisch RR. Successful surgery of multiple recurrent basal cell carcinomas guided by photodynamic diagnosis. *Aesthetic Plastic Surg.* (1997) 21:437–9. doi: 10.1007/s002669900153
42. de Leeuw J, van der Beek N, Neugebauer WD, Bjerring P, Neumann HA. Fluorescence detection and diagnosis of non-melanoma skin cancer at an early stage. *Lasers Surg Med.* (2009) 41:96–103. doi: 10.1002/lsm.20739
43. Redondo P, Marquina M, Pretel M, Aguado L, Iglesias ME. Methyl-ALA-induced fluorescence in photodynamic diagnosis of basal cell carcinoma prior to Mohs micrographic surgery. *Arch Dermatol.* (2008) 144:115–7. doi: 10.1001/archdermatol.2007.3
44. Martin A, Tope WD, Grevelink JM, Starr JC, Fewkes JL, Flotte TJ, et al. Lack of selectivity of protoporphyrin IX fluorescence for basal cell carcinoma after topical application of 5-aminolevulinic acid: implications for photodynamic treatment. *Arch Dermatol Res.* (1995) 287:665–74. doi: 10.1007/BF00371740
45. Ericson MB, Sandberg C, Gudmundson F, Rosen A, Larko O, Wennberg AM. Fluorescence contrast and threshold limit: implications for photodynamic diagnosis of basal cell carcinoma. *J Photochem Photobiol B Biol.* (2003) 69:121–7. doi: 10.1016/S1011-1344(02)00413-X
46. Fritsch C, Homey B, Stahl W, Lehmann P, Ruzicka T, Sies H. Preferential relative porphyrin enrichment in solar keratoses upon topical application of delta-aminolevulinic acid methylester. *Photochem Photobiol.* (1998) 68:218–21. doi: 10.1111/j.1751-1097.1998.tb02492.x
47. Tierney E, Petersen J, Hanke CW. Photodynamic diagnosis of tumor margins using methyl aminolevulinate before Mohs micrographic surgery. *J Am Acad Dermatol.* (2011) 64:911–8. doi: 10.1016/j.jaad.2010.03.045
48. Jeon SY, Kim KH, Song KH. Efficacy of photodynamic diagnosis-guided Mohs micrographic surgery in primary squamous cell carcinoma. *Dermatol Surg.* (2013) 39:1774–83. doi: 10.1111/dsu.12359
49. Pugliano-Mauro M, Goldman G. Mohs surgery is effective for high-risk cutaneous squamous cell carcinoma. *Dermatol Surg.* (2010) 36:1544–53. doi: 10.1111/j.1524-4725.2010.01576.x
50. Stenquist B, Ericson MB, Strandeberg C, Molne L, Rosen A, Larko O, et al. Bispectral fluorescence imaging of aggressive basal cell carcinoma combined

with histopathological mapping: a preliminary study indicating a possible adjunct to Mohs micrographic surgery. *Br J Dermatol.* (2006) 154:305–9. doi: 10.1111/j.1365-2133.2005.07035.x

51. Andersson-Engels S, Canti G, Cubeddu R, Eker C, af Klinteberg C, Pifferi A, et al. Preliminary evaluation of two fluorescence imaging methods for the detection and the delineation of basal cell carcinomas of the skin. *Lasers Surg Med.* (2000) 26:76–82. doi: 10.1002/(SICI)1096-9101(2000)26:1<76::AID-LSM11>3.0.CO;2-4
52. Na R, Stender IM, Wulf HC. Can autofluorescence demarcate basal cell carcinoma from normal skin? A comparison with protoporphyrin IX fluorescence. *Acta Dermato Venereol.* (2001) 81:246–9. doi: 10.1080/00015550152572859
53. Wan MT, Lin JY. Current evidence and applications of photodynamic therapy in dermatology. *Clin Cosmet Investig Dermatol.* (2014) 7:145–63. doi: 10.2147/CCID.S35334
54. Hillemanns P, Weingandt H, Stepp H, Baumgartner R, Xiang W, Korell M. Assessment of 5-aminolevulinic acid-induced porphyrin fluorescence in patients with peritoneal endometriosis. *Am J Obstetr Gynecol.* (2000) 183:52–7. doi: 10.1067/mob.2000.105897
55. Keefe KA, Chahine EB, DiSaia PJ, Krasieva TB, Lin F, Berns MW, et al. Fluorescence detection of cervical intraepithelial neoplasia for photodynamic therapy with the topical agents 5-aminolevulinic acid and benzoporphyrin-derivative monoacid ring. *Am J Obstetr Gynecol.* (2001) 184:1164–9. doi: 10.1067/mob.2001.113123
56. Helgesen AL, Gjersvik P, Peng Q, Vasovic V, Pripp AH, Jebsen P, et al. Biodistribution of protoporphyrin IX in female genital erosive lichen planus after topical application of hexaminolevulinate. *Photodiagn Photodyn Ther* (2014) 11:113–7. doi: 10.1016/j.pdpdt.2014.01.005
57. Wyss-Desserich MT, Sun CH, Wyss P, Kurlawalla CS, Haller U, Berns MW, et al. Accumulation of 5-aminolevulinic acid-induced protoporphyrin IX in normal and neoplastic human endometrial epithelial cells. Biochem Biophys *Res Commun.* (1996) 224:819–24. doi: 10.1006/bbrc.1996.1106
58. Degen A, Gabrecht T, Wagnieres G, Caduff R, Imthurn B, Wyss P. Influence of the menstrual cycle on aminolevulinic acid induced protoporphyrin IX fluorescence in the endometrium: *in vivo* study. *Lasers Surg Med.* (2005) 36:234–7. doi: 10.1002/lsm.20139
59. Loning M, Diddens H, Kupker W, Diedrich K, Huttmann G. Laparoscopic fluorescence detection of ovarian carcinoma metastases using 5-aminolevulinic acid-induced protoporphyrin IX. *Cancer.* (2004) 100:1650–6. doi: 10.1002/cncr.20155
60. Yonemura Y, Endo Y, Canbay E, Liu Y, Ishibashi H, Mizumoto A, et al. Photodynamic detection of peritoneal metastases using 5-Aminolevulinic acid (ALA). *Cancers (Basel).* (2017) 9:23. doi: 10.3390/cancers9030023
61. Leunig A, Rick K, Stepp H, Gutmann R, Alwin G, Baumgartner R, et al. Fluorescence imaging and spectroscopy of 5-aminolevulinic acid induced protoporphyrin IX for the detection of neoplastic lesions in the oral cavity. *Am J Surg.* (1996) 172:674–7. doi: 10.1016/S0002-9610(96)00312-1
62. Leunig A, Betz CS, Mehlmann M, Stepp H, Arbogast S, Grevers G, et al. Detection of squamous cell carcinoma of the oral cavity by imaging 5-aminolevulinic acid-induced protoporphyrin IX fluorescence. *Laryngoscope* (2000) 110:78–83. doi: 10.1097/00005537-200001000-00015
63. Zheng W, Olivo M, Soo KC. The use of digitized endoscopic imaging of 5-ALA-induced PPIX fluorescence to detect and diagnose oral premalignant and malignant lesions *in vivo*. *Int J Cancer.* (2004) 110:295–300. doi: 10.1002/ijc.20080
64. Mehlmann M, Betz CS, Stepp H, Arbogast S, Baumgartner R, Grevers G, et al. Fluorescence staining of laryngeal neoplasms after topical application of 5-aminolevulinic acid: preliminary results. *Lasers Surg Med.* (1999) 25:414–20. doi: 10.1002/(SICI)1096-9101(1999)25:5<414::AID-LSM8>3.0.CO;2-E
65. Csanady M, Kiss JG, Ivan L, Jori J, Czigner J. ALA (5-aminolevulinic acid)-induced protoporphyrin IX fluorescence in the endoscopic diagnostic and control of pharyngo-laryngeal cancer. *Eur Arch otorhinolaryngol.* (2004) 261:262–6. doi: 10.1007/s00405-003-0660-5
66. Suzuki T, Numata T, Shibuya M. Intraoperative photodynamic detection of normal parathyroid glands using 5-aminolevulinic acid. *Laryngoscope.* (2011) 121:1462–6. doi: 10.1002/lary.21857
67. Prosst RL, Gahlen J, Schnuelle P, Post S, Willeke F. Fluorescence-guided minimally invasive parathyroidectomy: a novel surgical therapy for secondary hyperparathyroidism. *Am J Kidney Dis.* (2006) 48:327–31. doi: 10.1053/j.ajkd.2006.05.002
68. Shahaf G, Pratt H. Thorough specification of the neurophysiologic processes underlying behavior and of their manifestation in EEG - demonstration with the go/no-go task. *Front Hum Neurosci.* (2013) 7:305. doi: 10.3389/fnhum.2013.00305
69. Quon H, Grossman CE, King RL, Putt M, Donaldson K, Kricka L, et al. Interference with the Jaffe method for creatinine following 5-aminolevulinic acid administration. *Photodiagn Photodyn Ther.* (2010) 7:268–74. doi: 10.1016/j.pdpdt.2010.07.008
70. Takeuchi S, Shimizu K, Shimizu K Jr, Akasu H, Okamura R. Identification of pathological and normal parathyroid tissue by fluorescent labeling with 5-aminolevulinic acid during endocrine neck surgery. *J Nippon Med Sch.* (2014) 81:84–93. doi: 10.1272/jnms.81.84
71. Betz CS, Stepp H, Janda P, Arbogast S, Grevers G, Baumgartner R, et al. A comparative study of normal inspection, autofluorescence and 5-ALA-induced PPIX fluorescence for oral cancer diagnosis. *Int J Cancer.* (2002) 97:245–52. doi: 10.1002/ijc.1596
72. Eker C, Montan S, Jaramillo E, Koizumi K, Rubio C, Andersson-Engels S, et al. Clinical spectral characterisation of colonic mucosal lesions using autofluorescence and delta aminolevulinic acid sensitisation. *Gut.* (1999) 44:511–8. doi: 10.1136/gut.44.4.511
73. Messmann H, Endlicher E, Freunek G, Rummele P, Scholmerich J, Knuchel R. Fluorescence endoscopy for the detection of low and high grade dysplasia in ulcerative colitis using systemic or local 5-aminolaevulinic acid sensitisation. *Gut.* (2003) 52:1003–7. doi: 10.1136/gut.52.7.1003
74. Namikawa T, Yatabe T, Inoue K, Shuin T, Hanazaki K. Clinical applications of 5-aminolevulinic acid-mediated fluorescence for gastric cancer. *World J Gastroenterol.* (2015) 21:8769–75. doi: 10.3748/wjg.v21.i29.8769
75. Brand S, Wang TD, Schomacker KT, Poneros JM, Lauwers GY, Compton CC, et al. Detection of high-grade dysplasia in Barrett's esophagus by spectroscopy measurement of 5-aminolevulinic acid-induced protoporphyrin IX fluorescence. *Gastrointest Endosc.* (2002) 56:479–87. doi: 10.1067/mge.2002.128172
76. Stepinac T, Felley C, Jornod P, Lange N, Gabrecht T, Fontolliet C, et al. Endoscopic fluorescence detection of intraepithelial neoplasia in Barrett's esophagus after oral administration of aminolevulinic acid. *Endoscopy.* (2003) 35:663–8. doi: 10.1055/s-2003-41514
77. Kishi K, Fujiwara Y, Yano M, Inoue M, Miyashiro I, Motoori M, et al. Staging laparoscopy using ALA-mediated photodynamic diagnosis improves the detection of peritoneal metastases in advanced gastric cancer. *J Surg Oncol.* (2012) 106:294–8. doi: 10.1002/jso.23075
78. Ushimaru Y, Fujiwara Y, Kishi K, Sugimura K, Omori T, Moon JH, et al. Prognostic significance of basing treatment strategy on the results of photodynamic diagnosis in advanced gastric cancer. *Ann Surg Oncol.* (2017) 24:983–9. doi: 10.1245/s10434-016-5660-y
79. Kaibori M, Matsui K, Ishizaki M, Iida H, Okumura T, Sakaguchi T, et al. Intraoperative detection of superficial liver tumors by fluorescence imaging using indocyanine green and 5-aminolevulinic acid. *Anticancer Res.* (2016) 36:1841–9.
80. Inoue Y, Tanaka R, Komeda K, Hirokawa F, Hayashi M, Uchiyama K. Fluorescence detection of malignant liver tumors using 5-aminolevulinic acid-mediated photodynamic diagnosis: principles, technique, and clinical experience. *World J Surg.* (2014) 38:1786–94. doi: 10.1007/s00268-014-2463-9
81. Baumgartner R, Huber RM, Schulz H, Stepp H, Rick K, Gamarra F, et al. Inhalation of 5-aminolevulinic acid: a new technique for fluorescence detection of early stage lung cancer. *J Photochem Photobiol B Biol.* (1996) 36:169–74. doi: 10.1016/S1011-1344(96)07365-4
82. Piotrowski WJ, Marczak J, Nawrocka A, Antczak A, Gorski P. Inhalations of 5-ALA in photodynamic diagnosis of bronchial cancer. *Monaldi Arch Chest Dis.* (2004) 61:86–93. doi: 10.4081/monaldi.2004.705
83. Baas P, Triesscheijn M, Burgers S, van Pel R, Stewart F, Aalders M. Fluorescence detection of pleural malignancies using 5-aminolaevulinic acid. *Chest.* (2006) 129:718–24. doi: 10.1378/chest.129.3.718
84. Pikin O, Filonenko E, Mironenko D, Vursol D, Amiraliev A. Fluorescence thoracoscopy in the detection of pleural malignancy. *Eur J Cardiothoracic Surg.* (2012) 41:649–52. doi: 10.1093/ejcts/ezr086

85. Hautmann H, Pichler JP, Stepp H, Baumgartner R, Gamarra F, Huber RM. *In-vivo* kinetics of inhaled 5-aminolevulinic acid-induced protoporphyrin IX fluorescence in bronchial tissue. *Respir Res.* (2007) 8:33. doi: 10.1186/1465-9921-8-33
86. Kitada M, Ohsaki Y, Matsuda Y, Hayashi S, Ishibashi K. Photodynamic diagnosis of pleural malignant lesions with a combination of 5-aminolevulinic acid and intrinsic fluorescence observation systems. *BMC Cancer.* (2015) 15:174. doi: 10.1186/s12885-015-1194-0
87. Moghissi K, Dixon K, Gibbins S. A surgical view of photodynamic therapy in oncology: a review. *Surg J.* (2015) 1:e1–15. doi: 10.1055/s-0035-1565246
88. Lipson RL, Baldes EJ, Olsen AM. Hematoporphyrin derivative: a new aid for endoscopic detection of malignant disease. *J Thoracic Cardiovasc Surg.* (1961) 42:623–9.
89. Hosek JE, Todd KS Jr, Kuhlenschmidt MS. Improved method for high-yield excystation and purification of infective sporozoites of *Eimeria* spp. *J Protozool.* (1988) 35:583–9. doi: 10.1111/j.1550-7408.1988.tb04156.x

20

The Probe Based Confocal Laser Endomicroscopy (pCLE) in Locally Advanced Gastric Cancer: A Powerful Technique for Real–Time Analysis of Vasculature

Alessandra Capuano[1†], *Eva Andreuzzi*[1†], *Eliana Pivetta*[1], *Roberto Doliana*[1], *Andrea Favero*[1], *Vincenzo Canzonieri*[2], *Stefania Maiero*[3], *Mara Fornasarig*[3], *Raffaella Magris*[3], *Renato Cannizzaro*[3*], *Maurizio Mongiat*[1‡] *and Paola Spessotto*[1‡]

[1] *Molecular Oncology, Centro di Riferimento Oncologico (CRO), IRCCS, Aviano, Italy,* [2] *Pathology, Centro di Riferimento Oncologico (CRO), IRCCS, Aviano, Italy,* [3] *Oncological Gastroenterology, Centro di Riferimento Oncologico (CRO), IRCCS, Aviano, Italy*

***Correspondence:**
Renato Cannizzaro
rcannizzaro@cro.it

† *These authors have contributed equally to this work*

‡ *These authors share co-last authorship*

Probe based confocal laser endomicroscopy (pCLE) is an advanced technique which provides imaging of gastrointestinal mucosa at subcellular resolution and, importantly, a valid tool for the evaluation of microvasculature during endoscopic examination. In order to assess intratumoral vascularization and the efficiency of blood flow in locally advanced gastric cancer, we examined 57 patients through pCLE imaging. The vascular alterations in gastric cancer were mainly characterized by leakage and by the presence of tortuous and large size vessels. Defects in blood flow were detected very rarely. No association between the angiogenic score and the gastric tumor site or histological type was observed. Interestingly, no correlation was also found with the tumor grading indicating that the vascular angiogenic anomalies in gastric cancer represent an early pathological event to be observed and detected. The majority of patients displayed unchanged vascular alterations following neoadjuvant chemotherapy and this positively correlated with stable or progressive disease, suggesting that an unaltered angiogenic score could *per se* be indicative of poor therapeutic efficacy. Different vascular parameters were evaluated by immunofluorescence using bioptic samples and the vessel density did not correlate with clinical staging, site or histologic type. Interestingly, only CD105, Multimerin-2 and GLUT1 were able to discriminate normal from tumoral gastric mucosa. Taken together, these findings indicate that functional and structural angiogenic parameters characteristic of tumor blood network were fully detectable by pCLE. Moreover, the evaluation of tumor vasculature by real-time assessment may provide useful information to achieve tailored therapeutic interventions for gastric cancer patients.

Keywords: pCLE, gastric cancer, angiogenesis, angiogenic score, CD31, CD34, CD105, MMRN2

INTRODUCTION

Gastric cancer is a major leading cause of cancer-related deaths and a relative common malignancy (1). Surgical resection of the tumor represents the approved option to improve patients' survival (2). At diagnosis, most of the patients display locally advanced or metastatic disease. To improve their chances they are treated with palliative chemotherapy, including cisplatin, docetaxel, oxaliplatin and 5FU, among other drugs (3–5). Unfortunately, at 5 years from the diagnosis only 10% of the patients affected by advanced or metastatic gastric cancer will survive and the median overall survival (OS) is only 1 year (6). Therefore, new therapeutic approaches and more specific targeted therapies are required for the treatment of this type of cancer. Angiogenesis, the development of new blood vessels from pre-existing vasculature, affects tumor growth and the metastatic dissemination of cancer cells and in the latest years has gained attention in gastric cancer research as a promising target (7–9). The angiogenic process is regulated by a plethora of cytokines and growth factors as well as by different cell types (10). Tumor cells will not grow beyond the size of few millimeters unless induce the secretion of angiogenic factors and the development of blood vessel for nutrients and oxygen supply. However, the erratic angiogenic stimulus leads to the formation of an abnormal and not fully functional vascular network (11). An attractive approach that has been advanced in the latest years is the normalization of the aberrant tumor-associated vessels for the induction of a more efficient vasculature. A normalized vasculature would allow an improved delivery of drugs within the tumor and hence a better therapy efficacy (12, 13). One of the major regulators of angiogenesis is the VEGFA/VEGFR2 signaling axis and represents a major target for anti-angiogenic therapy (13, 14). Interestingly, in gastric cancer patients high VEGFA levels have been associated with reduced survival and increased tumor aggressiveness (15). Anti-angiogenic therapy in gastric cancer patients did not so far meet the expectations despite some improvements have been observed (16). Thus, in order to improve the efficacy of anti-angiogenic therapy, it is of major importance to better characterize the vasculature associated with this tumor type.

The probe based Confocal Laser Endomicroscopy system (pCLE) is a highly enhanced endoscopic technique constituted by a confocal scanning microscope integrated into a conventional flexible endoscope. pCLE provides high quality imaging of the tissue, with a resolution of approximately 1 micron of the mucosal layer (17, 18). The main clinical application for which pCLE was developed includes the real-time histopathological diagnosis of gastrointestinal lesions. However, in recent years additional potential application have been proposed and gained attention such as cancer screening on the basis of cellular and vascular changes (19–22). In fact, by using intravenously administered fluorescein sodium (23), images of vascular network can be clearly detected offering the possibility to gain information on the characteristics of gastrointestinal tumor vessels in real time (24). Our group was among the pioneers in exploiting this new promising imaging tool to analyze the angiogenesis pattern in patients with gastric and rectal cancer (25). Unlike conventional immunohistochemistry, the aim was to provide a prompt and accurate evaluation of the pattern and efficiency of intratumoral vessels through a non-invasive technique. The analyses suggested that pCLE was exceptionally powerful tool to visualize and characterize the tumor-associated vasculature. Interestingly, we found that rectal and gastric cancers were highly angiogenic; however, rectal tumors displayed a higher percentage of dilated vessels and presence of defective flow (25).

With the aim of developing new strategies to achieve more efficacious gastric cancer patient-tailored treatments, in this study we thoroughly analyze the vascular characteristics of this type of tumor evaluating the employment of pCLE in the assessment of intratumoral angiogenesis.

MATERIALS AND METHODS

Patients

For this study 57 patients with locally advanced gastric cancer were enrolled to undergo endomicroscopy. Written informed consent was obtained from each patient on the day of the procedure. The methodologies conformed to the standards set by the Declaration of Helsinki. This study was approved by the Institutional Board of CRO-IRCCS, National Cancer Institute of Aviano (PN), Italy (IRB no. CRO-2014-03). The clinical evaluations are reported in **Table 1**. Patients underwent neoadjuvant multiregimen chemotherapy (oxaliplatin, capecitabine, and taxane) followed by surgical resection according to standard guidelines. Laboratory and pathological results were collected by means of the Hospital database.

TABLE 1 | Clinic-pathological characteristics of patients.

	N°	%
GENERAL INFORMATION		
All cases	57	100
Males	28	49
Mean age	62	
Females	29	51
Mean age	61	
HISTOLOGIC TYPE (LAUREN CLASSIFICATION)		
Diffuse	30	52.6
Intestinal	27	47.4
TUMOR SITE		
Body	35	61
Antrum	14	25
Fundus	5	9
Cardias	3	5
STAGING		
Ia-IIa	28	51
IIIa-IV	27	49

Endoscopy Procedures and pCLE Analyses

pCLE analyses were carried out with GastroFlex UHD probe (Cellvizio, Mauna Kea Technology, Paris, France) during gastroscopy (Olympus series 180) and immediately before endoscopic ultrasonography (Olympus series 160) as previously described (25). Patients were examined before chemotherapy or surgical intervention (first pCLE). 13 patients (corresponding to 23% of all patients) were also examined after chemotherapy treatment (second pCLE). Images and sequences of the normal and neoplastic mucosa were taken and the conventional bioptic samples obtained with macrobiopsy (COOK Medical, Ireland) at the end of examination. Images were recorded within the first 10 min following i.v. injection of fluorescein (5 ml of a 10% solution). pCLE images were collected at 12 frames per second to assure high video quality and a direct visualization on a single erythrocyte scale. pCLE recordings were performed for at least 3 min resulting in a real-time imaging of more than 2 thousand frames. Using the videomosaicing function provided by the analysis software, we also obtained the reconstruction of the scanned panoramas of the mucosa. The mucosal architecture, vessel morphology and the efficiency of the blood flow were evaluated. The images were digitally stored and reviewed with the dedicated software package (Cellvizio Viewer, Mauna Kea Technologies) by a single investigator who was blinded to any clinical, endoscopic, or histopathological information. The angiogenic score was assigned on the basis of the presence of tortuous and large sized vessels, the vessels' leakage and the presence of defective flow as previously described (25).

Immunofluorescence

For immunofluorescence (IF) analyses on bioptic samples, serial cryostat sections (7 μm) were collected on positively charged slides (BDH Superfrost Plus), air dried at room temperature (RT) and fixed with PFA for 15 min. After washing with phosphate-buffered saline (PBS), the slices were incubated with 0.5% Triton X-100 in PBS for 5 minutes at RT, saturated with 1% BSA–10% normal goat serum (DAKO) in PBS for 1 h at RT, and stained ON at 4 °C with the appropriate antibodies. Next, the samples were washed with PBS and incubated with the appropriate secondary antibodies and TO-PRO3 to stain the nuclei for 1 hour at RT. After washing with PBS, the slides were mounted in Mowiol containing 2.5% (w/v) of 1,4-diazabicyclo-(2,2,2)-octane (DABCO). Images were acquired with a Leica TCS SP8 Confocal system (Leica Microsystems Heidelberg, Mannheim, Germany), using the Leica Confocal Software (LCS). The monoclonal anti-human CD31, CD34, and CD105 antibodies were from Abcam (Cambridge, UK). The polyclonal anti-human Multimerin-2 (MMRN2) antibody was produced in our laboratories as previously described (26); the polyclonal anti-human GLUT 1 antibody was from Millipore (Temecula, CA, USA). The secondary antibodies conjugated with Alexa Fluor 488, 546 and TO-PRO-3 were from Invitrogen (Milan, Italy).

Quantification Analyses

Fluorescence intensity and quantification were evaluated by means of the Volocity software Version 6.1.1 (PerkinElmer Inc.,Waltham, MA, USA). The expression of CD31, CD34, CD105, MMRN2, and GLUT1 was calculated as pixel positive area of at least four 40x acquired fields. Corresponding values were expressed as mean ± SD.

Statistical Analysis

CD31, CD43, CD105, MMRN2, and GLUT1 expression levels between healthy and tumor mucosa of gastric cancer patients were compared by the Mann-Whitney non-parametric test. Relationships between positivity for vascular and angiogenesis markers and clinic-pathological features were evaluated using Spearman's rank correlation coefficient. Results were considered statistically significant for P-value < 0.05.

RESULTS

pCLE Is a Valuable Tool to Assess the Properties of Gastric Cancer-Associated Vasculature

pCLE has been used in the diagnosis of gastric lesions for the possibility to easily detect with high accuracy the typical morphological alterations of the mucosal architecture (27–33). In **Figure 1** we report representative reconstructions of the scanned panoramas of gastric mucosa obtained using the videomosaicing function which allows the alignment of the input frames. The differences in both morphological and vascular pattern between the normal (**Figure 1A**), atrophic (**Figure 1B**) and neoplastic (**Figure 1C**) gastric mucosa indicate that pCLE is a suitable tool not only for real time histopathological evaluations, but also for the assessment of the gastric cancer-associated vasculature. A thorough and prompt evaluation of the extent and quality of these vessels is in fact important to identify the patients that more likely will respond to anti-angiogenic treatment, as well as to develop new strategies to improve the efficacy of these treatments in non-responders. To this end we exploited the pCLE technology to evaluate the presence of tortuous and large-sized vessels, the presence of vascular leakage, and the efficiency of the vessels in terms of blood flow. We enrolled 57 patients affected by locally advanced gastric cancer and assigned an angiogenic score based on the pCLE analyses. The larger cohort of patients allowed us to confirm with statistical significance the observations gathered from few patients in a previous study aimed at comparing the vasculature of rectal and gastric tumors (25). Representative images of the vascular aberrations in gastric cancer patients characterized by different angiogenic scores are shown in **Figure 2A** (see also **Videos S1, S2**). A "3" angiogenic score was assigned to almost 50% of patients indicating that gastric tumors are characterized by a remarkably abnormal and unfunctional vasculature. In fact, a "1" angiogenic score was assigned to only the 11% of all the patients enrolled (**Figure 2B**). The most represented abnormalities were vessel leakage, which was detectable in 55 patients out of 57, the presence of tortuous vessels in 81% of the cases, and the presence of large diameter vessels in 67% of the patients. On the contrary, the presence of aberrant blood flow was detected only in 5% of the patients (**Figure 2C** and **Video S2**). To verify if the vascular pattern could depend on the clinical stage the

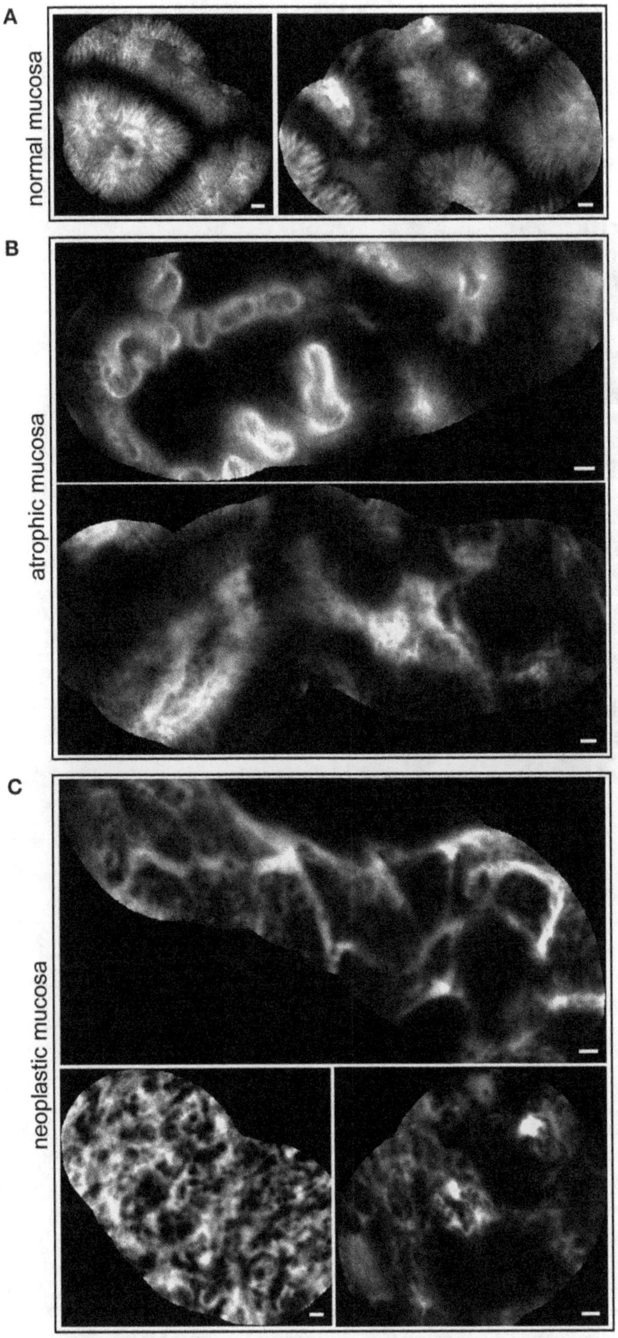

FIGURE 1 | pCLE imaging in gastric mucosa. Representative mosaic reconstructions obtained from scanned panoramas of normal **(A)**, atrophic **(B)**, and tumor **(C)** gastric mucosa. The morphology of regular glands is well defined in **(A)**; some mild to moderate alterations in morphological epithelium architecture as well as unstructured vessels are easily observed in **(B)**; complexity of mucosa with severe cell irregularity and very altered vascular network are shown in **(C)**. Scale bar = 20 μm.

patients were distributed into two categories: Ia-IIb and IIIa-IV. The statistical analyses indicated that there was no association between angiogenic score and staging (**Figure 3A**). In fact, the "2" and "3" angiogenic scores were homogenously distributed in both categories and the "1" and "4" angiogenic scores were not assigned to the low or high clinical stages, respectively. Next, we hypothesized that characteristics of the vasculature could depend on the tumor site or histological type according to Lauren classification (34, 35); however, we found that the angiogenic score did not correlate with these parameters (**Figures 3B,C**). A very high homogeneity was detected when we distributed the patients according to the histological type: no difference in angiogenic score distribution was observed between diffuse and intestinal type (**Figure 3C**). Although not statistically significant, the group characterized by lesions localized in the antrum displayed very frequently a "2" angiogenic score (**Figure 3D**). Taken together, the results from the pCLE analyses indicated that locally advanced gastric cancer is characterized by a remarkably abnormal and unfunctional vasculature.

Neoadjuvant Chemotherapy Does not Significantly Affect the Vascular Properties

Among the enrolled patients a total of 13 (9 with T3N+ and 4 with T3N0, as evaluated during the first endoscopy) completed the neoadjuvant chemotherapy program. The subjects were re-evaluated by pCLE before surgery. These analyses indicated that the chemotherapy treatment did not significantly affect the angiogenic score of the tumors, despite a slight improvement in tumor grading was observed in almost 70% of these patients (**Figure 4**). These results suggest that neodjuvant therapy halted primarily the proliferation of tumor cells without affecting the properties and extent of the vascular network. Interestingly, these findings are in line with the fact that no correlation was found between the results gathered through the pCLE analyses and the tumor staging (**Figure 3A**). Given that locally advanced gastric cancers are characterized by a highly abnormal vasculature, it can be speculated that the slight efficacy of the treatment may depend on a poor delivery of chemotherapy within the tumor of stable or progressive disease patients.

Gastric Cancer Vessels Are Poorly Efficient and Lead to Increased Intratumoral Hypoxia

In order to better define the quality of the gastric cancer associated vasculature we performed IF analyses employing different vascular markers i.e., CD31, CD34, CD105, Multimerin-2. Since Multimerin-2 was previously shown to affect HIF-1α expression (26) we also assessed the hypoxic levels in this tumor. To this end, we employed GLUT1 as a later maker of hypoxia, also in the light of the fact that it was recently reported to be a maker of poor prognosis (36, 37). To this end, during endoscopy and pCLE examination, bioptic samples of healthy and tumor mucosa of 33 patients were collected. First, we evaluated which marker could better detect the vascular density in normal and tumor gastric mucosa. These analyses are shown in **Figure 5** where we report the percentage of positivity relative to the mucosal area for each vascular marker. The results from these analyses indicated that, despite the staining for CD31 and CD34 were higher in the tumor mucosa compared to the normal counterpart, the differences were not statistically significant.

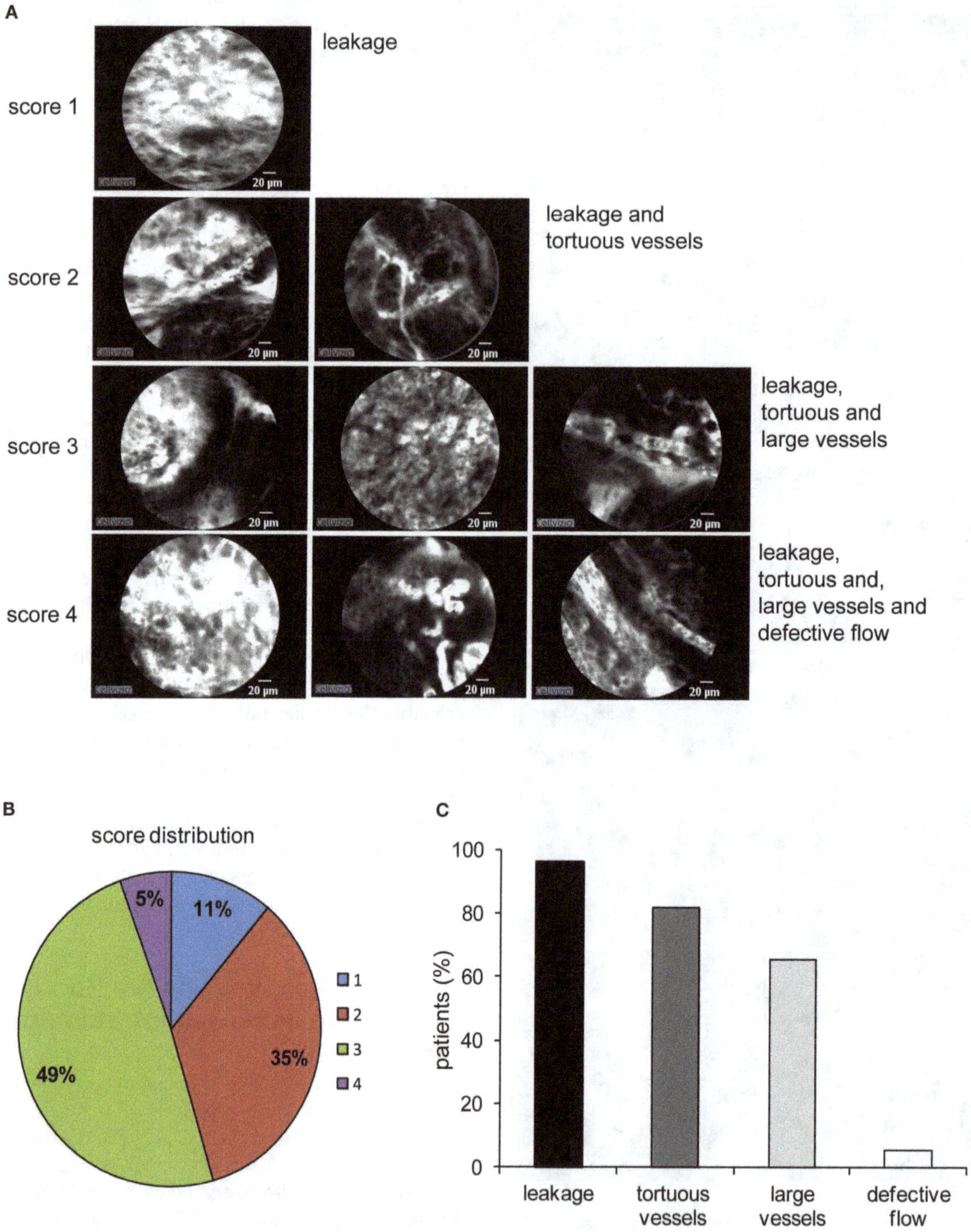

FIGURE 2 | Angiogenic score in gastric cancer. **(A)** Representative images from patients displaying different angiogenic scores (from 1 to 4). The altered features of the tumor vasculature taken into account (leakage, tortuous and large vessels, and aberrant blood flow) are displayed (see also **Videos S1**, **S2**). A value of "1" was assigned to indicate the presence of each vessel feature and a value of "0" for the absence. The angiogenic score is the result of the arithmetical sum of the single features. **(B)** Distribution of the angiogenic score among all 57 gastric cancers analyzed. **(C)** Percentage of gastric cancer patients displaying the morphological and functional features as defined for the angiogenic score assignment. Aberrant blood flow was rarely detectable whereas leakage and the presence of tortuous vessels were the most frequent.

On the other hand, CD105 staining was significantly higher in tumor tissues, suggesting that this marker could better measure the vascular density in gastric tumors. We next assessed the expression of Multimerin-2, an extracellular matrix glycoprotein specifically expressed by endothelial cells exerting an angiostatic and homeostatic function (26, 38–41). We found a striking loss

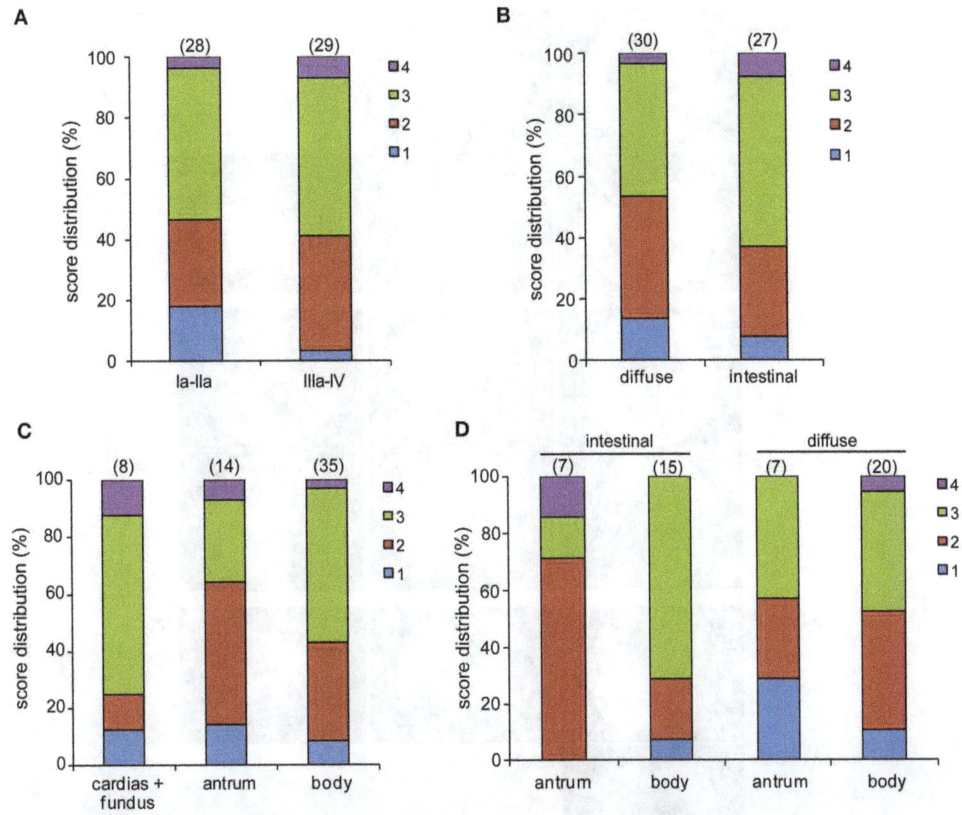

FIGURE 3 | pCLE analysis and patient clinical categories. No statistically significant differences were observed between the score distribution and the tumor staging **(A)**, histologic type **(B)**, or tumor site **(C)**. Although not statistically significant, the percentage of patients with an intestinal type of gastric cancer and a score "3" is more associated with a body than an antrum localization **(D)**.

of Multimerin-2 expression in many gastric tumor associated vessels (**Figure 5**). Another parameter to verify, even if indirectly, the vascular efficiency is to measure the extent of hypoxic regions. To this end, the bioptic samples were stained with GLUT1. As reported in **Figure 5**, most of the gastric cancer samples displayed an increased expression of GLUT1 compared to the normal counterpart. The relative expression of these markers was independent from the tumor staging (**Figure 6A**), similarly to what observed with the angiogenic score determined by pCLE analyses (**Figure 3A**). Also, no correlation between the markers' expression and the histological type and tumor site was detected (**Figures 6B,C**).

These findings encourage the use of pCLE as a powerful tool to detect functional aberrations and other anomalies of the tumor vasculature rather than a mere microscopic system for the assessment of the vascular density.

DISCUSSION

In this study we assessed the possible employment of pCLE as a valid clinical tool to evaluate the vascular properties in gastric cancer. The analyses indicated that this endoscopic technique is indispensable to provide structural and functional insights useful to better characterize the tumor vascular network in locally advanced gastric cancer. Unlike the conventional immunohistochemical approach, which provides a static portrayal of the vasculature, pCLE is a technique able to dynamically visualize the efficiency of the vessels evaluating the extent of vascular leakage and also the efficiency of blood flow within the vessels. Despite markers of vascular leakage are available, such as the erythrocyte marker Ter119, the staining is difficult to interpret and often not reliable. In fact, the use of the Ter119 on the gastric cancer samples did not lead to any detectable specific staining (data not shown). On the contrary, the use of pCLE allows a clear detection of the fluorescein staining outside the vascular wall. It is thus possible to identify the percentage of vessels whose functionality is compromised and characterized by increased leakage. An additional information that can be provided exclusively with the use of pCLE is the efficiency of blood vessels flow. Despite not very frequently, the pCLE analyses in some occasions detected the presence of defective blood flow characterized by an erratic non-directional cell stream. It is conceivable that such vessels are unable to efficiently transport and distribute the blood as well the therapeutic drugs within the tumor, thus leading to increased hypoxia and decreased therapy efficacy, respectively. We subsequently compared the results from the pCLE analyses with those obtained with the use of different vascular markers

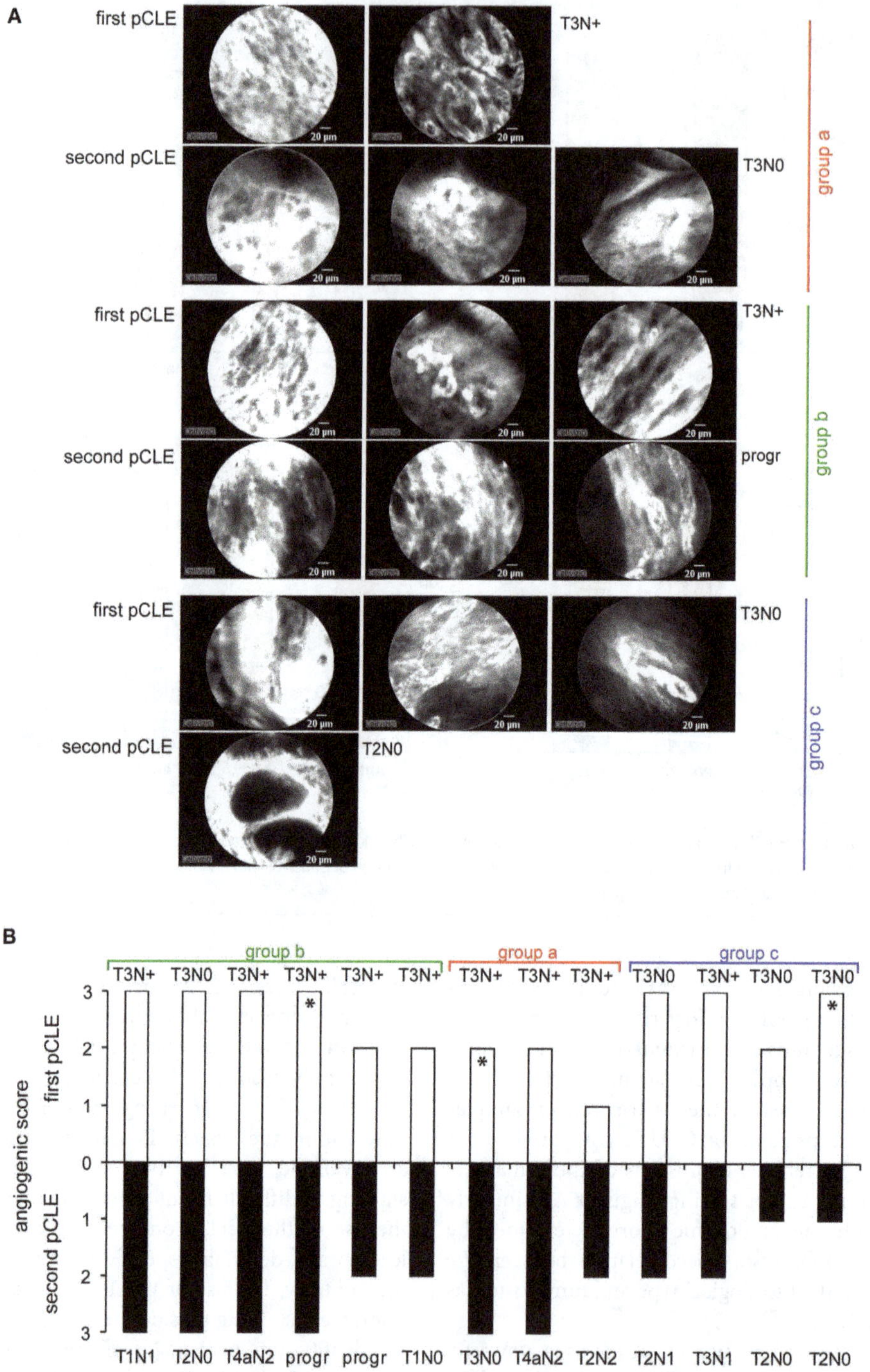

FIGURE 4 | pCLE in patients after chemotherapy treatment. **(A)** Representative pCLE images collected from three patients belonging to three different groups displaying increased (group a), equal (group b) or decreased (group c) angiogenic score after therapy (second pCLE). **(B)** Graph showing the angiogenic score assigned before (first pCLE) and after therapy in 13 gastric cancer patients. Asterisks in the graph indicate the patients whose pCLE images were chosen as representative in **(A)**. For each patients the corresponding tumor grading or disease progression (prog) before and after therapy is reported both in **(A,B)**.

following the immunohistochemical studies. We found that, unlike that of CD105, the analysis of the expression of CD31 and CD34 did not lead to a significant increased staining in gastric tumors, compared to the normal counterpart. Since CD105 is a marker of immature vessels, it is possible that these results depend on the fact that this maker is more appropriate for the detection of the newly formed vessels associated with tumors, as was previously suggested (42). In line with our

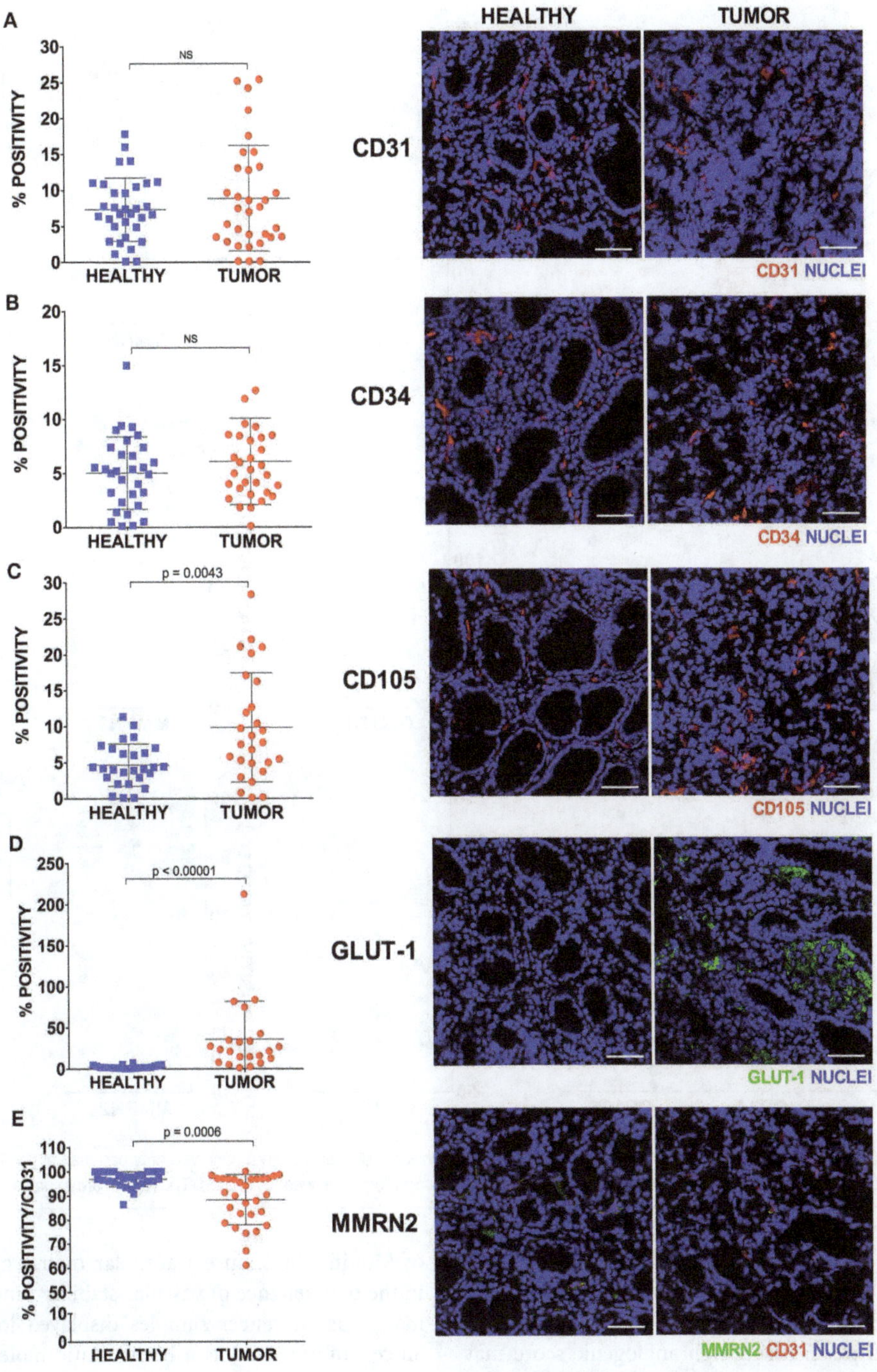

FIGURE 5 | Expression of endothelial cell markers in healthy and tumor gastric tissues. Representative images of healthy and tumor gastric mucosa stained with anti-vascular marker antibodies and scatter plots of the corresponding expression calculated as percentage of IF positive stained area [CD31, **(A)**; CD34, **(B)**; CD105, **(C)**; GLUT-1, **(D)**; MMRN2, **(E)**]. For each marker at least four 40x magnified fields were evaluated. The results are expressed as mean ± SD. Scale bar = 50 μm.

observations it was also reported that CD34 was universally expressed in blood vessels within benign and malignant tissues, whereas CD105 expression was barely detectable in benign tissues and high in gastric carcinoma (43, 44). No clear role for CD34 in angiogenesis has been reported so far (45–48). On the contrary, it has been shown that CD105, as a receptor as TGF-β, may regulate the role of this cytokine in the angiogenic process and be more suitable for detecting newborn blood vessels in gastric and colorectal cancer (49). CD105 expression is strongly upregulated in various tumor tissues, including colon, breast, brain, lung, prostate, and cervix (50, 51). Little is known about the clinical significance of CD105 in gastric carcinomas;

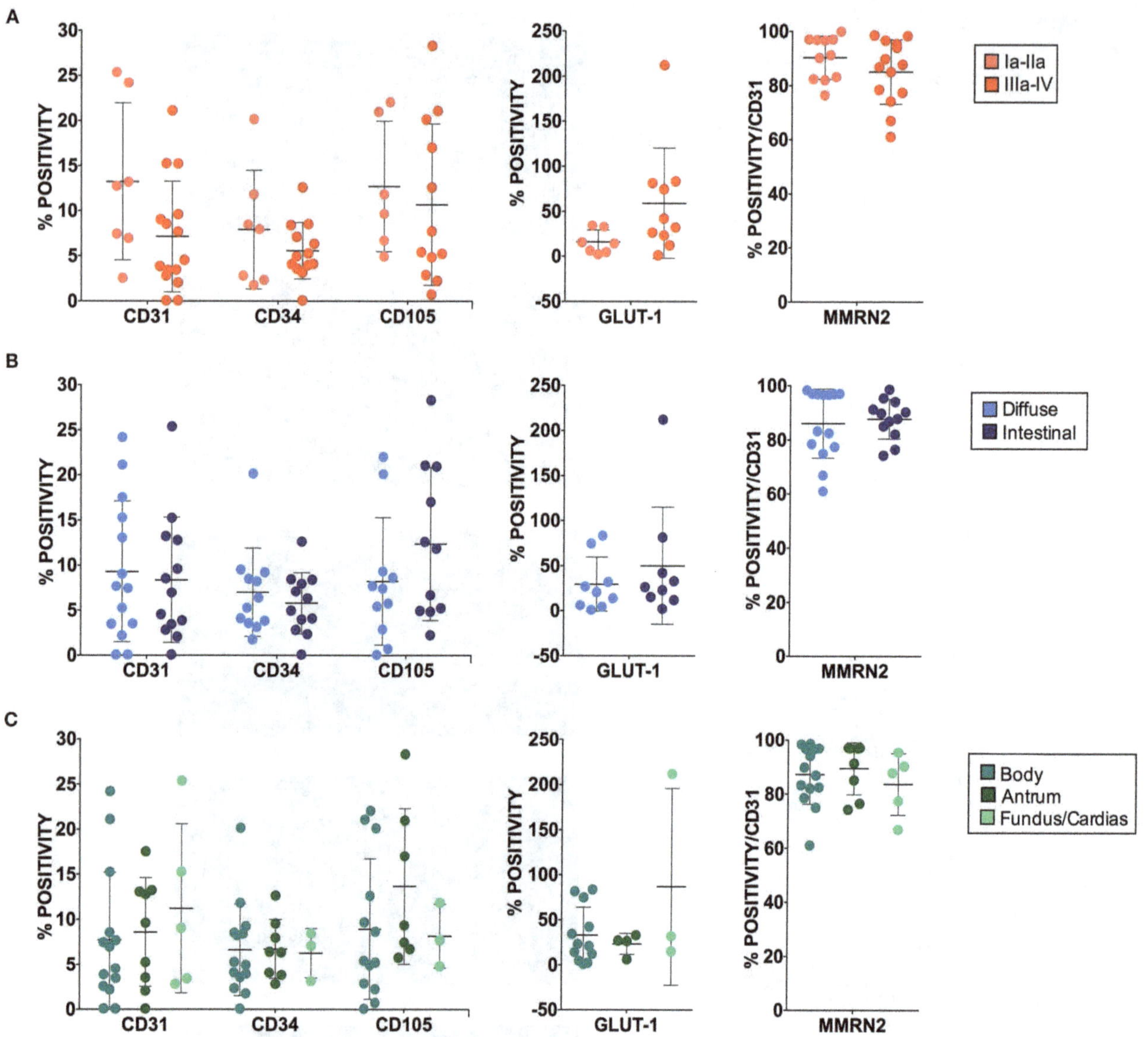

FIGURE 6 | Angiogenesis markers and patient clinical categories. No statistically significant differences were observed between marker positive staining and tumor staging **(A)**, histologic type **(B)**, or tumor site **(C)**. For each marker at least four 40x magnified fields were evaluated. The results are expressed as mean ± SD.

however, Nikiteas et al. have shown that VEGF and CD105 were involved in lymph node metastasis and acted as valuable indicators of the prognosis (52). The fact that high CD105 levels did not correlate with pCLE-based high angiogenic score may depend on the fact that vascular efficiency and stability is affected by several factors being controlled by cytokines, receptors and extracellular matrix components as well as mural cells. Thus, a comprehensive analysis of the proteins and pathways affecting vascular efficiency could be difficult and laborious to perform. On the contrary, the results obtained through the pCLE analyses provide information on the quality and efficiency of the vasculature independently from the molecular cause. In addition, an important advantage of the use of this tool is that the analyses precede the pathology investigations, thus providing a prompt information. We subsequently analyzed the expression of Multimerin-2, an extracellular matrix glycoprotein involved in the maintenance of vascular stability function. We found that many gastric cancer samples displayed loss of Multimerin-2. Since Multimerin-2 is a homeostatic molecule we hypothesize that vessels displaying low expression of this molecule are less efficient. However, no correlation was found between Multimerin-2 expression and the pCLE-based angiogenic score. This could be due to the fact that, as commented for the other vessel markers, vascular efficiency is affected by several molecules. In addition, the IF analyses are performed only in a small area of the tumor. Given the heterogeneity of the tumors it is likely that a more reliable analysis of the expression of the markers should be performed in several areas of the tumor. Interestingly, a stronger association was found between the results from the pCLE analyses and the expression of GLUT1.

Indeed, the presence of abnormal, leaky and poorly perfused vessels, independently from the molecular cause, and the consequent lack of sufficient oxygen supply lead to increased hypoxia and the establishment of an exacerbated mutagenic tumor microenvironment (13). The vascular alterations recorded by pCLE as well as the expression of angiogenic markers did not correlate with clinical staging, histological type and tumor site. Our previous observations indicated that high angiogenic scores as assessed by pCLE analyses associated with tumor progression more in rectal than in gastric cancer patients (25). The larger cohort taken into account in this study confirmed and reinforced these observations.

To better characterize the vasculature associated with gastric cancer is a required clinical need not only to predict which patients will respond to anti-angiogenic therapy, but also to develop new strategies to overcome resistance. The anti-angiogenic drugs employed in gastric cancer clinical trials mainly target VEGFA such as the monoclonal humanized antibody bevacizumab, or the VEGFR2, in particular ramucirumab and selective tyrosine kinase inhibitors such as sunitinib, sorafenib and apatinib. According to a very recent systematic review and meta-analysis the addition of anti-VEGFR2 targeting agents to the first- or second-line chemotherapy could prolong patient's OS and PFS in advanced or metastatic gastric cancer (16). The study also highlighted the inefficacy of anti-VEGFA therapy in this type of tumor, unlike what observed in other type of cancers (53–56). Thus, to better characterize the quality of the gastric cancer-associated vasculature by pCLE may grant the possibility to predict which patients will be more likely to respond to anti-angiogenic therapy, sparing the others from costly ineffective treatments and side effects. In addition, the comparative results from the pCLE and IF analysis may open new avenues toward the development of new strategies to circumvent anti-angiogenic therapy resistance.

ETHICS STATEMENT

This study was carried out in accordance with the recommendations of the Institutional Board of CRO-IRCCS, National Cancer Institute of Aviano (PN), Italy with written informed consent from all subjects. All subjects gave written informed consent in accordance with the Declaration of Helsinki. The protocol was approved by the Institutional Board of CRO-(IRB no. CRO-2014-03).

AUTHOR CONTRIBUTIONS

AC and EA developed the methodology, performed IF staining and graph editing, acquired data, and reviewed the manuscript. EP contributed to IF staining and analyses and critically reviewed the manuscript. RD collected, managed the bioptic samples, and reviewed the manuscript. AF collected data and helped for statistical analyses. VC provided final diagnosis and tumor staging. SM, MF, and RC identified and recruited patients and performed endoscopy and pCLE. RM helped in patient data managing. RC acquired funding, conceptualized the study and critically reviewed the manuscript. MM and PS conceptualized the study, reviewed as blinded investigators all pCLE videos, wrote original draft preparation and supervised investigation and analyses.

ACKNOWLEDGMENTS

The authors thank all patients that participated to this study.

REFERENCES

1. Bray F, Ferlay J, Soerjomataram I, Siegel RL, Torre LA, Jemal A. Global cancer statistics 2018: GLOBOCAN estimates of incidence and mortality worldwide for 36 cancers in 185 countries. *CA Cancer J Clin.* (2018) 68:394–424. doi: 10.3322/caac.21492
2. Rawicz-Pruszynski K, van Sandick JW, Mielko J, Ciseł B, Polkowski WP. Current challenges in gastric cancer surgery: European perspective. *Surg Oncol.* (2018) 27:650–6. doi: 10.1016/j.suronc.2018.08.004
3. Petrioli R, Francini E, Roviello F, Marrelli D, Fiaschi AI, Laera L, et al. Sequential treatment with epirubicin, oxaliplatin and 5FU (EOF) followed by docetaxel, oxaliplatin and 5FU (DOF) in patients with advanced gastric or gastroesophageal cancer: a single-institution experience. *Cancer Chemother Pharmacol.* (2015) 75:941–7. doi: 10.1007/s00280-015-2715-x
4. Buzzoni R, Bajetta E, Di Bartolomeo M, Miceli R, Beretta E, Ferrario E, et al. Pathological features as predictors of recurrence after radical resection of gastric cancer. *Br J Surg.* (2006) 93:205–9. doi: 10.1002/bjs.5225
5. Field K, Michael M, Leong T. Locally advanced and metastatic gastric cancer: current management and new treatment developments. *Drugs.* (2008) 68:299–317. doi: 10.2165/00003495-200868030-00004
6. Lordick F, Allum W, Carneiro F, Mitry E, Tabernero J, Tan P, et al. Unmet needs and challenges in gastric cancer: the way forward. *Cancer Treat Rev.* (2014) 40:692–700. doi: 10.1016/j.ctrv.2014.03.002
7. Pinto MP, Owen GI, Retamal I, Garrido M. Angiogenesis inhibitors in early development for gastric cancer. *Expert Opin Investig Drugs.* (2017) 26:1007–17. doi: 10.1080/13543784.2017.1361926
8. Roviello G, Petrioli R, Marano L, Polom K, Marrelli D, Perrella A, et al. Angiogenesis inhibitors in gastric and gastroesophageal junction cancer. *Gastric Cancer.* (2016) 19:31–41. doi: 10.1007/s10120-015-0537-5
9. Andreuzzi E, Capuano A, Pellicani R, Poletto E, Doliana R, Maiero S, et al. Loss of multimerin-2 and EMILIN-2 expression in gastric cancer associate with altered angiogenesis. *Int J Mol Sci.* (2018) 19:3983. doi: 10.3390/ijms19123983
10. Welti J, Loges S, Dimmeler S, Carmeliet P. Recent molecular discoveries in angiogenesis and antiangiogenic therapies in cancer. *J Clin Invest.* (2013) 123:3190–200. doi: 10.1172/JCI70212
11. Carmeliet P. Mechanisms of angiogenesis and arteriogenesis. *NatMed.* (2000) 6:389–95. doi: 10.1038/74651
12. Wong P-P, Demircioglu F, Ghazaly E, Alrawashdeh W, Stratford MRL, Scudamore CL, et al. Dual-action combination therapy enhances angiogenesis while reducing tumor growth and spread. *Cancer Cell.* (2015) 27:123–37. doi: 10.1016/j.ccell.2014.10.015
13. Jain RK. Antiangiogenesis strategies revisited: from starving tumors to alleviating hypoxia. *Cancer Cell.* (2014) 26:605–22. doi: 10.1016/j.ccell.2014.10.006
14. Park J-S, Kim I-K, Han S, Park I, Kim C, Bae J, et al. Normalization of tumor vessels by Tie2 activation and Ang2 inhibition enhances drug delivery and produces a favorable tumor microenvironment. *Cancer Cell.* (2016) 30:953–67. doi: 10.1016/j.ccell.2016.10.018
15. Park DJ, Seo AN, Yoon C, Ku GY, Coit DG, Strong VE, et al. Serum VEGF-A

and tumor vessel VEGFR-2 levels predict survival in caucasian but not asian patients undergoing resection for gastric adenocarcinoma. *Ann Surg Oncol.* (2015) 22(Suppl 3):S1508–15. doi: 10.1245/s10434-015-4790-y

16. Bai Z-G, Zhang Z-T. A systematic review and meta-analysis on the effect of angiogenesis blockade for the treatment of gastric cancer. *Onco Targets Ther.* (2018) 11:7077–87. doi: 10.2147/OTT.S169484
17. Kuiper T, van den Broek FJ, van ES, Fockens P, Dekker E. Feasibility and accuracy of confocal endomicroscopy in comparison with narrow-band imaging and chromoendoscopy for the differentiation of colorectal lesions. *AmJGastroenterol.* (2012) 107:543–50. doi: 10.1038/ajg.2012.14
18. Wallace MB, Fockens P. Probe-based confocal laser endomicroscopy. *Gastroenterology.* (2009) 136:1509–13. doi: 10.1053/j.gastro.2009.03.034
19. Wang KK, Carr-Locke DL, Singh SK, Neumann H, Bertani H, Galmiche JP, et al. Use of probe-based confocal laser endomicroscopy (pCLE) in gastrointestinal applications. a consensus report based on clinical evidence. *United Europ Gastroenterol J.* (2015) 3:230–54. doi: 10.1177/2050640614566066
20. De Palma GD. Confocal laser endomicroscopy in the "*in vivo*" histological diagnosis of the gastrointestinal tract. *World J Gastroenterol.* (2009) 15:5770–5. doi: 10.3748/wjg.15.5770
21. Shahid MW, Buchner AM, Heckman MG, Krishna M, Raimondo M, Woodward T, et al. Diagnostic accuracy of probe-based confocal laser endomicroscopy and narrow band imaging for small colorectal polyps: a feasibility study. *Am J Gastroenterol.* (2012) 107:231–9. doi: 10.1038/ajg.2011.376
22. Shahid MW, Buchner AM, Coron E, Woodward TA, Raimondo M, Dekker E, et al. Diagnostic accuracy of probe-based confocal laser endomicroscopy in detecting residual colorectal neoplasia after EMR: a prospective study. *Gastrointest Endosc.* (2012) 75:525–33. doi: 10.1016/j.gie.2011.08.024
23. Zhang YL, Bai L, Li Z, Ji R, Li CQ, Zuo XL, et al. Lower dose of fluorescein sodium is more suitable for confocal laser endomicroscopy: a feasibility study. *Gastrointest Endosc.* (2016) 84:917–23.e5. doi: 10.1016/j.gie.2016.05.011
24. Cannizzaro R, Mongiat M, Canzonieri V, Fornasarig M, Maiero S, De R V, et al. Endomicroscopy and cancer: a new approach to the visualization of neoangiogenesis. *Gastroenterol Res Pract.* (2012) 2012:537170. doi: 10.1155/2012/537170
25. Spessotto P, Fornasarig M, Pivetta E, Maiero S, Magris R, Mongiat M, et al. Probe-based confocal laser endomicroscopy for in vivo evaluation of the tumor vasculature in gastric and rectal carcinomas. *Sci Rep.* (2017) 7:9819. doi: 10.1038/s41598-017-10963-1
26. Colladel R, Pellicani R, Andreuzzi E, Paulitti A, Tarticchio G, Todaro F, et al. MULTIMERIN2 binds VEGF-A primarily via the carbohydrate chains exerting an angiostatic function and impairing tumor growth. *Oncotarget.* (2016) 7:2022–37. doi: 10.18632/oncotarget.6515
27. Ehling J, Lammers T, Kiessling F. Non-invasive imaging for studying anti-angiogenic therapy effects. *Thromb Haemost.* (2013) 109:375–90. doi: 10.1160/TH12-10-0721
28. Ehling J, Theek B, Gremse F, Baetke S, Mockel D, Maynard J, et al. Micro-CT imaging of tumor angiogenesis: quantitative measures describing micromorphology and vascularization. *Am J Pathol.* (2014) 184:431–41. doi: 10.1016/j.ajpath.2013.10.014
29. Li Z, Zuo XL, Li CQ, Liu ZY, Ji R, Liu J, et al. New classification of gastric pit patterns and vessel architecture using probe-based confocal laser endomicroscopy. *J Clin Gastroenterol.* (2016) 50:23–32. doi: 10.1097/MCG.0000000000000298
30. Safatle-Ribeiro AV, Ryoka Baba E, Corsato Scomparin R, Friedrich Faraj S, Simas de Lima M, Lenz L, et al. Probe-based confocal endomicroscopy is accurate for differentiating gastric lesions in patients in a Western center. *Chin J Cancer Res.* (2018) 30:546–52. doi: 10.21147/j.issn.1000-9604.2018.05.08
31. Goetz M. Characterization of lesions in the stomach: will confocal laser endomicroscopy replace the pathologist? *Best Pract Res Clin Gastroenterol.* (2015) 29:589–99. doi: 10.1016/j.bpg.2015.05.013
32. Goetz M, Malek NP, Kiesslich R. Microscopic imaging in endoscopy: endomicroscopy and endocytoscopy. *Nat Rev Gastroenterol Hepatol.* (2014) 11:11–8. doi: 10.1038/nrgastro.2013.134
33. Wallace M, Lauwers GY, Chen Y, Dekker E, Fockens P, Sharma P, et al. Miami classification for probe-based confocal laser endomicroscopy. *Endoscopy.* (2011) 43:882–91. doi: 10.1055/s-0030-1256632
34. Lauren P. The two histological main types of gastric carcinoma: diffuse and so-called intestinal-type carcinoma. an attempt at a histo-clinical classification. *Acta Pathol Microbiol Scand.* (1965) 64:31–49. doi: 10.1111/apm.1965.64.1.31
35. Zhao L-Y, Wang J-J, Zhao Y-L, Chen X-Z, Yang K, Chen X-L, et al. Superiority of tumor location-modified lauren classification system for gastric cancer: a multi-institutional validation analysis. *Ann Surg Oncol.* (2018) 25:3257–63. doi: 10.1245/s10434-018-6654-8
36. Boström PJ, Thoms J, Sykes J, Ahmed O, Evans A, van Rhijn BWG, et al. Hypoxia marker GLUT-1 (Glucose Transporter 1) is an independent prognostic factor for survival in bladder cancer patients treated with radical cystectomy. *Bladder Cancer.* (2016) 2:101–9. doi: 10.3233/BLC-150033
37. Airley RE, Loncaster J, Raleigh JA, Harris AL, Davidson SE, Hunter RD, et al. GLUT-1 and CAIX as intrinsic markers of hypoxia in carcinoma of the cervix: relationship to pimonidazole binding. *Int J Cancer.* (2003) 104:85–91. doi: 10.1002/ijc.10904
38. Lorenzon E, Colladel R, Andreuzzi E, Marastoni S, Todaro F, Schiappacassi M, et al. MULTIMERIN2 impairs tumor angiogenesis and growth by interfering with VEGF-A/VEGFR2 pathway. *Oncogene.* (2012) 31:3136–47. doi: 10.1038/onc.2011.487
39. Andreuzzi E, Colladel R, Pellicani R, Tarticchio G, Cannizzaro R, Spessotto P, et al. The angiostatic molecule Multimerin 2 is processed by MMP-9 to allow sprouting angiogenesis. *Matrix Biol.* (2017) 64:40–53. doi: 10.1016/j.matbio.2017.04.002
40. Galvagni F, Nardi F, Spiga O, Trezza A, Tarticchio G, Pellicani R, et al. Dissecting the CD93-Multimerin 2 interaction involved in cell adhesion and migration of the activated endothelium. *Matrix Biol.* (2017) 64:112–27. doi: 10.1016/j.matbio.2017.08.003
41. Mongiat M, Andreuzzi E, Tarticchio G, Paulitti A. Extracellular matrix, a hard player in angiogenesis. *Int J Mol Sci.* (2016) 17:1822. doi: 10.3390/ijms17111822
42. Nassiri F, Cusimano MD, Scheithauer BW, Rotondo F, Fazio A, Yousef GM, et al. Endoglin (CD105): a review of its role in angiogenesis and tumor diagnosis, progression and therapy. *Anticancer Res.* (2011) 31:2283–90.
43. Ding S, Li C, Lin S, Yang Y, Liu D, Han Y, et al. Comparative evaluation of microvessel density determined by CD34 or CD105 in benign and malignant gastric lesions. *Hum Pathol.* (2006) 37:861–6. doi: 10.1016/j.humpath.2006.02.006
44. Yu J-X, Zhang X-T, Liao Y-Q, Zhang Q-Y, Chen H, Lin M, et al. Relationship between expression of CD105 and growth factors in malignant tumors of gastrointestinal tract and its significance. *World J Gastroenterol.* (2003) 9:2866–9. doi: 10.3748/wjg.v9.i12.2866
45. Wang JM, Kumar S, Pye D, van Agthoven AJ, Krupinski J, Hunter RD. A monoclonal antibody detects heterogeneity in vascular endothelium of tumours and normal tissues. *Int J Cancer.* (1993) 54:363–70. doi: 10.1002/ijc.2910540303
46. Cheng J, Baumhueter S, Cacalano G, Carver-Moore K, Thibodeaux H, Thomas R, et al. Hematopoietic defects in mice lacking the sialomucin CD34. *Blood.* (1996) 87:479–90.
47. Tasev D, Konijnenberg LSF, Amado-Azevedo J, van Wijhe MH, Koolwijk P, van Hinsbergh VWM. CD34 expression modulates tube-forming capacity and barrier properties of peripheral blood-derived endothelial colony-forming cells (ECFCs). *Angiogenesis.* (2016) 19:325–38. doi: 10.1007/s10456-016-9506-9
48. Rakocevic J, Orlic D, Mitrovic-Ajtic O, Tomasevic M, Dobric M, Zlatic N, et al. Endothelial cell markers from clinician's perspective. *Exp Mol Pathol.* (2017) 102:303–13. doi: 10.1016/j.yexmp.2017.02.005
49. Minhajat R, Mori D, Yamasaki F, Sugita Y, Satoh T, Tokunaga O. Organ-specific endoglin (CD105) expression in the angiogenesis of human cancers. *Pathol Int.* (2006) 56:717–23. doi: 10.1111/j.1440-1827.2006.02037.x
50. Duff SE, Li C, Garland JM, Kumar S. CD105 is important for angiogenesis: evidence and potential applications. *FASEB J.* (2003) 17:984–92. doi: 10.1096/fj.02-0634rev
51. Fonsatti E, Altomonte M, Nicotra MR, Natali PG, Maio M. Endoglin (CD105): a powerful therapeutic target on tumor-associated angiogenetic blood vessels. *Oncogene.* (2003) 22:6557–63. doi: 10.1038/sj.onc.1206813

52. Nikiteas NI, Tzanakis N, Theodoropoulos G, Atsaves V, Christoni Z, Karakitsos P, et al. Vascular endothelial growth factor and endoglin (CD-105) in gastric cancer. *Gastric Cancer.* (2007) 10:12–7. doi: 10.1007/s10120-006-0401-8

53. Assoun S, Brosseau S, Steinmetz C, Gounant V, Zalcman G. Bevacizumab in advanced lung cancer: state of the art. *Future Oncol.* (2017) 13:2515–35. doi: 10.2217/fon-2017-030

54. Rossi L, Verrico M, Zaccarelli E, Papa A, Colonna M, Strudel M, et al. Bevacizumab in ovarian cancer: a critical review of phase III studies. *Oncotarget.* (2017) 8:12389–405. doi: 10.18632/oncotarget.13310

55. Alnimer Y, Hindi Z, Katato K. The effect of perioperative bevacizumab on disease-free and overall survival in locally advanced HER-2 negative breast cancer: a meta-analysis. *Breast Cancer.* (2018) 12:1178223418792250. doi: 10.1177/1178223418792250

56. Xu R, Xu C, Liu C, Cui C, Zhu J. Efficacy and safety of bevacizumab-based combination therapy for treatment of patients with metastatic colorectal cancer. *Onco Targets Ther.* (2018) 11:8605–21. doi: 10.2147/OTT.S171724

21

Fluorescence-Guided Surgery: A Review on Timing and Use in Brain Tumor Surgery

Alexander J. Schupper[1]*, Manasa Rao*[1]*, Nicki Mohammadi*[1]*, Rebecca Baron*[1]*,*
John Y. K. Lee[2]*, Francesco Acerbi*[3] *and Constantinos G. Hadjipanayis*[1*]

[1] *Department of Neurosurgery, Icahn School of Medicine at Mount Sinai, New York, NY, United States,* [2] *Department of Neurosurgery, University of Pennsylvania School of Medicine, Philadelphia, PA, United States,* [3] *Department of Neurosurgery, Fondazione Istituto Di Ricovero e Cura a Carattere Scientifico Istituto Neurologico Carlo Besta, Milan, Italy*

***Correspondence:**
Constantinos G. Hadjipanayis
constantinos.hadjipanayis@mountsinai.org

Fluorescence-guided surgery (FGS) allows surgeons to have improved visualization of tumor tissue in the operating room, enabling maximal safe resection of malignant brain tumors. Over the past two decades, multiple fluorescent agents have been studied for FGS, including 5-aminolevulinic acid (5-ALA), fluorescein sodium, and indocyanine green (ICG). Both non-targeted and targeted fluorescent agents are currently being used in clinical practice, as well as under investigation, for glioma visualization and resection. While the efficacy of intraoperative fluorescence in studied fluorophores has been well established in the literature, the effect of timing on fluorophore administration in glioma surgery has not been as well depicted. In the past year, recent studies of 5-ALA use have shown that intraoperative fluorescence may persist beyond the previously studied window used in prior multicenter trials. Additionally, the use of fluorophores for different brain tumor types is discussed in detail, including a discussion of choosing the right fluorophore based on tumor etiology. In the following review, the authors will describe the temporal nature of the various fluorophores used in glioma surgery, what remains uncertain in FGS, and provide a guide for using fluorescence as a surgical adjunct in brain tumor surgery.

Keywords: fluorescence-guided surgery, 5-ALA, fluorescein, ICG, extent of resection, timing

INTRODUCTION

The single best prognostic factor for patients diagnosed with high-grade gliomas (HGGs) is maximal resection, also known as gross total surgical resection (GTR) (1–3). HGG GTR has been associated with greater overall survival in addition to longer progression-free survival (PFS) (1, 4).In order to maximize the extent of resection (EOR), a number of visualization techniques have been introduced into the field of neurosurgery. Fluorescent agents, also known as fluorophores, aid in the delineation of normal and malignant tumor tissue (5, 6), permitting real-time image guided surgery that can maximize EOR (7).

There are a limited number of fluorophores currently used in clinical practice. Stummer first described the use of 5-aminolevulinic acid (5-ALA) and FGS in glioma patients in 1998. Based on the results of a landmark randomized, Phase III study confirming greater tumor resection and better patient outcomes in comparison to conventional microsurgery, 5-ALA (Gleolan) was approved as an oral intraoperative imaging agent for visualization of malignant tissue during glioma surgery (8–10). The fluorophores have various mechanisms of action, ranging from intracellular uptake with 5-ALA (11, 12) and ICG (13) to extracellular accumulation with fluorescein sodium (FS) and indocyanine-green (ICG), similar to the contrast enhancement found with gadolinium contrast enhancement found with MR imaging (14–16). FS is administered systemically after the induction of anesthesia while ICG and 5-ALA are given several hours before surgery (11, 15, 17, 18) (**Table 1**).

While each of these agents used for FGS are currently used in patients, there is still ongoing research on the pharmacokinetics of these molecules in order to understand the optimal timing of administration and fluorescence of tumors during surgery. Timing is important with fluorophore administration, as it can be impacted by patient and surgical delays, and may affect the efficacy of the agent. Other new targeted fluorophores are currently being investigated in HGG patients and also require better understanding of optimal administration for FGS. The purpose of this review is to elucidate the current evidence on the perspective of timing for the various fluorophores used in glioma patients for FGS and provide an outline of the literature on the use of the most currently used fluorophores for glioma surgery.

INDOCYANINE GREEN (ICG)

Indocyanine Green (ICG) has been used widely in medical applications, beginning with hepatic and cardiac function measurement, and expanding into ophthalmology indications where it is FDA approved (**Table 2**). Upon systemic administration, as an amphiphilic, tricarbocyanine iodide dye, ICG binds to plasma proteins yielding many advantages including its confinement to the vascular compartment (19). Additionally, it's light excitation and emission in the near-infrared (NIR), low toxicity, and rapid excretion leads to its popularity. ICG has been used as a cerebrovascular intraoperative contrast agent to confirm aneurysm occlusion during surgery. More recently, a more delayed administration of ICG has been described prior to glioma surgery (20). ICG works as a passive targeting agent and requires the breakdown of the BBB to concentrate at the tumor site (19). Unlike 5-ALA and fluorescein, two popular FDA-approved fluorophore agents, ICG is a near-infrared (NIR) fluorophore which presents unique utility in labeling tumor tissue (15, 21). NIR imaging affords higher resolution with increasing tissue penetration depths with excellent signal to noise ratio (SNR) (**Figure 1**).

Both preclinical and clinical studies report the use of ICG for glioma surgery albeit within a few minutes after systemic administration exploiting vascular permeability of glioma compared to normal brain (19, 22). Haglund et al. used ICG for enhanced optical imaging in human gliomas (23). Hansen et al. found that when ICG was injected intravenously into tumor-bearing rats, the tumor fluoresced intensely at 60–120 mg/kg for at least 1 h after injection (24). This study showed the ability of ICG to distinguish rat brain tumor from normal parenchyma with adequate tumor to normal brain background ratio, with minimal post-resection residual tumor cells (24).

ICG intrinsic properties include a plasma half-life of 3–4 min; in preclinical studies after 10 min only a small amount of originally injected ICG volume can be detected in the blood (25). Due to this short half-life, ICG is usually given as a bolus dose of <0.5–1 mg/kg and NIR imaging is performed shortly after (23). Haglund et al. found that ICG fluorescence of glioma tissue, unlike fluorescein, is time-dependent (23). Martirosyan et al. found tissue fluorescence when ICG was injected 15 min prior to visualization, while Haglund et al. found an optical signal between 5 and 10 min after ICG injection (23, 25). The dye uptake rate was shown to be faster in HGGs compared to low-grade gliomas, and this diversity in tumor cell population may explain the time-dependent nature of the ICG peak signal. Studies suggest that as ICG is rapidly being eliminated from the blood at 18–24% per minute, the dye is sequestered into the tumor (23).

More recently, ICG has been administered at higher doses and tumor visualization has been improved by exploiting the enhanced permeability and retention (EPR) of nanoparticle-sized ICG fluorophore within brain tumors (26). Zeh et al. administered doses above the FDA-approved limit of 2 mg/kg in rodents implanted with human glioma xenografts and demonstrated a broad plateau period extending up to 72 h, thus allowing for optimal imaging of glioma as compared to normal brain (20). With the SWIG approach, combining the natural permeability of the tumor vascularity with poor clearance allows for high doses of ICG to penetrate the tumor, a high dose (5 mg/kg) of intravenous ICG is given a day (24 h) prior to surgery, yielding improved intraoperative visualization of the tumor compared to white light (15, 27, 28). In a series of 15 gliomas featuring 11 HGG, sensitivity was 98% and specificity 45% (27).

FLUORESCEIN SODIUM

Fluorescein sodium (FS) is best known for its use in ophthalmology where it is FDA approved for angiography or angioscopy of the retina and iris vasculature (FDA approval letter). Recently, it has been reintroduced into neuro-oncologic surgery for HGG FGS. FS has a molecular weight of 376.27 and is the sodium salt of fluorescein. It was first used to visualize malignant brain tumor in 1948 (29). FS accumulates in HGGs where the BBB is disrupted and provides intra-operative visualization that is similar to pre-operative contrast-enhanced T1 images in which gadolinium accumulation is seen (30–33). FS can be viewed under white light, but the use of an operating microscope fitted with a dedicated filter allows to significantly reduce the dose needed to highlight tumoral tissue (**Figure 2**) (19, 30, 31, 34). FS is excited at 460–500 nm and emits a green, fluorescent emission wavelength at 540–690 nm (19, 35). FS is administered at the time of anesthesia prior to a craniotomy for HGG FGS. Immediately after systemic administration FS flows within the cerebral vasculature and afterwards accumulates in tumoral area where there is a damage of BBB. Fluorescence by FS can be visualized for up to 4 h after administration.

Both preclinical and clinical studies have confirmed that fluorescein, unlike other fluorophores, does not accumulate intracellularly but in the extracellular space in brain tumors (32, 35–37). Instead of tumor-specific uptake, it has been

TABLE 1 | Summary of the properties of fluorophores currently used in fluorescence-guided surgery.

Agent	Excitation (nm)	Emission (nm)	Targeting mode	Administration mode	Dosage (in humans)	Half-life	Time prior to visualization	Time to fluorescence disappearing in target tissue
ICG	778	700–850	Passive	IV	0.2–5 mg/kg	3–4 min	Seconds	Several minutes
Second Window ICG	778	700–850	Passive	IV	2.5–5.0 mg/kg		24 h	>72 h
Fluorescein	460–500	540–690	Passive	IV	2–20 mg/kg	23.5 min	2–4 h	2–4 h
5-ALA	375–440	640–710	Metabolic	Oral	20 mg/kg	1–3 h	2–8 h	22 h
BLZ-100	785	700–850	Molecular	IV	3–30 mg	30 min	3–29 h	48 h
CLR1501	500	517	Molecular	IV	16 mg/kg	4 days	4 days	–
CLR1502	760	778	Molecular	IV	2 mg/kg	4 days	4 days	–
IRDye800CW (EGFR)	–	794	Molecular	IV	Up to 24.5 mg/kg	15–20 min	1 h	3–4 days

ICG, indocyanine green; 5-ALA, 5-aminolevulinic acid; IV, intravenous.

TABLE 2 | Fluorophores currently used in brain tumor surgery and Food and Drug Administration (FDA) use approval.

Agent	Year of FDA approval	Use of FDA approval
ICG	1959	1. Determining cardiac output, hepatic function and liver blood flow. 2. For ophthalmic angiography.
Fluorescein	2006	1. Diagnostic fluorescein angiography or angioscopy of the retina and iris vasculature.
5-ALA	2017	1. Intraoperative optical imaging agent in patients with suspected high-grade gliomas

FDA, Food and Drug Administration; ICG, indocyanine green; 5-ALA, 5-aminolevulinic acid.

demonstrated that fluorescein sodium accumulates at disruptions of the BBB in areas with high- density tumor cells, thereby proving useful for HGG visualization (30–33, 36, 37). Fluorescein sodium has been found to have a sensitivity of 82–94% and a specificity of 90–91% for glioma visualization (19, 31, 32, 38). However, it has also been shown that FS fluorescence might not be limited to tumor tissue. As a matter of fact, some areas, such as dura mater, circumventricular organs and choroid plexus, due to the lack of BBB, appears intensively fluorescent (35). In addition, although the presence of FS fluorescence in normal brain parenchyma close to tumor tissue has been occasionally shown and considered a consequence of direct surgical manipulation (33, 39–41), it has been suggested that the application of a strict intraoperative protocol of FS injection could significantly limit this event (35).

Many studies have reported the safety, efficacy, and convenience of using fluorescein sodium during HGG resection (7, 16, 31, 35, 42–46). Maximal resection or gross-total resection (GTR) of tumors with FS has been reported with an increase in progression-free survival (PFS) (16, 19, 31–33, 35, 39, 40, 44, 45, 47). Additionally, due to concern that fluorescein is non-selective for tumor tissue, one study concluded that dual labeling with 5-ALA and fluorescein allowed for superior visualization in high-grade glioma resection because fluorescein sodium enhanced background tissue and 5-ALA enhanced tumor tissue (48).

Few studies have reported guidelines on when to administer FS for best visualization in the surgical field. Fluorescein distributes to tissues within 10 min and has a plasma half-life of 23.5 min (49). In clinical practice, FS is administered systemically in the operating room either immediately after anesthesia induction or prior to surgical resection (7, 16, 18, 31, 33, 35, 39, 42, 45, 49, 50). In order to elucidate whether fluorescein can be seen in non-tumor tissue, one study evaluated the pharmacokinetics of fluorescein sodium in different preclinical mouse models, without and with xenograft tumor (51). This study established that the majority (up to 70%) of injected fluorescein exists in circulating blood in the unbound form and that only up to 30% result to be protein-bound. Due to its low molecular weight, the circulating unbound form accumulates in normal mice brain tissue without xenograft tumor, with a peak timing of 30 min after injection, particularly if injected at human-equivalent high dosage, and that washout from normal brain seems to be completed 120 min after fluorescein injection. When used in orthotopic glioma models, the presence of unbound fluorescein in normal brain tissue 60 min after injection significantly reduces the tumor-to-normal contrast (51). The study also elucidated the fact that pegylated fluorescein sodium, which better matches gadolinium contrast in sizing, seems to provide more suitable kinetics and a higher ratio of tumor fluorescence compared to normal brain tissue in othotopic glioma models (51). There is a paucity of clinical data on the best timing of FS administration. Some studies have reported administration of fluorescein after incision of the dura with resection beginning as early as 10 or 20 min after injection (7, 16, 33, 39, 42, 44). However, in more recent

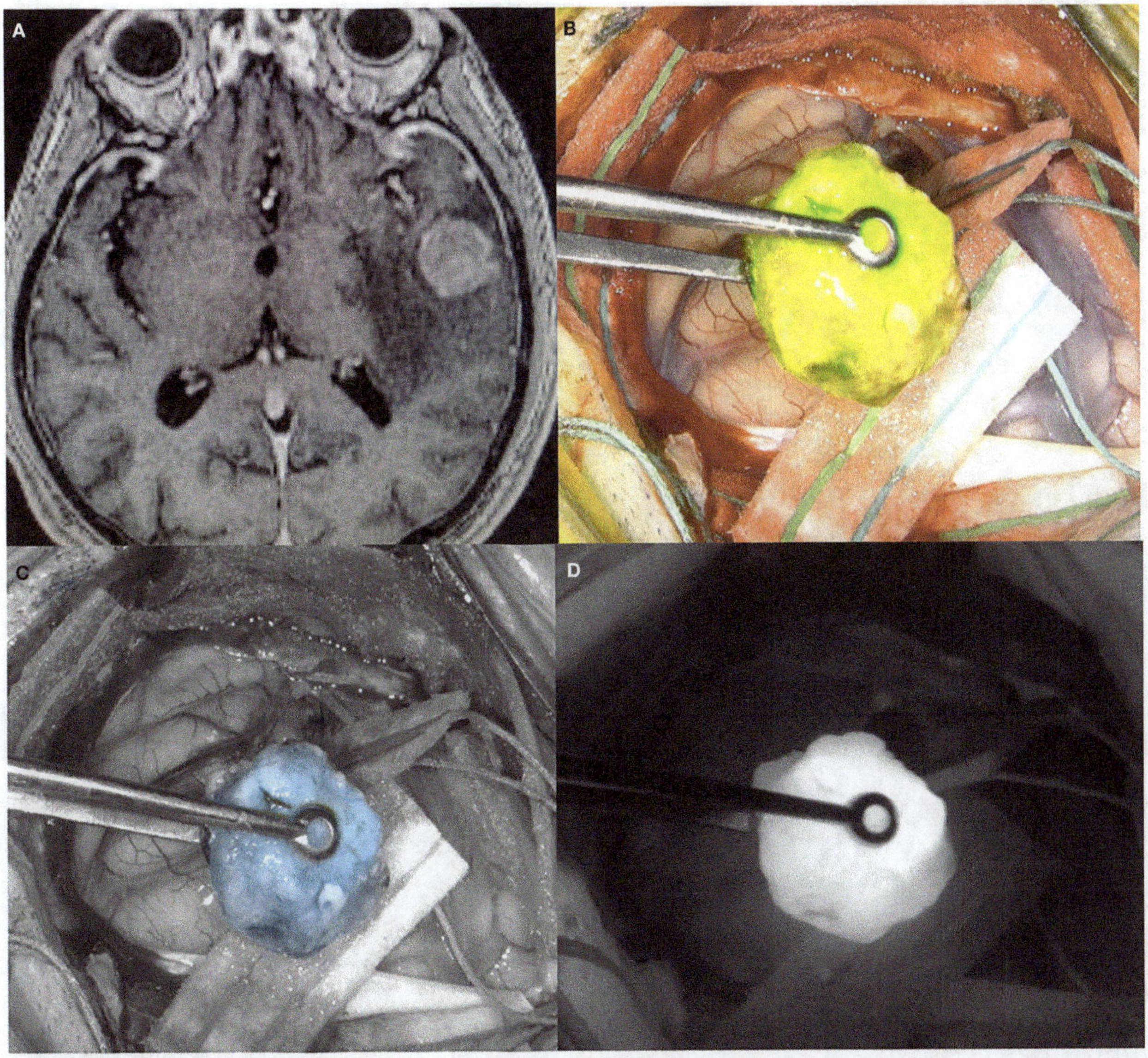

FIGURE 1 | (A) Pre-operative T1 post-contrast MR, showing a left temporal lesion with surrounding vasogenic edema. Histological diagnosis showed a metastatic lung adenocarcinoma. **(B)** Intraoperative picture during the surgical removal of the same case depicted in **(A)**, showing the ICG uptake by the tumor visualized with yellow-green excitation. **(C)** Intraoperative picture during the surgical removal of the same case depicted in **(A)**, showing the ICG uptake by the tumor with blue excitation. **(D)** Intraoperative picture during the surgical removal of the same case depicted in **(A)**, showing the ICG uptake by the tumor visualized with near-infrared excitation.

experiences it has been suggested to use low dose (5 mg/kg) of fluorescein, with intravenous injection performed after patient intubation, thus in most of the cases around 1 h before incision of dura mater (18, 31, 35). More specifically, it has been shown that the optimal strategy to optimize fluorescent contrast during surgery is to use lower dose (1–5 mg/kg) to minimize unspecific extravasation, administered 2–4 h before visualization, which corresponds to the wash-out period of the FLS (43). Surely, a need for further investigation of the clinically-relevant pharmacokinetics of optimal fluorescein sodium administration remains.

5-AMINOLEVULINIC ACID (5-ALA)

5-ALA, a precursor metabolized in the heme biosynthesis pathway to protoporphyrin (PPIX), accumulates intracellularly in tumor cells, and has a high affinity for high-grade glioma tissue (52). PPIX absorbs light between 375 and 440 nm and emits a violet-red fluorescence at 635 nm (**Figure 3**) (11) 5-ALA is the most well-studied fluorescent agent in glioma surgery that has been granted FDA approval (54, 55). A landmark randomized controlled study (RCT) was performed where HGG patients were randomized to FGS or conventional microsurgery (8) 5-ALA FGS

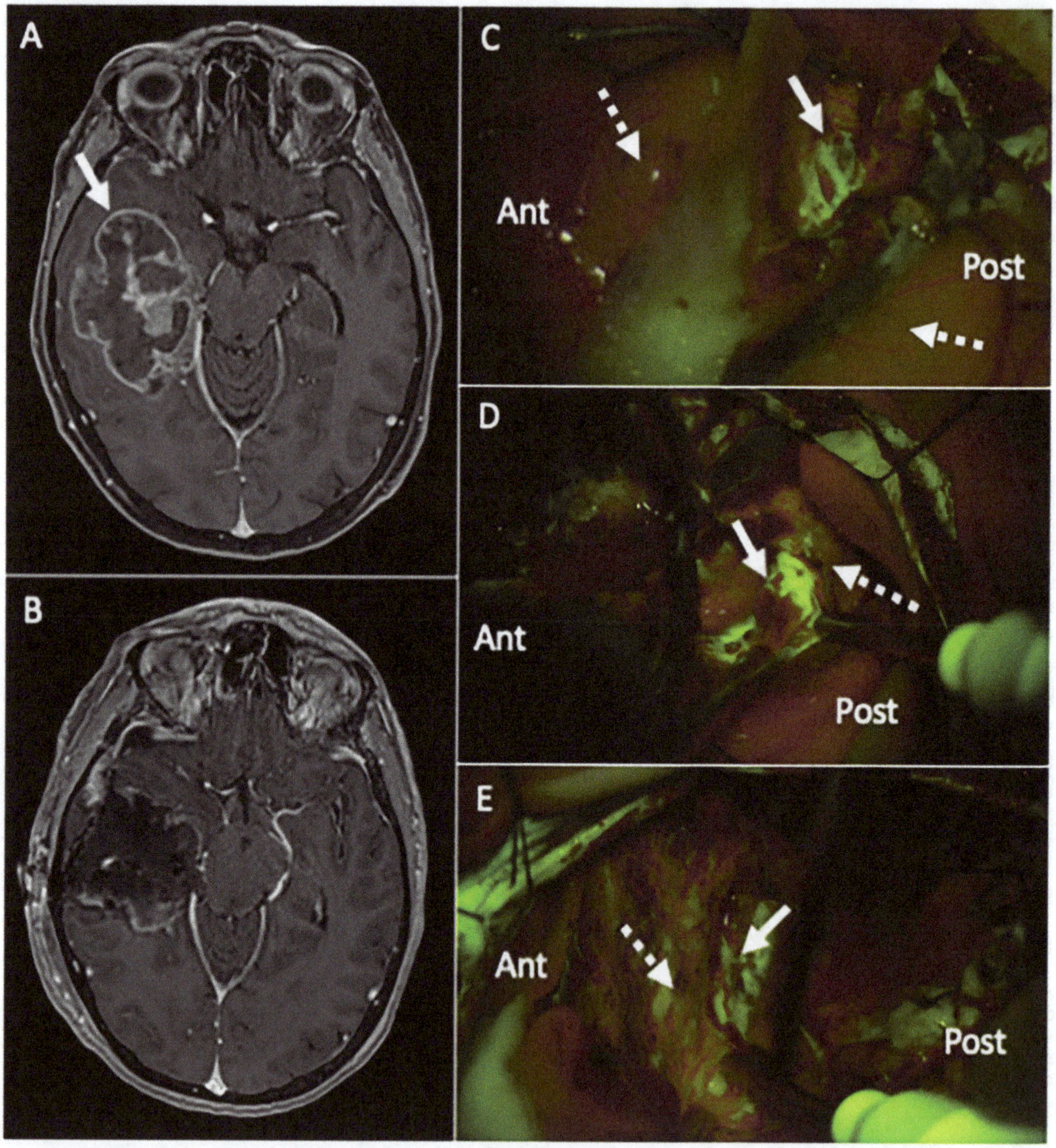

FIGURE 2 | (A) Pre-operative T1 post-contrast MR, showing a large right temporal lesion (white arrow), with irregular enhancement and mass effect, compatible with the suspect of high-grade glioma. **(B)** Post-operative T1 post-contrast MR, performed 24 h after surgery, confirming a gross-total resection (GTR) of the lesion (histological diagnosis showed a Glioblastoma, IDH wild-type). **(C–E)** Intraoperative picture during the surgical removal of the same case depicted in **(A)**, taken with the Y560 filter activated (Pentero 900 microscope, Carl Zeiss Meditec, Oberkochen, Germany): after a small corticectomy **(C)**, the pathological tissue is clearly visible as a bright green-yellow fluorescent area (white arrow), while the non-pathological temporal cortex (dotted white arrow) anteriorly and posteriorly is non-fluorescent (for orientation, Ant is anterior and Post is posterior temporal lobe); during surgical removal with ultrasonic aspirator (Sonoca 300, Soring, Quickborn, Germany), subcortical tumoral tissue is clearly discernible from normal peri-tumoral parenchyma by its bright green-yellow fluorescence (white arrow in **(D)** at the posterior border and in **(E)** at the anterior border), compared to pinkish peritumoral parenchyma (dotted white arrow).

was associated with improved progression-free survival (PFS) and greater overall tumor resection compared to white light control. 5-ALA FGS has been shown to be both safe and effective, with minimal side effects (8, 56, 57).

Since the publication of the RCT, the widespread use of 5-ALA globally has been based upon the same drug administration criteria used in the trial. An oral dose of ALA HCL solution of 20 mg/kg body weight, is administered 3 h (range 2–4 h) prior to induction of anesthesia (8) 5-ALA is rapidly absorbed into the blood after ingestion within 1 h and is metabolized quickly thereafter in brain tumors to its fluorescent PPIX metabolite. This dosing regimen was based upon rodent experiments in which there was a fluorescence peak observed 6 h after administration (10). The decision to have the patient ingest the medication at 3 h (with a range of 2–4 h) prior to surgery was recommended to allow ample time for anesthesia, monitoring and performing the craniotomy, in order for peak intraoperative PPIX fluorescence to be present during tumor resection (8, 56). As a result of this RCT and other European multicenter trials, the same administration criterion was used for the Food and Drug Administration (FDA) approval of 5-ALA (Gleolan®) in 2017 [(54); FDA approval] (58).

Recent studies have suggested that 5-ALA fluorescence may have a longer window of detection than previously described. In a prospective study of 68 patients and 201 tumor samples, Kaneko et al. found that maximal fluorescence intensity was observed 7–8 h following 5-ALA administration, and weak fluorescence peaked later than strong fluorescence, at 8–9 h (59). While prior animal studies have suggested an earlier fluorescence peak, there is now evidence that a longer latency time might lead to stronger fluorescence of HGG tissue. In a retrospective study of 16 patients who received 5-ALA over 4 h prior to anesthesia induction, our group found that adequate intraoperative fluorescence was seen up to almost 28 h post-ingestion, with no 5-ALA-related toxicity (53). Understanding the time window for 5-ALA PpIX fluorescence is clinically relevant, as surgeries are not uncommonly delayed due to emergent cases, staffing issues or other logistical challenges, and it is important to know if intraoperative fluorescence may be utilized despite delays in surgery. Unlike fluorescein and ICG which may be given in the operating room after induction of anesthesia, 5-ALA requires oral administration, and therefore there exists an element of anticipating time of surgery. Having a less narrow window of adequate intraoperative fluorescence allows surgeons greater flexibility with using 5-ALA for glioma surgery.

TARGETED FLUOROPHORES

In addition to the fluorophores mentioned above, there are current studies on fluorophores with more directed mechanisms of action, such as specific receptor targets. Below is a description of several targeted agents currently under clinical investigation.

BLZ-100

A conjugate of tumor-specific peptide chlorotoxin paired with a near-infrared fluorophore, BLZ-100 (tozuleristide, Blaze Bioscience Inc, Seattle, Washington) is visualized with a NIR camera (60). A recent phase I trial demonstrated safety and efficacy for the use of BLZ-100 in patients with primary and recurrent glioblastoma (60). Ongoing evaluation of the conjugate is currently being studied in both adult and pediatric brain tumors (NCT02234297, NCT02462629). BLZ-100 has the same benefits as ICG in the NIR spectrum, however, it adds further tumor specificity with chlorotoxin, a scorpion venom. Given intravenously, BLZ-100, also known as The Tumor Paint©, can safely be given to adults in doses ranging from 3 to 30 mg (60). In this trial, BLZ-100 was administered as a slow IV bolus injection over 1–5 min 3–29 h before surgery. It has a serum half-life of ~30 min, however, unlike 5-ALA, has been shown to be retained in tumors for over 24 h, particularly in doses over 9 mg or greater in World Health Organization (WHO) grade III and IV gliomas (60). Its length of time in tumor tissue is currently unknown. Further study is required on a larger patient sample, however, depending upon the sensitivity of specificity of BLZ-100, it may provide a useful fluorophore given its high intensity of fluorescence and prolonged retention in glioma tissue.

Alkyl Phosphocholine Analogs

Alkylphosphocholine analogs (APCs) are small synthetic phospholipid ether molecules, which may target specific tumors types, including osteosarcoma, pancreatic adenocarcinoma and glioblastoma (61). Due to lipid raft expression, APCs are able to remain intracellular for prolonged periods of time (61), providing a theoretical advantage for FGS. To date, there are no published clinical results on APC use in gliomas, however, in a proof-of-principle preclinical study, high glioblastoma cell selectivity has been shown with two APCs (CLR1501 and CLR1502, Cellectar Biosciences, Madison, Wisconsin) (62). In the xenograft model, the two APCs were given intravenously in doses ranging from 2 to 16 mg/kg 4 days prior to sacrifice. CLR1501 (green spectrum) showed a tumor to brain fluorescence ratio comparable to 5-ALA, while CLR1502 (NIR) had a superior tumor to brain fluorescence ratio (62).

Epidermal Growth Factor Receptor (EGFR) Targeted Fluorophores

Expressed as cell-surface receptors in many cancers including gliomas, epidermal growth factor receptor (EGFR) may be conjugated with fluorescent dyes, allowing for targeted cell-surface fluorescence (63). In an *in vivo* animal study of IRDye800CW labeled with anti-EGFR antibodies, there was a 100% sensitivity and specificity for distinguishing GBM-specific mutated EGFR positive from EGFR negative cell lines (64). While no clinical studies have been performed to date, preclinical studies have administered intravenous anti-EGFR fluorescence conjugates into rats, and observed safe doses up to 24.5 mg/kg of an IRDye800CW anti-EGFR antibody (ABY-029, Affibody, Sweden) (65). However, due to its short half-life it will need to be given during surgery in humans, and in preclinical investigation had poor fluorescent intensity in the brain (65). Based upon this preclinical trial, it was determined that ABY-029 can be administered within minutes to hours of the surgery start time, and fluorescence was still observed 48 h post-administration (66).

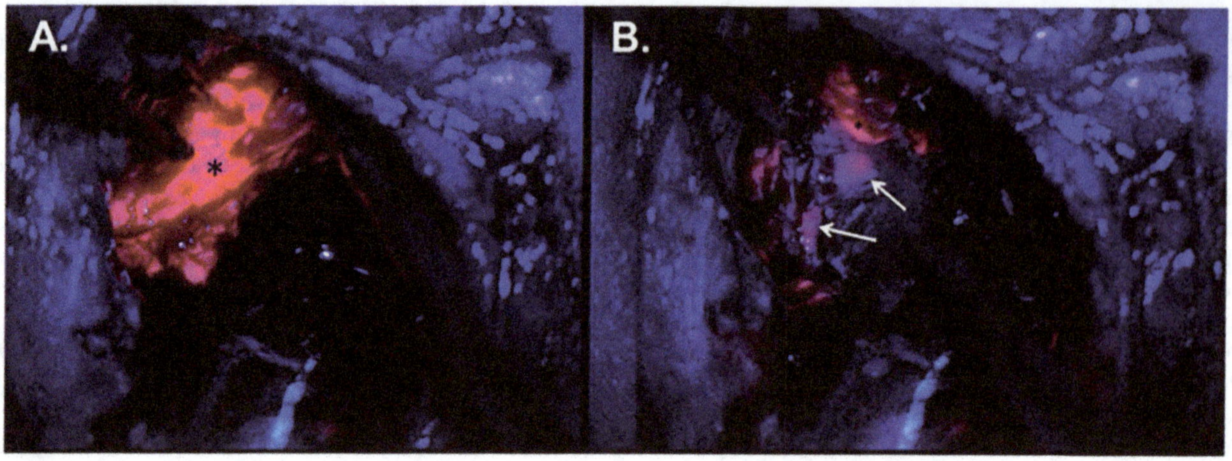

FIGURE 3 | Intraoperative imaging for case demonstration patient. **(A)** Tumor bulk fluorescence after 5-ALA administration (asterisk). **(B)** Infiltrative margin fluorescence after 5-ALA administration (white arrows). Taken with permission from Maragkos et al. (53).

Cetuximab, an EGFR monoclonal antibody, when conjugated with fluorescent IRDye 800CW, fluoresces in the NIR, and has been shown in preclinical studies to be effective for glioma surgery (67). In a first-in-human study, cetuximab-IRDye800 demonstrated both safety and efficacy, with high signal to background ration aiding in glioblastoma visualization (68). Larger studies are warranted to better underwent the use of cetuximab conjugates for FGS.

CHOOSING THE RIGHT FLUOROPHORES: PROPOSED SUGGESTIONS

While all fluorophores provide varying degrees of intraoperative fluorescence during brain tumor surgery, the various mechanisms of action make certain fluorophores better choices for different tumor types. Below is an outline for the different fluorophores currently available for use in FGS, based upon tumor pathology.

High-Grade Gliomas

High-grade gliomas (HGG) are the most widely studied tumor type in FGS. The three most commonly studied fluorophores, 5-ALA, fluorescein and ICG, have all been used in HGG surgery. 5-ALA has been the most robustly studied fluorophore in malignant gliomas. PPIX specifically accumulates in the tumor intracellular space, resulting in a robust red fluorescence in the tumor bulk, and a surrounding lighter pink fluorescence peripherally, representing surrounding infiltrative tumor cells (69, 70). This selective uptake in tumor cells results in high sensitivity and specficity, with prior studies showing mean sensitivity and specificity for delineating tumor tissue vs. surrounding brain to be 83–87% and 89–100%, respectively (6, 10, 71, 72). Additionally, 5-ALA has a strong positive predictive value, with multiple studies finding 100% PPV for solid fluorescence in both primary and recurrent HGG (70, 73, 74). Beyond histologic accuracy of 5-ALA PPIX fluorescence, correlations have been made between fluorescence intensity and histological grading, suggesting the ability to approximate grade by fluorescent signal (75, 76).

In addition to being safe for use in HGG surgery, 5-ALA has also shown to improve patient outcomes. In a phase III randomized controlled trial of 322 HGG patients randomized to 5-ALA FGS or white light surgery, Stummer et al. found that patients who received 5-ALA experience more complete resections of contrast-enhancing tumor (65 vs. 36%, $p < 0.0001$), and higher 6-month progression-free survival (41.0 vs. 21.1%, $p = 0.0003$) (8). In a retrospective study of glioblastoma patients that had undergone surgery with 5-ALA, those patients without residual tissue fluorescence had greater median overall survival compared to those with residual fluorescence (27 vs. 17.5 months, $p = 0.015$) (77).

Despite the advantages of 5-ALA for HGG surgery, the agent is expensive and not universally available. Following a series of successful clinical trials in 5-ALA, FGS researchers tested the safety and efficacy of other more widely accessible fluorophores for HGG resections. Several recent studies have assessed the use of fluorescein sodium, and found that fluorescein improves extent of resection and rates of gross total resection, with GTR rates up to 80% (7, 30, 31, 78). Despite being selective for areas of blood-brain barrier breakdown, rather than tumor tissue itself, fluorescein fluorescent signal has been shown to correlate with contrast-enhancement on preoperative MR imaging (32, 40). To date, there are no randomized controlled trials for fluorescein-guided tumor surgery, however, in a recent multicenter phase II study, Acerbi et al. found that fluorescein was safe and effective in HGG surgery, with a GTR rate of 82.6% and 6-month progression-free survival of 56.6% (35). ICG, a fluorophore used primarily in angiography, has recently been implemented in brain tumor surgery, for its enhanced permeability retention (EPR) effect as a result of BBB disruption. The second window ICG (SWIG) technique allows for ICG accumulation in HGG tissue, allowing for improved visualization (15, 28). While this technique has not yet been widely studies, in a recent case series of 11 HGG, SWIG was found to be highly sensitive for HGG tissue, and fluorescent signal correlated with MR imaging (27). While safely tolerated, the major disadvtange of ICG is that unlike 5-ALA and fluorescein, it emits in the near infrared spectrum, making it logistically difficult to operate while visualizing the signal.

Low-Grade Gliomas

Low-grade gliomas have created a larger challenge for FGS compared to HGG, as the lower grade tumors do not have as robust areas of BBB breakdown and contrast uptake compared to more infiltrative lesions. While historically "watch and wait" was the treatment paradigm for these lesions, there is now strong evidence for early, maximal safe resection (74, 79, 80). However, these tumors may be difficult to remove completely, as their appearance may only appear slightly different compared to normal brain, and therefore 5-ALA has been implemented. While initially researchers were doubtful that there would be any 5-ALA PPIX uptake in LGG cells due to less BBB breakdown, the differences appear quantitative, rather than qualitative (81). Although initial studies showed no fluorescence in LGG patients (82, 83). Widhalm et al. found a subset of non-contrast-enhancing LGG patients with 5-ALA-induced fluorescence (84). In the largest series to date, Jaber et al. found visible fluorescence in only 13 of 82 WHO grade II gliomas, and concluded that the majority of LGG do not show visible fluorescence (85). However, the value in use of 5-ALA for LGG surgery may be in the histological heterogeneity of these tumors, as areas of malignant transformation, or anaplastic foci, are characteristic for LGGs (86). By fluorescing areas of contrast-enhancement, 5-ALA can help identify areas of higher metabolic activity and subsequently greater proliferation (87).

Meningiomas

Meningiomas are the most common benign brain tumors, and with the propensity to enhance on contrasted imaging, they have been studied in the field of FGS. While the three major fluorophores, 5-ALA, ICG, and fluorescein, have all been studied in the visualization of meningiomas, 5-ALA has been most widely studied, with over 10 clinical studies to date (88). The largest study of FGS use in meningiomas is by Millesi et al., where after administration of 5-ALA to 204 meningioma patients, visible fluorescent signal was found in 91% of tumors, and 100% positive preductive value for bone infiltration (89). In a study of 12 meningioma patients, seven skull base and five convexity, Della Puppa et al. found 89% sensitivity and 100% specificity for 5-ALA detecting bone invasion (90). Additionally, in a small series of eight intradural spinal meningiomas using 5-ALA, there was a positive predictive value of 100% (91).

ICG and fluorescein have also been used in the resection of meningiomas. ICG in particular has been found to be helpful in cases where the tumor invades the dural sinuses, and helps visualize venous collaterals, the surrounding patent sinuses and the pial vascular supply (92–94). In these cases, however, ICG is being used as a vascular contrast agent with visualization within minutes of IV bolus dosing. In contrast, Lee et al., employed the high dose, delayed second window ICG technique found that 78% meningiomas exhibited more fluorescent signal than surrounding brain, with a sensitivity of 96.4%, but only 39% specificity (95). Fluorescein, like ICG, accumulates within tumor regions rapidly, however, the fluorescent signal may persist for hours, aiding in the visualization of meningiomas (54). In a recent study of 30 patients with meningiomas undergoing resection, Akcakaya et al. found that 88% of meningiomas demonstrate diffuse homogenous intraoperative enhancement, yielding a resection rate of 87% (96). With fluorescein, confocal microscopy can help illuminate meningiomas on the cellular level, with a confocal/histology concordance of 90%, with identification of dural invasion (97).

Brain Metastases

As the most common brain tumors in adults, the treatment paradigm for cerebral metastases has been widely studied. Depending on the size, location and quantity of CNS metastatic lesions, treatment options may include chemotherapy, radiation modalities such as stereotactic radiosurgery (SRS) and whole brain radiation therapy (WBRT), and surgical resection. For symptomatic tumors causing mass effect and cerebral compression, complete resection of metastatic lesions is always the goal when attainable (98). Despite the non-infiltrative nature of these lesions (compared to gliomas), 30% of resections are incomplete, which may explain the 60% local recurrence rate (99, 100), providing a rationale for use of an adjunct such as FGS.

5-ALA has been shown to fluoresce in metastatic lung, breast, colon, bladder, melanoma and other primary cancers with brain metastases (101–104). First studied in 2007, 5-ALA for brain metastases has not been widely studied, with only several large patient studies (54, 105). In the largest experience to date of 157 patients with known metastatic lesions undergoing resection with 5-ALA, Marhold et al. concluded that 66% of tumors exhibited fluorescence, with ductal breast cancer having the highest rate of fluorescence (106). In addition to having variable rates of fluorescence, 5-ALA has shown fluorescence in extra-tumoral edema in cases where the tumor core demonstrated poor fluorescence, making FGS less reliable in these cases (107). Further study is warranted on determining predictors of fluorescence among different primary cancers with brain metastases, as well as a more specified use for FGS in metastatic disease.

Fluorescein sodium has been broadly studied for its use in resection of brain metastases. In a series of 30 patients, Schebesch et al. found fluorescence in 90% of tumors, leading to an 83.3% GTR rate (108, 109). In a follow up study expanding upon this initial experience, Hohne et al. found a 95% fluorescence rate in 95 patients, with an 86% rate of no residual contrast enhancement. In this series, lung adenocarcinoma, melanoma and renal cell carcinoma were the only primary cancers that did not consistency exhibit fluorescein fluorescence (110). As part of the FLUOCERTUM Prospective Study, 25 metastastic lesions were included, of which 24 showed heterogenous enhancement (111). From these primary experiences and others, fluorescein appears to be a reliable fluorophore for brain metastasis surgery.

Second Window ICG technique appears to have advantages for visualization of brain metastasis as most of these tumors have a disrupted BBB and thus accumulate ICG (**Figure 1**). In a recent publication, Teng et al. demonstrated improved survival in patients with resection of all near infrared fluorescent signal in patients undergoing craniotomy for brain metastasis (112). In 47 patients who underwent resection of 51 metastatic lesions, all tumors demonstrated quantifiable NIR fluorescence with a mean SBR of 4.9. Diagnostic accuracy was improved by changing the threshold signal as compared to normal brain background, and a lack of residual NIR fluorescence not only predicted the postoperative MRI gadolinium findings but also predicted progression free survival at 1 year. ICG may prove to have its greatest role in resection of these tumors.

Pediatric Brain Tumors

Similar to the adult literature, maximal safe resection is the standard of care in pediatric HGG. However, unlike the adult literature, we lack randomized controlled trial data for using FGS in the treatment of pediatric brain tumors. The use of 5-ALA for brain tumor surgery in children was first reported by Ruge et al., where 5-ALA was used to resect in a 9-year-old with a right temporal lobe pleomorphic xantoastrocytoma (PXA) (113). There have been no large single center studies currently, however, in 78 patients among 20 European centers, Stummer et al. found that 85% HGG and 80% ependymomas showed fluorescence, and that most primitive neuro-ectodermal tumors (PNET), gangliogliomas, medulloblastomas and pilocytic astrocytomas did not fluoresce (70). Other studies have shown robust fluorescence in HGG, with inconsistent fluuoresence in medulloblastoma, which may be related to underlying subtype (21, 114). While the safety data for 5-ALA use has been well-established in the adult literature, it is less studied in pediatric patients, and there has prior suggestion of increased liver enzyme values with decreasing patient age (115). In a multicenter study of 24 pediatric patients, de Laurentis et al. found fluorescence in 77.8% of tumors, and found fluorescence to be "helpful" in half of the cases (116). BLZ-100 has recently shown to be safe and effective in the treatment of both HGG and LGG in adults, and is currently under investigation for pediatric brain tumors (60).

Spinal Cord Intramedullary Tumors

In the resection of intramedullary spinal cord tumors, establishing the margin between tumor and spinal cord is essential to minimize the risk of spinal cord injury. Ependymomas and astrocytomas, two of the most common intramedullary tumors, both have robust uptake of 5-ALA, and therefore it has studied for this use. Gross total resection of ependymomas is especially crucial, as it is a potentially curable lesion. The first series of intramedullary ependymomas using 5-ALA was published in 2013, when Inoue et al. found that 77% of ependymomas demonstrated fluorescence, leading to a GTR in 80% of cases (117). In a study of 52 patients with 55 spinal tumors including 12 ependymomas, Millesi et al. found 5-ALA to be a safe and effective adjunct in cases of ependymomas, meningiomas, hemangiopericytomas and drop metastases, with a GTR rate of 75% ependymomas (118). With spinal astrocytomas, the margins are less defined, and surgeons are faced with a more difficult situation in where to end a subtotal resection, at the expense of sensorimotor function. 5-ALA may help in identifying tumor margins, and to aid in deciding where to limit cytoreduction, to preserve high-level functionality.

Fluorescein sodium has been shown to be effective for intramedullary tumors in several studies. Acerbi et al. found fluorescence in 82% of tumors, including ependymomas, hemangioblastomas, astrocytoma, and a glioneuronal tumor forming rosettes (119). In a study of 34 intradural extramedullary and 15 intramedullary lesions, surgeons found fluorescein helpful in delineating tumor from surrounding tissue in 96% cases (120).

ICG has additionally been used for intramedullary tumors, specifically vascular spinal cord lesions, such as hemangioblastoma and cavernous angioma (54). In these cases, identifying the feeding and draining veins of these tumors can help surgeons safely remove the lesion. In the case of cavernous angiomas, the surrounding spinal cord takes up the ICG fluorescence, however, the angioma remains avascular, providing surgeons with a nice margin for resection (121).

Primary CNS Lymphoma and Stereotactic Biopsy

Safety and accuracy are the two most important objectives for stereotactic biopsy of cerebral lesions. Fluorescein has been shown to be effective in predicting tumor pathology, especially in contrast-enhancing lesions (122), and in a proof-of-concept study, Lynagh et al. found that *in vivo* fluorescein signal was strongly predictive of tumor tissue, and could be used to identify tumor prior to biopsy (123). Additionally, 5-ALA and ICG have been shown to be effective in identifying tumoral vessels, and 5-ALA, ICG and fluorescein can accurately detect tumor tissue prior to biopsy (124). By coupling fluorescence with confocal microscopy, identifying tumor tissue may now be feasible in real time without a frozen section (124), and may even increase the diagnostic yield, with Malinova et al. finding that 5-ALA fluorescence had a higher sensitivity and negative predictive value for unclear cerebral pathologies compared to frozen section (125). Second Window ICG has also been successfully used in stereotactic biopsy procedures, to assure the surgeon that the contrast-enhancing portion of the tumor has been biopsied (126).

Several case series have shown a potential role for 5-ALA PpIX fluorescence in primary CNS lympoma (127, 128). Lymphoma may mimic HGG radiographically, and therefore PpIX and other fluorophores have been used in cases of presumed HGG. However, the standard of care for primary CNS lymphoma is chemotherapy and radiotherapy following diagnostic biopsy (129), creating a potential role for 5-ALA in improving the diagnostic yield of lymphoma tissue. In the largest series to date on stereotactic biopsies for primary CNS lymphoma, Yamamoto et al. found that 34 of 41 lesions showed fluorescent signal, with a true-positive rate of 82.9% (128). Kiesel et al. found fluorescence in 79% primary lymphoma lesions, and it has recently been proposed that if a lesion demonstrates strong fluorescence, that it may not require intraoperative histopathology, potentially making biopsies safer by decreasing number of biopsy samples and reducing length of stay (130). Fluorescein has also been used to effectively delinate lymphoma tissue vs. normal brain in two case series, where lesions were preoperatively diagnosed as HGG (47, 108). Further study is required to better understand the role for fluorescein in primary CNS lymphoma. In addition, Second Window ICG accumulates dramatically as expected in primary CNS lymphoma, and may be effective in identifying this tissue for biopsy (131).

Other Tumors and Pathological Conditions Requiring Surgery

In addition to the aforementioned CNS tumors, there are several other tumor types that have been studied in the FGS literature.

Peripheral nerve sheath tumors (PNST), comprised of mostly schwannomas, may be difficult to distinguish from surrounding tissues, allowing for a potential role for FGS guidance. In a series of 25 PNST, Vetrano et al. found that fluorescein showed fluorescence in 13 of 14 schwannomas, and allowed for further resection leading to a GTR in six neurofibroma cases and one schwannoma case (132). In a series by Marbacher et al. of 458 tumors receiving 5-ALA PpIX, zero of seven schwannomas showed fluorescence (133). To our knowledge, there have not been studied conducted evaluating SWIG for these tumors.

Sellar tumors, in particular pituitary adenomas, have not been reported to demonstrate strong fluorescent signal, and therefore, not much research has been studied on these tumors. In the Marbacher et al. series, only one of 12 pituitary adenomas demonstrated fluorescence (133). Falco et al. found fluorescence in one of one patients studies in the FLUOCERTUM cohort (111). The role of SWIG in these lesions may be limited, as the pituitary gland is a normal structure that fluoresces with ICG (54). Despite this potential limitaions, ICG endoscopy has been proposed for resection of skull base surgery, and techniques for use have been described (134), with distinguishable margins able to be identified in both functional and non-functional pituitary lesions (135).

Hemangioblastomas may be an important tumor for FGS, as subtotal resection may lead to local recurrence, and FGS may help visualize the intramural nodule within the associated peritumoral cyst. As part of the FLUOCERTUM prospective study of 279 patients receiving fluorescein-guided tumor resection, seven patients with hemangioblastoma were included, all of which demonstrated fluorescence (111). Utsuki et al. used 5-ALA fluorescence, and showed strong fluorescence in all nine hemangioblastoma cases (136). The use of ICG has been rarely reported for both brain and intramedullary hemangioblastoma resections (137, 138).

Several other tumor types have shown potential promise in FGS, such as strong fluorescence observed in fourth ventricle subependymomas (139), germ cell tumors undergoing endoscopic biopsy (140). Further research is warranted on these rarer tumors, to better understand which fluorophores may be implored for use.

CONCLUSION

Understanding the administration and properties of the various fluorophores used in glioma surgery is essential for its use as a surgical adjunct. Fluorophores may target areas of blood-brain barrier breakdown, areas of inflammation, or specifically glioma cells. Fluorophores are administered by different routes, and surgeons should be aware of the relationship between fluorophore administration and tumor fluorescence. ICG and fluorescein work by passive targeting, and have the benefit of IV administration in the operating room within seconds (ICG as vascular angiography agent) to a couple hours (fluorescein), to the next day (Second Window ICG as an EPR accumulated agent). As an oral agent, 5-ALA is consumed prior to anesthseia, and is able to persist in target tissue for longer, allowing for logistical delays. Newly studied molecular targets, such as BLZ-100 and EGFR conjugates, are also given in the operating room, but may last in tumor tissue for up to several days.

AUTHOR CONTRIBUTIONS

AS and CH: conceptualization and investigation. AS, MR, NM, RB, JL, FA, and CH: writing—original draft preparation, writing—review, and editing. AS: visualization. CH: supervision and project. All authors have read and agreed to the published version of the manuscript.

REFERENCES

1. Brown TJ, Brennan MC, Li M, Church EW, Brandmeir NJ, Rakszawski KL, et al. Association of the extent of resection with survival in glioblastoma: a systematic review and meta-analysis. *JAMA Oncol.* (2016) 2:1460–9. doi: 10.1001/jamaoncol.2016.1373
2. Fernandes C, Costa A, Osório L, Lago RC, Linhares P, Carvalho B, et al. *Current Standards of Care in Glioblastoma Therapy.* Glioblastoma: Codon Publications. (2017).
3. Haj A, Doenitz C, Schebesch KM, Ehrensberger D, Hau P, Putnik K, et al. Extent of resection in newly diagnosed glioblastoma: impact of a specialized neuro-oncology care center. *Brain Sci.* (2018) 8:5. doi: 10.3390/brainsci8010005
4. Yamada S, Muragaki Y, Maruyama T, Komori T, Okada Y. Role of neurochemical navigation with 5-aminolevulinic acid during intraoperative MRI-guided resection of intracranial malignant gliomas. *Clin Neurol Neurosurg.* (2015) 130:134–9. doi: 10.1016/j.clineuro.2015.01.005
5. Zhang ZZ, Shields LB, Sun DA, Zhang YP, Hunt MA, Shields CB. The art of intraoperative glioma identification. *Front Oncol.* (2015) 5:175. doi: 10.3389/fonc.2015.00175
6. Su X, Huang Q-F, Chen H-L, Chen J. Fluorescence-guided resection of high-grade gliomas: a systematic review and meta-analysis. *Photodiagn Photodyn Therapy.* (2014) 11:451–8. doi: 10.1016/j.pdpdt.2014.08.001
7. Neira JA, Ung TH, Sims JS, Malone HR, Chow DS, Samanamud JL, et al. Aggressive resection at the infiltrative margins of glioblastoma facilitated by intraoperative fluorescein guidance. *J Neurosurg.* (2016) 127:111–22. doi: 10.3171/2016.7.JNS16232
8. Stummer W, Pichlmeier U, Meinel T, Wiestler OD, Zanella F, Reulen HJ, et al. Fluorescence-guided surgery with 5-aminolevulinic acid for resection of

malignant glioma: a randomised controlled multicentre phase III trial. *Lancet Oncol.* (2006) 7:392–401. doi: 10.1016/S1470-2045(06)70665-9
9. Hadjipanayis CG, Stummer W. *Fluorescence-Guided Neurosurgery: Neuro-Oncology and Cerebrovascular Applications.* New York, NY: Thieme. (2019). doi: 10.1055/b-0038-164181
10. Stummer W, Stocker S, Novotny A, Heimann A, Sauer O, Kempski O, et al. *In vitro* and *in vivo* porphyrin accumulation by C6 glioma cells after exposure to 5-aminolevulinic acid. *J Photochem Photobiol B.* (1998) 45:160–9. doi: 10.1016/S1011-1344(98)00176-6
11. Hadjipanayis CG, Widhalm G, Stummer W. What is the surgical benefit of utilizing 5-aminolevulinic acid for fluorescence-guided surgery of malignant gliomas? *Neurosurgery.* (2015) 77:663–73. doi: 10.1227/NEU.0000000000000929
12. Bottomley, S. S. Pathophysiology of heme synthesis. *Semin Hematol.* (1988) 25:282–302.
13. Onda N, Kimura M, Yoshida T, Shibutani M. Preferential tumor cellular uptake and retention of indocyanine green for *in vivo* tumor imaging. *Int J Cancer.* (2016) 139:673–82. doi: 10.1002/ijc.30102
14. Francaviglia N, Iacopino DG, Costantino G, Villa A, Impallaria P, Meli F, et al. Fluorescein for resection of high-grade gliomas: a safety study control in a single center and review of the literature. *Surg Neurol Int.* (2017) 8:17. doi: 10.4103/sni.sni_89_17
15. Cho SS, Salinas R, Lee JY. Indocyanine-green for fluorescence-guided surgery of brain tumors: evidence, techniques, and practical experience. *Front Surg.* (2019) 6:11. doi: 10.3389/fsurg.2019.00011
16. Okuda T, Yoshioka H, Kato A. Fluorescence-guided surgery for glioblastoma multiforme using high-dose fluorescein sodium with excitation and barrier filters. *J Clin Neurosci.* (2012) 19:1719–22. doi: 10.1016/j.jocn.2011.12.034
17. Haglund MM, Hochman DW, Spence AM, Berger MS. Enhanced optical imaging of rat gliomas and tumor margins. *Neurosurgery.* (1994) 35:930–41. doi: 10.1227/00006123-199411000-00019
18. Acerbi F, Broggi M, Broggi G, Ferroli P. What is the best timing for fluorescein injection during surgical removal of high-grade gliomas? *Acta Neurochir.* (2015) 157:1377–8. doi: 10.1007/s00701-015-2455-z
19. Senders JT, Muskens IS, Schnoor R, Karhade AV, Cote DJ, Smith TR, et al. Agents for fluorescence-guided glioma surgery: a systematic review of preclinical and clinical results. *Acta Neurochir.* (2017) 159:151–67. doi: 10.1007/s00701-016-3028-5
20. Zeh R, Sheikh S, Xia L, Pierce J, Newton A, Predina J, et al. The second window ICG technique demonstrates a broad plateau period for near infrared fluorescence tumor contrast in glioblastoma. *PLoS ONE.* (2017) 12:e0182034. doi: 10.1371/journal.pone.0182034
21. Zhang C, Boop FA, Ruge J. The use of 5-aminolevulinic acid in resection of pediatric brain tumors: a critical review. *J Neurooncol.* (2019) 141:567–73. doi: 10.1007/s11060-018-03004-y
22. Eyüpoglu IY, Hore N, Fan Z, Buslei R, Merkel A, Buchfelder M, et al. Intraoperative vascular DIVA surgery reveals angiogenic hotspots in tumor zones of malignant gliomas. *Sci Rep.* (2015) 5:1–7. doi: 10.1038/srep07958
23. Haglund MM, Berger MS, Hochman DW. Enhanced optical imaging of human gliomas and tumor margins. *Neurosurgery.* (1996) 38:308–17. doi: 10.1097/00006123-199602000-00015
24. Hansen DA, Spence AM, Carski T, Berger MS. Indocyanine green (ICG) staining and demarcation of tumor margins in a rat glioma model. *Surg. Neurol.* (1993) 40:451–6. doi: 10.1016/0090-3019(93)90046-4
25. Martirosyan NL, Cavalcanti DD, Eschbacher JM, Delaney PM, Scheck AC, Abdelwahab MG, et al. Use of *in vivo* near-infrared laser confocal endomicroscopy with indocyanine green to detect the boundary of infiltrative tumor: laboratory investigation. *J Neurosurg.* (2011) 115:1131–8. doi: 10.3171/2011.8.JNS11559
26. Maeda H, Tsukigawa K, Fang J. A retrospective 30 years after discovery of the enhanced permeability and retention effect of solid tumors: next-generation chemotherapeutics and photodynamic therapy–problems, solutions, and prospects. *Microcirculation.* (2016) 23:173–82. doi: 10.1111/micc.12228
27. Lee JY, Thawani JP, Pierce J, Zeh R, Martinez-Lage M, Chanin M, et al. Intraoperative near-infrared optical imaging can localize gadolinium-enhancing gliomas during surgery. *Neurosurgery.* (2016) 79:856–71. doi: 10.1227/NEU.0000000000001450
28. Cho SS, Salinas R, De Ravin E, Teng CW, Li C, Abdullah KG, et al. Near-infrared imaging with second-window indocyanine green in newly diagnosed high-grade gliomas predicts gadolinium enhancement on postoperative magnetic resonance imaging. *Mol Imaging Biol.* (2020) 22:1427–37. doi: 10.1007/s11307-019-01455-x
29. Moore GE, Peyton WT. The clinical use of fluorescein in neurosurgery; the localization of brain tumors. *J Neurosurg.* (1948) 5:392–8. doi: 10.3171/jns.1948.5.4.0392
30. Schebesch K, Brawanski A, Hohenberger C, Hohne J. Fluorescein sodium-guided surgery of malignant brain tumors: history, current concepts, and future projects. *Turkish Neurosurg.* (2016) 26:185–94. doi: 10.5137/1019-5149.JTN.16952-16.0
31. Acerbi F, Broggi M, Eoli M, Anghileri E, Cavallo C, Boffano C, et al. Is fluorescein-guided technique able to help in resection of high-grade gliomas? *Neurosurg Focus.* (2014) 36:E5. doi: 10.3171/2013.11.FOCUS13487
32. Diaz RJ, Dios RR, Hattab EM, Burrell K, Rakopoulos P, Sabha N, et al. Study of the biodistribution of fluorescein in glioma-infiltrated mouse brain and histopathological correlation of intraoperative findings in high-grade gliomas resected under fluorescein fluorescence guidance. *J Neurosurg.* (2015) 122:1360–9. doi: 10.3171/2015.2.JNS132507
33. Shinoda J, Yano H, Yoshimura S, Okumura A, Kaku Y, Iwama T, et al. Fluorescence-guided resection of glioblastoma multiforme by using high-dose fluorescein sodium: technical note. *J Neurosurg.* (2003) 99:597–603. doi: 10.3171/jns.2003.99.3.0597
34. Valli D, Belykh E, Zhao X, Gandhi S, Cavallo C, Martirosyan NL, et al. Development of a simulation model for fluorescence-guided brain tumor surgery. *Front Oncol.* (2019) 9:748. doi: 10.3389/fonc.2019.00748
35. Acerbi F, Broggi M, Schebesch KM, Höhne J, Cavallo C, De Laurentis C, et al. Fluorescein-guided surgery for resection of high-grade gliomas: a multicentric prospective phase II study (FLUOGLIO). *Clin Cancer Res.* (2018) 24:52–61. doi: 10.1158/1078-0432.CCR-17-1184
36. Belykh E, Miller EJ, Patel AA, Yazdanabadi MI, Martirosyan NL, Yagmurlu K, et al. Diagnostic accuracy of a confocal laser endomicroscope for *in vivo* differentiation between normal injured and tumor tissue during fluorescein-guided glioma resection: laboratory investigation. *World Neurosurg.* (2018) 115:e337–48. doi: 10.1016/j.wneu.2018.04.048
37. Ichioka T, Miyatake S, Asai N, Kajimoto Y, Nakagawa T, Hayashi H, et al. Enhanced detection of malignant glioma xenograft by fluorescein–human serum albumin conjugate. *J Neurooncol.* (2004) 67:47–52. doi: 10.1023/B:NEON.0000021783.62610.1b
38. Martirosyan NL, Eschbacher JM, Kalani MY, Turner JD, Belykh E, Spetzler RF, et al. Prospective evaluation of the utility of intraoperative confocal laser endomicroscopy in patients with brain neoplasms using fluorescein sodium: experience with 74 cases. *Neurosurg Focus.* (2016) 40:E11. doi: 10.3171/2016.1.FOCUS15559
39. Kuroiwa T, Kajimoto Y, Ohta T. Development of a fluorescein operative microscope for use during malignant glioma surgery: a technical note and preliminary report. *Surg Neurol.* (1998) 50:41–9. doi: 10.1016/S0090-3019(98)00055-X
40. Chen B, Wang H, Ge P, Zhao J, Li W, Gu H, et al. Gross total resection of glioma with the intraoperative fluorescence-guidance of fluorescein sodium. *Int J Med Sci.* (2012) 9:708–14. doi: 10.7150/ijms.4843
41. Roberts DW, Olson J. Fluorescein guidance in glioblastoma resection. *N Engl J Med.* (2017) 376:e36. doi: 10.1056/NEJMicm1611258
42. Bowden SG, Neira JA, Gill, B. J. A., Ung TH, Englander ZK, Zanazzi G, et al. Sodium fluorescein facilitates guided sampling of diagnostic tumor tissue in non-enhancing gliomas. *Neurosurgery.* (2018) 82:719–27. doi: 10.1093/neuros/nyx271
43. Belykh E, Shaffer KV, Lin C, Byvaltsev VA, Preul MC, Chen L. Blood-brain barrier, blood-brain tumor barrier, and fluorescence-guided neurosurgical oncology: delivering optical labels to brain tumors. *Front Oncol.* (2020) 10:739. doi: 10.3389/fonc.2020.00739
44. Koc K, Anik I, Cabuk B, Ceylan S. Fluorescein sodium-guided surgery in glioblastoma multiforme: a prospective evaluation. *Br J Neurosurg.* (2008) 22:99–103. doi: 10.1080/02688690701765524
45. Schebesch KM, Proescholdt M, Höhne J, Hohenberger C, Hansen E, Riemenschneider MJ, et al. Sodium fluorescein-guided resection under the YELLOW 560 nm surgical microscope filter in malignant brain

tumor surgery–a feasibility study. *Acta Neurochir.* (2013) 155:693–9. doi: 10.1007/s00701-013-1643-y

46. Zhang DY, Singhal S, Lee JYK. Optical principles of fluorescence-guided brain tumor surgery: a practical primer for the neurosurgeon. *Neurosurgery.* (2019) 85:312–24. doi: 10.1093/neuros/nyy315
47. Hamamcioglu MK, Akçakaya MO, Göker B, Kasimcan MÖ, Kiriş T. The use of the YELLOW 560 nm surgical microscope filter for sodium fluorescein-guided resection of brain tumors: our preliminary results in a series of 28 patients. *Clin Neurol Neurosurg.* (2016) 143:39–45. doi: 10.1016/j.clineuro.2016.02.006
48. Suero Molina E, Wölfer J, Ewelt C, Ehrhardt A, Brokinkel B, Stummer W. Dual-labeling with 5-aminolevulinic acid and fluorescein for fluorescence-guided resection of high-grade gliomas: technical note. *J Neurosurg.* (2018) 128:399–405. doi: 10.3171/2016.11.JNS161072
49. Ung TH, Kellner C, Neira JA, Wang SH, D'Amico R, Faust PL, et al. The use of fluorescein sodium in the biopsy and gross-total resection of a tectal plate glioma. *J Neurosurg Pediatr.* (2015) 16:732–5. doi: 10.3171/2015.5.PEDS15142
50. Xiang Y, Zhu XP, Zhao JN, Huang GH, Tang JH, Chen HR, et al. Blood-brain barrier disruption, sodium fluorescein, and fluorescence-guided surgery of gliomas. *Br J Neurosurg.* (2018) 32:141–8. doi: 10.1080/02688697.2018.1428731
51. Folaron M, Strawbridge R, Samkoe KS, Filan C, Roberts DW, Davis SC. Elucidating the kinetics of sodium fluorescein for fluorescence-guided surgery of glioma. *J Neurosurg.* (2018) 131:724–34. doi: 10.3171/2018.4.JNS172644
52. Stummer W, Tonn JC, Goetz C, Ullrich W, Stepp H, Bink A, et al. 5-Aminolevulinic acid-derived tumor fluorescence: the diagnostic accuracy of visible fluorescence qualities as corroborated by spectrometry and histology and postoperative imaging. *Neurosurgery.* (2014) 74:310–9. doi: 10.1227/NEU.0000000000000267
53. Maragkos GA, Schupper AJ, Lakomkin N, Sideras P, Price G, Baron RB, et al. Fluorescence-guided high-grade glioma surgery more than 4 h after 5-aminolevulinic acid administration. *Front Neurol.* (2021) 2021:644804. doi: 10.3389/fneur.2021.644804
54. Hadjipanayis CG, Stummer W. Fluorescence-guided neurosurgery: neuro-oncology and cerebrovascular applications. *Thieme.* (2019).
55. Hadjipanayis CG, Stummer W. 5-ALA and FDA approval for glioma surgery. *Neurooncol.* (2019) 141:479–86. doi: 10.1007/s11060-019-03098-y
56. Stummer W, Novotny A, Stepp H, Goetz C, Bise K, Reulen HJ. Fluorescence-guided resection of glioblastoma multiforme by using 5-aminolevulinic acid-induced porphyrins: a prospective study in 52 consecutive patients. *J Neurosurg.* (2000) 93:1003–13. doi: 10.3171/jns.2000.93.6.1003
57. Teixidor P, Arráez MÁ, Villalba G, Garcia R, Tardáguila M, González JJ, et al. Safety and efficacy of 5-aminolevulinic acid for high grade glioma in usual clinical practice: a prospective cohort study. *PLoS ONE.* (2016) 11:e0149244. doi: 10.1371/journal.pone.0149244
58. Center for Drug Evaluation and Research. *Aminolevulinic Acid Hydrochloride, Known as ALA HCl (Gleolan, NX Development Corp.) as an Optical Imaging Agent Indicated in Patients With Gliomas.* (2017). Available online at: https://www.fda.gov/drugs/resources-information-approved-drugs/aminolevulinic-acid-hydrochloride-known-ala-hcl-gleolan-nx-development-corp-optical-imaging-agent (accessed June 3, 2020).
59. Kaneko S, Suero Molina E, Ewelt C, Warneke N, Stummer W. Fluorescence-based measurement of real-time kinetics of protoporphyrin IX after 5-aminolevulinic acid administration in human *in situ* malignant gliomas. *Neurosurgery.* (2019) 85:E739–46. doi: 10.1093/neuros/nyz129
60. Patil CG, Walker DG, Miller DM, Butte P, Morrison B, Kittle DS, et al. Phase 1 safety, pharmacokinetics, and fluorescence imaging study of tozuleristide (BLZ-100) in adults with newly diagnosed or recurrent gliomas. *Neurosurgery.* (2019) 85:E641–9. doi: 10.1093/neuros/nyz125
61. Weichert JP, Clark PA, Kandela IK, Vaccaro AM, Clarke W, Longino MA, et al. Alkylphosphocholine analogs for broad-spectrum cancer imaging and therapy. *Sci Transl Med.* (2014) 6:240ra75. doi: 10.1126/scitranslmed.3007646
62. Swanson KI, Clark PA, Zhang RR, Kandela IK, Farhoud M, Weichert JP, et al. Fluorescent cancer-selective alkylphosphocholine analogs for intraoperative glioma detection. *Neurosurgery.* (2015) 76:115–24. doi: 10.1227/NEU.0000000000000622
63. Seekell K, Lewis S, Wilson C, Li S, Grant G, Wax A. Feasibility study of brain tumor delineation using immunolabeled gold nanorods. *Biomed. Opt. Express.* (2013) 4:2284–95. doi: 10.1364/BOE.4.002284
64. Davis SC, Samkoe KS, O'Hara JA, Gibbs-Strauss SL, Payne HL, Hoopes PJW, et al. MRI-coupled fluorescence tomography quantifies EGFR activity in brain tumors. *Acad Radiol.* (2010) 17:271–6. doi: 10.1016/j.acra.2009.11.001
65. Samkoe KS, Gunn JR, Marra K, Hull SM, Moodie KL, Feldwisch J, et al. Toxicity and pharmacokinetic profile for single-dose injection of ABY-029: a fluorescent anti-EGFR synthetic affibody molecule for human use. *Mol Imaging Biol.* (2017) 19:512–21. doi: 10.1007/s11307-016-1033-y
66. de Souza AL, Marra K, Gunn J, Samkoe KS, Hoopes PJ, Feldwisch J, et al. Fluorescent affibody molecule administered *in vivo* at a microdose level labels EGFR expressing glioma tumor regions. *Mol Imaging Biol.* (2017) 19:41–8. doi: 10.1007/s11307-016-0980-7
67. Warram JM, de Boer E, Korb M, Hartman Y, Kovar J, Markert JM, et al. Fluorescence-guided resection of experimental malignant glioma using cetuximab-IRDye 800 CW. *Br J Neurosurg.* (2015) 29:850–8. doi: 10.3109/02688697.2015.1056090
68. Miller SE, Tummers WS, Teraphongphom N, van den Berg NS, Hasan A, Ertsey RD, et al. First-in-human intraoperative near-infrared fluorescence imaging of glioblastoma using cetuximab-IRDye800. *J Neurooncol.* (2018) 139:135–43. doi: 10.1007/s11060-018-2854-0
69. Schipmann S, Schwake M, Suero Molina E, Stummer W. Markers for identifying and targeting glioblastoma cells during surgery. *J Neurol Surg A Cent Eur Neurosurg.* (2019) 80:475–87. doi: 10.1055/s-0039-1692976
70. Stummer W, Rodrigues F, Schucht P, et al. Predicting the "usefulness" of 5-ALA-derived tumor fluorescence for fluorescence-guided resections in pediatric brain tumors: a European survey. *Acta Neurochir.* (2014) 156:2315–24. doi: 10.1007/s00701-014-2234-2
71. Zhao S, Wu J, Wang C, Liu H, Dong X, Shi C, et al. Intraoperative fluorescence-guided resection of high-grade malignant gliomas using 5-aminolevulinic acid-induced porphyrins: a systematic review and meta-analysis of prospective studies. *PLoS ONE.* (2013) 8:e63682. doi: 10.1371/journal.pone.0063682
72. Eljamel S. 5-ALA fluorescence image guided resection of glioblastoma multiforme: a meta-analysis of the literature. *Int J Mol Sci.* (2015) 16:10443–56. doi: 10.3390/ijms160510443
73. Diez Valle R, Tejada Solis S, Idoate Gastearena MA, Garcia de Eulate R, Dominguez Echavarri P, and Aristu Mendiroz, J. Surgery guided by 5-aminolevulinic fluorescence in glioblastoma: volumetric analysis of extent of resection in single-center experience. *J Neurooncol.* (2011) 102:105–13. doi: 10.1007/s11060-010-0296-4
74. Lau D, Hervey-Jumper SL, Chang S, Molinaro AM, McDermott MW, Phillips JJ, et al. A prospective Phase II clinical trial of 5-aminolevulinic acid to assess the correlation of intraoperative fluorescence intensity and degree of histologic cellularity during resection of high-grade gliomas. *J Neurosurg.* (2016) 124:1300–9. doi: 10.3171/2015.5.JNS1577
75. Idoate MA, Diez Valle R, Echeveste J, Tejada S. Pathological characterization of the glioblastoma border as shown during surgery using 5-aminolevulinic acid-induced fluorescence. *Neuropathology.* (2011) 31:575–82. doi: 10.1111/j.1440-1789.2011.01202.x
76. Roberts DW, Valdés PA, Harris BT, Fontaine KM, Hartov A, Fan X, et al. Coregistered fluorescence-enhanced tumor resection of malignant glioma: relationships between delta-aminolevulinic acid-induced protoporphyrin IX fluorescence, magnetic resonance imaging enhancement, and neuropathological parameters. Clinical article. *J Neurosurg.* (2011) 114:595–603. doi: 10.3171/2010.2.JNS091322
77. Aldave G, Tejada S, Pay E, Marigil M, Bejarano B, Idoate MA, et al. Prognostic value of residual fluorescent tissue in glioblastoma patients after gross total resection in 5-aminolevulinic Acid-guided surgery. *Neurosurgery.* (2013) 72:915–20. doi: 10.1227/NEU.0b013e31828c3974
78. Rey-Dios R, Hattab EM, Cohen-Gadol AA. Use of intraoperative fluorescein sodium fluorescence to improve the accuracy of tissue diagnosis during stereotactic needle biopsy of high-grade gliomas. *Acta Neurochir.* (2014) 156:1071–5. doi: 10.1007/s00701-014-2097-6

79. Jakola AS, Myrmel KS, Kloster R, Torp SH, Lindal S, Unsgård G, et al. Comparison of a strategy favoring early surgical resection vs. a strategy favoring watchful waiting in low-grade gliomas. *JAMA.* (2012) 308:1881–8. doi: 10.1001/jama.2012.12807
80. Smith JS, Chang EF, Lamborn KR, Chang SM, Prados MD, Cha S, et al. Role of extent of resection in the longterm outcome of low-grade hemispheric gliomas. *J Clin Oncol.* (2008) 26: 1338–45. doi: 10.1200/JCO.2007.13.9337
81. Teng L, Nakada M, Zhao SG, Endo Y, Furuyama N, Nambu E, et al. Silencing of ferrochelatase enhances 5-aminolevulinic acid-based fluorescence and photodynamic therapy efficacy. *Br J Cancer.* (2011) 104:798–807. doi: 10.1038/bjc.2011.12
82. Hefti M, von Campe G, Moschopulos M, Siegner A, Looser H, Landolt H. 5-aminolevulinic acid induced protoporphyrin IX fluorescence in high-grade glioma surgery: a one-year experience at a single institutuion. *Swiss Med Wkly.* (2008) 138:180–5.
83. Utsuki S, Oka H, Sato S, Suzuki S, Shimizu S, Tanaka S, et al. Possibility of using laser spectroscopy for the intraoperative detection of non-fluorescing brain tumors and the boundaries of brain tumor infiltrates. Technical note. *J Neurosurg.* (2006) 104:618–20. doi: 10.3171/jns.2006.104.4.618
84. Widhalm G, Wolfsberger S, Minchev G, Woehrer A, Krssak M, Czech T, et al. 5-Aminolevulinic acid is a promising marker for detection of anaplastic foci in diffusely infiltrating gliomas with non-significant contrast enhancement. *Cancer.* (2010) 116:1545–52. doi: 10.1002/cncr.24903
85. Jaber M, Wölfer J, Ewelt C, Holling M, Hasselblatt M, Niederstadt T, et al. The value of 5-aminolevulinic acid in lowgrade gliomas and high-grade gliomas lacking glioblastoma imaging features: an analysis based on fluorescence, magnetic resonance imaging, 18F-fluoroethyl tyrosine positron emission tomography, and tumor molecular factors. *Neurosurgery.* (2016) 78:401–11. doi: 10.1227/NEU.0000000000001020
86. Paulus W, Peiffer J. Intratumoral histologic heterogeneity of gliomas. A quantitative study. *Cancer.* (1989) 64:442–7. doi: 10.1002/1097-0142(19890715)64:2<442::AID-CNCR2820640217>3.0.CO;2-S
87. Widhalm G, Kiesel B, Woehrer A, Traub-Weidinger T, Preusser M, Marosi C, et al. 5-Aminolevulinic acid induced fluorescence is a powerful intraoperative marker for precise histopathological grading of gliomas with non-significant contrast-enhancement. *PLoS ONE.* (2013) 8:e76988. doi: 10.1371/journal.pone.0076988
88. Kamp MA, Krause Molle Z, Munoz-Bendix C, Rapp M, Sabel M, Steiger HJ, et al. Various shades of red-a systematic analysis of qualitative estimation of ALA-derived fluorescence in neurosurgery. *Neurosurg Rev.* (2018) 41:3–18. doi: 10.1007/s10143-016-0745-4
89. Millesi M, Kiesel B, Mischkulnig M, Martínez-Moreno M, Wöhrer A, Wolfsberger S, et al. Analysis of the surgical benefits of 5-ALA-induced fluorescence in intracranial meningiomas: experience in 204 meningiomas. *J Neurosurg.* (2016) 125:1408–19. doi: 10.3171/2015.12.JNS151513
90. Della Puppa A, Rustemi O, Gioffrè G, Troncon I, Lombardi G, Rolma G, et al. Predictive value of intraoperative 5-aminolevulinic acid-induced fluorescence for detecting bone invasion in meningioma surgery. *J Neurosurg.* (2014) 120:840–5. doi: 10.3171/2013.12.JNS131642
91. Eicker SO, Floeth FW, Kamp M, Steiger HJ, Hänggi D. The impact of fluorescence guidance on spinal intradural tumour surgery. *Eur Spine J.* (2013) 22:1394–401. doi: 10.1007/s00586-013-2657-0
92. d'Avella E, Volpin F, Manara R, Scienza R, Della Puppa A. Indocyanine green videoangiography (ICGV)-guided surgery of parasagittal meningiomas occluding the superior sagittal sinus (SSS). *Acta Neurochir.* (2013) 155:415–20. doi: 10.1007/s00701-012-1617-5
93. Ueba T, Okawa M, Abe H, Nonaka M, Iwaasa M, Higashi T, et al. Identification of venous sinus, tumor location, and pial supply during meningioma surgery by transdural indocyanine green videography. *J Neurosurg.* (2013) 118:632–6. doi: 10.3171/2012.11.JNS121113
94. Han SJ, Magill ST, Tarapore PE, Horton JC, McDermott MW. Direct visualization of improved optic nerve pial vascular supply following tuberculum meningioma resection: case report. *J Neurosurg.* (2016) 125:565–9. doi: 10.3171/2015.6.JNS15765
95. Lee JYK, Pierce JT, Thawani JP, Zeh R, Nie S, Martinez-Lage M, et al. Near-infrared fluorescent image-guided surgery for intracranial meningioma. *J Neurosurg.* (2018) 128:380–90. doi: 10.3171/2016.10.JNS161636
96. Akçakaya MO, Göker B, Kasimcan MÖ, Hamamcioglu MK, Kiriş T. Use of sodium fluorescein in meningioma surgery performed under the YELLOW-560 nm surgical microscope filter: feasibility and preliminary results. *World Neurosurg.* (2017) 107:966–73. doi: 10.1016/j.wneu.2017.07.103
97. Eschbacher J, Martirosyan NL, Nakaji P, Sanai N, Preul MC, Smith KA, et al. *In vivo* intraoperative confocal microscopy for real-time histopathological imaging of brain tumors. *J Neurosurg.* (2012) 116:854–60. doi: 10.3171/2011.12.JNS11696
98. Al-Shamy G, Sawaya R. Management of brain metastases: the indispensable role of surgery. *J Neurooncol.* (2009) 92:275–82. doi: 10.1007/s11060-009-9839-y
99. Kamp MA, Rapp M, Bühner J, Slotty PJ, Reichelt D, Sadat H, et al. Early postoperative magnet resonance tomography after resection of cerebral metastases. *Acta Neurochir.* (2015) 157:1573–80. doi: 10.1007/s00701-015-2479-4
100. Patchell RA, Tibbs PA, Walsh JW, Dempsey RJ, Maruyama Y, Kryscio RJ, et al. A randomized trial of surgery in the treatment of single metastases to the brain. *N Engl J Med.* (1990) 322:494–500. doi: 10.1056/NEJM199002223220802
101. Gamarra F, Lingk P, Marmarova A, Edelmann M, Hautmann H, Stepp H, et al. 5-Aminolevulinic acid-induced fluorescence in bronchial tumours: dependency on the patterns of tumour invasion. *J Photochem Photobiol B.* (2004) 73:35–42. doi: 10.1016/j.jphotobiol.2003.09.009
102. Moan J, Bech O, Gaullier JM, Stokke T, Steen HB, Ma LW, et al. Protoporphyrin IX accumulation in cells treated with 5-aminolevulinic acid: dependence on cell density, cell size and cell cycle. *Int J Cancer.* (1998) 75:134–9. doi: 10.1002/(SICI)1097-0215(19980105)75:1<134::AID-IJC20>3.0.CO;2-F
103. Riedl CR, Daniltchenko D, Koenig F, Simak R, Loening SA, Pflueger H. Fluorescence endoscopy with 5-aminolevulinic acid reduces early recurrence rate in superficial bladder cancer. *J Urol.* (2001) 165:1121–3. doi: 10.1016/S0022-5347(05)66442-7
104. Tsai T, Ji HT, Chiang PC, Chou RH, Chang WS, Chen CT. ALA-PDT results in phenotypic changes and decreased cellular invasion in surviving cancer cells. *Lasers Surg Med.* (2009) 41:305–15. doi: 10.1002/lsm.20761
105. Utsuki S, Miyoshi N, Oka H, Miyajima Y, Shimizu S, Suzuki S, et al. Fluorescence-guided resection of metastatic brain tumors using a 5-aminolevulinic acid-induced protoporphyrin IX: pathological study. *Brain Tumor Pathol.* (2007) 24:53–5. doi: 10.1007/s10014-007-0223-3
106. Marhold F, Mercea PA, Scheichel F, Berghoff AS, Heicappell P, Kiesel B, et al. Detailed analysis of 5-aminolevulinic acid induced fluorescence in different brain metastases at two specialized neurosurgical centers: experience in 157 cases. *J Neurosurg.* (2019) 27:1–12. doi: 10.3171/2019.6.JNS1997
107. Kamp MA, Grosser P, Felsberg J, Slotty PJ, Steiger HJ, Reifenberger G, et al. 5-aminolevulinic acid (5-ALA)-induced fluorescence in intracerebral metastases: a retrospective study. *Acta Neurochir.* (2012) 154:223–8. doi: 10.1007/s00701-011-1200-5
108. Schebesch KM, Hoehne J, Hohenberger C, Acerbi F, Broggi M, Proescholdt M, et al. Fluorescein sodium-guided surgery in cerebral lymphoma. *Clin Neurol Neurosurg.* (2015) 139:125–8. doi: 10.1016/j.clineuro.2015.09.015
109. Schebesch KM, Hoehne J, Hohenberger C, Proescholdt M, Riemenschneider MJ, Wendl C, et al. Fluorescein sodium-guided resection of cerebral metastases—experience with the first 30 patients. *Acta Neurochir.* (2015) 157:899–904. doi: 10.1007/s00701-015-2395-7
110. Höhne J, Hohenberger C, Proescholdt M, Riemenschneider MJ, Wendl C, Brawanski A, et al. Fluorescein sodium-guided resection of cerebral metastases-an update. *Acta Neurochir.* (2017) 159:363–7. doi: 10.1007/s00701-016-3054-3
111. Falco J, Cavallo C, Vetrano IG, de Laurentis C, Siozos L, Schiariti M, et al. Fluorescein application in cranial and spinal tumors enhancing at preoperative MRI and operated with a dedicated filter on the surgical microscope: preliminary results in 279 patients enrolled in the FLUOCERTUM prospective study. *Front Surg.* (2019) 6:49. doi: 10.3389/fsurg.2019.00049
112. Teng CW, Cho SS, Singh Y, De Ravin E, Somers K, Buch L, et al. Second window ICG predicts gross-total resection and progression-free survival during brain metastasis surgery. *J Neurosurg.* (2021) 2:1–10. doi: 10.3171/2020.8.JNS201810

113. Ruge JR, Liu J. Use of 5-aminolevulinic acid for visualization and resection of a benign pediatric brain tumor. *J Neurosurg Pediatr.* (2009) 4:484–6. doi: 10.3171/2009.6.PEDS08428
114. Preuss M, Renner C, Krupp W, Christiansen H, Fischer L, Merkenschlager A, et al. The use of 5-aminolevulinic acid fluorescence guidance in resection of pediatric brain tumors. *Childs Nerv Syst.* (2013) 29:1263–7. doi: 10.1007/s00381-013-2159-8
115. Offersen CM, Skjoeth-Rasmussen J. Evaluation of the risk of liver damage from the use of 5-aminolevulinic acid for intra-operative identification and resection in patients with malignant gliomas. *Acta Neurochir.* (2017) 159:145–50. doi: 10.1007/s00701-016-3014-y
116. de Laurentis C, Höhne J, Cavallo C, Restelli F, Falco J, Broggi M, et al. The impact of fluorescein-guided technique in the surgical removal of CNS tumors in a pediatric population: results from a multicentric observational study. *J Neurosurg Sci.* (2019) 63:679–87. doi: 10.23736/S0390-5616.19.04601-0
117. Inoue T, Endo T, Nagamatsu K, Watanabe M, Tominaga T. 5-aminolevulinic acid fluorescence-guided resection of intramedullary ependymoma: report of 9 cases. *Neurosurgery.* (2013) 72:ons159–68. doi: 10.1227/NEU.0b013e31827bc7a3
118. Millesi M, Kiesel B, Woehrer A, Hainfellner JA, Novak K, Martínez-Moreno M, et al. Analysis of 5-aminolevulinic acid-induced fluorescence in 55 different spinal tumors. *Neurosurg Focus.* (2014) 36:E11. doi: 10.3171/2013.12.FOCUS13485
119. Acerbi F, Cavallo C, Schebesch KM, Akçakaya MO, de Laurentis C, Hamamcioglu MK, et al. Fluorescein-guided resection of intramedullary spinal cord tumors: results from a preliminary, multicentric, retrospective study. *World Neurosurg.* (2017) 108:603–9. doi: 10.1016/j.wneu.2017.09.061
120. Olguner SK, Arslan A, Açik V, Istemen I, Can M, Gezercan Y, et al. Sodium fluorescein for spinal intradural tumors. *Front Oncol.* (2021) 10:618579. doi: 10.3389/fonc.2020.618579
121. Endo T, Aizawa-Kohama M, Nagamatsu K, Murakami K, Takahashi A, Tominaga T. Use of microscope-integrated near-infrared indocyanine green videoangiography in the surgical treatment of intramedullary cavernous malformations: report of eight cases. *J Neurosurg Spine.* (2013) 18:443–9. doi: 10.3171/2013.1.SPINE12482
122. Nevzati E, Chatain GP, Hoffman J, Kleinschmidt-DeMasters BK, Lillehei KO, Ormond DR. Reliability of fluorescein-assisted stereotactic brain biopsies in predicting conclusive tissue diagnosis. *Acta Neurochir.* (2020) 162:1941–7. doi: 10.1007/s00701-020-04318-5
123. Lynagh R, Ishak M, Georges J, Lopez D, Osman H, Kakareka M, et al. Fluorescence-guided stereotactic biopsy: a proof-of-concept study. *J Neurosurg.* (2019) 1–7.
124. Akshulakov SK, Kerimbayev TT, Biryuchkov MY, Urunbayev YA, Farhadi DS, Byvaltsev VA. Current Trends for improving safety of stereotactic brain biopsies: advanced optical methods for vessel avoidance and tumor detection. *Front Oncol.* (2019) 9:947. doi: 10.3389/fonc.2019.00947
125. Malinova V, von Eckardstein K, Mielke D, Rohde V. Diagnostic yield of fluorescence-assisted frame-based stereotactic biopsies of intracerebral lesions in comparison with frozen-section analysis. *J Neurooncol.* (2020) 149:315–23. doi: 10.1007/s11060-020-03608-3
126. Li C, Sullivan PZ, Cho S, Nasrallah MP, Buch L, Isaac Chen HC, et al. Intraoperative molecular imaging with second window indocyanine green facilitates confirmation of contrast-enhancing tissue during intracranial stereotactic needle biopsy: a case series. *World Neurosurg.* (2019) 126:e1211–8. doi: 10.1016/j.wneu.2019.02.231
127. Evers G, Kamp M, Warneke N, Berdel W, Sabel M, Stummer W, et al. 5-aminolaevulinic acid-induced fluorescence in primary central nervous system lymphoma. *World Neurosurg.* (2017) 98:375–80. doi: 10.1016/j.wneu.2016.11.011
128. Yamamoto T, Ishikawa E, Miki S, Sakamoto N, Zaboronok A, Matsuda M, et al. Photodynamic diagnosis using 5-aminolevulinic acid in 41 biopsies for primary central nervous system lymphoma. *Photochem Photobiol.* (2015) 91:1452–7. doi: 10.1111/php.12510
129. Batchelor T, Loeffler JS. Primary CNS lymphoma. *J Clin Oncol.* (2006) 24:1281–8. doi: 10.1200/JCO.2005.04.8819
130. Millesi M, Kiesel B, Wöhrer A, Mercea PA, Bissolo M, Roetzer T, et al. Is intraoperative pathology needed if 5-aminolevulinic-acid-induced tissue fluorescence is found in stereotactic brain tumor biopsy? *Neurosurgery.* (2020) 86:366–73. doi: 10.1093/neuros/nyz086
131. Henderson F Jr, Brem S, Hussain J, Buch L, Maloney E, Singhal S, et al. Second window indocyanine green localizes CNS lymphoma in real time in the operating room: report of two cases. *Br J Neurosurg.* (2020) 3:1–5. doi: 10.1080/02688697.2020.1716945
132. Vetrano IG, Acerbi F, Falco J, Devigili G, Rinaldo S, Messina G, et al. Fluorescein-guided removal of peripheral nerve sheath tumors: a preliminary analysis of 20 cases. *J Neurosurg.* (2019) 6:1–10. doi: 10.3171/2019.9.JNS19970
133. Marbacher S, Klinger E, Schwyzer L, Fischer I, Nevzati E, Diepers M, et al. Use of fluorescence to guide resection or biopsy of primary brain tumors and brain metastases. *Neurosurg Focus.* (2014) 36:E10. doi: 10.3171/2013.12.FOCUS13464
134. Inoue A, Kohno S, Ohnishi T, Nishida N, Suehiro S, Nakamura Y, et al. Tricks and traps of ICG endoscopy for effectively applying endoscopic transsphenoidal surgery to pituitary adenoma. *Neurosurg Rev.* (2020). doi: 10.1007/s10143-020-01382-4
135. Amano K, Aihara Y, Tsuzuki S, Okada Y, Kawamata T. Application of indocyanine green fluorescence endoscopic system in transsphenoidal surgery for pituitary tumors. *Acta Neurochir.* (2019) 161:695–706. doi: 10.1007/s00701-018-03778-0
136. Utsuki S, Oka H, Kijima C, Miyajima Y, Hagiwara H, Fujii K. Utility of intraoperative fluorescent diagnosis of residual hemangioblastoma using 5- aminolevulinic acid. *Neurol India.* (2011) 59:612–5. doi: 10.4103/0028-3886.84349
137. Molina CA, Pennington Z, Ahmed AK, Westbroek E, Goodwin ML, Tamargo R, et al. Use of intraoperative indocyanine green angiography for feeder vessel ligation and en bloc resection of intramedullary hemangioblastoma. *Oper Neurosurg.* (2019) 17:573–9. doi: 10.1093/ons/opz053
138. Singh YB, Cho SS, Blue R, Teng CW, De Ravin E, Buch L, et al. Second-window indocyanine green for visualization of hemangioblastoma: a case report with two-dimensional operative video. *Oper Neurosurg.* (2021) 20:E229–33. doi: 10.1093/ons/opaa392
139. Bernal García LM, Cabezudo Artero JM, Marcelo Zamorano MB, Gilete Tejero, I. Fluorescence-guided resection with 5-aminolevulinic acid of subependymomas of the fourth ventricle: report of 2 cases: technical case report. *Neurosurgery.* (2015) 11(suppl.2):E364–71. doi: 10.1227/NEU.0000000000000682
140. Takeda J, Nonaka M, Li Y, et al. 5-ALA fluorescence-guided endoscopic surgery for mixed germ cell tumors. *J Neurooncol.* (2017). 134:119–24. doi: 10.1007/s11060-017-2494-9

22

The Second Near-Infrared Window Indocyanine Green Angiography in Giant Mediastinal Tumor Resection

Jiahui Mi [1], Ganwei Liu [1], Liyang Lu [1], Feng Yang [1], Hui Zhao [1], Yun Li [1], Guanchao Jiang [1], Fan Yang [1], Zhenhua Hu [2] and Jian Zhou [1*]*

[1] *Department of Thoracic Surgery, Peking University People's Hospital, Beijing, China,* [2] *Key Laboratory of Molecular Imaging of Chinese Academy of Sciences, Institute of Automation, Chinese Academy of Sciences, Beijing, China*

Correspondence:
Zhenhua Hu
zhenhua.hu@ia.ac.cn
Jian Zhou
zhoujian@bjmu.edu.cn

Giant mediastinal tumors are often accompanied by the abundant blood supply and have an unclear border with adjacent vessels, making surgical resection difficult. Failure to distinguish the complex vessels during the operation often results in vascular injury or hemorrhage, which severely increases the operation time and perioperative risk. At present, surgeons can only determine the vessel's location and course by preoperative imaging and intraoperative exploration in visible light. Therefore, we report a case of a giant anterosuperior mediastinal tumor resection assisted by near-infrared (NIR) indocyanine green (ICG) angiography. Furthermore, we applied the second near-infrared window (NIR-II, 1,000–1,700 nm) to detect the fluorescence signals in the clinic for the first time. The NIR-II window is able to explore deeper tissues in centimeters and obtain higher resolution in millimeters than the traditional first near-infrared window (NIR-I, 700–900 nm). Finally, NIR-II ICG angiography shows the clear location and course of the vessels, which can help surgeons reduce unnecessary blood vessel injury and increase the safety of mediastinal tumor resection.

Keywords: second near-infrared window, indocyanine green, angiography, mediastinal tumor, intraoperative imaging

INTRODUCTION

Resection of a giant mediastinal tumor is complicated in thoracic surgery because the thorax encompasses vital and complex vascular structures. At present, surgeons can only determine the vessel's location and course by preoperative imaging and intraoperative exploration in visible light. Although digital subtraction angiography can clearly show blood vessels, it is rarely used in open surgery because of its complicated operation and continuous X-ray exposure. Therefore, an appropriate real-time vascular imaging technique is needed to help surgeons identify blood vessels in mediastinal tumor resection.

Fluorescence imaging has shown several advantages with a high temporal and spatial resolution (1). First, near-infrared (NIR-I, 700–900 nm) indocyanine green (ICG) angiography has been applied in real-time vascular imaging in various surgical scenarios (2, 3). In addition, recent advances have shown that the second near-infrared window (NIR-II, 1,000–1,700 nm) can reduce light scattering by tissues and increase penetration depth, surpassing the NIR-I window's performance (1). To date, no clinical application has been reported for NIR-II ICG angiography.

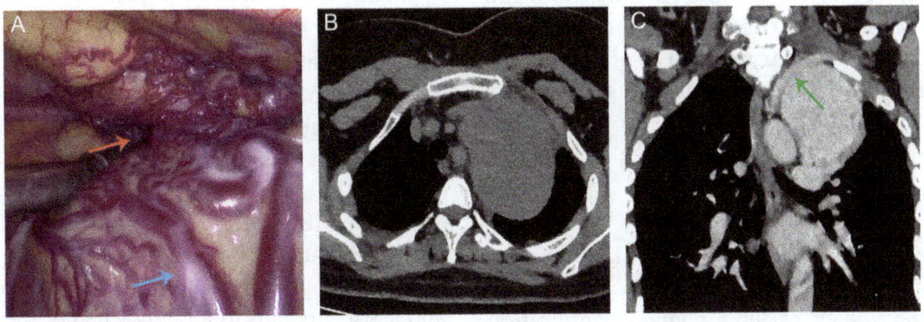

FIGURE 1 | (A) Intraoperative photograph showing abundant tortuous blood vessels on the surface of the tumor (blue arrow) and an unclear border at the top of the chest (red arrow). **(B)** A CT scan revealed a giant anterosuperior mediastinal tumor (6.7 × 9.8 × 9.7 cm) near the left side of the aortic arch. **(C)** Contrast-enhanced CT scan showed that the tumor was surrounded by tortuous vessels and was poorly demarcated from the left subclavian artery (green arrow).

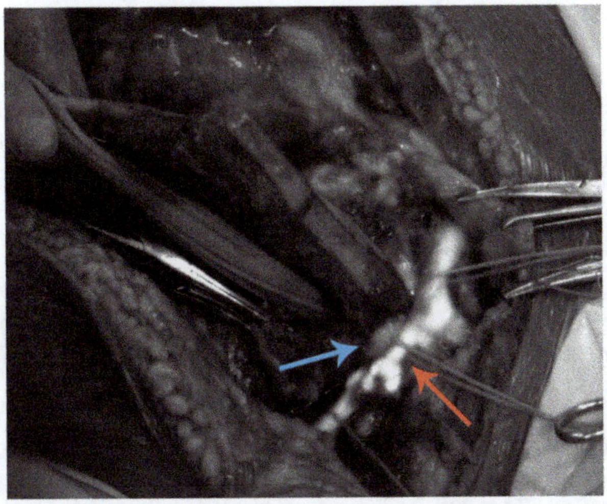

FIGURE 2 | Second near-infrared (NIR-II) indocyanine green (ICG) angiography of the left subclavian vein (red arrow) and the left subclavian artery (blue arrow) during the operation.

Herein, we report a patient with a mediastinal tumor adjacent to the subclavian artery and vein who underwent a successful operation assisted by NIR-II ICG angiography for the first time.

CASE REPORT

A 36-year-old woman presented with chest discomfort, wherein an anterosuperior mediastinal tumor had been diagnosed 3 weeks prior in the local hospital. Intraoperative exploration found abundant tortuous blood vessels on the surface of the tumor, and the surrounding tissue structure was unclear (**Figure 1A**), which easily caused uncontrollable bleeding. Therefore, the operation had to be terminated early.

Upon referral, she was admitted to our hospital for further treatment. Chest CT scan showed a giant anterosuperior mediastinal tumor (6.7 × 9.8 × 9.7 cm) near the left side of the aortic arch (**Figure 1B**). The tumor was surrounded by tortuous vessels on a contrast-enhanced CT scan and was poorly demarcated from the left subclavian artery (**Figure 1C**). A multidisciplinary discussion led to the decision to perform interventional embolization to decrease the tumor volume and the blood supply to the tumor in preparation for the subsequent surgical resection.

A contrast-enhanced CT scan was reviewed 7 days after interventional embolization, and the volume and blood supply of the mediastinal tumor were slightly reduced compared with before. After preoperative inspection, no contraindication was found in this patient, and we decided to perform mediastinal tumor resection.

The patient was anesthetized in the supine position. We split the sternum in the middle, disconnected the sternoclavicular joint, and removed half of the left clavicle to sufficiently expose the tumor. Intraoperative exploration found that the upper pole of the tumor was located at the entrance of the thorax and was closely adhered to the surrounding tissues. To distinguish the subclavian artery and vein from the surrounding tissues, the upper pole of the tumor was imaged in real-time by a NIR-II imaging system. The NIR-II imaging system contained a camera (Cheetah 640, Xenics, Belgium) using an InGaAs detector with 640 x 512-pixel resolution, a lens specially designed for high-performance shortwave infrared imaging (SWIRON 2.8/50, Schneider Kreuznach, Germany), and a spectral filter (FELH1000, Thorlabs, USA). A 792-nm laser (Bosheng Optoelectronics Co. Ltd., China) beam was coupled to a collimator and expanded by a lens to provide uniform illumination on the upper pole of the tumor. Then, 25 mg (5 mg/ml) ICG (Dandong Yichuang Pharmaceutical Co. Ltd., China) was injected into the patient's left radial vein in 10 s. The left subclavian vein and the left subclavian artery showed obvious fluorescence signals (**Figure 2**) and displayed a clear boundary of 3 and 17 s after the initial injection of ICG, respectively (**Supplementary Video 1**). With the help of NIR-II ICG angiography, we could recognize the deeper position of the subclavian vein and artery and avoid vascular damage during the operation. In addition, the clear blood vessel borders visualized by NIR-II ICG angiography ensured that the subclavian vein and artery were dissected free of all surrounding tissue without any vascular injury.

No allergic symptoms occurred after the ICG injection, and no severe nausea or vomiting occurred after the operation. Histologic examination of the tumor revealed a solitary fibrous tumor, and this patient's postoperative course was uneventful at follow-up.

DISCUSSION

Real-time NIR-I fluorescence imaging *in vivo* has received significant recognition as a powerful technique. It has been used in thoracic surgery, such as lung nodule identification (4). However, there is growing interest in NIR-II fluorescence imaging research due to reducing light scattering by tissues and increasing penetration depth compared to NIR-I fluorescence imaging (1). In addition, ICG as a non-targeting fluorescence agent has been approved for clinical use by the US Food and Drug Administration (FDA) for more than six decades and has been proven to be suitable for NIR-II imaging (5). Although animal experiments have proven that NIR-II ICG angiography has advantages over NIR-I ICG angiography (6), NIR-II ICG angiography has not yet been applied in clinical practice.

In our patient, the subclavian vein began to show fluorescence signals 3 s after ICG was injected into the radial vein. The subclavian artery began to show fluorescence signals 17 s after the blood combined with ICG passed through the pulmonary circulation and flowed into the subclavian artery. Therefore, intravenous injection of ICG from the upper limb had quick feedback for vascular fluorescence imaging in the mediastinum. In addition, NIR-II fluorescence imaging can show a more apparent vascular boundary by the characteristics of diminishing tissue autofluorescence, reducing photon scattering, and exhibiting lower levels of photon absorption at longer wavelengths (7), which could help surgeons identify complex vascular structures and reduce the risk of vascular injury.

The video demonstrated that the fluorescence signal intensity in the subclavian vein was not homogeneous at the beginning. Fluorescence imaging of the subclavian vein even showed apparent blood flow turbulence and vortex in the vascular bifurcation. This phenomenon is due to ICG being injected only into the radial vein. In other veins, such as the superior scapular vein, internal jugular vein, and external jugular vein, blood without ICG flowed into the subclavian vein together. The precise blood flow imaging proved that NIR-II ICG angiography has a relatively high resolution, consistent with previous research (8). Therefore, if the blood vessels had to be reconstructed due to severe injury or tumor invasion during the operation, NIR-II ICG angiography could also monitor the vessels' blood flow and assist surgeons in judging whether the reconstructed vessels were unobstructed in real-time. Compared with traditional X-ray vascular imaging, NIR-II ICG angiography can show blood flow continuously without considering radiation damage to patients and medical personnel.

CONCLUSION

Our case is the first reported clinical application of NIR-II ICG angiography in mediastinal tumor surgery and showed that NIR-II ICG angiography, as a new clinical imaging technique, is a safe, convenient, and efficient real-time method to help surgeons deal with vital vessels in mediastinal tumor operations in the future.

ETHICS STATEMENT

Written informed consent was obtained from the individual(s) for the publication of any potentially identifiable images or data included in this article.

AUTHOR CONTRIBUTIONS

JM reviewed the literature and drafted the manuscript. GL and LL collected the analyzed the data. FeY, HZ, and YL provided technical support. GJ and FaY contributed to the conception and design of the study. ZH and JZ reviewed the manuscript. All authors issued approval of the final version.

REFERENCES

1. Hu Z, Fang C, Li B, Zhang Z, Cao C, Cai M, et al. First-in-human liver-tumour surgery guided by multispectral fluorescence imaging in the visible and near-infrared-I/II windows. *Nat Biomed Eng.* (2020) 4:259–71. doi: 10.1038/s41551-019-0494-0
2. Aiba T, Uehara K, Ogura A, Tanaka A, Yonekawa Y, Hattori N, et al. The significance of the time to arterial perfusion in intraoperative ICG angiography during colorectal surgery. *Surg Endosc.* (2021) 35:7227–35. doi: 10.1007/s00464-020-08185-0
3. Maser C, Kohlbrenner AH, Dirks R. Use of indocyanine green and fluorescence angiography in parathyroid surgery: a feasibility study. *Surg Innov.* (2020) 27:587–93. doi: 10.1177/1553350620956437
4. Okusanya OT, Holt D, Heitjan D, Deshpande C, Venegas O, Jiang J, et al. Intraoperative near-infrared imaging can identify pulmonary nodules. *Ann Thorac Surg.* (2014) 98:1223–30. doi: 10.1016/j.athoracsur.2014.05.026
5. Wu D, Xue D, Zhou J, Wang Y, Feng Z, Xu J, et al. Extrahepatic cholangiography in near-infrared II window with the clinically approved fluorescence agent indocyanine green: a promising imaging technology for intraoperative diagnosis. *Theranostics.* (2020) 10:3636–51. doi: 10.7150/thno.41127
6. Bhavane R, Starosolski Z, Stupin I, Ghaghada KB, Annapragada A. NIR-II fluorescence imaging using indocyanine green nanoparticles. *Sci Rep.* (2018) 8:14455. doi: 10.1038/s41598-018-32754-y
7. Hong G, Antaris AL, Dai H. Near-infrared fluorophores for biomedical imaging. *Nat Biomed Eng.* (2017) 1:0010. doi: 10.1038/s41551-016-0010
8. He S, Song J, Qu J, Cheng Z. Crucial breakthrough of second near-infrared biological window fluorophores: design and synthesis toward multimodal imaging and theranostics. *Chem Soc Rev.* (2018) 47:4258–78. doi: 10.1039/c8cs00234g

Permissions

All chapters in this book were first published by Frontiers; hereby published with permission under the Creative Commons Attribution License or equivalent. Every chapter published in this book has been scrutinized by our experts. Their significance has been extensively debated. The topics covered herein carry significant findings which will fuel the growth of the discipline. They may even be implemented as practical applications or may be referred to as a beginning point for another development.

The contributors of this book come from diverse backgrounds, making this book a truly international effort. This book will bring forth new frontiers with its revolutionizing research information and detailed analysis of the nascent developments around the world.

We would like to thank all the contributing authors for lending their expertise to make the book truly unique. They have played a crucial role in the development of this book. Without their invaluable contributions this book wouldn't have been possible. They have made vital efforts to compile up to date information on the varied aspects of this subject to make this book a valuable addition to the collection of many professionals and students.

This book was conceptualized with the vision of imparting up-to-date information and advanced data in this field. To ensure the same, a matchless editorial board was set up. Every individual on the board went through rigorous rounds of assessment to prove their worth. After which they invested a large part of their time researching and compiling the most relevant data for our readers.

The editorial board has been involved in producing this book since its inception. They have spent rigorous hours researching and exploring the diverse topics which have resulted in the successful publishing of this book. They have passed on their knowledge of decades through this book. To expedite this challenging task, the publisher supported the team at every step. A small team of assistant editors was also appointed to further simplify the editing procedure and attain best results for the readers.

Apart from the editorial board, the designing team has also invested a significant amount of their time in understanding the subject and creating the most relevant covers. They scrutinized every image to scout for the most suitable representation of the subject and create an appropriate cover for the book.

The publishing team has been an ardent support to the editorial, designing and production team. Their endless efforts to recruit the best for this project, has resulted in the accomplishment of this book. They are a veteran in the field of academics and their pool of knowledge is as vast as their experience in printing. Their expertise and guidance has proved useful at every step. Their uncompromising quality standards have made this book an exceptional effort. Their encouragement from time to time has been an inspiration for everyone.

The publisher and the editorial board hope that this book will prove to be a valuable piece of knowledge for researchers, students, practitioners and scholars across the globe.

List of Contributors

Mark Bradley
EaStChem School of Chemistry, University of Edinburgh, Edinburgh, United Kingdom

Gavin P. Birch
EaStChem School of Chemistry, University of Edinburgh, Edinburgh, United Kingdom

Thane Campbell and Kevin Dhaliwal
Centre for Inflammation Research, University of Edinburgh, Edinburgh, United Kingdom

Sergey A. Goryaynov, Vladimir A. Okhlopkov, Denis A. Golbin, Artem Batalov, Nikolay A. Konovalov, Petr V. Zelenkov and Alexandr A. Potapov
N. N. Burdenko National Medical Research Center of Neurosurgery of the Ministry of Health of the Russian Federation, Moscow, Russia

Konstantin A. Chernyshov
I. M. Sechenov First Moscow State Medical University of the Ministry of Health of the Russian Federation, Moscow, Russia

Dmitrij V. Svistov and Boris V. Martynov
S. M. Kirov Military Medical Academy of the Ministry of Defense of the Russian Federation, St-Petersburg, Russia

Alexandr V. Kim
V. A. Almazov Federal North-West Medical Research Centre of the Ministry of Health of the Russian Federation, St-Petersburg, Russia

Vadim A. Byvaltsev
Laboratory of Neurosurgery, Irkutsk Scientific Center of Surgery and Traumatology, Irkutsk, Russia
Department of Neurosurgery, Irkutsk State Medical University, Irkutsk, Russia

Galina V. Pavlova
Institute of Gene Biology, Russian Academy of Science, Moscow, Russia

Victor B. Loschenov
Prokhorov General Physics Institute of the Russian Academy of Science, Moscow, Russia
National Research Nuclear University MEPhI, Moscow, Russia

Steve S. Cho
Perelman School of Medicine at the University of Pennsylvania, Philadelphia, PA, United States
Department of Neurosurgery at the Hospital of the University of Pennsylvania, Philadelphia, PA, United States

Ryan Salinas and John Y. K. Lee
Department of Neurosurgery at the Hospital of the University of Pennsylvania, Philadelphia, PA, United States

Shinjiro Fukami, Megumi Ichikawa and Michihiro Kohno
Department of Neurosurgery, Tokyo Medical University, Tokyo, Japan

Jiro Akimoto
Department of Neurosurgery, Tokyo Medical University, Tokyo, Japan
Department of Neurosurgery, Kohsei Chuo General Hospital, Tokyo, Japan

Awad Mohamed
Department of Neurosurgery, Tokyo Medical University, Tokyo, Japan
Department of Neurosurgery, Sohag University, Sohag, Egypt

Konstantin S. Yashin, Igor A. Medyanik and Leonid Ya. Kravets
Microneurosurgery Group, University Clinic, Privolzhsky Research Medical University, Nizhny Novgorod, Russia

Elena B. Kiseleva, Ekaterina V. Gubarkova and Natalia D. Gladkova
Laboratory of Optical Coherence Tomography, Research Institute of Experimental Oncology and Biomedical Technologies, Privolzhsky Research Medical University, Nizhny Novgorod, Russia

Pavel A. Shilyagin, Grigory V. Gelikonov and Alexander A. Moiseev
Laboratory of High-Sensitivity Optical Measurements, Institute of Applied Physics, Russian Academy of Sciences, Nizhny Novgorod, Russia

Sergey S. Kuznetsov
Department of Anatomical Pathology, Privolzhsky Research Medical University, Nizhny Novgorod, Russia

Alexander A. Potapov
Federal State Autonomous Institution "N.N.Burdenko National Scientific and Practical Center for Neurosurgery" of the Ministry of Healthcare of the Russian Federation, Moscow, Russia

Elena V. Zagaynova
Research Institute of Experimental Oncology and Biomedical Technologies, Privolzhsky Research Medical University, Nizhny Novgorod, Russia

Hugues Duffau
Department of Neurosurgery, Montpellier University Medical Center, Gui de Chauliac Hospital, Montpellier, France
Team "Plasticity of Central Nervous System, Stem Cells and Glial Tumors," U1051 Laboratory, National Institute for Health and Medical Research (INSERM), Institute for Neurosciences of Montpellier, Montpellier University Medical Center, Montpellier, France

Danil Chelushkin, Marina Ryzhova, Ludmila Shishkina and Vadim Jukov
N. N. Burdenko Scientific Research Neurosurgery Institute, Moscow, Russia

Georg Widhalm
Department of Neurosurgery, Medical University of Vienna, Vienna, Austria

Maria F. Goldberg and Kosta A. Chernyshov
I.M. Sechenov First Moscow State Medical University, Moscow, Russia

Aldo Spallone
NCL-Institute of Neurological Sciences, Rome, Italy
Department of Biomedicine, University of Rome Tor Vergata, Rome, Italy

Galina Pavlova and Alexander Revischin
Institute of Gene Biology, Russian Academy of Science, Moscow, Russia

Loschenov Victor and Alexander Potapov
Prokhorov General Physics Institute, Russian Academy of Sciences, Moscow, Russia

Tatyana Savelieva
Prokhorov General Physics Institute, Russian Academy of Sciences, Moscow, Russia
National Research Nuclear University, Moscow Engineering Physics Institute, Moscow, Russia

Nikita Lakomkin and Constantinos G. Hadjipanayis
Department of Neurosurgery, Mount Sinai Health System, Icahn School of Medicine at Mount Sinai, New York, NY, United States
Department of Neurosurgery, Mount Sinai Health System, Icahn School of Medicine, New York, NY, United States

Pablo A. Valdes, Parikshit Juvekar, Nathalie Y. R. Agar and Alexandra J. Golby
Department of Neurosurgery, Harvard Medical School, Brigham and Women's Hospital, Boston, MA, United States

Sylvain Gioux
ICube Laboratory, University of Strasbourg, Télécom Physique Strasbourg, Alsace, France

Alessandra Capuano, Eva Andreuzzi, Eliana Pivetta, Roberto Doliana, Andrea Favero, Maurizio Mongiat and Paola Spessotto
Molecular Oncology, Centro di Riferimento Oncologico (CRO), IRCCS, Aviano, Italy

Vincenzo Canzonieri
Pathology, Centro di Riferimento Oncologico (CRO), IRCCS, Aviano, Italy

Stefania Maiero, Mara Fornasarig, Raffaella Magris and Renato Cannizzaro
Oncological Gastroenterology, Centro di Riferimento Oncologico (CRO), IRCCS, Aviano, Italy

Pedro Norat, Sauson Soldozy, Mazin Elsarrag, Jennifer Sokolowski, Kaan Yağmurlu, Min S. Park, Petr Tvrdik and M. Yashar S. Kalani
Department of Neurological Surgery, University of Virginia Health System, Charlottesville, VA, United States

Yezhou Yang
School of Computing, Informatics, and Decision System Engineering, Arizona State University, Tempe, AZ, United States

Mohammadhassan Izadyyazdanabadi
School of Computing, Informatics, and Decision System Engineering, Arizona State University, Tempe, AZ, United States
The Loyal and Edith Davis Neurosurgery Research Laboratory, Department of Neurosurgery, St. Joseph's Hospital and Medical Center, Barrow Neurological Institute, Phoenix, AZ, United States

Xiaochun Zhao, Leandro Borba Moreira, Sirin Gandhi, Claudio Cavallo and Mark C. Preul
The Loyal and Edith Davis Neurosurgery Research Laboratory, Department of Neurosurgery, St. Joseph's Hospital and Medical Center, Barrow Neurological Institute, Phoenix, AZ, United States

Evgenii Belykh
Department of Neurosurgery, Barrow Neurological Institute, St. Joseph's Hospital and Medical Center, Phoenix, AZ, United States
Department of Neurosurgery, Irkutsk State Medical University, Irkutsk, Russia

Ingo Ludolph, Raymund E. Horch, Andreas Arkudas and Marweh Schmitz
Department of Plastic and Hand Surgery and Laboratory for Tissue Engineering and Regenerative Medicine, University Hospital of Erlangen, Friedrich-Alexander-University of Erlangen-Nuernberg FAU, Erlangen, Germany

Bin Xu and Ming Chen
Department of Urology, Affiliated Zhongda Hospital of Southeast University, Nanjing, China

Yuqing Wu and Jibo Jing
Department of Urology, Affiliated Zhongda Hospital of Southeast University, Nanjing, China
Surgical Research Center, School of Medicine, Institute of Urology, Southeast University, Nanjing, China

Jinfeng Wang
Department of Urology, School of Medicine, Affiliated Yancheng Hospital, Southeast University, Yancheng, China

Mulong Du
Jiangsu Key Laboratory of Cancer Biomarkers, Department of Environmental Genomics, Prevention and Treatment, Collaborative Innovation Center for Cancer Personalized Medicine, Nanjing Medical University, Nanjing, China
Department of Biostatistics, Center for Global Health, School of Public Health, Nanjing Medical University, Nanjing, China

Eric J. Miller, Alessandro Carotenuto, Arpan A. Patel, Nikolay L. Martirosyan, Michael T. Lawton
Department of Neurosurgery, Barrow Neurological Institute, St. Joseph's Hospital and Medical Center, Phoenix, AZ, United States

Debbie R. Healey and Adrienne C. Scheck
Department of Neuro-Oncology Research, Barrow Neurological Institute, St. Joseph's Hospital and Medical Center, Phoenix, AZ, United States

Jennifer M. Eschbacher
Department of Neuropathology, Barrow Neurological Institute, St. Joseph's Hospital and Medical Center, Phoenix, AZ, United States

Linpeng Wei
Department of Mechanical Engineering, University of Washington, Seattle, WA, United States

Yoko Fujita and Nader Sanai
Department of Neurological Surgery, Barrow Neurological Institute, Phoenix, AZ, United States

Jonathan T. C. Liu
Department of Mechanical Engineering, University of Washington, Seattle, WA, United States
Department of Pathology, University of Washington School of Medicine, Seattle, WA, United States

Dana Ferrari-Light, Travis C. Geraci, Prabhu Sasankan and Robert J. Cerfolio
Department of Cardiothoracic Surgery, New York University Langone Health, New York, NY, United States
School of Medicine, New York University Langone Health, New York, NY, United States

Ignazio G. Vetrano, Camilla de Laurentis, Lampros Siozos, Marco Schiariti, Morgan Broggi and Paolo Ferroli
Department of Neurosurgery, Fondazione IRCCS Istituto Neurologico Carlo Besta, Milan, Italy

Jacopo Falco
Department of Neurosurgery, Fondazione IRCCS Istituto Neurologico Carlo Besta, Milan, Italy
Department of Neurosurgery, Barrow Neurological Institute, St. Joseph's Hospital and Medical Center, Phoenix, AZ, United States

Francesco Acerbi
Department of Neurosurgery, Fondazione Istituto Di Ricovero e Cura a Carattere Scientifico Istituto Neurologico Carlo Besta, Milan, Italy

Daniel Valli
Department of Neurosurgery, Barrow Neurological Institute, St. Joseph's Hospital and Medical Center, Phoenix, AZ, United States

Joseph F. Georges, Amber Valeri, Aaron Brooking and Michael Kakareka
Department of Neurosurgery, Philadelphia College of Osteopathic Medicine, Philadelphia, PA, United States
Department of Neurosurgery, Cooper University Healthcare, Philadelphia, PA, United States

Steven Yocom
Department of Neurosurgery, Cooper University Healthcare, Philadelphia, PA, United States

Huan Wang and Si Yu
School of Medicine, Cooper Medical School of Rowan University, Camden, NJ, United States,

Carrie Li
Perelman School of Medicine, University of Pennsylvania, Philadelphia, PA, United States

Steve S. Cho
Perelman School of Medicine, University of Pennsylvania, Philadelphia, PA, United States
Department of Neurosurgery, Hospital of the University of Pennsylvania, Philadelphia, PA, United States

Zein Al-Atrache, Michael Bamimore and Joseph Ifrach
School of Medicine, Philadelphia College of Osteopathic Medicine, Philadelphia, PA, United States

Hany Osman
Wellman Center for Photomedicine, Massachusetts General Hospital, Boston, MA, United States

Kristin Brill
Department of Surgery, MD Anderson Cancer Center at Cooper Health Systems, Camden, NJ, United States

Alexander J. Schupper, Manasa Rao, Nicki Mohammadi and Rebecca Baron
Department of Neurosurgery, Icahn School of Medicine at Mount Sinai, New York, NY, United States

Jiahui Mi, Ganwei Liu, Liyang Lu, Feng Yang, Hui Zhao, Yun Li, Guanchao Jiang, Fan Yang and Jian Zhou
Department of Thoracic Surgery, Peking University People's Hospital, Beijing, China

Zhenhua Hu
Key Laboratory of Molecular Imaging of Chinese Academy of Sciences, Institute of Automation, Chinese Academy of Sciences, Beijing, China

Index

www.ingramcontent.com/pod-product-compliance
Lightning Source LLC
LaVergne TN
LVHW082155200926
848484LV00008B/2163